Small Animal Laparoscopy and Thoracoscopy

To my husband Claude for inspiration and support in every aspect of life. To my daughters Selma and Ella for providing endless joy, life balance, and perspective. To the surgical residents who make me grow as a mentor and a surgeon. And to my parents, Sivert and Anita, whose unconditional love and support formed my foundation.

— BAF

To my parents Alan and Hildegard for their unwavering support, kindness, and generosity. To my wife Kelli and my children Reece, Aidan, and Brynn for making life so rich and rewarding and full of joy and laughter.

— PDM

Small Animal Laparoscopy and Thoracoscopy

Edited by

Boel A. Fransson, DVM, PhD, DACVS

Associate Professor of Small Animal Surgery
Washington State University
Pullman, WA
USA

Philipp D. Mayhew, BVM&S, MRCVS, DACVS

Associate Professor of Small Animal Surgery
University of California-Davis
School of Veterinary Medicine
Davis, CA
USA

WILEY Blackwell

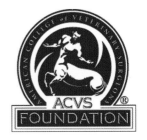

Editorial offices: 1606 Golden Aspen Drive, Suites 103 and 104, Ames, Iowa 50010, USA
The Atrium, Southern Gate, Chichester, West Sussex, PO19 8SQ, UK
9600 Garsington Road, Oxford, OX4 2DQ, UK

For details of our global editorial offices, for customer services and for information about how to apply for permission to reuse the copyright material in this book please see our website at www.wiley.com/wiley-blackwell.

Authorization to photocopy items for internal or personal use, or the internal or personal use of specific clients, is granted by Blackwell Publishing, provided that the base fee is paid directly to the Copyright Clearance Center, 222 Rosewood Drive, Danvers, MA 01923. For those organizations that have been granted a photocopy license by CCC, a separate system of payments has been arranged. The fee codes for users of the Transactional Reporting Service are ISBN-13: 978-1-1188-4596-7/2015.

Designations used by companies to distinguish their products are often claimed as trademarks. All brand names and product names used in this book are trade names, service marks, trademarks or registered trademarks of their respective owners. The publisher is not associated with any product or vendor mentioned in this book.

The contents of this work are intended to further general scientific research, understanding, and discussion only and are not intended and should not be relied upon as recommending or promoting a specific method, diagnosis, or treatment by health science practitioners for any particular patient. The publisher and the author make no representations or warranties with respect to the accuracy or completeness of the contents of this work and specifically disclaim all warranties, including without limitation any implied warranties of fitness for a particular purpose. In view of ongoing research, equipment modifications, changes in governmental regulations, and the constant flow of information relating to the use of medicines, equipment, and devices, the reader is urged to review and evaluate the information provided in the package insert or instructions for each medicine, equipment, or device for, among other things, any changes in the instructions or indication of usage and for added warnings and precautions. Readers should consult with a specialist where appropriate. The fact that an organization or Website is referred to in this work as a citation and/or a potential source of further information does not mean that the author or the publisher endorses the information the organization or Website may provide or recommendations it may make. Further, readers should be aware that Internet Websites listed in this work may have changed or disappeared between when this work was written and when it is read. No warranty may be created or extended by any promotional statements for this work. Neither the publisher nor the author shall be liable for any damages arising herefrom.

A catalogue record for this book is available from the Library of Congress.

Wiley also publishes its books in a variety of electronic formats. Some content that appears in print may not be available in electronic books.

Main cover image: © 2014 KARL STORZ GmbH & Co. KG

Set in 9/11pt Minion Pro by Aptara Inc., New Delhi, India
Printed and bound in Singapore by Markono Print Media Pte Ltd

1   2015

Contents

Contributors

Jessica K. Baron, DVM
Resident
Small Animal Surgery
Cummings School of Veterinary Medicine at Tufts
University
North Grafton, MA

Fausto Brandão, DVM, MSc,
Cert. Spec. VEaMIS
Karl Storz GmbH & Co.
Lisbon, Portugal

Floryne O. Buishand, DVM
ECVS, Resident Small Animal Surgery
Department of Clinical Sciences of Companion Animals
Faculty of Veterinary Medicine, Utrecht University
Utrecht, The Netherlands

Nicole J. Buote, DVM, DACVS
Chief of Surgery
VCA West Los Angeles
Los Angeles, CA

J. Brad Case, DVM, MS, DACVS
Assistant Professor
Department of Small Animal Clinical Sciences
College of Veterinary Medicine
University of Florida
Gainesville, FL

Christopher Chamness, DVM
Global Director, Veterinary
Karl Storz GmbH & Co.
Santa Barbara, CA

Kayla M. Corriveau, DVM
Resident, Small Animal Surgery
Small Animal Clinical Sciences
Texas A&M University
College Station, TX

William T.N. Culp, VMD, DACVS
ACVS Founding Fellow, Surgical Oncology
Assistant Professor

Department of Surgical and Radiological Sciences
School of Veterinary Medicine,
University of California-Davis
Davis, CA

Marlis L. de Rezende, DVM, PhD,
DACVAA
Assistant Professor, Anesthesiology
Department of Clinical Sciences
Colorado State University
Fort Collins, CO

Gilles Dupre, Univ. Prof. Dr. med. vet.,
Dipl. ECVS
Head of Small Animal Surgery, Ophthalmology,
Dentistry and Rehabilitation
University of Veterinary Medicine, Vienna
Vienna, Austria

Gary W. Ellison, DVM, MS, DACVS
Professor
Department of Small Animal Clinical Sciences
College of Veterinary Medicine
University of Florida
Gainesville, FL

Boel A. Fransson, DVM, PhD, Dipl.
ACVS
Associate Professor Small Animal Surgery
Washington State University
Department Veterinary Clinical Sciences
Pullman, WA

Lynetta Freeman DVM, MS, DACVS
Associate Professor of Small Animal Surgery and
Biomechanical Engineering
Department of Veterinary Clinical Sciences
Purdue University College of Veterinary Medicine
West Lafayette, IN

John C. Huhn DVM, MS
Medical Director
Covidien Animal Health
Salem, CT

Geraldine B. Hunt, BVSc, MVetClinStud,
PhD
Professor
Department of Surgical and Radiological Sciences
School of Veterinary Medicine
University of California-Davis
Davis, CA

Katie C. Kennedy, DVM, MS,
DACVS-SA
June Harper Fellow Candidate in Surgical Oncology
Flint Animal Cancer Center
Colorado State University
Fort Collins, CO

Jolle Kirpensteijn, DVM, PhD,
DACVS, DECVS
Professor
Department of Clinical Sciences of Companion
Animals
Faculty of Veterinary Medicine
Utrecht University
Utrecht, The Netherlands;
Chief Professional Relations Officer
Hills Pet Nutrition
Topeka, KS

Janet Kovak McClaran,
DVM, DACVS
Section Head
Department of Surgery
Animal Medical Center
New York, NY

Stephane Libermann, DVM
Department of Surgery
Centre Hospitalier Veterinaire des Cordeliers
Meaux, France

Khursheed Mama, DVM, DACVAA
Professor, Anesthesiology
Department of Clinical Sciences
Colorado State University
Fort Collins, CO

Sarah Marvel, DVM, MS, DACVS-SA
ACVS Fellow, Surgical Oncology
Staff Surgeon
Southern Arizona Veterinary Specialty
and Emergency
Tuscon, AZ

Philipp D. Mayhew, BVM&S, DACVS
Associate Professor
Department of Surgical and Radiological Sciences
School of Veterinary Medicine
University of California-Davis
Davis, CA

Eric Monnet, DVM, PhD, DACVS, DECVS
Professor, Small Animal Surgery
Colorado State University
Fort Collins, CO

Peter J. Pascoe BVSc, DVA, DACVA, DECVAA
Professor of Anesthesiology
Department of Surgical and Radiological Sciences
School of Veterinary Medicine
University of California, Davis
Davis, CA

MaryAnn Radlinsky, DVM, MS, DACVS
Associate Professor of Soft Tissue Surgery
Department of Small Animal Medicine & Surgery
College of Veterinary Medicine
The University of Georgia
Athens, GA

Claude A. Ragle, DVM, Dipl. ACVS, DABVP-EP
Associate Professor Equine Surgery
Washington State University
Department of Veterinary Clinical Sciences
Pullman, WA

Clarence A. Rawlings, DVM, PhD, DACVS
Professor Emeritus
College of Veterinary Medicine
University of Georgia
Athens, GA

Keith Richter, DVM, DACVIM
Hospital Director
Veterinary Specialty Hospital of San Diego
San Diego, CA

Sheri Ross, DVM, PhD, DACVIM
Coordinator Hemodialysis, Nephrology, and Urology
University of California Veterinary Medical Center, San Diego
San Diego, CA

Jeffrey J. Runge DVM, DACVS
Assistant Professor of Minimally Invasive Surgery
Department of Clinical Studies, Section of Surgery
School of Veterinary Medicine
University of Pennsylvania
Philadelphia, PA

Stephanie L. Shaver, DVM
Staff Surgeon
VCA Douglas County Animal Hospital
Castle Rock, CO

Ameet Singh, DVM, DVSc, DACVS
Assistant Professor, Small Animal Surgery
Department of Clinical Studies
Ontario Veterinary College, University of Guelph
Guelph, ON, Canada

Michele A. Steffey, DVM, DACVS
ACVS Founding Fellow, Surgical Oncology
Assistant Professor
Department of Surgical and Radiological Sciences
University of California-Davis
Davis, CA

Elizabeth A. Swanson, DVM, MS, DACVS-SA
Assistant Professor, Small Animal Surgery
Department of Clinical Sciences
College of Veterinary Medicine
Mississippi State University
Mississippi State, MS

Heather A. Towle Millard, DVM, MS, DACVS-SA
Staff Surgeon
BluePearl Specialty and Emergency Medicine for Pets
Overland Park, KS

Sebastiaan A. van Nimwegen, DVM, PhD, DECVS
Staff Member
Small Animal Surgery
Department of Clinical Sciences of Companion Animals
Faculty of Veterinary Medicine
Utrecht University
Utrecht, The Netherlands

Chloe Wormser VMD
Lecturer
Section of Surgery
School of Veterinary Medicine
University of Pennsylvania
Philadelphia, PA

Foreword

The American College of Veterinary Surgeons (ACVS) Foundation is excited to present *Small Animal Laparoscopy and Thoracoscopy* in the book series titled *Advances in Veterinary Surgery*. The ACVS Foundation is an independently charted philanthropic organization devoted to advancing the charitable, educational, and scientific goals of the ACVS. Founded in 1965, the ACVS sets the standards for the specialty of veterinary surgery. The ACVS, which is approved by the American Veterinary Medical Association, administers the board certification process for Diplomates in veterinary surgery and advances veterinary surgery and education. One of the principal goals of the ACVS Foundation is to foster the advancement of the art and science of veterinary surgery. The Foundation achieves these goals by supporting investigations in the diagnosis and treatment of surgical diseases; increasing educational opportunities for surgeons, surgical residents, and veterinary practitioners; improving surgical training of residents and veterinary students;

and bettering animal patients' care, treatment, and welfare. This collaboration with Wiley-Blackwell will benefit all who are interested in veterinary surgery by presenting the latest evidence-based information on a particular surgical topic.

Small Animal Laparoscopy and Thoracoscopy is edited by Drs. Boel Fransson and Philipp Mayhew, both of whom are Diplomates of the ACVS. They have assembled the leaders in this field presenting sections on technical skills, equipment, fundamental techniques, and suggested procedures where these modalities can best be used. The ACVS Foundation is proud to partner with Wiley-Blackwell in this important series and is honored to present this book in the series.

Mark D. Markel
Chair, Board of Trustees
ACVS Foundation

Foreword

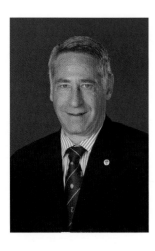

Minimal access surgery has revolutionized surgical care by providing precise, effective, and durable surgical interventions with minimal injury from access to body cavities. These techniques have expanded from the abdominal cavity and pelvis to the retroperitoneum, thoracic cavity, and joint spaces. The impact of this novel approach has been enormous, whether applied in the urban area, rural environments, or the developing world. Extensive published data confirm the recovery benefits and the reduction in complications associated with these novel surgical approaches.

The challenge in minimal access surgery has been to train surgeons to overcome the technical demands of these techniques. These involve primarily working with a monocular optical system while doing surgery in three dimensions, using long instruments constrained by trocars working across a fulcrum, decreased tactile feedback, and reduced range of motion. Suturing and knot tying, fundamental to most surgical procedures, can be especially difficult for new laparoscopists. However, these skills can be readily learned and applied clinically.

The response to these technical challenges has led to a new and better approach to surgical education using simulation-based principles. Programs such as the Fundamentals of Laparoscopic Surgery™ have been proven to be highly effective, efficient, and durable to train surgeons and to verify their technical skills before they apply these approaches to patient care.

These same advantages have been clearly demonstrated in veterinary surgery. *Small Animal Laparoscopy and Thoracoscopy*, by Drs. Boel Fransson and Philipp Mayhew, should be required reading for veterinary surgeons and veterinary surgical students who practice or plan to practice minimally invasive surgical techniques. This textbook provides an eloquent, well-illustrated, and up-to-date description of the applications of minimal access surgery in veterinary medicine, including specific recommendations for perioperative care. Furthermore, the authors address the educational opportunities for veterinary surgeons wishing to acquire the minimally invasive surgical skills required to perform these innovative procedures. *Small Animal Laparoscopy and Thoracoscopy* is a beautifully written and valuable resource for veterinary surgeons.

Gerald M. Fried, MD, CM, FRCSC, FACS, FCAHS
Edward W. Archibald Professor and Chairman, Department of
Surgery, McGill University
Surgeon-in-Chief, McGill University Health Centre
Past President, Society of American Gastrointestinal and Endoscopic
Surgeons (2013–2014)

Preface

Minimally invasive surgery (MIS) started in veterinary medicine around 20 years ago as a diagnostic tool, and now more than 100 publications already exist about different surgical techniques available to small animal surgeons. This book is the witness of the exponential development of MIS in veterinary practice over the past 5 years. All of the techniques described and illustrated in this textbook are currently used in veterinary practice. This book, edited by Drs. Boel Fransson and Philipp Mayhew, is the first textbook exclusively dedicated to veterinary MIS. The two editors recruited the most experienced authors in their own field to write different chapters. Each chapter is well illustrated to represent a solid base for general practitioners, surgeons in training, and board-certified surgeons.

Eric Monnet, DVM, PhD, FAHA, DACVS, DECVS
Professor of Small Animal Surgery
Colorado State University

Approximately 25 years ago, a paradigm shift to minimally invasive surgical techniques occurred with the introduction of laparoscopy and thoracoscopy in human medicine. Although the world of veterinary surgery has taken somewhat longer to follow suit, it is now changing at a rapid pace driven in part by the introduction of new technology and the abundant opportunities for further training in advanced procedures. The previous textbook entirely dedicated to small animal laparoscopy and thoracoscopy was published a decade and a half ago. Since then, more than 200 articles have been published in peer-reviewed journals, and minimally invasive surgery has moved from being mainly a diagnostic tool in specialty practice into therapeutic applications in general and specialty veterinary practice.

This book is the first one entirely dedicated to laparoscopy and thoracoscopy, and it has brought together the most experienced surgeons from around the world in a joint mission to create an instructive review of minimally invasive surgical techniques. It is also the first book on the subject to be written by authors with significant experience of MIS in clinical populations of small animal patients. A strongly contributing factor to this community of veterinary surgeons has been the Veterinary Endoscopy Society (VES). Founded in 2003 by Dr. Eric Monnet, VES has brought veterinarians from around the world interested in endoscopic surgery together to share their ideas and experiences in the field of veterinary endoscopy. From this platform, a network of dedicated veterinarians formed, sharing a passion for surgical endoscopy. The editors are indebted to these experts and fine colleagues for their willingness to share their expertise and for their time and effort spent in the undertaking of this project. It is because of these authors we can share the most current information with the readership.

Although the editors believe that this book represents a certain "coming of age" for the field of veterinary laparoscopy and thoracoscopy, there is no doubt that this represents perhaps the end of the beginning. It is our hope that in the years to come the procedures described in the book will be performed more frequently. We also hope for that expansion to be paralleled with an appreciation for the value of critical scientific evaluation of results and outcomes. Although much data exists in the human literature to validate the benefits of many minimally invasive approaches we should not be complacent in the knowledge that if it is better in people, it must be better in our small animal patients. Ongoing and future studies performed using the principles of evidence-based medicine should form the bedrock of this subspecialty, and the results of these studies should guide our recommendations and indications for MIS in the future.

Boel A. Fransson, DVM, PhD, DACVS
Associate Professor of Small Animal Surgery
Washington State University

Philipp D. Mayhew, BVM&S, MRCVS, DACVS
Associate Professor of Small Animal Surgery
University of California-Davis

Acknowledgments

We are indebted to the skilled work of our medical illustrator, John Doval, whose tireless hours of work were performed with relentless good humor and enthusiasm. He was responsible for creating all of the animations in the book as well as editing many of the figures. We also would like to extend a special word of gratitude to the companies that play a huge role in driving forward the development of MIS in veterinary medicine through innovation and education. In particular, Karl Storz Endoscopy and Covidien, Inc. have been ever present supporters of both the Veterinary Endoscopy Society and other hands-on educational offerings in the field.

In addition, we thank Erica Judisch, Wiley, for initiating the development of this book and for her expertise and support in the field of publishing. We also appreciate the assistance extended by her colleagues Nancy Turner and Catriona Cooper.

Finally, we want to express our gratitude to the ACVS Foundation who, in collaboration with Wiley-Blackwell, made production of this book possible.

BAF
PDM

About the Companion Website

This book is accompanied by a companion website:

www.wiley.com/go/fransson/laparoscopy

The website includes:
- Videos (indicated by an "eye" icon in the margin)
- PowerPoint figures from the book

History of Small Animal Laparoscopy and Thoracoscopy

Boel A. Fransson

Veterinary minimally invasive surgery (MIS) as a surgical technique is unique because it had its origin in human application. Other biomedical techniques were traditionally developed in animal models and later applied to human patients. Therefore, the history of small animal MIS has to start with the overall history of laparoscopy. Parallel with the developments in laparoscopy were work in the chest cavity, but because much of the development were driven by urologists and gynecologists, the text below will often use the term laparoscopy interchangeably with *MIS*.

Endoscopy in the 19th Century

A variety of opinions exist on who should be credited with the invention of endoscopy. Some suggest to go back to Hippocrates (460–377 BC), who performed rectal examinations with a speculum.[7,8]

More consistently, the German physician Philipp Bozzini (1773–1809) has received credit for clinical use of his invention, the "Lichtleiter," the light conductor, a primitive endoscope for inspection of the ears, mouth, nasal cavity, urethra, rectum, bladder, and cervix. The Bozzini family was a well-to-do Italian family, but they had to leave Italy for Germany because of a lost duel by the father. Bozzini dedicated the last 5 years of his life, which was cut short by contracting typhus from his patients, to development of his instrument, a vase-shaped, leather-covered tin lantern using a wax candle light source (Figure 0-1).[3] Although the Austrian contemporary health authorities were satisfied with the instrument, a second opinion by the Vienna medical school, likely negatively influenced by the church, concluded that such an instrument should not be used.

In the latter part of the 19th century, interest was again renewed in using endoscopy. A French urologist, Antoine Jean Desormeaux (1815–1882), modified Bozzini's lichtleiter such that a mirror would reflect light from a kerosene lamp through a long metal channel, referring to his instrument as an "endoscope." Desormeaux is considered a leader in early endoscopy development and perhaps the first to successfully use the new technology for diagnostic and therapeutic use in clinical practice. Desormeaux's endoscope was certainly not without its flaws—the required positioning of the device entailed risks of burning the face of the physician or the thighs of the patient. Also, because catheter systems were not yet in use, urine would often "extinguish the flame, ruining the examination".[8]

The 1930s: The Glory Days

The 20th century saw rapid technology development, which led to more widespread promotion of endoscopy. Paralleled with this development were improvements in safety and operating procedures provided by antibiotics, better anesthesia, and blood

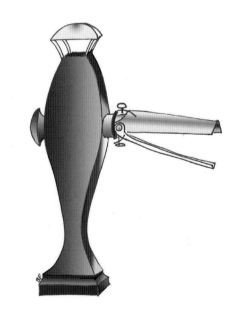

Figure 0-1 Bozzini's Lichtleiter, a vase-shaped, leather-covered tin lantern using a wax candle light source. (Courtesy of Dr. David C. Twedt.)

transfusions. By the 1930s, endo-urologists had embraced endoscopic technology with giddy enthusiasm, but surgical application was still lagging behind. Inadequate optics has been stated as one of the major reasons for this stall in progress.

Enter the German gastroenterologist Heinz Kalk (1895–1973), who in 1929 introduced a foreoblique lens system, which effectively increased the field of vision. Kalk is considered by many to be one of the greatest clinical laparoscopists of all time. He was disturbed by the contemporary high fatality rates associated with liver biopsies, and he was the first to introduce a safe and accurate method of endoscopic biopsies of the liver, gallbladder, and kidney. With Kalk's improvements, the increased usefulness of the endoscope invigorated surgeons to start using the technology. Before Kalk, endoscopy had mainly been applied by gynecologists and urologists. Kalk was fortunate to, just barely, make it out alive during the Stalingrad invasion of 1943. His survival was fortuitous for the development of laparoscopy because the highly productive physician continued his prolific scientific publishing and research well into the 1950s. During the 1950s, he began collaborating with Karl Storz in the development of instrumentation.

Another landmark in the 1930s occurred when the Hungarian physician Janos Veress developed a novel spring-loaded needle in 1937. The needle was originally used to perform therapeutic pneumothorax to treat patients with tuberculosis. However, laparoscopists quickly realized its potential for safe creation of pneumoperitoneum.[8]

Meanwhile, back in America, John Ruddock (1891–1961), an internist from Los Angeles, was most likely the principal driving force behind the acceptance of laparoscopy in the United States during the 1930s and beyond. Ruddock was known to work tirelessly to advocate for the laparoscope and to make a plea to internists and surgeons to work more cooperatively toward the goal of bringing minimally invasive care to patients. With his "peritoneoscope," he was able to diagnose patients with metastatic gastric carcinoma by minimally invasive means, sparing them a nontherapeutic and thus wasted laparotomy because metastatic disease was considered non-operable at the time.

By the end of the 1930s, operative laparoscopic procedures were finally in more general clinical use and were no longer restricted to a few dedicated centers. However, parallel with this development were rising death rates from endoscopy complications. Some of the early pioneer physicians were visionary enough to comment on "the need for doctors to essentially retrain themselves" as an important impediment to general acceptance of laparoscopy.

Out in the Cold: The 1940s to the Mid 1960s

The increasing rate of deadly complications associated with rising use of laparoscopy was likely the reason that a 25-year gap in development took place in the United States between 1939 and 1966.[8] Fortunately, the development continued in Europe, with the Swedish-born French gynecologist Raoul Palmer (1904–1985) achieving brilliant milestones. During the early 1940s, in occupied Paris during World War II, he discovered the benefits of the Trendelenburg position for pelvic visualization. He developed safer administration of insufflation gases; video capture of procedures; and not least, excelled in the training of innumerable disciples from all over the world. Many of the great laparoscopists of the 1960s through the 1980s were trained by Palmer, who apparently was a generous and beloved teacher and mentor.

Unfortunately, the development of laparoscopy was not straightforward. In 1961, it suffered a great fall from grace when its use was banned in Germany as a "prohibitively hazardous procedure," a result of faulty insufflator and electrocautery units. By 1964, the ban was lifted because of improvements in component technology, but its reputation was nonetheless damaged.

Controversy Galore: The 1970s to the 1990s

For 21st century laparoscopic surgeons, the controversy surrounding laparoscopy as late as the 1980s and 1990s seems unbelievable. One of the remarkable pioneers, who persevered despite a massive storm of criticism, was the gynecologist Kurt Semm (1927–2003). In the 1970s, his innovations included the electronic insufflator, whose capability to precisely monitor intraabdominal pressures greatly increased the safety of pneumoperitoneum. He all but eliminated thermal injuries by improving radiofrequency electrosurgical techniques. He pioneered extra- and intracorporeal knot tying and invented the loop applicator.

In 1980, he performed the first laparoscopic appendectomy. No one could believe this was possible, and he was accused of pathological hoaxing. At the time, the gap between surgeons and gynecologists was immense. Semm's entrance into general surgery was seen as an attempt by a gynecologist to bolster his "operation ego".[1,6] All of his attempts to publish on his surgical technique were refused with the reasoning that such "nonsense will never belong to general surgery" or that it was "unethical." Even Semm's gynecologic colleagues thought he had gone too far and attacked his publications as being faulty and biased. The insulting criticism often went to extremes; the projector was unplugged during his presentations, with the motivation that unethical surgery was presented. After Semm lectured on laparoscopic appendectomy, the president of the German Surgical Society wrote to the Board of Directors of the German Gynecological Society suggesting suspension of Semm's license to practice medicine.

Camran Nezhat (1947–), a laparoscopic surgeon affiliated with Stanford University Medical Center in Palo Alto, California, and with the University of California San Francisco, is another such persevering pioneer.[2] He developed video laparoscopy, which removed the need for the surgeon to look directly through the eyepiece of the scope (Figure 0-2). This was a milestone and a pre-

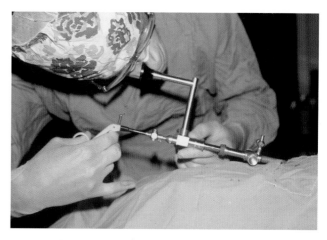

Figure 0-2 Laparoscopy performed in 1974, before the introduction of video laparoscopy. (Courtesy of Dr. David C. Twedt.)

requisite for the laparoscopic revolution that followed; a surgeon simply cannot perform advanced procedures crouched over an eyepiece. His development also made him one of the most controversial figures in the movement of minimally invasive technology. Opponents of MIS accused laparoscopists like Nezhat of hiding their complication rates and advancing dangerous methods for personal gain. A couple of high-profile lawsuits in the early 2000s triggered nationwide media coverage, as Nezhat was accused of medical malpractice and racketeering. Both suits were dismissed, and the allegations were considered frivolous lawsuits in the one case; the attorney in the second was subsequently charged with contempt of court. Allegations of research fraud were made against Nezhat, all which were found to be unsubstantiated.

Fortunately, some surgeons saw these hard-earned achievements for their true value, and by the early 1990s, laparoscopic appendectomies were performed by these early adaptors in vast numbers. Shortly thereafter, the "laparoscopic revolution" broke out, and suddenly Semm's and Nezhat's expertise and publications were in great demand. Finally, in 2002, Semm received the Pioneer in Endoscopy Award from the Society of American Gastrointestinal Endoscopic Surgeons.[1] Nezhat also has won numerous awards and honors from prestigious societies such as the American College of Obstetricians and Gynecologists, American College of Surgeons, and Society of Laparoendoscopic Surgeons.

Small Animal Minimally Invasive Surgery

With the human laparoscopic physicians leading the way, small animal MIS has not been nearly as controversial as its human counterpart. Similar to the case in the medical field, MIS was fairly slow to be incorporated in general veterinary clinical practice. Our development appears to parallel that of human surgery but with an approximately 20-year delay. A "laparoscopic revolution" like that in the human medical field cannot yet be claimed by veterinary surgeons, but MIS is steadily moving the stakes forward with increasing use and improved surgical technique.

Early Work: The 1970s

The first reports on laparoscopy in small animals were conducted on dogs in the early 1900s, but these were mainly experimental models before application in humans. Similar to gynecologists, theriogenologists were among the earliest clinical adapters of MIS in research and clinical veterinary medicine during the 1950s and 1960s. However, in the early 1970s, work with diagnostic laparoscopy was emerging in the small animal field. Surgical application was sparse, but David E. Wildt, a non-DVM PhD affiliated with the Division of Research Services at National Institutes of Health, reported on male and female sterilization by occlusion of the vas deferens and uterine horn, respectively, in the early 1980s. Dr. Wildt coedited the first textbook in 1980 on animal laparoscopy together with Richard Harrison, PhD, at Tulane University.[4]

In 1977, the DVM Drs. Gerald F. Johnson and David C. Twedt (Figure 0-3), both at the time affiliated with the Animal Medical Center in New York, presented the first review of small animal laparoscopy for clinical use.[5] At that time, laparoscopy was exclusively a diagnostic tool (Figure 0-4), and nitrous oxide was the pneumoperitoneum gas of choice, especially if performed without general anesthesia. Air and carbon dioxide were also recommended,

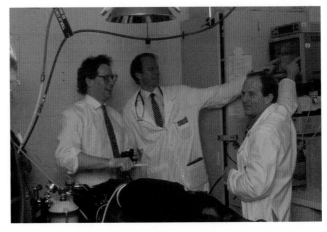

Figure 0-3 From left to right, Drs. Todd Tams, Steve Hill, and David Twedt are enjoying video laparoscopy in 1995. (Courtesy of Dr. David C. Twedt.)

and the authors mention their preferred use of a Corkmaster (Figure 0-5), a carbon dioxide dispenser intended for opening wine bottles, adapted for generation of pneumoperitoneum.[5]

Minimally Invasive Surgery Takes Off in Small Animal Surgery: The 2000s and Beyond

Arthroscopy was globally embraced by small animal veterinarians several years before the use of laparoscopy became widespread. From those early investigations in the late 1970s and 1980s, it would take another 2 decades before MIS would be commonly used for soft tissue applications in small animal surgery, the principal focus of this textbook. In 2009, the American College of Veterinary Surgeons added a requirement for MIS in resident training programs.

In 1999, Dr. Lynetta J. Freeman published *Veterinary Endosurgery*, the first textbook dedicated to application of MIS in small animals. To this day, this text remains a pioneering work because at that time, few clinical procedures had been described in dogs or cats, and the editor and her colleagues (Figure 0-6) shared their extensive clinical research and training experience

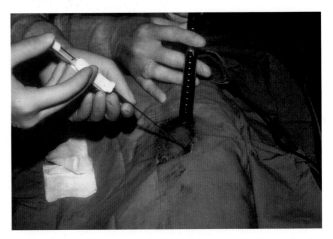

Figure 0-4 A proctoscope is used as a low-cost laparoscope for visualization of a liver biopsy in the 1970s. (Courtesy of Dr. David C. Twedt.)

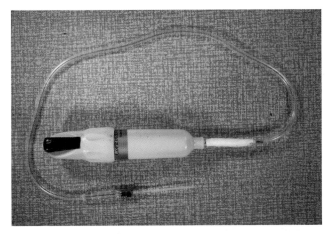

Figure 0-5 A Corkmaster, a carbon dioxide dispenser intended for opening wine bottles, adapted for generation of capnoperitoneum used by Drs. Twedt and Johnson in the 1970s. (Courtesy of Dr. David C. Twedt.)

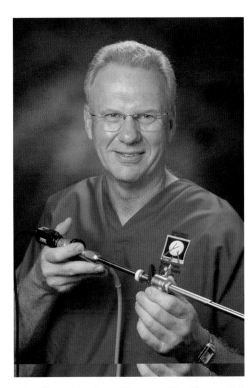

Figure 0-7 Dr. Clarence Rawlings. (Courtesy of Dr. Clarence A. Rawlings.)

from the research and development section of Ethicon Endosurgery.

Dr. Clarence A. Rawlings (Figure 0-7) and coworkers presented a series of publications in the early 2000s describing use of different laparoscopic-assisted surgical techniques. These continue to serve an important function today, bridging the gap between open and fully laparoscopic procedures. Dr. Rawlings is a pioneer of veterinary MIS and has been a dedicated instructor to hundreds of veterinarians interested in the field.

Small animal MIS has benefitted from an important advocate in Dr. Eric Monnet over the past 20 years. His contributions to the field have been imperative to clinical adaptation and development of laparoscopic and thoracoscopic techniques. In addition, Dr. Monnet's contributions also include founding the Veterinary Endoscopy Society (VES) (Figure 0-8) in 2003, bringing American veterinarians together with a common mission

of promoting and developing minimally invasive techniques. Recently, the VES has reached out internationally, with the hope of expanding into a multinational community of veterinarians interested in the field.

Development of increasingly advanced clinical techniques is currently ongoing at a fast pace, and important contributions over the past decade have been made by Drs. Gilles Dupre, Philipp Mayhew, Jolle Kirpensteijn, Mary-Ann Radlinsky, Eric Viguier, and many others.

Lack of skills was noted as an important impediment to MIS development among our predecessors in the human field. Our research group at Washington State University has made important contributions to the veterinary MIS field within the area of assessment and training of veterinarians' manual skills.

A number of talented clinicians and researchers are currently active within small animal MIS. We anticipate further milestone achievements by these great men and women of our profession in the near future.

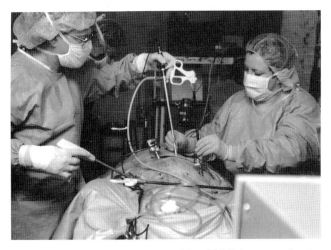

Figure 0-6 Drs. Lynnetta J. Freeman and Ronald J. Kolata are performing laparoscopy on a lion at the Audubon Zoo. (Courtesy of Dr. Lynneta J. Freeman.)

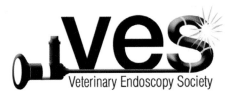

Figure 0-8 The Veterinary Endoscopy Society was founded by Dr. Eric Monnet in 2003.

Acknowledgements

Regretfully, many important contributors to the field were not mentioned in this text for the sake of brevity. Many pioneers contributed milestone developments and achieved glorious things despite technological limitations and often in a skeptical environment. To them, we collectively want to express our gratitude for their hard work paving the road to contemporary MIS. Thank you!

References

1 Bhattacharya, K. (2007) Kurt Semm: a laparoscopic crusader. J Minim Access Surg 3(1), 35-36.

2 Carter, J.E. (2006) Biography of Camran Nezhat, MD, FACOG, FACS. JSLS 10(2), 275-280.

3 Harrison, R.M. (1980) Historical Development of Laparoscopy in Animals. In: Harrison, R.M., Wildt, D.E. (eds.) Animal Laparoscopy. Williams & Wilkins, Baltimore, pp. 1-14.

4 Harrison, R.M., Wildt, D.E. (1980) Animal Laparoscopy. Williams & Wilkins, Baltimore.

5 Johnson, G.F., Twedt, D.C. (1977) Endoscopy and laparoscopy in the diagnosis and management of neoplasia in small animals. Vet Clin North Am 7(1), 77-92.

6 Litynski, G.S. (1998) Kurt Semm and the fight against skepticism: endoscopic hemostasis, laparoscopic appendectomy, and Semm's impact on the "laparoscopic revolution." JSLS 2(3), 309-313.

7 Mishra, R.K. (2009) Chronological advances in minimal access surgery. In: Mishra RK (ed.) Textbook of Practical Laparoscopic Surgery. 2nd edn. Jaypee Brothers Medical Publishers, , pp. 3-8.

8 Nezhat, C. (2011) Nezhat's History of Endoscopy: A Historical Analysis of Endoscopy's Ascension Since Antiquity. EndoPress, Tuttlingen, Germany.

SECTION I

Laparoscopic Skills

1 Surgeons' Skills Training

Boel A. Fransson, Heather A. Towle Millard, and Claude A. Ragle

Adding Minimally Invasive Surgery to the Surgical Repertoire

Since the introduction of laparoscopy and thoracoscopy in small animal surgery in the mid 1970s, the main focus has been on the development of surgical techniques and equipment. Not until recently has veterinary medicine recognized the importance of skills development for surgeons who want to incorporate minimally invasive surgery (MIS) in their clinical practice.

Even for surgeons with considerable expertise in traditional open surgery, it will be readily apparent when approaching MIS that some laparoscopic skills are distinctly different from those of open surgery. The challenges and differences include the use of long instruments, which magnifies any tremor and limits tactile sensation, often referred to as haptic feedback. When the instrument movement is limited by a portal into the body cavity, the surgeon needs to handle the resulting fulcrum effect and the loss of freedom to simply alter an approaching angle. But even more important, the normal binocular vision becomes monocular; as a result, the associated depth perception is lost. Other challenges include the loss of a readily accessible bird's eye view of the entire body cavity. The advantage of magnification may be perceived as offset by a reduced field of view, and any instrument activity outside the view becomes a liability.

Understandably, a surgeon who has performed hundreds or more of any given procedure, with good success and minimal time expenditure, may initially be reluctant to take on the challenges of MIS. This may be especially conspicuous in small animal laparoscopy, in which the conventional surgical approach provides excellent and easy access to all intraabdominal organs. A budding small animal laparoscopic surgeon may meet resistance from referring veterinarians and even staff members when converting open procedures to laparoscopic because costs and surgery time, at least initially, tend to be higher. Educating the referral base, clients, and staff in the advantages of laparoscopy may alleviate but not remove the initial resistance.

The solution to minimizing the surgeon's pains of transitioning from open to laparoscopic surgery consists of pretraining. The basic laparoscopic skills of ambidexterity, optimizing instrument interaction; observing cues for depth perception; and precise, deliberate movements need to be achieved early in the skills development for the benefit of patient safety and surgeon's confidence in the operating room (OR).

Basic Laparoscopic Skills

The basic skills required for laparoscopic surgery include ambidexterity, hand–eye coordination, instrument targeting accuracy, and recognition of cues to provide a sense of depth.[1,2]

Although these skills are used, and therefore trained, in clinical practice, the surgeon should not rely on caseload for training. The Institute of Medicine reported in "To Err Is Human" that approximately 100,000 humans die each year as a result of medical errors and that approximately 57% of these deaths are secondary to surgical mistakes.[3] Despite efforts to prevent surgery-related human deaths, the cost of training one surgical resident in an OR throughout the course of his or her residency is estimated to cost nearly $50,000.[4,5] and this is becoming cost prohibitive for teaching institutions. In addition, medical surgery residents are now limited to working 80 hours per week,[6] which further limits their exposure to clinical cases.

Although the number of surgical-related deaths in veterinary medicine in the United States is not known, they do occur. In addition, even though OR costs do not equal those of training a human surgical resident and we currently do not have limits on the work week of veterinary students or veterinary surgery residents, veterinary medicine has its own set of dilemmas. Veterinary training curricula are also faced with financial limitations, as well as increasing external and internal ethical concerns regarding the use of research animals for surgical training; increasing number of veterinary students being admitted to programs and subsequent decreased

Small Animal Laparoscopy and Thoracoscopy, First Edition. Edited by Boel A. Fransson and Philipp D. Mayhew.
© 2015 by ACVS Foundation. Published 2015 by John Wiley & Sons, Inc.
Companion website: www.wiley.com/go/fransson/laparoscopy

exposure to laboratory and clinical cases; lack of sustainability of cadavers because of problems with availability, storage, and limited usefulness because of decay; and the drive to reduce errors made by inexperienced surgeons on actual patients.[7,8] For these reasons, both human and veterinary educators are being compelled to develop innovative teaching methods for surgical skill instruction.

Beside the ethical and cost issues, it is likely that a training program built on practice in live patients becomes limited and inconsistent. Interestingly, we have noticed in our work that even experienced veterinary laparoscopic surgeons tend to lag in efficient use of their nondominant hands, something easily rectified by simulation training.[9] In fact, the basic skills are most efficiently trained through simulation training.[10] This has been recognized for more than a decade among medical doctors, and since 2008, laparoscopic simulation training curricula have been a requirement for surgery residency programs in the United States.[11] Robust evidence has been presented to demonstrate that skills developed by simulation indeed transfer into improved OR performance.[12-16]

Simulation Training Models

A number of simulation models have been presented and can currently be divided into three main categories: physical; virtual reality (VR); and hybrid, or augmented reality (AR), models.

Physical Simulation Models: Box Trainers

Box trainers have in common that tasks are performed using regular laparoscopic instruments in a box containing a camera, which projects onto a computer or TV screen. A number of box trainers are commercially available (Figure 1-1) and carry the advantages of being portable and highly versatile. As web cam technology has improved within recent years, homemade trainers can be a very cost-effective alternative if portability is not a requirement. An example of a homemade trainer used in the author's Veterinary Applied Laparoscopic Training (VALT) laboratory is presented in Figures 1-2 to 1-4. Homemade versions are used solely for practice and not for skills assessments.

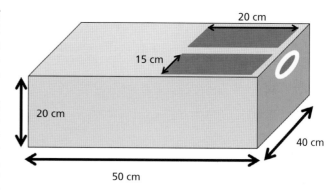

Figure 1-2 Commonly used dimensions in laparoscopic training boxes.

Box training can be considered low-fidelity simulation (i.e., less lifelike but nonetheless highly efficient training tools). A number of practice drills have been developed and validated. In the 1990s, several structured training tasks were described, including the Dr. Rosser's station tasks developed at Yale University, which are part of the popular "Top-Gun Shoot-Out" competition at national meetings for physicians. The physical training task system with the most solid validation to date is the McGill Inanimate Simulator for Training and Evaluation of Laparoscopic Skills (MISTELS).[10,17-19] At present, MISTELS includes peg transfer, pattern cutting, ligature loop placement, and intra- and extracorporeal suturing. An additional cannulation task is currently being incorporated.[20]

We have considerable experience of MISTELS-type training of veterinarians in our simulation training facility, the VALT laboratory

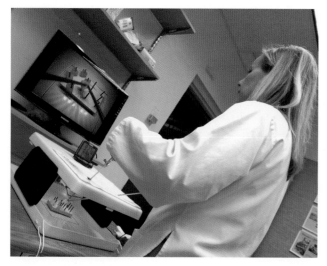

Figure 1-1 A number of laparoscopic skills training boxes are commercially available. Most are portable, and many have cameras that connect to a computer by USB connections. Some, including the official box for Fundamentals of Laparoscopic Surgery, require a TV screen. (Photo courtesy of Henry Moore, Jr., Washington State University, College of Veterinary Medicine.)

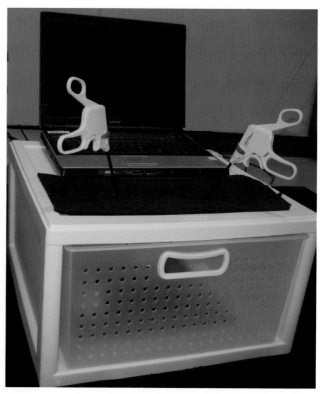

Figure 1-3 An example of a homemade training box.

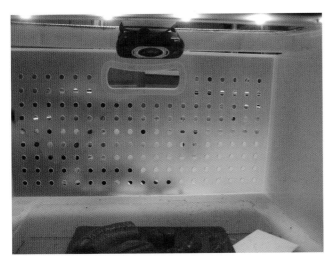

Figure 1-4 Recent advances in web cameras enable real-time imaging to a low cost.

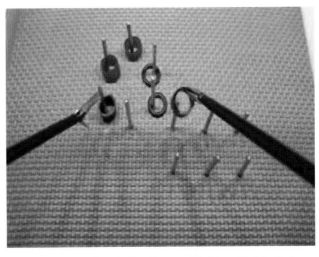

Figure 1-6 Peg transfer task. Six objects are lifted from the left-sided pegs with nondominant grasper, transferred midair to the dominant hand grasper, and then placed on a right-sided peg. The exercise is then reversed.

(Figure 1-5) at Washington State University. The adaptation of MIS-TELS for the VALT laboratory has been described in detail elsewhere,[9,21] and currently, the tasks we use include:

1 **Pegboard transfer:** Laparoscopic grasping forceps in the nondominant hand is used to lift each of six pegs from a pegboard, transfer them to a grasper in the dominant hand, place them on a second pegboard, and finally reverse the exercise (Figure 1-6).

2 **Pattern cutting:** This task involves cutting a 4-cm diameter circular pattern out of a 10 × 15-cm piece of instrument wrapping material or a gauze suspended between alligator clips (Figure 1-7).

3 **Ligature loop placement:** The task involves placing a ligature loop pretied with a laparoscopic slip knot over a mark placed on a foam appendix and cinching it down with a disposable-type knot pusher (Figure 1-8).

4 **Extracorporeal suturing:** A simple interrupted suture using long (90-cm) suture on a taper point needle is placed through marked needle entry and exit points in a slitted Penrose drain segment. The first throw in the knot is tied extracorporeally with a slip knot and cinched down by use of a knot pusher. Thereafter, three single square throws are placed by use of laparoscopic needle holders and the suture is cut (Figure 1-9).

5 **Intracorporeal suturing:** A simple interrupted suture is placed using short (12- to 15-cm-long) suture on a taper point needle through marked needle entry and exit points in a slitted Penrose drain segment. Three throws are placed, the first being a surgeon's (double) throw, by use of laparoscopic needle holders. The exercise is completed when the suture is cut (Figure 1-10).

In addition to the MISTELS exercises, we have found important benefits in the VALT laboratory of a variety of exercises, which have been presented.[9] We find that exercises performed in a simulated canine abdomen (Mayo Endoscopy Simulated Image, Sawbones,

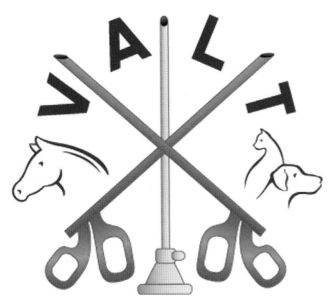

Figure 1-5 Logotype for the Veterinary Applied Laparoscopic Training laboratory at Washington State University.

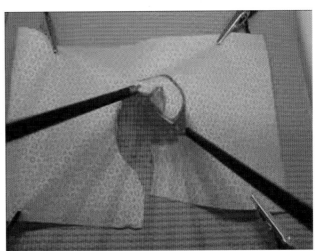

Figure 1-7 Pattern cut task. A 4-cm circle is cut, with a penalty applied if the cut is outside the mark.

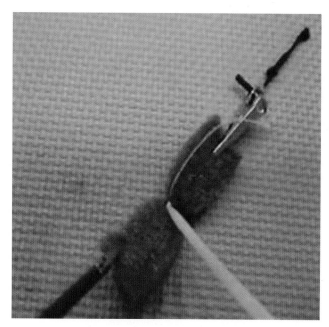

Figure 1-8 Ligature loop application task.

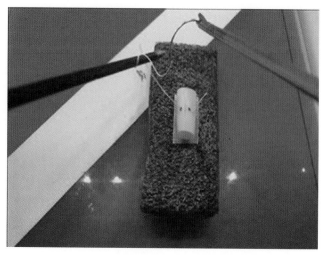

Figure 1-10 Intracorporeal suture task.

Vashon, WA; Figure 1-11) can be helpful in practicing camera manipulation and mirroring situations (i.e., camera facing surgeon) and can help prepare the surgeon for the confines of a canine abdomen.

The one major disadvantage with box training is the lack of instant feedback. Without automated feedback, an experienced surgeon needs to be available to critique the performance of the trainee, which becomes an important limitation because of the busy schedules of most surgeons. However, proficiency goals have been defined for MISTELS such that the trainee can monitor his or her progress by simple metrics such as time and errors.[22] With these goals in mind, the trainee can practice independently for the basic tasks of peg transfer, pattern cutting, and ligature loop placement. Laparoscopic suturing requires instructive sessions with an experienced surgeon. When suturing technique has been learned, the trainee can continue to practice independently to reach an expert level of performance, as defined by the proficiency goals.

Another disadvantage of box training is the current lack of veterinary high-fidelity surgery procedural models. Physical models

for cholecystectomy, appendectomy, and so on are commercially available, but they are all fairly expensive. In addition, they are all based on human anatomy and physiology and thus are less relevant for veterinary surgeons. A physical model, which can often be used only once, may not be feasible for most residency training programs if the cost is more than $100/each. Research into construction of low-cost yet higher fidelity physical models is ongoing at our institution, which may provide increased access to veterinary procedure models in the future.

Virtual Reality Simulation

Highly realistic VR simulation (Figure 1-12) is commercially available for both basic skills as well as entire simulated surgical procedures. In fact, one of the main advantages with VR training is realistic simulation of surgical procedures, which is hard to achieve to a reasonable cost in box training. For veterinarians, this advantage is somewhat limited, though, because anatomy and surgical procedures are all based on human anatomy.

Basic task simulations give the trainee opportunity to experience a variety of surgical complications, such as bleeding, dropping clips, and repercussion from rough tissue handling while benefiting from

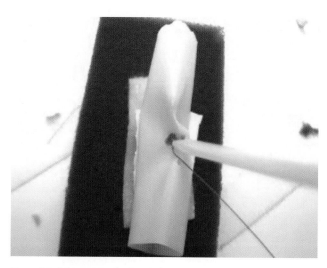

Figure 1-9 Extracorporeal suture task.

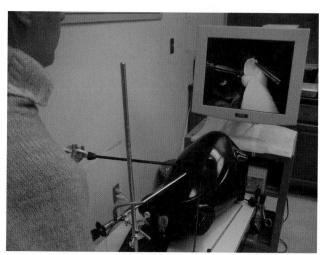

Figure 1-11 The Mayo Endoscopic Simulated Image (MESI) canine model (Sawbones, Vashon, WA) for laparoscopic and endoscopic practice.

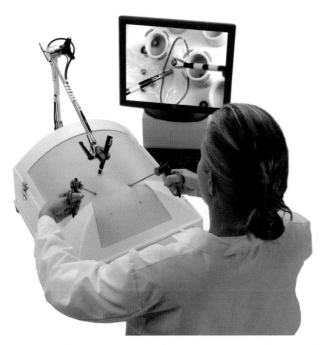

Figure 1-12 The ProMis augmented reality trainer is a combination of a physical box trainer and a virtual reality overlay used in many surgical exercises. (Photo courtesy of CAE Healthcare, © 2014 CAE Healthcare.)

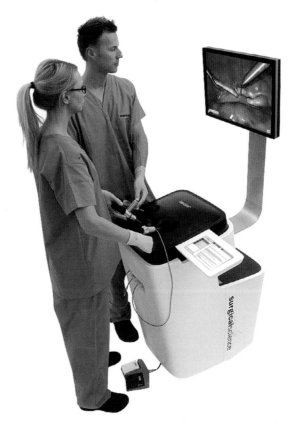

Figure 1-13 The LapSimHaptic system virtual reality trainer is combining high-technological virtual reality exercises with haptic feedback. (© Surgical Science Inc. Reproduced with permission from Surgical Science Inc.)

instant feedback and suggestions on how to proceed. Other advantages of VR simulation are that modules contain detailed instruction for performance of all tasks and summative feedback comparing the overall performance with an expert level. The summative performance is also broken down into a number of performance metrics, such as time, instrument path length for the dominant and nondominant hands, and errors, giving objective information about the performance. Therefore, the provided feedback of VR gives the trainee opportunity to practice without the need for an instructor. We have found that this instant feedback also serves as motivation because most surgeons and residents have competitive personalities and enjoy the comparison with expert level.

At present, a number of VR simulators are commercially available, but they all carry the disadvantage of being expensive. For example, a haptic LapSim (Surgical Science, Minneapolis, MN) unit currently cost a little over $90,000 (personal communication, Tony Rubin, VP, Surgical Science, Inc., September 2013), and software updates are also expensive. Another disadvantage is that, as mentioned, all VR simulation is based on human anatomy, and developing software for veterinary simulation is expensive; such models may not become available, at least not in the near future.

Because of the high cost of VR training, investigations have tried to determine if VR training can be justified by being more effective than box training. A recent systematic review through the Cochrane Institute found that VR procedural training shows some advantage over box training in operating time and performance.[23] Some controversy seems to exist: a similar review concluded that VR and box training both are valid teaching models and that both methods are recommended in surgical curricula but with no definitive superiority of VR.[24] Important for veterinary conditions, VR procedural training may not be superior unless it is procedure specific,[25] and thus it likely needs to be species specific.

Currently, the VALT laboratory group is studying the effects of incorporating VR basic skills or surgical procedural skills into the physical training curriculum, and this information will be available in the near future. Preliminary data do not support that VR cholecystectomy training translates to performance on a physical cholecystectomy model.

Hybrid Training Models: Augmented Reality

Virtual reality simulation has been criticized for the lack of realistic haptic feedback[26]; therefore, hybrid, or AR, simulators were developed that combine a live and a virtual environment. A number of AR simulators are commercially available.[27] To date, the most validated system is the ProMIS simulator (CAE Healthcare, Montreal, Quebec; Figure 1-13), which has been used in the VALT laboratory since 2010. Tasks are performed in a box trainer using real instruments, but a virtual interface can be placed over the image of the camera. Three cameras are used for motion tracking of the physical instruments in three planes. Therefore, objective metrics such as instrument path and economy of movement (i.e., velocity and directional changes over time, also expressed as motion smoothness) are provided. The metrics used have showed construct validity in suturing tasks and in the ability to separate expert colorectal surgeons from experienced laparoscopic, but novice colorectal, surgeons.[28,29]

In our experience, the use of surgical instruments adds realism to the simulation, which is in agreement with a study comparing AR with VR simulation.[30] However, an even bigger advantage for veterinary surgery is the ability to use novel physical models for simulation. Species-specific models can be custom made and used in the ProMIS, obtaining motion metrics feedback. Until species-specific simulation in VR is developed, this will likely be the most useful procedural simulation training device. The VALT laboratory is currently working on development of realistic simulation models made from materials of reasonable costs. Unfortunately, availability of the ProMIS simulator is currently reduced because the manufacturing company recently changed, and production is temporarily on hold.

Video Games in Laparoscopic Skills Training

Bench-top models, VR simulators, medical simulators, and robotic surgical systems have been investigated extensively in the human medical field. Although these systems have proven effective, they can be costly and time consuming to set up and maintain. Video gaming is a multi-billion dollar industry. In 2014, it was estimated that 59% of Americans play video games, with 52% of gamers being male and 42% of gamers being female. Twenty-nine percent of gamers are younger than 18 years old, 32% are 18 to 35 years old, and 39% are older than 36 years old.[31] This surge in the availability and the creation of new video games that have motion-sensing interfaces that allow gamers to move the controllers through three dimensions have led to an increasing interest in the usability of video games to aid in surgical training. Video games are portable, do not necessitate the use of a specialized skills laboratory, are easy to set up and use, and can be used within small spaces, and no consumables are associated with their use.

Contemporary video game consoles use similar skills as laparoscopic surgery in that they improve precision and accuracy of hand movements, two-hand coordination, and conversion of three-dimensional movements to a two-dimensional screen.[32] They require depth perception, timing, visual-motor dexterity, and quick reflexes.[33] Studies have shown that individuals who grew up playing video games have faster reaction times and improved performance on hand–eye coordinative tasks, spatial visualization tasks, and neuropsychological tests.[6,34-37] Video games have also been proven to enhance visual selective attention capacity[37] and to increase response time to visual stimuli.[38] Green and Bavalier[37] found that gamers have improved abilities to take in peripheral detail while still focusing on the specific task at hand; this is called "flanker compatibility task." Compared with nongamers, they also found that gamers have greater attention to detail as task difficulty increases and an increased ability to perform better at task switching and enumeration tasks. Green and Bavelier questioned if students who played video games had a natural inclination toward these skill sets or if playing video games actually increased performance. To test this, they had nongamers play video games for 1 hour per day for 10 days. Nongamers were able to improve their visuospatial task scores, thus rejecting the notion that video gamers do better because of a natural aptitude.[37] Last, video games have the added benefit of reducing stress among students while also being competitive and entertaining.[8,38]

Proof of Utility of Video Games

The positive correlation of performance with laparoscopic box trainers and surgical simulators to improved operative laparoscopic performance has been demonstrated repeatedly in human medicine.[14,22,33,39] Although hands-on training is ultimately required for complete training, video games may provide a useful precursor or adjunct to laparoscopic box trainers and surgical simulators. However, proof of the utility of video games must be demonstrated before incorporating video games into surgical training programs. Within the past decade, the human field has also published numerous studies demonstrating the positive correlation between video

game performance and laparoscopic box trainers, surgical simulators, and actual OR performance. Few studies currently exist in veterinary medicine. The following studies are just a glimpse of the benefits of using video games.

Badurdeen et al.[40] recruited 20 medical students and junior doctors with minimal laparoscopic surgical or video game experience. They found a positive correlation with video game scores and laparoscopic box-training skills (r = 0.78). In fact, participants scoring in the top tertile for video games scored 60.3% higher on laparoscopic box trainers than the bottom tertile ($P <0.01$).

Boyle et al.[41] recruited 22 medical students without previous laparoscopic or video game experience. Baseline laparoscopic box-training skills were obtained. Then half of the students were allocated to continue to not play video games while the other half was allocated to play for 3 hours. All participants then returned in 5 to 7 days to retest their laparoscopic skills. Those with just 3 hours of video game experience scored better than those that did not play.

Adams et al.[6] obtained baseline laparoscopic simulator scores and then randomly allocated 31 surgical residents to 6 weeks of practice on a laparoscopic simulator, XBOX 360 (Microsoft Corp., Redmond, WA) or Nintendo Wii (Nintendo of America, Redmond, WA). At the end of the 6 weeks, all participants were retested on the laparoscopic simulator. Quite interestingly, participants who played the XBOX 360 or Nintendo Wii improved the most.

Grantcharov et al.[42] surveyed 25 surgical residents with and without past video game experience. Those with past video game experience of varying levels made fewer errors than nonusers in the OR ($P = 0.035$).

Shane et al.[43] found that fourth-year medical students who played more than 3 hours of video games per week had improved laparoscopic simulator scores and shorter learner curves than nongamers.

Rosser et al.[44] found that surgeons who play video games for more than 3 hours each week were 27% faster, made 37% fewer errors, and scored 42% better overall than surgeons who had no video game exposure with laparoscopic operative skills and suturing. Current video game players were 24% faster, made 32% fewer errors, and scored 26% better overall than their nonplayer colleagues. Past and current video game skill not only increased speed but also decreased errors.

Towle Millard et al.[8] published the first veterinary study correlating video game performance and laparoscopic skills. Twenty-nine third-year veterinary students volunteered to participate in the study; they all had varying levels of past video game experience. However, none of the participants had previous experience with the three test video games or the three laparoscopic box-trainer tasks. The study clearly demonstrated a positive correlation between video game proficiency and laparoscopic box-trainer proficiency (rs = +0.40, $P = 0.031$).[8]

Future Incorporation of Video Games Into Training Programs

The studies just discussed are just a few of the many studies that demonstrate the positive correlation between past and current video game experience and improved scores on laparoscopic box trainers, laparoscopic surgical simulators, and laparoscopic operative performance. Additional veterinary studies are needed, but one could surmise that the results will likely be similar to those in the human medical field. Now that the link has been made, educators can explore methods to incorporate video games into helping students discover natural aptitudes and advancing surgical training before they enter the OR.

Kennedy et al.[36] recently proposed that video games may be useful for identifying and assessing natural aptitudes. Studies have been conducted on high school students, medical students, medical surgery residents, and veterinary students. Video games may be a method to help direct students into discovering hidden talents and help direct them to future career paths. Towle Millard and Freeman[45] surveyed 68 third-year veterinary students. They found that the 38 students with a higher interest in surgery had higher video game scores ($P = 0.023$) than the 30 students with a higher interest in internal medicine. Interestingly, Fanning et al.[46] found that teenagers with video gaming experience performed better on laparoscopy simulators than medical surgery residents with no gaming experience. Kennedy et al.[36] found that medical students who average 7 hours of video gaming per week had better psychomotor skills than those who did not play regularly. Shane et al.[43] found that medical students and first-year surgery residents with previous and current video gaming experience took fewer trials to gain proficiency on a laparoscopic simulator than did nongamers. Badurdeen et al.[40] suggested that the surgical residents who perform better on video games could be viewed more positively when selecting suitable surgery candidates to advance to laparoscopic training programs.

Besides helping identify promising young students and incorporating video games into training programs before entering the OR, video games may also be used as a "warm-up" method before starting surgeries to decrease the number of OR complications. Gallagher et al.[47] and Gallagher and Satava[48] demonstrated that 15 to 20 minutes of warm-up with simulators resulted in fewer OR errors in both fresh and fatigued surgeons. Rosser et al.[34] demonstrated that the use of video games just before performing surgery resulted in faster surgeons who made fewer errors versus surgeons who did not warm up. Using video games as a warm-up method is just another benefit of this cost-effective, motivational, and highly available resource.

Conclusion

Medical and veterinary educators are compelled to develop innovative methods to teach surgery as they are faced with expanding curricula, more students, financial constraints, limited time, and increasing ethical concerns of inexperience students and surgeons operating on actual patients. The traditional approach of "learning by doing" in a clinical arena is falling out of favor in both human and veterinary surgery.[49] The current social climate in human medicine is that novices should not gain their basic skills on actual patients, and this is extending to veterinary medicine as more and more veterinary owners think of their small animal pets as family members.

Although box trainers and surgical simulators are obvious training modalities, video games are an underused modality that is inexpensive and has been shown to directly correlate with box trainers, surgical simulators, and OR performance. As the technology advances, video games can be designed that directly simulate laparoscopic surgery. These modalities will not completely replicate actual OR experiences, but using them could be part of the solution of improving patient outcomes and addressing the dilemmas faced by teaching institutions.

The Optimal Training Program

Extensive amounts of research have provided comprehensive information on training program design. What follows is a brief discussion of current evidence-based information, with

comparative aspects with our experience of veterinary training in the VALT laboratory.

Ideally, training initially focuses on basic skills task training before progressing to specific surgical procedure training. More important than the type of simulation model one has access to is that the practice is deliberate.[50] Expertise is not gained by simply spending time practicing but by engaging in a specific type of practice. The concept of deliberate practice[50] outlines the critical elements of optimal learning, that is, tasks with (1) well-defined goals, (2) motivation to learn, (3) feedback, and (4) opportunities for repetition and refinement.

Tasks and Goals

Training tasks can be selected based on construct validity (i.e., tasks in which performance has been demonstrated to correlate with higher skill levels). However, face value is also important (i.e., experienced surgeons confirming that a training task is using the same skill sets as those required in clinical practice). All tasks need to be demonstrated clearly and effectively for superior learning. Ideally, trainees have unlimited access to high-quality video tutorials and demonstrations, complementing and significantly decreasing the need for expert instructor involvement.[51]

Training goals in form of performance targets are generally accepted as superior to time-based training because individuals may differ considerably in how fast the target is reached. For MISTELS-based training, performance goals have been clearly defined.[22] For other practice tasks, speed, accuracy, or even motion metrics have shown severe limitations, and appropriate training goals for trainees at different levels of training remain work in progress.[51] A training study in the VALT laboratory failed to document advantages of proficiency goals compared with time control,[9] and this observation has also been made by others.[52] Perhaps as the medical field learns more about simulation training, we will become increasingly successful in setting appropriate goals. Despite our experiences in the VALT laboratory, we consider proficiency goals valuable because we have noted that training goals appear to add motivation to practice.

Motivation

Internal motivation is a prerequisite for learning but cannot be relied on as the sole driving source for a successful training program. Surgical residents and practicing surgeons are affected by long working hours, limited free time, and seemingly endless clinical responsibilities. Not surprisingly, studies on voluntary participation of skills training in a busy residency showed the participation rate as between 6% and 14%.[53,54] These studies showed that providing dedicated regular time for mandatory training, known ahead of time to trainees and their faculty, greatly improved participation. For a laboratory with limited resources, this may be hard to accomplish. In the VALT laboratory, we have had success with mandatory training sessions but with timing flexibility through an online sign-up policy, so each trainee can choose the time that works best for him or her without affecting the clinic or crowding the laboratory. The importance of dedicated laboratory personnel, keeping track of the trainees' sessions, and the commitment from faculty in supporting the training cannot be stressed enough. In addition, external motivation can be gained from training feedback and scheduled skills assessments. Further external motivation may be gained by performance requirements on simulators before OR participation,[51] but we have not yet felt a need for that at the VALT laboratory. Importantly, we have found an inverse relationship between motivation for simulation training and clinical experience,[9] under-scoring the importance of initiating simulation training early in a laparoscopic surgeon's career.

Feedback

Regular feedback during simulation training is not only a tool for motivation but is also essential for skills acquisition and retention. As already discussed, motion metrics serve as instant feedback during VR training and are likely one of the most important advantages to that type of simulation training. However, verbal feedback from experts has been shown more effective than motion metrics.[55] Specific and individualized feedback and subsequent training tailored to address that feedback have recently been shown to greatly improve OR performance.[56]

Opportunity to Practice

Currently, the opportunity for simulation training is severely limited for veterinary surgeons and residents. Hopefully, veterinary surgery will show a similar development to that occurring over the past decade among MD surgeons. In 2006, only 55% of residency programs had training laboratories,[57] but by 2008, such laboratories became a requirement.[11] Currently, the VALT laboratory offers training for external DVMs, but ideally, residents should have easy access to simulation training at their home institutions and practices. This preference is based on the fact that distributed practice leads to better skills acquisition compared with intense extended practice.[51] The optimal distribution is presently considered to be 1-hour sessions with a maximum of two sessions per day interspersed by a rest period, allowing the brain the opportunity to internalize the learning.[58] Approximately 10 hours of practice has been demonstrated to lead to fundamentals of laparoscopic surgery (FLS) competency,[22] but mastery within any given field requires approximately 10,000 hours of deliberate practice.[58] Skill decay will ensue after rigorous training, but with ongoing practice in small amounts at 6-months intervals, performance has been shown to be maintained at a high level.[58]

Self-training

Most veterinarians in practice do not and will not have easy access to simulation training curricula. Fortunately, MISTELS type exercises lend themselves well to self-study because there are well-defined training goals that are easy to monitor. Self-study guidelines based on performance time have been demonstrated, showing that reliable achievement of 53-s peg transfer, 50-s pattern cut, 87-s ligature loop, 99-s extracorporeal suturing, and 96-s intracorporeal suturing times are associated with an 84% chance of passing the FLS test,[59] thus demonstrating basic skills competency. Laparoscopic suturing will likely require training proctored by experienced surgeons, and we encourage self-study trainees to seek instruction for those exercises. Presently, there is a move to make video-tutorial training material and a manual skills test, Veterinary Assessment of Laparoscopic skills (VALS), also available for veterinarians. The VALS program is based on the rigorously validated MISTELS program for training and assessment of skills. The goal is to create a readily available training program for all veterinary surgeons, leading to improved OR performance. A 5-week systematic video game training program showed a positive impact on subsequent performance on complex surgical simulator tasks.[60] Such a rigorous video gaming program could be readily available to surgeons, and if routinely incorporated into VALS, constitute an inexpensive precursor or concurrent training modality.

References

1 Derossis, A.M., Fried, G.M., Abrahamowicz, M., Sigman, H.H., Barkun, J.S., Meakins, J.L. (1998) Development of a model for training and evaluation of laparoscopic skills. Am J Surg 175(6), 482-487.
2 Rosser, J.C. Jr, Rosser, L.E., Savalgi, R.S. (1998) Objective evaluation of a laparoscopic surgical skill program for residents and senior surgeons. Arch Surg 133(6), 657-661.
3 Kohn, L.T.C.J., Donaldson, M.S. (2000) Institute of Medicine: To Err Is Human: Building a Safer Health System. National Academies Press, Washington, DC.
4 Van Hove, C., Perry, K.A., Spight, D.H., et al. (2008) Predictors of technical skill acquisition among resident trainees in a laparoscopic skills education program. World J Surg 32(9), 1917-1921.
5 Bridges, M., Diamond, D.L. (1999) The financial impact of teaching surgical residents in the operating room. Am J Surg 177(1), 28-32.
6 Adams, B.J., Margaron, F., Kaplan, B.J. (2012) Comparing video games and laparoscopic simulators in the development of laparoscopic skills in surgical residents. J Surg Educ 69(6), 714-717.
7 Langebaek, R., Berendt, M., Pedersen, L.T., Jensen, A.L., Eika, B. (2012) Features that contribute to the usefulness of low-fidelity models for surgical skills training. Vet Rec 170(14), 361.
8 Millard, H.A., Millard, R.P., Constable, P.D., Freeman, L.J. (2014) Relationships among video gaming proficiency and spatial orientation, laparoscopic, and traditional surgical skills of third-year veterinary students. J Am Vet Med Assoc 244(3), 357-362.
9 Fransson, B.A., Ragle, C.A. (2012) Effects of two training curricula on basic laparoscopic skills and surgical performance. J Am Vet Med Assoc 240(9), 451-460.
10 Fried, G.M., Feldman, L.S., Vassiliou, M.C., et al. (2004) Proving the value of simulation in laparoscopic surgery. Ann Surg 240(3), 518-525; discussion 25-28.
11 Scott, D.J., Dunnington, G.L. (2008) The new ACS/APDS Skills Curriculum: moving the learning curve out of the operating room. J Gastrointest Surg 12(2), 213-221.
12 Stefanidis, D., Acker, C., Heniford, B.T. (2008) Proficiency-based laparoscopic simulator training leads to improved operating room skill that is resistant to decay. Surg Innov 15(1), 69-73.
13 Stelzer, M.K., Abdel, M.P., Sloan, M.P., Gould, J.C. (2009) Dry lab practice leads to improved laparoscopic performance in the operating room. J Surg Res 154(1), 163-166.
14 Korndorffer, J.R. Jr, Stefanidis, D., Scott, D.J. (2006) Laparoscopic skills laboratories: current assessment and a call for resident training standards. Am J Surg 191(1), 17-22.
15 Buckley, C.E., Kavanagh, D.O., Traynor, O., Neary, P.C. (2014) Is the skillset obtained in surgical simulation transferable to the operating theatre? Am J Surg 207(1), 1461-1457.
16 Dawe, S.R., Windsor, J.A., Broeders, J.A., Cregan, P.C., Hewett, P.J., Maddern, G.J. (2014) A systematic review of surgical skills transfer after simulation-based training: laparoscopic cholecystectomy and endoscopy. Ann Surg 259(2), 236-248.
17 Vassiliou, M.C., Ghitulescu, G.A., Feldman, L.S., et al. (2006) The MISTELS program to measure technical skill in laparoscopic surgery: evidence for reliability. Surg Endosc. 20(5), 744-747.
18 Dauster, B., Steinberg, A.P., Vassiliou, M.C., et al. (2005) Validity of the MISTELS simulator for laparoscopy training in urology. J Endourol 19(5), 541-545.
19 Fraser, S.A., Klassen, D.R., Feldman, L.S., Ghitulescu, G.A., Stanbridge, D., Fried, G.M. (2003) Evaluating laparoscopic skills: setting the pass/fail score for the MISTELS system. Surg Endosc 17(6), 964-967.
20 Soper, N.J., Fried, G.M. (2008) The fundamentals of laparoscopic surgery: its time has come. Bull Am Coll Surg 93(9), 30-32.
21 Fransson, B.A., Ragle, C.A. (2010) Assessment of laparoscopic skills before and after simulation training with a canine abdominal model. J Am Vet Med Assoc 236(10), 1079-1084.
22 Scott, D.J., Ritter, E.M., Tesfay, S.T., Pimentel, E.A., Nagji, A., Fried, G.M. (2008) Certification pass rate of 100% for fundamentals of laparoscopic surgery skills after proficiency-based training. Surg Endosc 22(8), 1887-1893.
23 Nagendran, M., Gurusamy, K.S., Aggarwal, R., Loizidou, M., Davidson, B.R. (2013) Virtual reality training for surgical trainees in laparoscopic surgery. Cochrane Database Syst Rev 8:CD006575.
24 Willaert, W., Van De Putte, D., Van Renterghem, K., Van Nieuwenhove, Y., Ceelen, W., Pattyn, P. (2013) Training models in laparoscopy: a systematic review comparing their effectiveness in learning surgical skills. Acta Chir Belg 113(2), 77-95.
25 Jensen, K., Ringsted, C., Hansen, H.J., Petersen, R.H., Konge, L. (2014) Simulation-based training for thoracoscopic lobectomy: a randomized controlled trial: virtual-reality versus black-box simulation. Surg Endosc 28(6), 1821-1829.
26 Panait, L., Akkary, E., Bell, R.L., Roberts, K.E., Dudrick, S.J., Duffy, A.J. (2009) The role of haptic feedback in laparoscopic simulation training. J Surg Res 156(2), 312 316.

27 Botden, S.M., Buzink, S.N., Schijven, M.P., Jakimowicz, J.J. (2007) Augmented versus virtual reality laparoscopic simulation: what is the difference? A comparison of the ProMIS augmented reality laparoscopic simulator versus LapSim virtual reality laparoscopic simulator. World J Surg 31(4), 764-772.

28 Neary, P.C., Boyle, E., Delaney, C.P., Senagore, A.J., Keane, F.B., Gallagher, A.G. (2008) Construct validation of a novel hybrid virtual-reality simulator for training and assessing laparoscopic colectomy; results from the first course for experienced senior laparoscopic surgeons. Surg Endosc 22(10), 2301-2309.

29 Van Sickle, K.R., McClusky, D.A. 3rd, Gallagher, A.G., Smith, C.D. (2005) Construct validation of the ProMIS simulator using a novel laparoscopic suturing task. Surg Endosc 19(9), 1227-12231.

30 Botden, S.M., Jakimowicz, J.J. (2009). What is going on in augmented reality simulation in laparoscopic surgery? Surg Endosc 23(8), 1693-1700.

31 Entertainment Software Association. (2014) Sales, demographic, and usage data: essential facts about the computer and video game industry. 2014 [cited 2014 April 27]; Available from: http://www.theesa.com/about-esa/industry-facts/.

32 Giannotti, D., Patrizi, G., Di Rocco, G., et al. (2013) Play to become a surgeon: impact of Nintendo Wii training on laparoscopic skills. PLoS One 8(2), e57372.

33 Ju, R., Chang, P.L., Buckley, A.P., Wang, K.C. (2012) Comparison of Nintendo Wii and PlayStation2 for enhancing laparoscopic skills. JSLS 16(4), 612-618.

34 Rosser, J.C. Jr, Gentile, D.A., Hanigan, K., Danner, O.K. (2012) The effect of video game "warm-up" on performance of laparoscopic surgery tasks. JSLS 16(1), 3-9.

35 Griffith, J.L., Voloschin, P., Gibb, G.D., Bailey, J.R. (1983) Differences in eye-hand motor coordination of video-game users and non-users. Percept Mot Skills 57(1), 155-158.

36 Kennedy, A.M., Boyle, E.M., Traynor, O., Walsh, T., Hill, A.D. (2011) Video gaming enhances psychomotor skills but not visuospatial and perceptual abilities in surgical trainees. J Surg Educ 68(5), 414-420.

37 Green, C.S., Bavelier, D. (2003) Action video game modifies visual selective attention. Nature 423(6939), 534-537.

38 Castel, A.D., Pratt, J., Drummond, E. (2005) The effects of action video game experience on the time course of inhibition of return and the efficiency of visual search. Acta Psychol (Amst) 119(2), 217-230.

39 Diesen, D.L., Erhunmwunsee, L., Bennett, K.M., et al. (2011) Effectiveness of laparoscopic computer simulator versus usage of box trainer for endoscopic surgery training of novices. J Surg Educ 68(4), 282-289.

40 Badurdeen, S., Abdul-Samad, O., Story, G., Wilson, C., Down, S., Harris, A. (2010) Nintendo Wii video-gaming ability predicts laparoscopic skill. Surg Endosc 24(8), 1824-1828.

41 Boyle, E., Kennedy, A.M., Traynor, O., Hill, A.D. (2011) Training surgical skills using nonsurgical tasks—can Nintendo Wii improve surgical performance? J Surg Educ 68(2), 148-154.

42 Grantcharov, T.P., Funch-Jensen, P. (2009) Can everyone achieve proficiency with the laparoscopic technique? Learning curve patterns in technical skills acquisition. Am J Surg 197(4), 447-449.

43 Shane, M.D., Pettitt, B.J., Morgenthal, C.B., Smith, C.D. (2008) Should surgical novices trade their retractors for joysticks? Videogame experience decreases the time needed to acquire surgical skills. Surg Endosc 22(5), 1294-1297.

44 Rosser, J.C. Jr, Lynch, P.J., Cuddihy, L., Gentile, D.A., Klonsky, J., Merrell, R. (2007) The impact of video games on training surgeons in the 21st century. Arch Surg 142(2), 181-186; discussion 186.

45 Towle Millard, H.A.M.R., Freeman, L.J. (2014) Association between Wii video-gaming ability, 3-D spatial analysis skills, and laparoscopic performance and the level of surgical interest and gender in third year veterinary students. Presented at the 11th Annual Scientific Meeting of the Veterinary Endoscopy Society, Florence, Italy, May 15 to 17, 2014.

46 Fanning, J., Fenton, B., Johnson, C., Johnson, J., Rehman, S. (2011) Comparison of teenaged video gamers vs PGY-I residents in obstetrics and gynecology on a laparoscopic simulator. J Minim Invasive Gynecol 18(2), 169-172.

47 Gallagher, A.G., Satava, R.M. (2002) Virtual reality as a metric for the assessment of laparoscopic psychomotor skills. Learning curves and reliability measures. Surg Endosc 16(12), 1746-1752.

48 Gallagher, A.G., Smith, C.D., Bowers, S.P., et al. (2003) Psychomotor skills assessment in practicing surgeons experienced in performing advanced laparoscopic procedures. J Am Coll Surg 197(3), 479-488.

49 Kneebone, R.L., Scott, W., Darzi, A., Horrocks, M. (2004) Simulation and clinical practice: strengthening the relationship. Med Educ 38(10), 1095-1102.

50 Ericsson, K.A. (2004) Deliberate practice and the acquisition and maintenance of expert performance in medicine and related domains. Acad Med 79(10 suppl), S70-S81.

51 Stefanidis, D., Heniford, B.T. (2009) The formula for a successful laparoscopic skills curriculum. Arch Surg 144(1), 77-82; discussion.

52 Gonzalez, R., Bowers, S.P., Smith, C.D., Ramshaw, B.J. (2004) Does setting specific goals and providing feedback during training result in better acquisition of laparoscopic skills? Am Surg 70(1), 35-39.

53 Chang, L., Petros, J., Hess, D.T., Rotondi, C., Babineau, T.J. (2007) Integrating simulation into a surgical residency program: is voluntary participation effective? Surg Endosc 21(3), 418-421.

54 Stefanidis, D., Acker, C.E., Swiderski, D., Heniford, B.T., Greene, F.L. (2008b) Challenges during the implementation of a laparoscopic skills curriculum in a busy general surgery residency program. J Surg Educ 65(1), 4-7.

55 Porte, M.C., Xeroulis, G., Reznick, R.K., Dubrowski, A. (2007) Verbal feedback from an expert is more effective than self-accessed feedback about motion efficiency in learning new surgical skills. Am J Surg 193(1), 105-110.

56 Palter, V.N., Grantcharov, T.P. (2014) Individualized deliberate practice on a virtual reality simulator improves technical performance of surgical novices in the operating room: a randomized controlled trial. Ann Surg 259(3), 443-448.

57 Korndorffer, J.R. Jr, Dunne, J.B., Sierra, R., Stefanidis, D., Touchard, C.L., Scott, D.J. (2005) Simulator training for laparoscopic suturing using performance goals translates to the operating room. J Am Coll Surg 201(1), 23-29.

58 Swanström, L.L., Soper, N.J. (2014) Mastery of Endoscopic and Laparoscopic Surgery. 4th ed. Lippincott Williams & Wilkins, Philadelphia.

59 Cassera, M.A., Zheng, B., Swanstrom, L.L. (2012) Data-based self-study guidelines for the fundamentals of laparoscopic surgery examination. Surg Endosc 26(12), 3426-3429.

60 Kolga Schlickum, M., Hedman, L, Enochsson, L., Kjellin, A., Fellander-Tsai, L. (2008) Transfer of systematic computer game training in surgical novices on performance in virtual reality image guided surgical simulators. Stud Health Technol Inform 132:210-215.

2 Minimally Invasive Suturing Techniques

Boel A. Fransson and John C. Huhn

Key Points

- Laparoscopic intracorporeal suturing requires simulator training until the motion is fluent and automatic. There will be added challenges in the operating room (OR), and if the skill is not fluent in the simulator, clinical suturing will be near impossible.
- Sutures longer than 30 cm (12 in) are extremely challenging for intracorporeal suturing.
- Learn to identify clockwise and counterclockwise wrapping of suture to ensure square knots during intracorporeal suturing.
- For intracorporeal continuous suturing, barbed sutures are outstanding.
- Extracorporeal suturing requires a long suture, ideally exceeding 75 cm (30 in), and a knot pusher in addition to needle driver and grasper.
- For braided sutures, the knot is complete with three throws. However, for monofilament sutures, four to six throws are required for knot security.
- The ability to tie one or more types of slip knots for extracorporeal use is a useful skill for minimally invasive surgeons. As with intracorporeal suturing, the conditions in the OR tend to be more challenging, so make sure you make the slip knots with ease outside the OR.
- Most extracorporeal slip knots require added throws performed with intra- or extracorporeal technique to be secure.
- Automated suturing devices, including the Endo Stitch and the SILS (single incision laparoscopic surgery) Stitch device, are preferred by many surgeons.

Introduction to Laparoscopic Suturing

In the early years of minimally invasive surgery (MIS), controversy existed regarding the need for suturing skills. Many practicing surgeons thought that laparoscopic suturing was too difficult to ever be considered a realistic requirement.[1] However, in the early 1990s, a consensus was built: laparoscopic surgeons had to learn and apply basic suturing skills unless the development of laparoscopic surgery was to be impeded.[2] Soon it was recognized that these complex skills had to be practiced with other methods than the classical "see one, do one, teach one" paradigm of conventional residency training. As a result, simulation training became a requirement.

Currently, veterinary medicine is facing the same dilemma. The introduction of MIS into small animal surgery has resulted in MIS technology being available at most specialized and many nonspecialized practices. For progressive evolution of small animal MIS, we need to embrace suturing techniques. Because of the challenge of suturing, many replacement devices have been introduced, but most are expensive and not always as versatile or secure as desired. With suturing skills, many open surgical techniques can be replaced with minimally invasive counterparts for the benefit of our patients. Having suturing skills also increases the surgeon's confidence to deal with emergent situations during a surgical procedure without the need for conversion to open surgery.

This chapter is intended to give novice laparoscopic surgeons a foundation, enabling them to start practicing suturing in a simulator in preparation for clinical application. With suturing skills developed in the simulator, we have found that the step to intracorporeal clinical suturing is small for most trainees.

Needle Holders for Laparoscopic Suturing

Conventional laparoscopic needle holders differ from most other laparoscopic instruments in that they do not rotate around the axis of the instruments in order to provide stability. Articulating and rotating needle drivers have been introduced but have been criticized for creating imprecision in needle exit and for being more difficult to learn to use than conventional needle drivers.[3]

The handles are often of a straight axial design, placing the needle in line with the surgeon's hands to allow greater maneuverability and more natural motion of the wrist when suturing. The jaws are often single action and are usually operated by means of an ergonomic spring-loaded palm grip on the handle.

Small Animal Laparoscopy and Thoracoscopy, First Edition. Edited by Boel A. Fransson and Philipp D. Mayhew.

© 2015 by ACVS Foundation. Published 2015 by John Wiley & Sons, Inc.

Companion website: www.wiley.com/go/fransson/laparoscopy

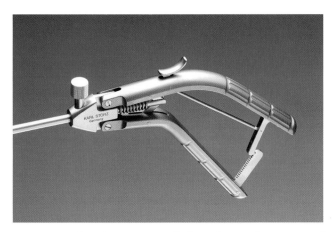

Figure 2-1 Pistol grip laparoscopic needle driver. (© 2014 Photo courtesy of KARL STORZ GmbH & Co. KG.)

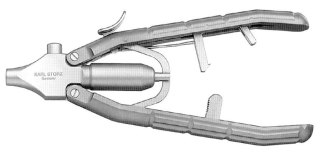

Figure 2-3 For novice laparoscopic surgeons, we recommend needle drivers that are sturdy, with straight handles, ribbed grips, and conveniently located needle release buttons on the grips. (© 2014 Photo courtesy of KARL STORZ GmbH & Co. KG.)

Several handle types are available, and the efficacies of four of them were compared.[4] It was found that a pistol grip (Figure 2-1) was superior for experienced operators but not for novices, who preferred a palmed straight grip. Neither experienced or novice users performed well nor preferred a thumb–ring finger grip (Figure 2-2).[4]

For novice laparoscopic surgeons, we recommend a needle driver that is sturdy, with straight handle, a ribbed grip, and a conveniently located needle release button on the grip (Figure 2-3). Hand size differs among surgeons; therefore, the preferred position of the release button may differ. When the release button is placed in the axis of the instrument, it can be used with either hand.

Needle driver jaws may be straight, curved left, or curved right (Figure 2-4). They can also be self-righting. Straight jaws are this author's (BAF) preference because they can be used in both left and right positions. The jaws are designed for a particular range of needle sizes, which is important to note before purchase. Self-righting needle drivers force the needle into a fixed position, usually at 90-degree angle to the instrument shaft. The limitations of self-righting needle drivers is that they should not be used to grasp the suture because they may damage or weaken the material. In addi-

tion, they reduce the surgeon's freedom to position the needle in different angles.

Suture Materials for Minimally Invasive Suturing

Conventional Sutures

Conventional suture materials are routinely used in MIS (Table 2.1). Braided synthetic absorbable sutures are often favored over monofilament synthetic absorbable sutures for intracorporeal suturing. The primary reason for this preference is the ease of handling that follows from the decreased memory of braided versus monofilament sutures. Furthermore, braided sutures are more resistant to instrument-induced damage during the knotting process. As knots are formed, there is significant interstrand friction, commonly known as chatter. This friction can induce significant damage to suture materials, particularly monofilaments. Braided materials are less vulnerable to this damage because their strength is distributed over many fibers similar to the cables of a suspension bridge. Braided materials are not without their downside, however. They have considerably more tissue drag than monofilament sutures, and they can harbor and potentiate bacterial infections. To minimize these effects, suture manufacturers have devised two solutions. First, application of coating agents, such as silicone, wax,

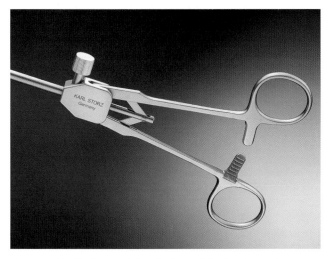

Figure 2-2 Needle driver with handle designed for thumb–ring finger grip. These did not perform as well as other designs.[4] (© 2014 Photo courtesy of KARL STORZ GmbH & Co. KG.)

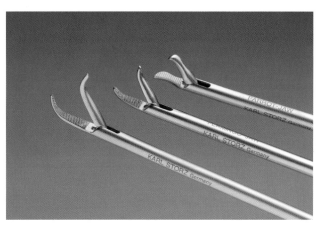

Figure 2-4 Different configurations of needle driver jaws. From top to bottom: "parrot jaw" curved left, "flamingo jaw" curved right for a 6-mm cannula, and "flamingo jaw" curved right for an 11-mm cannula. (© 2014 Photo courtesy of KARL STORZ GmbH & Co. KG.)

	Tensile Strength	Memory	Absorption Profile[22,23]	Throws Required[5]
Braided				
Polysorb	++++	–		3–4
Vicryl	++++	–		3–4
Monofilament				
Monocryl	++	–		3–4
Biosyn	+++	—	90–110 d	4–5
Polydioxanone (PDS)	++	–		3–4
Maxon	+++	—	180 d	4–5

Table 2-1 Conventional Sutures Used in Minimally Invasive Surgery

polytetrafluoroethylene (PTFE), caprolactone, and calcium stearate, fills in the gaps in the interstices of the braid and decreases friction during tissue passage. Second, some manufacturers use antimicrobial coatings on their materials to preemptively address suture-potentiated infections.

Knot security is a function of suture interstrand friction. Braided suture materials have a higher coefficient of friction than monofilament sutures. As such, braided sutures can form secure knots with fewer throws than monofilament sutures. In general, whereas braided sutures require three or four throws to form a secure knot, monofilament sutures require four or five throws.[5] Coated braided materials have less interstrand friction than their uncoated counterparts but still require fewer throws than monofilaments for stable knot formation.

Suture Needles

Conventional 1/2 and 3/8 suture needles are commonly used in MIS. Specialized half-curved ("ski") needles can be advantageous when operative space is limited. The J needle may be beneficial when closing port incisions. Straight needles can be used in special circumstances, but limited access precludes their general usage (Figure 2-5).

It is helpful to use needles that are flattened along their bodies to allow stable grasping with an endoscopic needle holder. Taper or tapercut points are best. Reverse cutting needles may be used, but one must be conscious of the cutting edge on the convex surface. Inadvertent cutting of vascular structures is possible because of poor visualization of the back side of the reverse cutting needle. Usage of cutting needles should be avoided because the sharp concave edge cuts through tissue during needle passage. This can lead to suture "pull-through" as well as increased hemorrhage.

Suture needles used in MIS should be strong enough to resist the increased forces placed on them during intracorporeal suturing. Suture needles are made of stainless steel alloys containing chromium and nickel. Chromium confers corrosion resistance, and nickel imparts strength to the needle. With the optimal component ratios, suture needles demonstrate the ability to deform without fracture, a property known as ductility.[6] Major suture manufacturers commonly produce standard and premium grade suture needles as part of their suture line. There is a premium to be paid for higher quality suture needles, which can be custom manufactured in combination with any suture material. Proprietary coatings are applied to suture needles to facilitate their tissue passage.

Barbed Suture

Two of the most difficult aspects of intracorporeal suturing are square knot formation and maintaining suture tension during continuous pattern suturing. The incorporation of barbed suture technology into MIS has made a significant impact in alleviating these difficulties.

In 2007, absorbable and nonabsorbable bidirectional barbed sutures (Quill SRS; Angiotech Pharmaceuticals, Vancouver, British Columbia, Canada) received U.S. Food and Drug Administration (FDA) clearance for use in approximating soft tissues.[7] These materials were cut from poliglecaprone and polydioxanone for absorbable sutures and polypropylene and nylon for nonabsorbable sutures. Quill SRS sutures feature a helically barbed strand with bidirectional barbs (10 barbs/cm) emanating from a central unbarbed segment. The strand itself is double armed and is meant to be applied so that the suturing process commences at the midpoint of the surgical incision. Suturing proceeds with each arm proceeding 180 degrees away from the center toward the opposite edges of the incision. At the end of the incision, the respective suture needles are directed 90 degrees laterally to the sutured line and cut flush with the tissue. With Quill sutures, the suture size naming convention is such that the size of the suture is a function of the parent strand from which it was barbed. For example, a 3/0 Quill suture is derived from a 3/0 parent strand. However, the strength of this suture more closely approximates a 4/0 USP suture.[8] This is important for the surgeon to bear in mind when using these products.

In 2009, absorbable unidirectional barbed sutures (V-Loc 90/180, Covidien, Mansfield, MA) were FDA approved for soft tissue approximation. These materials were produced from absorbable glycolide–dioxanone–trimethylene carbonate polyester (V-Loc 90) and absorbable polyglyconate (V-Loc 180). More recently, a nonabsorbable polybutester (V-Loc PBT) has become available. V-Loc sutures feature a single-armed strand with

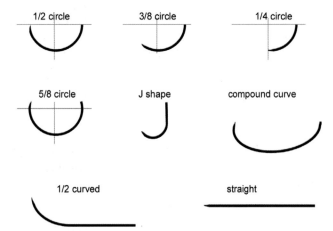

1/2 circle   3/8 circle   1/4 circle

5/8 circle   J shape   compound curve

1/2 curved   straight

Figure 2-5 Numerous needle configurations can be used for intracorporeal suturing. In general, whereas shorter needle arcs allow easier needle retrieval, longer needle arcs facilitate working where access is limited.

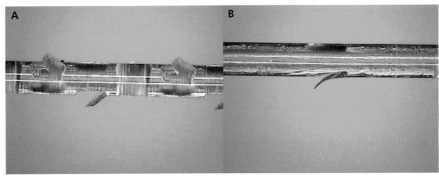

Figure 2-6 V-Loc 90 (**A**) and Quill Monoderm (**B**) barbed suture materials. V-Loc 180 sutures feature unidirectional dual-angle barbs with a suture needle on one end and a terminal welded loop on the other. Quill Monoderm sutures are double armed and feature bidirectional, helical, single-angle barbs that emanate from the center of the strand. (Reproduced with permission from J. Zaruby.)

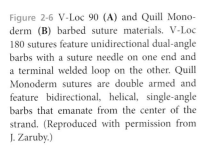

unidirectional helical barbs (20 barbs/cm) that proceed from the swage toward the terminal end of the strand, which is welded into a loop. V-Loc suturing begins with advancement of the suture needle through the tissue on one side of the incision until the base of the terminal loop is reached. The suture needle is then passed through the tissue on the opposite side of the incision, leaving the terminal loop on the contralateral side. Before taking a third tissue bite, the suture needle tip is advanced through the terminal loop. The following suture bites may be performed in either a vertical or horizontal pattern to affect a simple continuous or mattress closure respectively. The suture size naming convention used with V-Loc sutures is such that the suture size is a function of USP tensile strength.[8] As such, 3/0 V-Loc suture has a tensile strength that is close to that of a conventional monofilament 3/0 suture. This eliminates the "mental gymnastics" that the surgeon might encounter when deciding an appropriate suture size for the tissue application. V-Loc sutures are available in sizes 0 to 4/0 and in 6-, 9-, 12-, 18-, and 24-inch strand lengths (Figure 2-6).

Barbed sutures can greatly simplify intracorporeal suturing. A notable example is in laparoscopic gastropexy. Maintaining suture tension during stomach suspension is greatly facilitated with barbed sutures.[9] Another example is in intrapelvic herniorrhaphy, in which suture approximation is difficult because of space limitations.[10] Other uses for barbed suture remain to be determined but are developing with MIS implementation in veterinary surgery.

Intracorporeal Suturing Technique

Please note that most descriptions in this section refer to right-handed surgeons, preparing to take a right to left suture bite, for the purpose of increased readability. The instruments involved usually consist of a needle driver in the dominant hand (right in the examples here) and either a good-quality grasper or a second needle driver in the nondominant (left) hand.

Cannula Placement

A fundamental difference between laparoscopic and open suturing is the restricted instrument mobility. The surgeon is confined by the cannula placement to a single arc of rotation perpendicular to the axis of the instrument. The cannula placement has to be as ideal as possible to make suturing easier. An intercannula distance of at least 5 cm is desirable for the needle driver and accessory instrument. The working tips of these instruments should meet at oblique angles with each other at a relatively wide angle of 60 degrees or more. If possible, the cannula for the right needle driver should be parallel to the suture

line. The distance between cannula entrance and operative field should be approximately half of the length of the instrument (e.g., for 30-cm instruments, the cannula should be placed 15 cm [~6 in] from the target field).[2] The instruments and camera need to be directed in the same axis as the surgeon's view toward the screen to avoid mirrored vision.

Needle Introduction

The needle introduction method used depends on the type and size of needle, the size of the cannulas used, and the animal's size in relation to needle size. If the body wall thickness and needle size allow, the needle can simply be passed transcutaneously into the abdominal cavity anywhere in the surgically prepared area and be grasped intracorporeally with the needle driver. If so, the needle is ideally passed perpendicular to the dominant hand instrument axis so the needle can simply be grasped at the midpoint, and suturing ensues.

Often the needle and suture need to be passed through the cannula or the cannula site. If the needle size is compatible with cannula size, which usually requires a 10- to 12-mm cannula, the easiest introduction for a right-handed surgeon is to grasp the suture 2 to 3 cm from the swaged on end of the needle with the left instrument and pass it through the cannula. The suture is grasped with the needle tip pointing toward the left (Figure 2-7) and thus is ready to be grasped with the right hand instrument. If the needle position is not good, it can easily be corrected by applying gentle traction to the suture material (Figure 2-8). An alternative is to backload the needle and introduce through the cannula, and when intracorporeal, reposition the needle as described in detail later (Figures 2-9 and 2-10).[11] The cannula valve may need to be released when introducing to avoid disrupting the needle position or damaging the valve.

If the needle size is larger than the cannula allows, it may have to be passed through the cannula site with the cannula temporarily removed. The cannula is removed from the site while the assistant blocks gas exit, usually by placing a finger in the defect. The instrument is placed through the cannula, and when it is exiting through the cannula end, the needle is either backloaded or the suture is grasped 2 cm from the swaged end and introduced into the abdomen through the cannula site. The cannula through which the instrument is positioned is then immediately replaced in the site to minimize gas leakage.

Needle Positioning

For surgeons experienced in traditional open suturing, the challenge of obtaining correct needle positioning in the needle driver often becomes a surprise. In fact, it has been shown that for novice laparoscopic surgeons, needle grasping and positioning within the

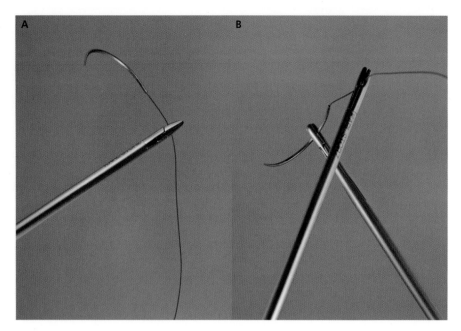

Figure 2-7 Needle introduction through a cannula. **A.** The suture is grasped with the left-hand instrument (for the right-handed surgeon) 2 to 3 cm from the swaged on end. The needle is then passed through the cannula. The cannula valve may need to be released when introducing to avoid disrupting the needle position. **B.** When visible in the field, the right needle driver is grasping the needle. The left instrument is maintaining grasp on the suture until needle position is as desired for the suture bite.

needle driver are the most difficult and time-consuming laparoscopic tasks.[4]

In our experience, the limitation of the two-dimensional view in determining if an acceptable perpendicular position has been obtained is one of the major challenges. Novices often do not understand the magnitude of the needle displacement until suturing is attempted and found to be near impossible. Self-righting needle drivers may be an important aid, but we have found that most trainees will learn the cues for needle positioning reasonably fast. If using a standard 3/8 circle needle, one cue to correct perpendicular needle positioning is that the light source is reflected along the side of the needle.

In the Veterinary Applied Laparoscopic Training (VALT) curriculum, we practice two varieties of needle positioning, the needle "dance" and a backloading technique described by Brody and coworkers.[11]

With either of the two techniques, if grasping the needle has resulted in a nonperpendicular position, the displacement is most easily corrected by unlocking the ratchet of the needle driver, and while still stabilizing and not letting go of the needle, using the ancillary instrument to grasp the suture 1 or 2 cm from the

swaged on end of the needle and by manipulating the suture until a more perpendicular needle position is obtained (Figure 2-8, Video Clip 2-1).

When a perpendicular or near-perpendicular needle position has been achieved, the suture bite is performed very similar to open surgery. Clockwise rotation of the instrument handle will allow tissue purchase within the arc of the needle.

Needle Dance

The "needle dance" is commonly used when a left instrument has inserted the needle by grasping the suture. As the needle is visualized in the field, the convex part of the needle is allowed to lightly touch an organ surface, and the grasping instrument is "dancing the needle" by letting it pivot around the organ contact point until a position is reached where the needle driver can grasp the needle in a perpendicular position and be ready for a suture bite (Figure 2-11, Video Clip 2-2). Doing the "dance" mid-air is seldom successful; the surface contact is usually needed to manipulate the needle. If no suitable surface is available in the clinical situation, the alternative needle positioning method is called for.

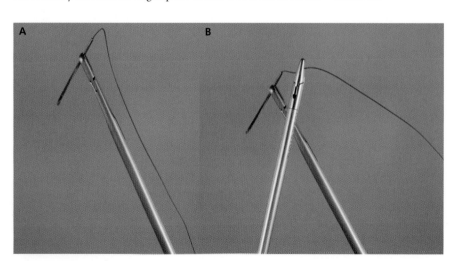

Figure 2-8 Needle position correction. **A.** The needle is not perpendicular in the jaw of the needle driver. **B.** The left-hand instrument grasps the suture, and the right hand is releasing the ratchet to loosen up the grasp of the needle without letting go of it. Now the suture can be gently manipulated until the needle is in a more optimal position.

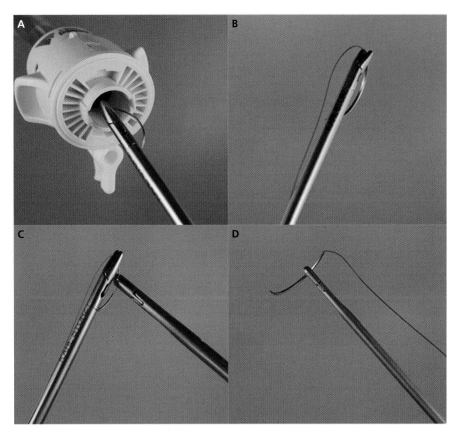

Figure 2-9 Needle introduction through a left-sided cannula according to Brody et al.[11] **A.** The needle is grasped with the left hand instrument backloaded (i.e., with the needle tip pointing in toward the shaft of the instrument). The convex part of the needle is positioned at 3 o'clock. **B.** The instrument is rotated clockwise 90 degrees so the convexity points toward 6 o'clock. **C.** The right needle driver can grasp the needle, one third to half the distance from the swaged on end, and the place the suture bite. **D.** The needle is well positioned for a right-to-left suture bite.

Brady Needle Introduction

The needle can be introduced backloaded on the left instrument,[11] with convexity to the right (Figure 2-9, Video Clip 2-1). If the angle between the instruments is less than 90 degrees, the left instrument needs to sway toward the lower right part of the visual field to allow a perpendicular grasping.

If the introducing cannula is located on the right, a backload technique can also be used (Figure 2-10, Video Clip 2-3).[11] This technique preferably is used with a needle driver in the right hand and a grasping forceps in the left, as the grasping forceps rotate around the instrument axis, making the 180-degree turn more ergonomic.

Techniques for Knot Tying: Simple Interrupted Sutures

Similar to open surgery, many knot-tying techniques are available in laparoscopic suturing. Here we will provide detailed instructions for two alternative techniques used in the VALT curriculum to successfully train a great number of novices.

After obtaining an appropriate needle position as described earlier, the ratchet is engaged with a firm grasp of the needle as the bite is initiated.

Knot Tying Using a Vertical Plane: The "Rosser Technique"

(Figure 2-12, Video Clip 2-4)
With this method, the right-hand instrument (needle driver) is always creating the throws around the left-hand instrument. When maximal driving along the arc of the needle has occurred, the right-hand needle driver is used to grasp the tip of the needle to disengage it from the tissue.

If a short (8–15 cm) suture is used, for interrupted suturing, our preference is to maintain this grip on the needle throughout the entire creation of the knot. Grasping the needle helps to control the suture memory to aid in the throws. If the suture is longer, the right needle driver has to release the needle and grasp the suture material closer to the incision during tightening of the knot and then regrasp the needle for creation of the next throw. It is important to realize that intracorporeally tied knots have a tendency to be less tight than knots tied under direct vision,[12] and it is necessary for the surgeon to counteract this tendency by ensuring that appropriate tension is applied.

Both instruments are located in the vertical plane above the suture site. A common novice mistake is to move the instrument tips from the suture site closer toward the surgeon, which will make knot tying harder.

For braided suture, the knot is complete with these three throws. However, for monofilament suture, two or three more single throws are required for knot security.

Paying attention to in which direction one is wrapping the suture material around the instrument needs to become second nature. Alternating between clockwise and counterclockwise wrappings (Figure 2-13) ensures that square knots are formed.

Knot Tying with Horizontal C-Loops as Described by Szabo *et al.*[13,14] (Figure 2-14, Video Clip 2-5)

If vertical space is limited, the instruments can work in a horizontal plane as described later (Figure 2-14). This technique also differs from the earlier one in that the throws are wrapped around the ipsilateral instrument (i.e., the throws are alternately made around the

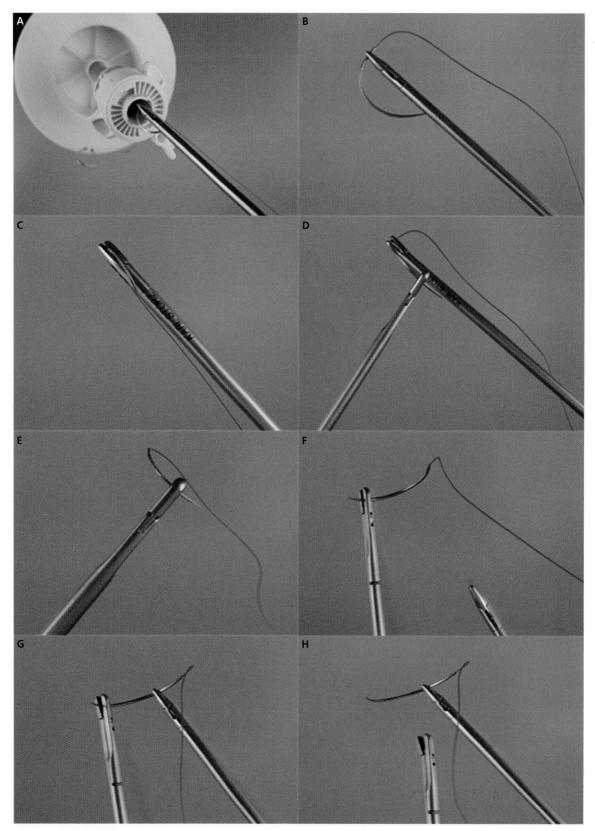

Figure 2-10 Needle introduction through a right-sided cannula according to Brody et al. [11]**A.** The needle is backloaded on the right hand instrument (i.e., with the needle tip pointing in toward the shaft of the instrument) and introduced with the convexity to the left at 9 o'clock. **B.** Needle visible in the field at the 9 o'clock position. **C.** The right instrument is rotated clockwise 90 degrees so the needle convexity now points to 12 o'clock. **D.** The left instrument is grasping the needle. **E.** The left instrument has grasped the needle with the convexity still 12 o'clock. **F.** The left instrument is rotated counterclockwise 180 degrees so the convexity points to 6 o'clock. This technique preferably is used with a needle driver in the right hand and a grasping forceps in the left, as the grasping forceps rotate around the instrument axis, making the 180-degree turn more ergonomic. **G.** The needle can now be grasped at the appropriate position. **H.** The needle is positioned for a right-to-left suture bite.

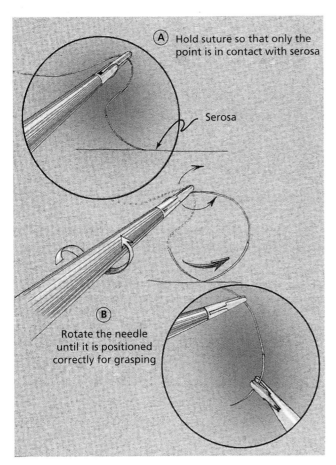

(A) Hold suture so that only the point is in contact with serosa

Serosa

(B) Rotate the needle until it is positioned correctly for grasping

Figure 2-11 The "needle dance" for needle positioning (**A** and **B**). (From Stoloff DA. Laparoscopic suturing and knot tying techniques. In: Freeman LJ (ed). *Veterinary Endosurgery*. St. Louis: Mosby; 1999. Reproduced with permission from Elsevier.)

left and the right instrument). Traditionally, this suturing is performed with two needle drivers, with a right and a left curved jaw, respectively. Note that with this technique, the instruments should never cross during tensioning because their positions are shifted with each throw.

Continuous Suture Patterns

The intracorporeal continuous suture starts with similar technique as the interrupted pattern described earlier. Again, any suture longer than 30 cm is difficult to control. Alternatively, a jamming starter knot can be construed in the loop end before the suture material is introduced. Szabo's jamming anchor knot is easy to construct (Figure 2-15) and can be used for this purpose.[13]

The major challenge with conventional suture is to maintain tension on the long limb of the suture as the next suture bite is placed. If any tension exists across the defect being sutured, the suture line will slack and the defect open. An assistant may use a grasper to maintain the tension, but this requires additional cannulas. The laparoscopic surgeon really benefit from using barbed suture for continuous suturing because tension is maintained by the barbs, hindering the tissue sliding along the suture.

The next challenge with conventional suture material is to finish a continuous suture line. Tying a knot in the long limb to the loosened last loop of the running suture usually results in loss of tension on the suture line and a weak knot.[5] Clips are not secure enough to serve as an anchor for a suture line.[2] A separate interrupted suture or an opposing continuous suture can be used and the two ends tied intracorporeally as described earlier. Alternatively, an Aberdeen knot can be used. Barbed suture is designed for knotless suturing, which again is a great advantage for the laparoscopic surgeon.

Extracorporeal Suturing

Indications

Extracorporeal knot tying is indicated when the maneuvering space is insufficient for intracorporeal suturing. Another indication is if the tension on the defect exceeds what an intracorporeal surgeon's throw, or a tumbled square knot used as a sliding half-hitch knot, can withstand because a high-strength jamming knot tied extracorporeally is stronger. Extracorporeal knot tying is also useful for placing ligatures without the need to divide the structure before ligation.

Technique

In extracorporeal suturing, a long suture is required, with 75 to 90 cm (30–36 in) or longer being ideal in a large breed dog. The needle is introduced into the body cavity while the end of the suture is secured outside the cannula. If the valves cannot hinder CO_2 leak with the suture in place, an introducer is necessary. Needle introduction, suture bite, and needle removal are performed as described in intracorporeal suturing. Importantly, the needle end of the suture is exteriorized through the same cannula as it was introduced through (Figure 2-16). When both ends of the suture are available at equal length, a slip knot is tied by hand. The knot is cinched down using a knot pusher while the surgeon maintains tension on one or both ends of the suture, depending on knot type.

Knot pushers are available with either a slotted end or a closed end. The disadvantage with a slotted design is that they may disengage from the suture during cinching. Closed end designs need to be threaded onto the post suture, which can be a disadvantage if inadequate suture length is used. As an alternative to knot pushers, an autraumatic Babcock clamp can be used as depicted in Figure 2-17.[15]

The knot type used depends on the indication for using an extracorporeal knot. If paucity of intracorporeal space is the main reason, regular square throws can be tied extracorporeally, with each throw being cinched with a knot pusher while both suture ends are secured outside the body. These throws should be applied with proper one-handed technique to avoid that identical half hitches are placed, resulting in granny knots.

However, if a stronger starting knot is needed to overcome tension, a more complex slip knot is needed. With few exceptions, these slip knots need additional throws for security. Some of these slip knots do not accept any tension placed on the loop end while being cinched, and it is more practical to cinch them into the abdomen along the post end of the suture, with a short loop end, and the remainder of the throws are placed with intracorporeal technique.

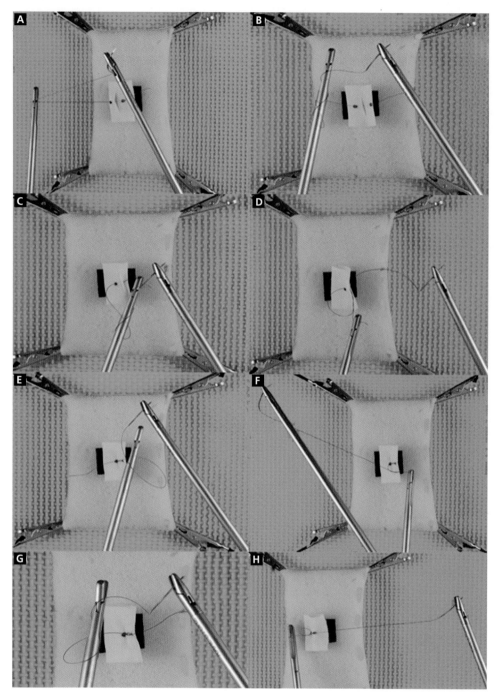

Figure 2-12 Knot tying in a vertical plane: the Rosser technique. **A.** A suture bite has been taken from right to left. With the tip of the needle pointing upward (convexity to the left) or toward the surgeon's right (convexity upwards), the left instrument is used as a "pulley" to gently pull the suture through, forming a C-shaped loop in a vertical plane. A short tag, 2 to 3 cm, is left on the contralateral incision side. **B.** The right instrument is positioned above the left and wrapping the suture close to the needle around the shaft of the left, in a clockwise direction, twice for a surgeon's throw. *This is in contrast to open suturing in which the instrument often is rotated around the suture to form the throws.* Partially opened jaws on the left hand instrument may help to avoid a recently formed throw from falling off the instrument tip prematurely. **C.** The two instruments are moved together toward the loop end (the short tag), and the left instrument grasps the end. If the novice fails to move the instruments together, the throws may be tightened on the left-hand instrument, which tends to either cinch the suture down in the box-lock where it will get stuck or to tighten around the jaws, hindering them from opening to grasp the tag. **D.** The two throws are slid off the left-hand instrument *before* tension is applied to the two ends in order to not get stuck in the box lock. The left instrument is mainly stabilizing the end, and the majority of tension is applied on the needle end in order to not pull the loop end longer. *If so, the tag will lengthen, which both wastes important suture length needed for the next C-loop and requires a wider travel to grab the tag on the following throw, making suturing harder.* If the suture is longer than 10 to 15 cm, the right hand will have to let go of the needle and grasp the suture material closer to the knot one or more times until appropriate tension has been applied to the knot. **E.** The right instrument either maintains the grip on the needle if suture is short or regrasp it if the suture is longer and is wrapping the suture material in a counterclockwise direction around the shaft of the left instrument. The position of both instrument tips is located vertical to the knot. **F.** Tension is applied to both ends, and the right instrument path crosses over the left at this time. **G.** The third and final throw is applied in the same fashion as the initial throw but is at this time a single throw in clockwise fashion. **H.** Tension is applied, without crossing of instruments.

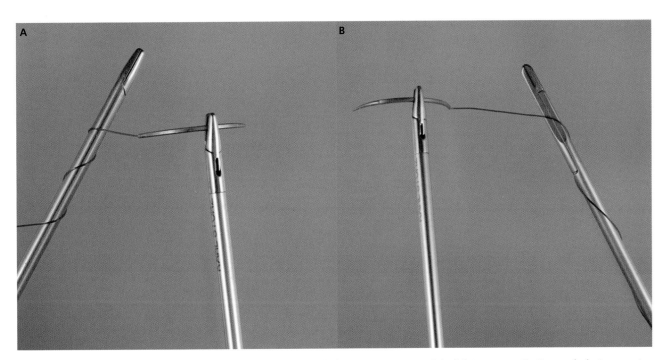

Figure 2-13 Clockwise and counter-clockwise wrapping of suture. **A.** Clockwise wrapping around the left instrument. **B.** Counterclockwise wrapping around the right instrument.

Figure 2-14 Knot tying with horizontal C-loops, as described by Szabo.[14] **A.** A suture bite has been taken from right to left. The left instrument is used as a "pulley" to gently pull the suture through, forming a horizontal C-shaped loop. **B.** A horizontal C-loop has been formed on the left side, and the left instrument is placed on top of the C-loop close to the needle. **C.** The right-hand instrument has wrapped the suture twice around the shaft of the left instrument in a counter-clockwise fashion. **D.** The two instruments moves together to pick up the short loop end with the left instrument. **E.** Tension is applied, with care taken to not pull hard on the short end and thus lengthen the tag. The tag should remain 2 to 3 cm throughout. **F.** The left instrument picks up the needle and forms a reversed C-shaped loop, again in a horizontal plane, and the right instrument is placed on top of the loop close to the needle end. **G.** The suture is wrapped around the right instrument once in clockwise direction, the wraps are moved over the needle driver, and tension is applied to the suture bilaterally. Note that crossing of instrument paths is not occurring with this technique. **H.** The third and final throw is applied similar to the first, but only a single throw is required, in counterclockwise direction. **I.** Tension is applied.

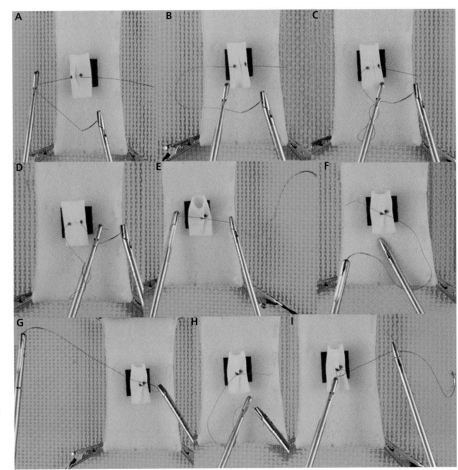

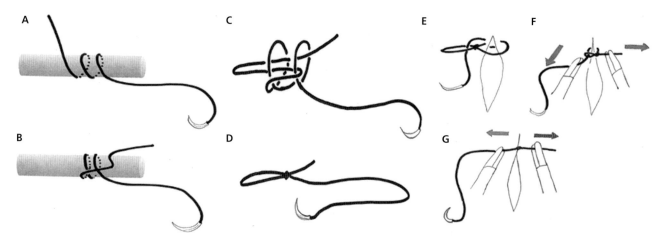

Figure 2-15 Szabo's (2008) jamming anchor knot. **A.** Wrap the suture end two turns around an instrument or the surgeon's finger. **B.** Bring the suture end forward, folding it on itself. **C.** Bring the folded suture end through the two loops. **D.** Tighten the knot while maintaining the loop. **E.** After placing the suture, the needle is placed through the loop. **F.** Tension is applied on the suture and the end of the anchor knot until the knot is tightened and the loop has disappeared. **G.** Finally, the anchor knot is jammed by application of opposing tension.

Slip Knots

The simplest of slip knots is a regular single throw advanced and cinched down with the knot pusher, but this does not withstand any tension on the suture line. A great number of more complex knots have been described, and the veterinary literature has evaluated the performance of a number of these, including the 4S modified Roeder (4SMR), modified Roeder, and Weston and Brooks knots.[16] The 4SMR knot was significantly stronger than the other knots, but these did not have the recommended added throws.[16] The 4SMR and Weston knots have also been compared in smaller suture size, 3-0 polyglactin and polydioxanone (PDS). The 4SMR, a complex knot without added throws, performed comparable to a Weston with three additional square throws in 3-0 PDS but tended to slip with the braided polyglactin. The Weston knot performed well in both braided and monofilament suture.[17]

 Weston Knot (Figure 2-18, Video Clip 2-6)
The Weston knot has been advocated as the knot of choice[18] for ease of tying and knot strength. The Weston knot performs well in

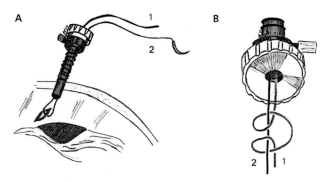

Figure 2-16 Extracorporeal suture concepts. **A.** A long suture enters and exits the same cannula. Slip knots are tied with the loop end (1) around the post (2), which most often constitutes the needle end of the suture. **B.** A tumbled square knot is one of the simplest slip knots. The loop end (1) slides along the post (2). Knots are cinched into place with a knot pusher applied to the post end.

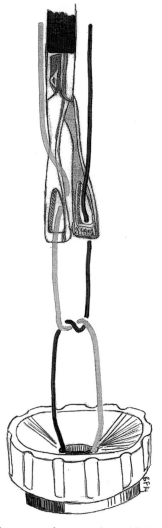

Figure 2-17 A Duvall atraumatic forceps can be used for knot pushing. The extracorporeally tied suture throw is threaded lateral to medial through the holes in the instrument jaws. With closed jaws, the instrument is pushing the throw into place, and when cinched, the jaws are gently opened to additionally tighten the throw.

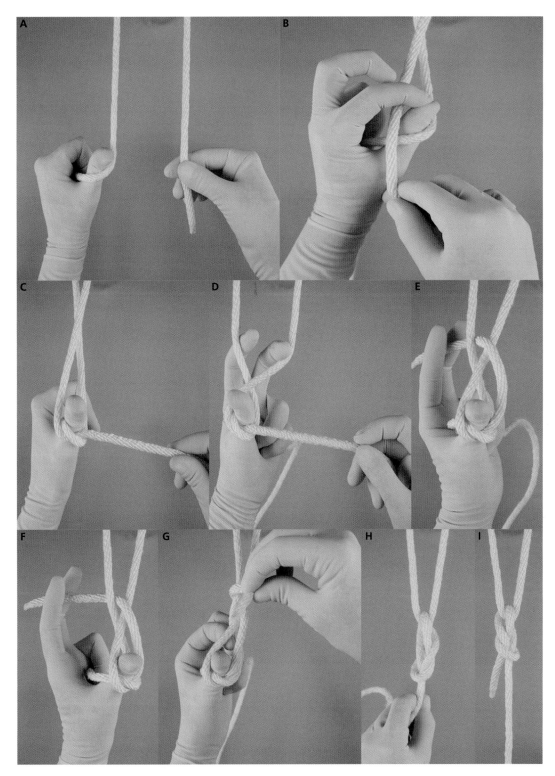

Figure 2-18 Weston knot tying. **A.** A right-to-left bite has been simulated. The needle end (left) is the post; the short (right) constitutes the loop end. The left hand is wrapping the suture around the dorsal thumb. **B.** The loop end has crossed over the post, and the thumb and index finger meet and rotate down through the loop, grasping the loop end and bringing it up (posterior to anterior) through the loop to create a single throw. **C.** The thumb remains positioned in the loop and the throw is maintained at the dorsal thumb. **D.** The left hand index and middle fingers, pointing upward (posterior to anterior direction), cross the strands by pushing the post from right to left and the loop from left to right. **E.** The loop end is grasped by the left index and middle finger, which are used to pull the loop end in an anterior to posterior direction. **F.** The loop end is passed under the left strand (post), and then it is grasped by the right hand and moved up again (posterior to anterior). **G.** The right hand passes the loop end into the small triangular space that is formed by the two strands on the right of the thumb and the one strand to the left of the thumb. The thumb and index finger of the left hand grasp the loop end. **H.** The figure 8–shaped knot is pulled tighter by applying gentle and equal tension on both the post and the loop end. **I.** Excessive tension on the loop (short) end will make the knot tumble, which will lock it, and the knot will not slip. Ensure that the loop end is not overtightened. The knot can now be slipped down and cinched with a knot pusher, which will tumble the knot and lock it. Additional throws are applied with intracorporeal knot-tying technique.

monofilament as well as braided suture but requires three added throws for security. The Weston knot tumbles and locks if tension is applied to the (short) loop end and therefore needs to be cinched without any tension on the loop end. Thus, it cannot be tied with both ends remaining extracorporeally unless very long suture is used. Most often the added throws are made with intracorporeal technique, which may be a disadvantage to this knot if intracorporeal space is limited.

 ### 4S Modified Roeder Knot (Figure 2-19, Video Clip 2-7)
The 4SMR knot is a Roeder knot modified by one added throw and one added half hitch, and it is a very complex knot. The main advantage with this knot is that if tied properly, it does not require additional throws for security. After cinching this knot down with the knot pusher, it may be beneficial to apply additional tension on the loop end (short end) for added knot security.[17]

Automated Suturing Devices
Needle passage during tissue approximation and suture knot formation is one of the most difficult challenges in conventional intracorporeal suturing. Automated suturing devices (ASDs) have been developed to address this challenge. ASDs facilitate intracorporeal suturing and reduce laparoscopic suturing time by 45% to 70% compared with conventional suturing techniques. One such ASD is the Endo Stitch (Covidien, Mansfield, MA), which received FDA 510K approval in 1994 after its development by United States Surgical Corporation (Figure 2-20). Since that time, the Endo Stitch device has been successfully used in thousands of human surgical procedures. The most notable usage has been in the areas of bariatric gastrointestinal and female urogenital surgery.

The mechanics and function of the Endo Stitch are noteworthy. The tip of the instrument features apposing jaws with holes on each side to accept a 9-mm double-taperpoint suture needle. The suture material is swaged on to the center of the needle and is supplied in a plastic cartridge for loading into the Endo Stitch. The shaft of the device is 10 mm in diameter and is available in short (23-cm) and long (38-cm) lengths for open and laparoscopic procedures, respectively. The handle portion of the Endo Stitch fits comfortably into the surgeon's dominant hand and is used to control the instrument tips. A centrally located loading button is used to initially arm the Endo Stitch device with suture material. A swiveling toggle button located within reach of the index finger is used to transfer the suture needle from one jaw (armed jaw) to the other (unarmed jaw) following tissue passage and closure of the instrument tips. Suture materials available for use with the Endo Stitch include braided lactomer, silk, nylon, and polyester in 4/0 to 0 USP sizes and lengths of 7 in (18 cm) to 48 in (122 cm). Whereas short lengths are for intracorporeal use, longer sutures are used for extracorporeal knots, wherein the Endo Stitch device can be used as a knot pusher.[19]

 ### Using the Endo Stitch (Video Clip 2-8)
Suture knot formation with the Endo Stitch is easy to learn. After the suture disposable loading unit has been loaded into the Endo Stitch, the instrument is placed in the palm of the dominant hand. For the following description, we will assume a right-handed surgeon.

The instrument handles are squeezed together, and the blue toggle button is advanced to place the suture needle in the right arm of the Endo Stitch. The left arm (unarmed jaw) of the instrument is placed into the wound, and the handles are squeezed. This causes the needle to pass through the tissue between the jaws and engage the hole in the opposite jaw. The blue toggle lever is again advanced to transfer the needle to the left jaw. When the handles are now allowed to open, the surgeon will see that the suture needle is seated in the left jaw of the Endo Stitch. The surgeon then axially rotates the Endo Stitch 180 degrees so that the armed jaw of the instrument is now on the right. The needle is again placed into the center of the wound, and the handles are squeezed to allow the needle to penetrate the left wound margin. At this point, the Endo Stitch is axially rotated 180 degrees in a clockwise direction. This leaves the instrument armed in such a fashion that the armed jaw is on the surgeon's right, and the unarmed jaw is on the left. An atraumatic grasper is introduced from the left port and is advanced in order to grasp the free end of the suture in the left hand. A short segment (3–5 cm) of the free end is held vertically in the operative field for subsequent knot-tying maneuvers. This short segment will be designated "the post" in the following description.[19]

In knot formation, it is important to note that the armed jaw of the Endo Stitch is always advanced toward the post. In so doing, a reversed D is formed with the suture material. The unarmed jaw is always inserted into the center of the reversed D, and the instrument is toggled in order to transfer the needle around the post and into the other jaw. The handles are squeezed, and the Endo Stitch instrument is then pulled axially toward the surgeon to form the first suture throw. Pressure is then released from the handles, and the suture needle will now lie in the left jaw of the instrument. Again, moving the armed jaw toward the post, allow the unarmed jaw to pass into the center of the inverted D and transfer the needle around the post. Squeeze the instrument handles and pull the Endo Stitch axially toward the surgeon. This will form the second throw of the suture knot. Repeat this process to achieve the desired number of suture throws. It is helpful to visualize an inverted V when considering the direction of axial pull on the suture. This alternation of pulling directions along the arms of the V keeps the surgeon forming square knots, all while the post remains stationary, held by the left hand grasper.[19] The use of Endo Stitch is demonstrated at http://www.covidien.com/videos/pages.aspx?page=videodetail&video=327.

A significant advance in Endo Stitch technology came with the availability of V-Loc reloads for use with the device (Figure 2-21). Use of V-Loc sutures with the Endo Stitch simplifies two common difficulties of intracorporeal suturing: (1) knot tying and (2) maintaining suture line tension between suture bites.[20]

V-Loc reloads are supplied as glycolide–trimethylene carbonate (V-Loc 180) or polybutester (V-Loc PBT) versions. V-Loc 180 reloads are absorbable and have an absorption profile similar to Maxon suture. V-Loc PBT reloads are nonabsorbable and are composed of the same material as Novafil suture. V-Loc reloads are available in sizes 3/0 to 0 and 4-in (10-cm), 6-in (15-cm), and 8 in (20-cm) lengths.

A further advance in ASD came with the recent introduction of the SILS (single incision laparoscopic surgery) Stitch device. This device represents a modification of the Endo Stitch device and is ideally suited for use with the SILS system. The SILS Stitch is essentially a roticulating Endo Stitch (Figure 2-22). It is ideally suited for use with the SILS port because working space is limited and two or

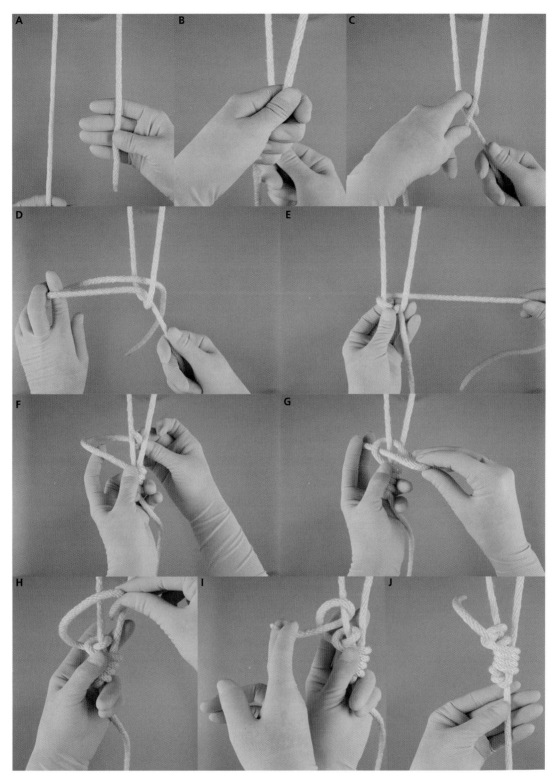

Figure 2-19 . 4S modified Roeder (4SMR) knot tying.[23] **A.** A right-to-left bite has been simulated. The needle end (left) is the post; the short (right) constitutes the loop end. **B.** The left hand grasps the loop end, and the right hand grasps the post end, with the loop end on top. This is surgeon's choice, and if hand repositioning is not desired, the knot can still be tied but "upside down." **C.** The left index finger is placed through the loop formed by the crossing suture strands. **D.** This finger is then flexed around the post end of the suture, with the dorsal index finger anterior to the loop end, which is flipped up using the dorsal index finger and pulled through to form a single throw. **E.** The left hand stabilizes the throw formed, and the right hand wraps the loop end of the suture around both suture strands in a counterclockwise fashion for four full turns. The loop end is passed up (posterior to anterior) between the strands (**F**) and down through the loop formed, creating a half hitch around the (left)post end of the suture **(G). H.** The loop end is passed anterior to posterior (down) between the strands for a second half hitch. **I.** The loop end is passed through the second half-hitch loop. **J.** The completed 4SMR knot ready to be cinched down with a knot pusher. This knot does not require additional throws, but tension applied to the loop end intracorporeally will be beneficial: and add knot security.[17]

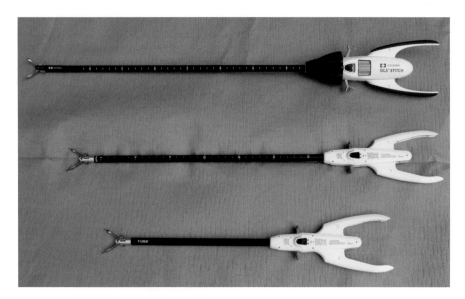

Figure 2-20 Automated suturing devices. Small and standard Endo Stitch devices (bottom and center) and SILS (single incision laparoscopic surgery) Stitch (top). Both devices use monofilament and braided sutures as well as barbed sutures available on specially designed loading units.

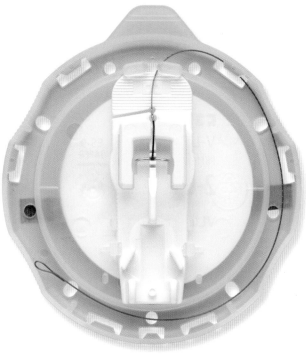

Figure 2-21 V-Loc 180 automated suture loading unit, 7-inch length with a terminal welded loop. Shorter suture lengths facilitate ligation and limited suturing. (Copyright © 2013 Covidien. All rights reserved. Used with the permission of Covidien.)

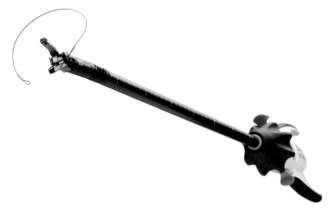

Figure 2-22 SILS (single incision laparoscopic surgery) Stitch automated suture device loaded with 7-inch V-Loc 180 reload. The SILS Stitch device allows angular articulation of the distal 5 cm of the instrument, which affords greater versatility in suture needle placement. (Copyright © 2013 Covidien. All rights reserved. Used with the permission of Covidien.)

References

1 Wolfe, B.M., Szabo, Z., Moran, M.E., Chan, P., Hunter, J.G. (1993) Training for minimally invasive surgery. Need for surgical skills. Surg Endosc 7(2), 93-95.

2 Soper, N.J., Hunter, J.G. (1992) Suturing and knot tying in laparoscopy. Surg Clin North Am 72(5), 1139-1152.

3 Tuncel, A., Lucas, S., Bensalah, K., et al. (2008) A randomized comparison of conventional vs articulating laparoscopic needle-drivers for performing standardized suturing tasks by laparoscopy-naive subjects. BJU Int 101(6), 727-730.

4 Ramani, A.P., Braasch, M., Botnaru, A., et al. (2008) Evaluation of efficacy of four laparoscopic needle drivers. JSLS 12(1), 77-80.

5 Marturello, D.M., McFadden, M.S., Bennett, R.A., Ragetly, G.R., Horn, G. (2014) Knot security and tensile strength of suture materials. Vet Surg 43(1), 73-79.

6 Venugopalan, R., Wu, M. (2005) Medical device materials III: Materials & Processes for Medical Devices Conference. In: Venugopalan, R., Wu, M. (eds.). Materials & Processes for Medical Devices Conference, Boston, November 14 to 16, 2005, pp. 93-98.

7 Ruff, G.L. (2013) The history of barbed sutures. Aesthet Surg J 33(3 suppl), 12S-16S.

8 Zaruby, J., Gingras, K., Taylor, J., Maul, D. (2011) An in vivo comparison of barbed suture devices and conventional monofilament sutures for cosmetic skin closure: biomechanical wound strength and histology. Aesthet Surg J 31(2), 232-240.

9 Spah, C.E., Elkins, A.D., Wehrenberg, A., et al. (2013) Evaluation of two novel self-anchoring barbed sutures in a prophylactic laparoscopic gastropexy compared with intracorporeal tied knots. Vet Surg 42(8), 932-942.

three instruments and telescope are in close proximity. The SILS Stitch has a difficult learning curve, but suturing principles with this device are similar to those with the Endo Stitch. The challenge lies in mastering three-dimensional manipulation while viewing a two-dimensional operative field. Use of the SILS port is described elsewhere in this textbook.

All videos cited in this chapter can be found on the book's companion website at **www.wiley.com/go/fransson/ laparoscopy**.

10 Ragle, C.A., Yiannikouris, S., Tibary, A.A., Fransson, B.A. (2013) Use of a barbed suture for laparoscopic closure of the internal inguinal rings in a horse. J Am Vet Med Assoc 242(2), 249-253.

11 Brody, F., Rehm, J., Ponsky, J., Holzman, M. (1999) A reliable and efficient technique for laparoscopic needle positioning. Surg Endosc 13 (10), 1053-1054.

12 Kadirkamanathan, S.S., Shelton, J.C., Hepworth, C.C., Laufer, J.G., Swain, C.P. (1996) A comparison of the strength of knots tied by hand and at laparoscopy. J Am Coll Surg 182 (1), 46-54.

13 Szabo, Z. (2008) Laparoscopic Suturing System with Szabo-Berci Needle Driver Set. Karl Storz GmbH & Co, Tuttlingen, Germany, pp. 11-13.

14 Szabo, Z., Hunter, J., Berci, G., Sackier, J., Cuschieri, A. (1994) Analysis of surgical movements during suturing in laparoscopy. Endosc Surg Allied Technol 2(1), 55-61.

15 Puttick, M.I., Nduka, C.C., Darzi, A. (1994) Extracorporeal knot tying using an atraumatic Babcock clamp. J Laparoendosc Surg 4(5), 339-341.

16 Shettko, D.L., Frisbie, D.D., Hendrickson, D.A. (2004) A comparison of knot security of commonly used hand-tied laparoscopic slipknots. Vet Surg 33(5), 521-524.

17 Fugazzi, R.W., Fransson, B.A., Curran, K.M., Davis, H.M., Gay, J.M. (2013) A biomechanical study of laparoscopic 4S-modified Roeder and Weston knot strength in 3-0 polyglactin 910 and 3-0 polydioxanone. Vet Surg 42 (2), 198-204.

18 Gantert, W.A., Bhoyrul, S., Way, L.W. (2008) Suturing and Knot Tying. Advanced Videoscopic Surgery for the General Surgeon. University of California San Francisco, San Francisco.

19 Covidien. (2008) Endo Stitch™ Suturing instrument intracorporeal knot tying manual. [cited 2014 August 21]; Available from: http://surgical.covidien.com/content/dam/covidien/library/global/english/product/hand-instruments-and-ligation/endoscopic-suturing-devices/endo-stitch-knot-tying-manual.pdf.

20 Wang, K.C. (2012) Alternative suture and technologies used in gynecologic laparoscopy. Presented at the 41st AAGL Global Congress on Minimally Invasive Gynecology, November 5 to 9, 2012, Las Vegas, pp. 19-23.

21 Covidien. (2014) Wound closure absorbable sutures. [cited 2014 August 21]; Available from: http://surgical.covidien.com/products/wound-closure/absorbable-sutures.

22 Catalog EP. (2014) Sutures absorbable. [cited 2014 August 21]; Available from: http://www.ecatalog.ethicon.com/sutures-absorbable.

23 Sharp, H.T., Dorsey, J.H. (1997) The 4-S modification of the Roeder knot: how to tie it. Obstet Gynecol 90(6), 1004-1006.

SECTION II

Equipment

3 Imaging Equipment and Operating Room Setup

Fausto Brandão and Christopher Chamness

Key Points

- The most basic video endoscopy imaging system consists of a light source, light-transmitting cable, endoscope, camera, and monitor. The resulting endoscopic image can only be as good as the weakest link in the chain.
- An carbon dioxide insufflator is also essential to laparoscopic surgeons.
- An operating laparoscope contains optics of a 5-mm telescope but has an integrated working channel allowing passage of 5-mm instruments. These can be used for certain routine procedures.

Imaging Equipment

While human medicine has defined the major trends and achievements in minimally invasive surgery (MIS) over the past 2 decades, veterinary medicine has followed in its path and developed specialized techniques and instrumentation. The high costs and enormously diverse options of equipment sets available may seem discouraging to many veterinary practices. The goal of this chapter is to help practitioners to make rational choices for a fully equipped MIS operating room (OR). Careful selection of the most versatile, durable, and modular devices is often the best choice for veterinary practitioners.

Imaging Chain

The most basic video endoscopy imaging system consists of a *light source, light-transmitting cable, endoscope, camera,* and *monitor* (Figure 3-1). Each component is essential, and the resulting endoscopic image can only be as good as the weakest link in the chain. For example, if a surgeon has a very high-quality camera, telescope, and light cable but chooses to use a low-resolution consumer-grade television as a monitor, the resulting image quality will be limited by the monitor. Even an old, damaged, or dirty light cable can degrade the image quality of an otherwise high-end

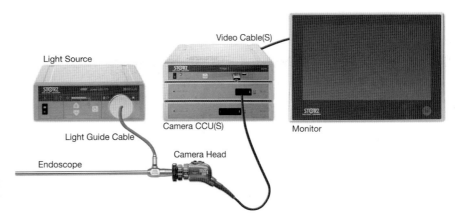

Figure 3-1 The basic endoscopic imaging chain. (© 2014 Photo Courtesy of KARL STORZ GmbH & Co. KG.)

Small Animal Laparoscopy and Thoracoscopy, First Edition. Edited by Boel A. Fransson and Philipp D. Mayhew.
© 2015 by ACVS Foundation. Published 2015 by John Wiley & Sons, Inc.
Companion website: www.wiley.com/go/fransson/laparoscopy

Table 3-1 Image Troubleshooting Guide

Problem	Possible Cause	Resolution
Image is not clear	Fogged or dirty lens	Blot distal lens of telescope on live tissue or apply antifog agent to lens.
	Fogged distal lens	Immerse telescope in warm sterile water or apply antifog agent to lens.
	Dirty eyepiece, camera, or adapter	Clean using cotton swab moistened with sterile water.
	Lens not adjusted to operator's eyesight	Rotate focus adjustment ring on camera head until image is clear.
	Internal fluid damage or cracked rod lens	Moisture within telescope will permanently cloud lens in distal end or eyepiece (repair by manufacturer).
	Misconnected camera on telescope eyepiece	Check for proper coupling and positioning of camera head to telescope by adjusting adapter.
Image is too dark or too bright	Dirty light guide	Clean light-guide connector and distal tip using gauze moistened with sterile water.
	Improper light source or camera settings	Adjust brightness control knob, camera gain, or manual aperture setting.
	Old or improperly installed lamp	Properly install lamp; replace old lamp.
Image is too blue	White balance improperly done or not done before telescope insertion into patient	Remove telescope from patient, clean distal lens, and perform white balance correctly.
Deficient illumination	Bulb lifespan ending	Check working hours on light source; replace bulb or activate alternate bulb inside light source.
	Improperly connected light cable	Check for correct and full insertion of light-transmitting cable.
	Worn light cable (broken fibers)	If >30% of light-transmitting capacity is lost, then substitute cable.
	Light source on stand-by mode	Check and press stand-by button to activate light output.
	Light source is turned down	Increase light source output.
Loss of pneumoperitoneum	Empty tank or closed valve from gas supply	Check gas remaining in tank; replace tank; open valves of general gas supply.
	Open Luer-lock on one or more trocars, leaking gas	Check and close all stopcocks except the one coming from insufflator.
	Blockage of line going to patient	Be sure tip of Veress needle is not blocked by tissue and that the valve on the Veress needle or gas input cannula is open to incoming gas.
	Leaky cannula valve or sealing cap	Assure proper assembly and functioning of each cannula and replace any worn sealing caps.
	Leakage around portal sites	Check for leakage around wounds and suture closed where necessary.
No image on screen or monitor or black and white image only	Connector into front of the camera control unit (CCU) is not fully inserted, dirty, or wet	Clean and dry the connector and replace securely.
	Video cables between the CCU and monitor are faulty or not tightly connected	Tighten connections and replace cables, if necessary.
	Camera head cable that connects to CCU is damaged	Send to manufacturer for repair.
	One or more devices in the video chain are not activated or damaged	Check that all devices in the video chain are turned on and have proper and tightly connected power cords.

endoscopic imaging system.[1-4] An image troubleshooting guide is presented in Table 3-1.

The light generated by the light source is transmitted by the fiberoptic light cable, and farther down the telescope, by fiberoptics to illuminate the anatomy being observed. The image is transmitted through a series of lenses from the distal end of the telescope to the eyepiece, where the chip in the video *camera head* senses the image and transmits it to the *camera control unit* (CCU), which processes the endoscopic image and transmits it to a monitor for viewing. This video projection enables the surgeon to maintain an ergonomic posture and to share the visual information with observers. Furthermore, video imaging facilitates documentation of procedures, in several formats, valuable for client education, medical records, teaching, or consultation purposes.[1-4] Video imaging also enables remote access to a live procedure via streaming video.[5]

Telescopes

Rigid endoscopes are more convenient than flexible endoscopes for examining and performing procedures in body cavities.[6-8] Rigid scopes (i.e., telescopes) are also much simpler in design and less expensive than flexible endoscopes. Despite containing lenses and fiber optics, they do not contain flexible materials, are easier to clean and maintain, and have a longer working lifespan.[9] Some models may include a working channel, integrated instrument, or a variable viewing angle, which allows a wider viewing field. State-of-the-art rigid telescopes are constructed with high-quality optical glass rod lenses (Hopkins rod lenses), producing high-quality images that are bright, magnified, wide angle, and of high resolution and contrast.[1-4,8] No single model of rigid endoscope is universally suitable. The appropriate sized telescope should be selected based on the surgical procedure, size and morphology of the patient and ultimately by the preference and experience of the surgeon. Although smaller scopes tend to be more versatile, they are also more prone to breakage, and their illumination capacity is limited when used in larger, more light-absorptive cavities such as the abdomen or thorax of large breed dogs.

Standard surgical telescopes come in a variety of sizes (Figure 3-2). The most versatile and popular rigid telescopes used in small animal laparoscopy and thoracoscopy are 5 mm in diameter and approximately 30 cm in length. Smaller rigid

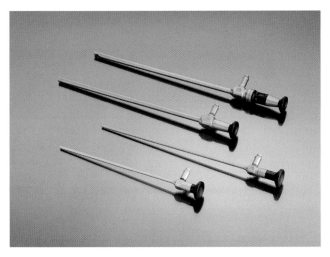

Figure 3-2 Rigid endoscopes. From top to bottom: 10-mm ENDOCAMEL-EON, 10 mm, 5 mm, and 4 mm. (© 2014 Photo Courtesy of KARL STORZ GmbH & Co. KG.)

endoscopes, 2.7 or 3 mm in diameter and 14 to 18 cm long are ideal for cats, puppies and toy breeds. With a smaller diameter and shorter shaft, these are easier to maneuver in smaller patients but too short in larger patients, and light-carrying capacity may be inadequate in larger cavities. Telescopes larger than 5 mm in diameter have decreased in popularity, mostly because of the improvements in image size and brightness of 5-mm telescopes.[1-4,7,8]

Conversely, the 10-mm-diameter *operating laparoscope* has become popular. It contains optics similar to that of a 5-mm

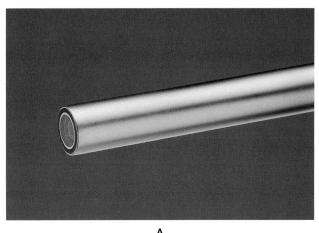

A

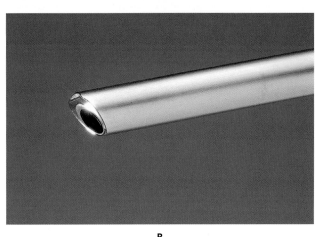

B

Figure 3-4 Telescope viewing angles. **A.** Zero degree. **B.** 30 degree. (© 2014 Photo Courtesy of KARL STORZ GmbH & Co. KG.)

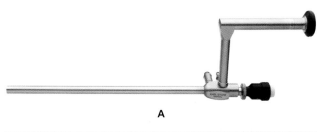

A

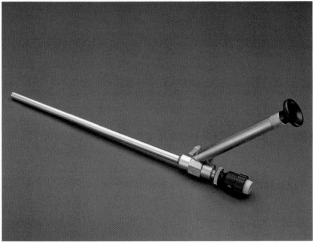

B

Figure 3-3 Operating laparoscopes. **A.** Right angled. **B.** Oblique. (© 2014 Photo Courtesy of KARL STORZ GmbH & Co. KG.)

telescope but has an integrated working channel that allows passage of 5-mm instruments down the same shaft. Operating scopes are available in two types, right angled or oblique (Figure 3-3). Some surgeons prefer this style of telescope for certain routine procedures such as biopsies and ovariectomies because the instruments are always under visual control. For this reason, an operating telescope may also be recommended for novice endoscopic surgeons.[1-4]

The viewing angle of a telescope is an important consideration because it affects both orientation and visual access (Figure 3-4). Standard forward-viewing telescopes (0 degree) provide the simplest spatial orientation, centered on the axis of the telescope, but they present a relatively limited viewing field. A 30-degree viewing angle allows the surgeon to view a larger area by simply rotating the shaft of the telescope on its longitudinal axis.[7,8] With experience, the operator becomes proficient at using angled telescopes and gaining a wider viewing field. Telescopes with more acute tip angulations are also available (70, 90, and 120 degrees), but they are rarely used in small animal laparoscopy and thoracoscopy.[1-4]

New 10-mm-diameter rigid telescopes are available with a *variable* viewing angle, allowing the surgeon to control angulation from 0 to 120 degrees, with a mechanical twisting mechanism near the eyepiece (ENDOCAMELEON; Karl Storz GmbH & Co., Goleta,

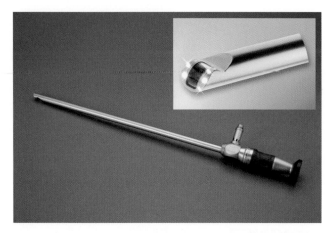

Figure 3-5 Telescope with variable viewing angle, adjusted by turning the collar on the eyepiece. (© 2014 Photo Courtesy of KARL STORZ GmbH & Co. KG.)

CA; Figure 3-5). These newer telescopes are only beginning to gain popularity among veterinary surgeons, mainly because of cost and large diameters.

Using a telescope and instruments of the same diameter (i.e., 5 mm) is convenient for maximum flexibility during surgery and allows exchanging location of the telescope and instruments during a procedure without exchanging ports.[1-4,8] Nevertheless, trocar cannulae can be fitted with a reducer (Figure 3-6) to accommodate smaller diameter instrumentation without loss of pneumoperitoneum.[8]

Light Sources

The power (expressed in watts) and type of a light source are two of the main factors determining the brightness, clarity, and color accuracy of an endoscopic image. Condition and quality of light-transmitting cables, cleanliness of lens surfaces, light sensitivity of the camera, and monitor type also contribute to image brightness and quality.[1-4,7,10-13]

The most common types of high-quality light sources today are Xenon, Hi-Lux, and LED, typically ranging in power from 50 to 300 W. The wattage of a light source is not necessarily indicative of its brightness but indicates the energy required to power it, which does not directly correlate to brightness (expressed in lumens). Therefore, wattage alone is not valid for comparison of light sources of different types. As a general rule Xenon, Hi Lux, and LED light sources produce brighter, whiter light (~6000–6500° Kelvin) than older halogen light sources (3400° Kelvin). For example, a 50-W Hi-Lux light source emits an amount of light similar to a 125- to 175-W Xenon light source.[1,2,3,4]

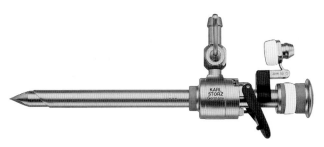

Figure 3-6 A 10-mm trocar and cannula fitted with a 10/5 reducer that can be flipped into place for 5-mm instruments. (© 2014 Photo Courtesy of KARL STORZ GmbH & Co. KG.)

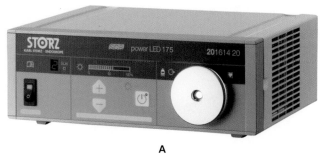

A

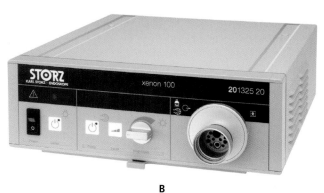

B

Figure 3-7 Light sources. **A.** LED light source with connector for standard light cable. **B.** Xenon light source with connector for gastroscope. (© 2014 Photo Courtesy of KARL STORZ GmbH & Co. KG.)

Currently, the Xenon light source is the most popular because it offers excellent tissue color reproduction with light closely approximating that of pure sunlight (5800° Kelvin). However, LED technology is increasingly used because of greater efficiency, long lifetime, small size, and light weight. An LED bulb will last approximately 30,000 hours, 30 times that of a xenon light bulb. Spare bulbs should always be available, or a light source equipped with two bulbs should be considered.[1-4,10,12]

When selecting a light source for multidisciplinary endoscopy services, including flexible endoscopy, the compatibility with a modular pump for insufflation and irrigation, and attachment of endoscope to the light source are important (Figure 3-7). Although the initial cost of a versatile, high-power light source may be high, it could represent considerable savings later, if it prevents the purchase of multiple light sources. When not in use, the light source should always be in stand-by mode or completely turned off, to avoid any thermal injuries to the patient or surgical drapes.[1-4,6,7]

Light Cables

A fiberoptic *light guide cable* transmits the light from the light source to the telescope. The light cable consists of a bundle of thousands of optical glass fibers ranging in size from 30 μm to several hundred microns, surrounded by a protective jacket, and equipped with metal fittings at each end. Cables with additional armoring last longer than ones without this protection. The cable is inserted into the light source at one end and attached to the light post of the telescope at the other end. Light cables are available in various styles and diameters, depending on the diameter of the telescope. Correct matching prevents overheating or underillumination. Generally,

Table 3-2 Matching Diameter of Telescope and Light Cable for Optimal Illumination and to Avoid Overheating

Telescope Diameter (mm)	Recommended Cable Diameter (mm)
6.5–12	4.8–5.0
3.0–6.5	3.0–3.5
0.8–2.9	2.0–2.5

a smaller scope requires a smaller light cable. The most common cable used with 5-mm telescopes for small animal MIS is 3.5 mm in diameter and 230 cm long (Table 3-2).[1-4]

Careful handling of a light cable will prolong its life span, avoiding discoloration of the ends and breakage of individual fibers. Light cable integrity is assessed by looking through one end of the cable toward a room light or window. Discoloration reduces light transmission and can change the color of the light that is emitted. Broken fibers will appear as small black or gray areas. When more than 30% of the fibers are broken, replacement of the cable is recommended. Excessive bending, twisting, or crushing of light cables should be avoided to minimize fiber breakage.

Contemporary light cables are autoclaveable, but manufacturers' recommendations for time and cycle should be carefully followed. Light cables should always be stored in a loosely coiled position because this minimizes stresses on the glass fibers.[1-4,7,10]

Endoscopic Video Cameras

The video camera system consists of the adapter, camera head, CCU, and monitor. Generally, modern cameras have integrated adapter and camera head, although camera heads exist with separate adapters, which screw into the head. Adapters have different focal lengths, determining the displayed image size. However, image size and magnification can more conveniently be changed with integrated *optical zoom* adjustment located on the camera head. Optical zoom produces a true magnified image without compromising the resolution, unlike digital zoom, which merely increases pixel size.[1-4,7,10]

An important consideration may be the flexibility of the chosen camera for different procedures and different endoscopes. It may be prudent to consider both a variable focal distance head as well as a CCU that is compatible with all the types of scopes that might be used in the practice (fiberscopes, videoendoscopes, and rigid telescopes). Multidisciplinary and versatile systems may permit a broad endoscopy service at reasonable cost. Larger practices may, however, wish to have separate systems for different services.[1-4]

Medical cameras contain a computer "chip" (i.e., a semiconductor sensor, or charge-coupled device [CCD]), which transforms the optical image into an electronic signal transmitted to the CCU. Recent improvements in quality and miniaturization of CMOS (complementary metal-oxide-semiconductor) "chips" have led to development of CMOS cameras, whose performance and image quality are competitive with CCD cameras.[1-4]

Although endoscopic camera quality has previously been defined by single-chip or three-chip technology, it is currently more relevant to refer to *high-definition* (HD) image technology. An HD image can be produced with either a single chip or three-chip camera, which provides a wide screen display (Figure 3-8). The HD aspect ratio of 16:9 more closely approximates the human visual field than the historical standard 4:3 and allows the surgeon

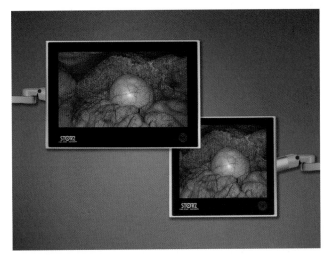

Figure 3-8 Monitors. Left: aspect ratio, 16:9. Right: aspect ratio, 4:3. (© 2014 Photo Courtesy of KARL STORZ GmbH & Co. KG.)

to see instruments entering the surgical field sooner than with a traditional monitor.[1-4]

However, HD cameras differ in resolution and light sensitivity, performance characteristics that affect detail recognition, color, features, and price. Some newer cameras, for example, have integrated image capturing capabilities or image processing options that enhance contrast or brighten dark areas. *Full HD* cameras deliver the superior picture 1080p (i.e., 1920 × 1080) pixel resolution and *progressive scanning*, as opposed to "i" for *interlaced*. The progressive scanning method simultaneously displays all 1080 lines on every frame, thus producing the smoothest, clearest image, especially when the video content is motion intensive.

New generation full HD camera heads have titanium bodies, making them robust and autoclavable. In contrast, older models were only sterilizable by gas or soaking.[1-4,9] Newer camera heads provide intraoperative access to preset functions such as white balance, image capture, video recording, and image enhancement. Importantly, for endoscopic images to be displayed in HD, each component of the imaging chain must be HD compatible, from the camera head to the transmission media and systems (CCU and cables) to the monitor.[1-4,10,14]

Display Monitors, Auxiliary Screens, and "All-in-One" Video Systems

To achieve superior live images during surgery, the quality of the display monitors and auxiliary screens is as important as any other part of the video chain. They vary in size, resolution, inputs and other features. Monitors 17 to 26 inches are the most common. Flat screen monitors have replaced the old CRT monitors, as in consumer electronics. The resolution of the monitor should match or surpass the resolution of the other elements of the imaging chain. Surgical display monitors should have a minimum of 500 lines for standard definition single-chip cameras, 750 lines for standard definition three-chip cameras, and 1080p to obtain maximum benefit from a full HD camera system.[1-4]

Ideally, multiple mobile monitors should be situated opposite the surgeon and surgeon's assistants so that each surgical team member has a straightforward view.[8] Compact "all-in-one" units typically

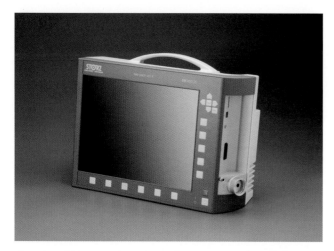

Figure 3-9 All-in-one unit consisting of a camera control unit, light source, monitor, digital capture system, and insufflation pump (for gastrointestinal endoscopy). (© 2014 Photo Courtesy of KARL STORZ GmbH & Co. KG.)

include a CCU, light source, monitor, insufflation pump (for flexible endoscopy), screen, and image capture module (Figure 3-9). A dedicated keyboard can be attached, allowing the surgical team to enter patient data and to send it to a hospital network by means of USB cable or flash drives.[1-4,7,10,11]

Insufflators

A CO_2 insufflator is used to create and maintain a working space between the telescope and the target tissues (Figure 3-10).[15,16] The insufflator automatically controls CO_2 flow rate and pressure throughout the procedure.

The carbon dioxide source is typically a pressurized tank connected to the insufflator with a high-pressure hose. However, in referral facilities an in-house gas delivery system may be available. The reduced pressure CO_2 gas is delivered to the patient via sterilized tubing that connects from the front panel of the insufflator to the hub of a Veress needle or Luer-lock connector on a cannula.

An antibacterial sterile filter should be coupled inline, which prevents contamination from the CO_2 tank or in case reflux fluid moves from the patient to the insufflator, which can occur when a sudden fall in pressure is observed because of tank emptying.[1-4,7,15,16]

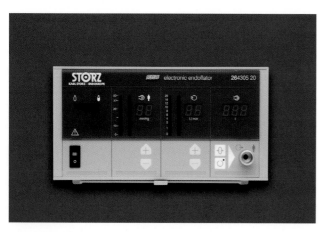

Figure 3-10 An electronic insufflator regulates the flow of CO_2 gas into the patient, maintaining pneumoperitoneum automatically at a preset pressure. (© 2014 Photo Courtesy of KARL STORZ GmbH & Co. KG.)

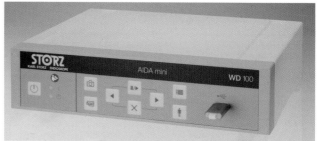

Figure 3-11 Miniature version of an advanced image data archiving system. (© 2014 Photo Courtesy of KARL STORZ GmbH & Co. KG.)

Electronic insufflators with gas heating are available to minimize hypothermia.[8]

Capture and Storage of Images and Video

Over the past decade, digital image capturing systems have effectively made SLR cameras, video cassette recorders (VCRs), and video printers obsolete. When trying to capture images directly to a computer, most practitioners face some limitations directly related to the outputs on the CCU and monitor and the inputs of the computer itself. Software compatibility may also become an issue. The ultimate image quality and user friendliness are critical factors.[1-4,10]

Newer sophisticated digital capture systems (Figure 3-11) offer high image quality and easy export of data to the hospital network or patient files. Most units also have an internal storage of limited volume, including patient-related information. Still images and videos are captured and stored on the unit's hard drive or alternatively recorded onto USB flash drives or external devices.

Some endoscopic camera systems contain an integrated capture system (Figures 3-9 and 3-12). These integrated systems lack some of the features of independent image capture and archiving systems[1-4]

Video Carts and Ceiling Booms

Mobile equipment carts (see Figure 3-12) are essential for MIS. A multi-shelf wheeled cart is a common choice, which contains multiple electrical outlets for the equipment and insulated wheels to fulfill the electrical safety standards for medical equipment. The cart may also accommodate peripheral arms or stands for auxiliary screens and other devices (e.g., touch screen for digital capture or integrated software platforms) and drawers to store accessory instrumentation such as cables, filters, tubing, and so on.[1-4,7]

New hardware and design concepts help organize the OR, keeping flooring free from cables and easing cleaning and sterilization (Figure 3-13). Ceiling-mounted movable arms or tracks can conveniently position equipment near the patient while freeing the floor space around the operating table. Ceiling booms can be fixed or movable by means of suspended racks and are highly advantageous in the OR. They provide integrated electrical connection as well as access to gas lines and suction, and they provide shelves and drawers. Other less complex ceiling booms support surgical illumination and auxiliary screens, which are standard in modern MIS suites. Disadvantages mainly include cost and specific installation requirements.

Integrated and Intelligent Operating Rooms

As the number of devices has increased in MIS, access to each equipment piece has become a challenge, risking excessive circulation near

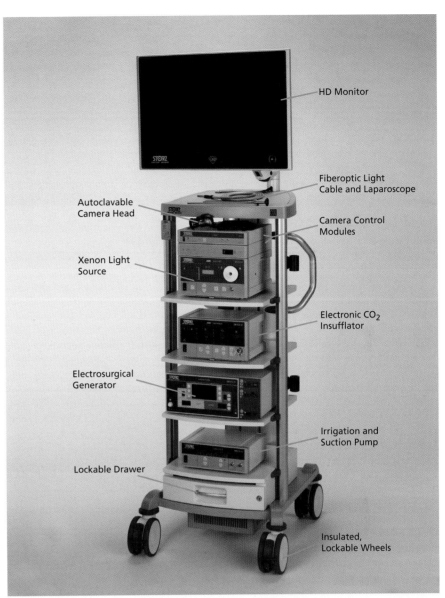

HD Monitor

Fiberoptic Light
Cable and Laparoscope

Autoclavable
Camera Head

Camera Control
Modules

Xenon Light
Source

Electronic CO$_2$
Insufflator

Electrosurgical
Generator

Irrigation and
Suction Pump

Lockable Drawer

Insulated,
Lockable Wheels

Figure 3-12 Mobile cart fully equipped for laparoscopy and thoracoscopy. (© 2014 Photo Courtesy of KARL STORZ GmbH & Co. KG.)

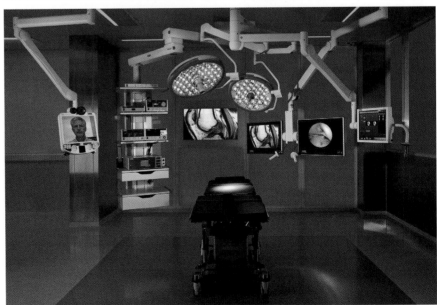

Figure 3-13 An integrated operating room with ceiling booms and shelving holding all hardware, including lighting, devices, display monitors, and auxiliary screens. (© 2014 Photo Courtesy of KARL STORZ GmbH & Co. KG.)

or within the sterile area. This challenge led to the development of integrative software and hardware platforms, or the *integrated room*. The integrated OR's concept is based on a single-post control station near the limit of the sterile area, which allows a single operator to coordinate, manipulate, manage, and access all information by a network connectivity and integration software that is displayed on one or multiple screens.[18]

These integrative platforms optimize the space in the OR while establishing capabilities to teleconferencing and teaching. The internal connection with hospital data management programs and other imaging platforms such as PACS (Picture Archiving and Communication System) also permits surgeons inside the OR to access other diagnostic images simultaneously for navigation or decision making during procedures. Although costly, the ease of accessing and producing medical reports, data exchange, and storage can be advantageous in hospitals with large caseloads.[19]

Operating Room Setup

The optimum design of an OR has been widely discussed, and standards for OR construction have been published by the American College of Surgeons on the Operating Room Environment and the American Institute of Architects Committee on Architecture for Health. In veterinary medicine, no specific guidelines exist, so common sense and translations from human surgery are used. Several solutions are commonly proposed to reduce equipment crowding and cables or lines crossing the floor in the OR.[20-22]

Preparation for Open Surgery

All instrumentation for open surgery should be available if conversion becomes necessary. The entire surgical team should be prepared for a smooth and expedient transition.[8,23-29]

Considerations for a Minimally Invasive Theater or Suite

The room must accommodate at least two equipment towers (endoscopy and anesthesia), and space must allow for free movement of these to either end of the surgical table. Also, adequate clearance from the patient is required to avoid breaks in sterile technique. Ideally, two to three monitors are positioned either on booms, the equipment towers, or separate wheeled stands.[21-24]

Ergonomic Considerations

Endoscopic surgery challenges the surgeon's natural view of the operating field. One basic ergonomic consideration—the correct position of the video display relative to the user's eyes—is often ignored in veterinary endoscopy. It has been shown that the preferred viewing angle for video displays is between 10 and 25 degrees *below* the line of sight. Excessive height of monitors may cause neck and back pain for the surgeon. Ceiling booms and mobile stands allow the surgeon to place the monitor at the ideal position.[20,37,38]

Endoscopic surgery is associated with ergonomic challenges. Laparoscopic and thoracoscopic instruments require four to six times more force than open surgery instruments to complete the same task. It is therefore not surprising that surgeons report increased fatigue after endoscopic surgery. Furthermore, endoscopic surgery has changed the surgeon's posture to an axial skeletal posture, more upright during laparoscopic surgery than during open surgery. This upright posture, however, seems to be accompanied by substantially less body movement and weight shifting than during open surgery. Increased static postural fatigue may occur during laparoscopic surgery. With incorrect movements and incorrect postures, surgeons significantly increase the physical load on the shoulder, neck, and arm musculature.[22,38,42]

As with the monitor positioning, awareness of some basic ergonomic rules that affect the surgeon's posture, such as lowering the height of the OR table to accommodate the increased length of rigid instruments, is lacking in veterinary medicine. The choice of surgical table is of utmost importance in addressing these ergonomic challenges. Electrically adjustable hydraulic tables allowing Trendelenburg to reverse-Trendelenburg positioning and lateral side tilt are ideal. V-top tables are also highly acceptable because they permit smooth tilting of the patient from one side to the other, facilitating access to different organs during a surgical procedure.[39-42]

Planning Coordination and Efficiency

The entire surgical team is involved in planning for MIS procedures. A surgical checklist may facilitate preparation. Adequate function and availability of equipment needs to be confirmed by the surgeon before anesthesia of the patient.

A sample checklist of MIS room assessment is:
- Confirm light source working properly and check bulb life (expended hours).
- Turn insufflator on and check for gas availability and spare tank.
- Check image capture devices for appropriate functioning and storage capacity.
- Turn on electrosurgical unit and check for proper function.
- Check suction and irrigation equipment and confirm for sterile containers and parts.
- Confirm availability of additional hemostasis devices, Gelfoam, and so on.
- Confirm availability of other disposables necessary (e.g., staplers, graspers, trocars, surgical loops).
- Confirm availability of trays and instrumentation needed for MIS and conventional surgery.[22,24,31,43-45]

In general, thoracoscopic procedures should be scheduled first because of challenges of anesthesia, such as one-lung ventilation, as well as the increased potential for complications. Clean laparoscopic procedures are often scheduled after thoracic procedures, and clean-contaminated procedures that lead to contamination of instrumentation should be scheduled last.[46-50]

Fully Equipped Minimally Invasive Surgery Suite: Hybrid Rooms

The combination of endoscopy and fluoroscopy led to the establishment of interventional endoscopy and radiology. In recent years, the concept has been adopted in the veterinary field. Multipurpose MIS rooms integrating interventional endoscopy and interventional radiology led to the concept of *hybrid rooms*.

These require fluoroscopy equipment (C-arm), either a floor-wheeled unit or ceiling boom suspended. Radiation protection is required. Endo-ultrasonography is also a modality commonly available in human medical hybrid settings, but its use has not yet been established in veterinary medicine.[51-55] In human hospitals, complex hybrid rooms also contain interventional computed tomography or interventional magnetic resonance units for intraoperative imaging, navigation, planning and reconstruction, often mounted on suspended racks.[37,56]

References

1 Chamness, C.J. (1999) Endoscopic instrumentation. In: Tams, T.R. (ed.) Small Animal Endoscopy, 2nd ed. Mosby, St. Louis, pp. 1-16.

2 Chamness, C.J. (2011) Endoscopic instrumentation and documentation for flexible and rigid endoscopy. In: Tams, T.R. (ed.) Small Animal Endoscopy, 3rd edn. Mosby, St. Louis, pp. 3-26.

3 Chamness, C.J. (2008) Instrumentation. In: Lhermette, P., Sobel, D. (eds.) BSAVA Manual of Canine and Feline Endoscopy and Endosurgery. British Small Animal Veterinary Association, Quedgeley, UK, pp. 11-30.

4 Chamness, C.J. (2005) Introduction to veterinary endoscopy and endoscopic instrumentation. In: McCarthy, T.C. (ed.) Veterinary Endoscopy for the Small Animal Practitioner. Saunders, St. Louis, pp. 1-20.

5 Goldstein, D.S., Chandhoke, P.S. Kavoussi, L.R., et al. (1994) Laparoscopic equipment. In: Sopper, N.J., Clayman, R.V. Odem, R., et al. (eds.) Essentials of Laparoscopy. Quality Medical Publishing, St. Louis, pp. 104-147.

6 Buyalos, R.P. (1997) Principles of endoscopic optics and lighting. In: Practical Manual of Operative Laparoscopy and Hysteroscopy. Springer, New York, pp. 23-31.

7 Coller, J.A., Murray, J.J. (1994) Equipment. In: Ballantyne, G.H., Leahy, P.F., Modlin, I.M. (eds.) Laparoscopic Surgery. Saunders, Philadelphia.

8 Monnet, E., Twedt, D.C. (2003) Laparoscopy. Vet Clin North Am Small Anim Pract 33, 1147-1163.

9 Stasi, K., Melendez, L. (2001) Care and cleaning of the endoscope. Vet Clin North Am Small Anim Pract 31 (4), 589-603.

10 Cartmill, J., Aamodt, D. (1993) Video systems in laparoscopy. In: Graber, J.N., et al. (eds.) Laparoscopic Abdominal Surgery. McGraw-Hill, New York.

11 Doppler, D.W. (1992) Laparoscopic instrumentation, videoimaging, and equipment disinfection and sterilization. Surg Clin North Am 72, 1021-1031.

12 Radlinsky, M.G. (2009) Endoscopy. Vet Clin North Am Small Anim Pract 39 (5), 817-837.

13 Van Lue, S.J., Van Lue, A.P. (2009) Equipment and instrumentation in veterinary endoscopy. Vet Clin North Am Small Anim Pract 39, 817-837.

14 Nissen, N.N., Menon, V.G., Colquhoun, S.D., Williams, J., Berci, G. (2013) Universal multifunctional HD video system for minimally invasive, [corrected] open and microsurgery. Surg Endosc 27 (3), 782-787.

15 La Chapelle, C.F., Bemelman, W.A., Rademaker, B.M.P., Van Barneveld, T.A., Jansen, F.W. (2012) A multidisciplinary evidence-based guideline for minimally invasive surgery. Part 1: entry techniques and the pneumoperitoneum. Gynecol Surg 9 (3), 271-282.

16 Magne, M.L., Tams, T.R. (1999) Laparoscopy: instrumentation and technique. In: Tams, T.R. (ed.) Small Animal Endoscopy. Mosby, St. Louis, pp. 397-408.

17 Sanfilippo, J.S., Indman, P.D. (1995) Photo documentation in laparoscopic surgery. In: Vitale, G.C., Sanfilippo, J.S., Perissat, J. (eds.) Laparoscopic Surgery: An Atlas for General Surgeons. Lippincott, Philadelphia.

18 Wichert, A., Marcos-Suarez, P., Vereczkei, A., et al. (2004) Improvement of the ergonomic situation in the integrated operating room for laparoscopic operations. In: International Congress Series, Vol. 1268. Elsevier, St. Louis.

19 Wickham, J.E. (1994) Minimally invasive surgery. Future developments. BMJ 308 (6922), 193-196.

20 Berguer, R. (1999) Surgery and ergonomics. Arch Surg 134 (9), 1011-1016.

21 Birch, D.W., Misra, M., Farrokhyar, F. (2007) The feasibility of introducing advanced minimally invasive surgery into surgical practice. Can J Surg 50 (4), 256-260.

22 Clayman, R.V., Winfield, H.N. (1994) Room set-up and patient positioning. In: Soper, N.J., et al. (eds.) Essentials of Laparoscopy. Quality Medical Publishing, St. Louis.

23 Bailey, J.E., Pablo, L.S. (1998) Anesthetic and physiologic considerations for veterinary endosurgery. In: Freeman, L.J. (ed.) Veterinary Endosurgery. Mosby, St. Louis, pp. 24-43.

24 Connor, S. (2013) Checklists are not only for the operating room. ANZ J Surg 83 (10), 704-705.

25 Freeman, L.J. (1999) Operation room setup, equipment and instrumentation. In: Freeman, L.J. (ed.) Veterinary Endosurgery. Mosby, St. Louis, pp. 3-23.

26 Mayhew, P.D. (2009) Advanced laparoscopic procedures in dogs and cats. Vet Clin North Am Small Anim Pract 3, 925-939.

27 Mayhew, P.D., Freeman, L.J., Kwan, T., Brown, D.C. (2009) Prospective comparison of post-operative wound infection rates after minimally invasive versus open surgery. Proceedings of the Veterinary Endoscopy Society Annual Meeting, Vancouver, British Columbia, March 7.

28 Skinner, A.C. (1994) Minimally invasive surgery. BMJ 308 (6927), 532-533.

29 Twedt, D.C., Monnet, E. (2005) Laparoscopy: technique and clinical experience. In: McCarthy, T.C. (ed.) Veterinary Endoscopy for the Small Animal Practitioner. Elsevier Saunders, St. Louis, pp. 357-385.

30 Freeman, L.J., Pader , K. (2012) NOTES applications in veterinary medicine. In: Kalloo, A.N., Marescaux, J., Zorron, R. (eds.) Natural Orifice Translumenal Endoscopic Surgery: Textbook and Video Atlas, Wiley, Hoboken, NJ, pp. 215-231.

31 Guinet, A., Chaabane, S. (2003) Operating theatre planning. Int J Prod Econom 85 (1), 69-81.

32 Kenyon, T.A.G., Lenker, M.P., Bax, T.W., Swanstrom, L.L. (1997) Cost and benefit of the trained laparoscopic team. Surg Endosc 11 (8), 812-814.

33 Meijer, D.W. (2003) Safety of the laparoscopy setup. Minim Invasive Ther Allied Technol 12 (3-4), 125-128.

34 Quandt, J.E. (1999) Anesthetic considerations for laser, laparoscopy, and thoracoscopy procedures. Clin Tech Small Anim Pract 14, 50-55.

35 Richter, K.P. (2001) Laparoscopy in dogs and cats. Vet Clin North Am Small Anim Pract 31, 707-727.

36 Weisse, C., Mayhew, P. (2012) Minimally invasive operating room equipment. In: Tobias, K.M., Johnston, S.A. (eds.) Veterinary Surgery Small Animal. Elsevier, Saunders, Philadelphia, pp. 291-303.

37 Cook, R.I., Woods, D.D. (1996) Special section: adapting to new technology in the operating room. human factors. J Hum Factors Ergonom Soc 38 (4), 593-613.

38 Healey, A.N., Sevdalis, N., Vincent, C.A. (2006) Measuring intra-operative interference from distraction and interruption observed in the operating theatre. Ergonomics 49 (5-6), 589-604.

39 Lenoir, C., Steinbrecher, H. (2010) Ergonomics, surgeon comfort, and theater checklists in pediatric laparoscopy. J Laparoendosc Adv Surg Tech A 20 (3), 281-291.

40 Maclean, A.R., Dixon, E., Ball, C.G. (2013) Effect of noise on auditory processing in the operating room. J Am Coll Surg 216 (5), 933-938.

41 Nguyen, N.T., Ho, H.S., Smith, W.D., et al. (2001) An ergonomic evaluation of surgeons' axial skeletal and upper extremity movements during laparoscopic and open surgery. Am J Surg 182 (6), 720-724.

42 Van Det, M.J., Meijerink, W.J.H.J., Hoff, C., Totté, E.R., Pierie, J.P.E.N. (2009) Optimal ergonomics for laparoscopic surgery in minimally invasive surgery suites: a review and guidelines. Surg Endosc 23 (6), 1279-1285.

43 Alarcon, A., Berguer, R. (1996) A comparison of operating room crowding between open and laparoscopic operations. Surg Endosc 10 (9), 916-919.

44 Cardoen, B., Demeulemeester, E., Beliën, J. (2010) Operating room planning and scheduling: a literature review. Eur J Oper Res 201 (3), 921-932.

45 Farrokhi, F.R., Gunther, M., Williams, B., Blackmore, C.C. (2013) Application of lean methodology for improved quality and efficiency in operating room instrument availability. J Healthc Qual Sep 24. doi: 10.1111/jhq.12053. [Epub ahead of print].

46 Hsiao, K.C., Machaidze, Z., Pattaras, J.G. (2004) Time management in the operating room: an analysis of the dedicated minimally invasive surgery suite. JSLS 8 (4), 300-303.

47 Kazemier, G., Van Veen-Berkx, E. (2013) Comment on "Identification and use of operating room efficiency indicators: the problem of definition." Can J Surg 56 (5), E103-E104.

48 Kenyon, T.A.G., Urbach, D.R., Speer, J.B., et al. (2001) Dedicated minimally invasive surgery suites increase operating room efficiency. Surg Endosc 15 (10), 1140-1143.

49 Low, D., Walker, I., Heitmiller, E.S., Kurth, D. (2012) Implementing checklists in the operating room. Paediatr Anaesth 22 (10), 1025-1031.

50 Papaconstantinou, H.T., Smythe, W.R., Reznik, S.I., Sibbitt, S., Wehbe-Janek, H. (2013) Surgical safety checklist and operating room efficiency: results from a large multispecialty tertiary care hospital. Am J Surg 206 (6), 853-860.

51 Gould, S.W.T., Darzi, A. (1997) The interventional magnetic resonance unit: the minimal access operating theatre of the future? Br J Radiol 70 (Suppl.), S89-S97.

52 Herron, D.M., Gagner, M., Kenyon, T.L., Swanström, L.L. (2001) The minimally invasive surgical suite enters the 21st century. Surg Endosc 15 (4), 415-422.

53 Santambrogio, R., Montorsi, M., Bianchi, P., Mantovani, A., Ghelma, F., Mezzetti, M. (1999) Intraoperative ultrasound during thoracoscopic procedures for solitary pulmonary nodules. Ann Thorac Surg 68 (1), 218-222.

54 Varu, V.N., Greenberg, J.I., Lee, J.T. (2013) Improved efficiency and safety for EVAR with utilization of a hybrid room. Eur J Vasc Endovasc Surg 46 (6), 675-679.

55 Weisse, C.W., Berent, A.C., Todd, K.L., Solomon, J.A. (2008) Potential applications of interventional radiology in veterinary medicine. J Am Vet Med Assoc 233, 1564-1574.

56 Yamada, K., Morimoto, M., Kishimoto, M., Wisner, E. (2007) Virtual endoscopy of dogs using multi-detector row CT. Vet Radiol Ultrasound 48 (4), 318-322.

Suggested Reading

Ad Hoc Committee on Infection Control in the Handling of Endoscopic Equipment (Association for Practitioners in Infection Control). (1980) Guidelines for preparation of laparoscopic instrumentation. AOR N J 32, 65-76.

Auyang, E.D., Santos, B.F., Enter, D.H., Hungness, E.S., Soper, N.J. (2011) Natural orifice translumenal endoscopic surgery (NOTES(*)): a technical review. Surg Endosc 25 (10), 3135-3148.

Barlow, D.E. (1990) Fiberoptic instrument technology. In: Tams, T.R. (ed.) Small Animal Endoscopy. Mosby. St. Louis, p. 1.

Beale, B.S., Hulse, D.A., Schulz, K.S., Withney, W.O. (2003) Arthroscopic instrumentation. In: Small Animal Arthroscopy. Elsevier Science, Philadelphia, pp. 15-21.

Blacker, A.J.R. (2005) How to build your own laparoscopic trainer. J Endourol 19 (6), 748-752.

Choll, W.K., Yu-Po, L., Taylor, W., Oygar, A., Kim, W.K. (2008) Use of navigation-assisted fluoroscopy to decrease radiation exposure during minimally invasive spine surgery. Spine J 8 (4), 584-590.

Clark, M.P., Qayed, E.S., Kooby, D.A., Maithel, S.K., Willingham, F.F. (2012) Natural orifice translumenal endoscopic surgery in humans: a review. Minim Invasive Surg 2012, 189296.

García, F., Prandi, D., Peña, T., Franch, J., Trasserra, O., De La Fuente, J. (1998) Examination of the thoracic cavity and lung lobectomy by means of thoracoscopy in dogs. Can Vet J 39 (5), 285-291.

Hashizume, M., Shimada, M., Tomikawa, M., et al. (2002) Early experiences of endoscopic procedures in general surgery assisted by a computer-enhanced surgical system. Surg Endosc 16 (8), 1187-1191.

Hill, D.L. (1993) The basis of laparoscopy. In: Gravber, J.N., Schultz, L., Pietrafitta, J., et al. (eds.) Laparoscopic Abdominal Surgery. McGraw-Hill, New York.

Kavoussi, L.R., Moore, R.G., Adams, J.B., Partin, A.W. (1995) Comparison of robotic versus human laparoscopic camera control. J Urol 154 (6), 2134–2136.

Korndorffer, J.R. Jr, Dunne, J.B., Sierra, R., Stefanidis, D., Touchard, C.L., Scott, D.J. (2005) Simulator training for laparoscopic suturing using performance goals translates to the operating room. J Am Coll Surg 201 (1), 23–29.

Mack, M.J. (2001) Minimally invasive and robotic surgery. JAMA 285 (5), 568-572.

Mamelak, A.N., Danielpour, M., Black, K.L., Hagike, M., Berci, G. (2008) A high-definition exoscope system for neurosurgery and other microsurgical disciplines: preliminary report. Surg Innov 15 (1), 38-46.

Mamelak, A.N., Nobuto, T., Berci, G. (2010) Initial clinical experience with a high-definition exoscope system for microneurosurgery. Neurosurgery 67 (2), 476-483.

Nahai, F. (1995) Instrumentation and setup for endoscopic plastic surgery. Clin Plast Surg 22 (4), 591-603.

Rahmathulla, G., Recinos, P.F., Traul, D.E., et al. (2012) Surgical briefings, checklists, and the creation of an environment of safety in the neurosurgical intraoperative magnetic resonance imaging suite. Neurosurg Focus 33 (5), E12.

Seymour, N.E., Gallagher, A.G., Roman, S.A., et al. (2002) Virtual reality training improves operating room performance. Ann Surg 236 (4), 458–464.

Smyth, E.T.M., Stacey, A., Taylor, E.W., Hoffman, P., Bannister, G. (2005) Survey of operating theatre ventilation facilities for minimally invasive surgery in Great Britain and Northern Ireland: current practice and considerations for the future. J Hosp Infect 61(2), 112-122.

Talamini, M.A., Gadacz, T.R. (1991) Laparoscopic equipment and Instrumentation. In: Zucker, K.A. (ed.) Surgical Laparoscopy. Quality Medical Publishing, St. Louis, pp. 23-27.

Weil, A.B. (2009) Anesthesia for endoscopy in small animals. Vet Clin North Am Small Anim Pract 39, 839-848.

4 Surgical Instrumentation

4.1 Surgical Instrumentation
Elizabeth A. Swanson and Heather A. Towle Millard

4.2 Trocars and Cannulas
Nicole J. Buote

4.3 Miscellaneous Surgical Instrumentation
Jessica K. Baron and Jeffrey J. Runge

4.1 Surgical Instrumentation

Elizabeth A. Swanson and Heather A. Towle Millard

Key Points

- Endoscopic instruments are modified basic surgical instruments and include forceps, scissors, tissue retractors, and needle holders.
- Types of forceps include grasping, dissection, and biopsy.
- The working end has a single- or double-action mechanism.
- For most surgical application in small animals, 5-mm instruments are adequate.
- Endoscopic instrument packs should include traditional open surgical instruments for securing of drapes and initial port entry and possible for conversion to open surgery.

Instrument Design

Endoscopic surgical instruments are designed to have the same functions as traditional open surgical instruments and thus are simply modifications of the basic instrument categories, including forceps (grasping, dissecting, and biopsy), scissors, tissue retractors, and needle holders. Several manufacturers provide a wide variety of minimally invasive instrumentation for use in both human and veterinary endoscopic surgery. In this section, we will focus on instruments most commonly used in small animal laparoscopic and thoracoscopic procedures. We will also discuss some instruments used in human surgery with potential for veterinary application.

Instruments for minimally invasive surgery (MIS) consist of the same basic parts as traditional instruments (Figure 4-1). Their shafts are long and thin to allow them to pass through an instrument portal into a body cavity. Some shafts are insulated to allow for monopolar or bipolar electrosurgical applications. If using an insulated shaft with electrosurgery, it is very important to regularly inspect the shafts for cracks or wear. Defects in the shaft insulation may lead to inadvertent electrical burns to other tissues. Shafts come in straight, articulating, and roticulating designs. Straight instruments are the basic instruments for MIS and are most commonly used for novice surgeons and in multiple-port surgery. Whereas articulating shafts bend in a single plane, roticulating shafts are able to rotate and bend in multiple planes, more accurately mimicking the motion of the human wrist. Articulating and roticulating instruments are used with multiple-port surgery but are also particularly advantageous

for single-port surgery because they allow for easier visualization of tissues and avoid conflict with the telescope and with each other.

Most instruments have either ratcheted or nonratcheted ringed handles (Figure 4-2). Ratcheted handles lock via one of several ratchet mechanisms, depending on the manufacturer. Laparoscopic needle holders, however, have a straight handle design with either a hemostat-style or a disengageable ratchet locking mechanism to allow for easier manipulation of suture and needle within a body cavity. Ringed handles are held in the same tripod manner as traditional instruments, with the thumb and ring finger in the rings and the index finger stabilizing the shaft. A dial that is easily reached by the index finger allows for 360-degree rotation of the shaft around

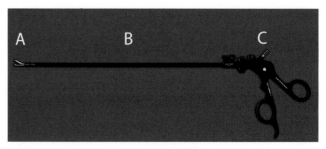

Figure 4-1 Endoscopic surgical instrument components. **A.** Working end (jaws of the instrument). **B.** Shaft. **C.** Handles. (© 2014 Photo courtesy of KARL STORZ GmbH & Co. KG.)

Small Animal Laparoscopy and Thoracoscopy, First Edition. Edited by Boel A. Fransson and Philipp D. Mayhew.

© 2015 by ACVS Foundation. Published 2015 by John Wiley & Sons, Inc.

Companion website: www.wiley.com/go/fransson/laparoscopy

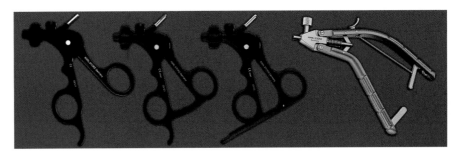

Figure 4-2 Minimally invasive surgical instrument handle types (from left to right): nonlocking (nonratcheted) rings, locking rings with a hemostat ratchet, locking rings with a Manhes ratchet, and straight handle with ratchet for certain endoscopic needle holders. (© 2014 Photo courtesy of KARL STORZ GmbH & Co. KG.)

its longitudinal axis. Shaft rotation allows for optimal positioning of the instrument jaws when working within a confined space. Handles intended for use with insulated shafts for monopolar or bipolar electrocoagulation also have a high-frequency connector for application of an electrical current from an electrosurgical generator. Monopolar and bipolar handles and shafts are distinct from one another and cannot be interchanged.

Instrument jaws come in a variety of shapes and sizes according to their intended function as graspers, dissectors, scissors, retractors, biopsy forceps, or needle holders. The working end of an endoscopic instrument may have a single- or double-action mechanism (Figure 4-3). With single-action instruments, one side of the jaw is hinged so that it opens and closes against a stationary opposing jaw. Double-action working ends are hinged in both jaws, allowing both sides to open and close and resulting in a wider and often stronger grasp.

Both disposable, single-use instruments and reusable instruments are available. For veterinary practice, reusable instruments are more economical. Early instrument designs may be more difficult to adequately clean and sterilize than more current designs, a fact that should be considered when purchasing laparoscopic equipment. Instruments are available as single-piece or as modular units, depending on the manufacturer, and can be made of high-grade plastic or stainless steel. There are benefits for each design type. Single-piece instruments avoid the possibility of mismatching components; however, as mentioned previously, older models may be difficult to decontaminate. Newer designs have portals that allow for cleaning of the shaft lumen. They also avoid nooks and crevices that are difficult to reach, making cleaning and decontamination easier. Modular units allow for the use of a variety of shafts and working ends with the same handles.

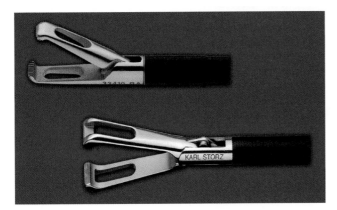

Figure 4-3 Examples of a single-action jaw mechanism (left) and a double-action jaw mechanism (right). (© 2014 Photo courtesy of KARL STORZ GmbH & Co. KG.)

Additionally, individual components are easier to thoroughly clean, can be sterilized separately or as a complete instrument, and can be replaced if they break rather than replacing the entire instrument.

Regular endoscopic instruments come in 5- and 10-mm diameters. For most small animal applications, 5-mm instruments are adequate. Common exceptions are the use of 10-mm Babcock or Duval forceps for grasping thicker tissues such as the stomach wall. Mini-laparoscopic instrumentation is now available for small dogs and cats weighing less than 10 kg. These come in 2-, 2.3-, and 3-mm-diameter sizes, depending on the manufacturer. The available shaft length depends on the instrument diameter and should be chosen based on patient size, with shorter shafts used for small patients and longer shafts for large or obese patients. Using a shaft that is either too long or too short for the patient can be awkward for the operator and can inhibit the ability to reach tissues inside the body cavity. Short and long shaft lengths vary by manufacturer but are similar. In general, 5- and 10-mm instruments range from 33 to 36 cm for the short length and from 43 to 45 cm for the long length. Mini-laparoscopy instruments range from 20 to 30 cm in length.

Forceps

Laparoscopic forceps can be divided into three categories: grasping forceps, dissecting forceps, and biopsy forceps. Just as in open surgery, the type of forceps selected will depend on its intended use. The jaws of laparoscopic forceps can be crushing or noncrushing, straight or curved, and long or short. Some forceps are designed as either graspers or dissectors; others may be used simultaneously for both functions. In addition, graspers can be used as tissue retractors.

Grasping forceps are used to grasp tissue for stabilization, relocation, or hemostasis. Noncrushing forceps most commonly used in small animal laparoscopy and thoracoscopy are Babcock and Duval forceps (Figure 4-4). The jaws of endoscopic Babcock forceps are identical to their open surgical counterparts. They are most commonly used to grasp and manipulate the pyloric antrum during laparoscopic-assisted gastropexy. Duval forceps are similar to Babcock forceps except that the jaws are slightly longer and offer a more aggressive grasp. For both Babcock and Duval forceps, a double-action mechanism allows for a wider grasp to include more tissue and better prevent slipping.

Many other types of grasping instruments are provided by the different manufacturers (Figure 4-5A). Basic designs include toothed graspers (varying number of teeth at the end of the instrument jaw), fenestrated graspers (a fenestrated slit is present down the length of the jaw), DeBakey graspers, Allis graspers, alligator graspers (pronounced transverse serrations for a stronger tissue grip), bowel graspers (longitudinal serrations, similar to a

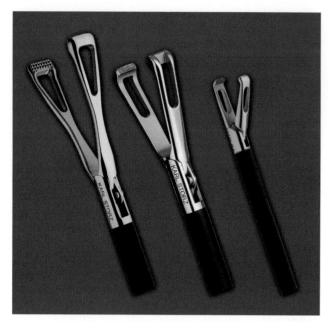

Figure 4-4 Duvall and Babcock forceps (from left to right): 10-mm, double-action Duvall forceps; 10-mm, double-action Babcock forceps; and 5-mm single-action Babcock forceps. (© 2014 Photo courtesy of KARL STORZ GmbH & Co. KG.)

DeBakey), straight and curved atraumatic graspers (for grasping and removing hollow organs), and bullet-nosed graspers (blunt-nosed, atraumatic jaws for grasping delicate tissues). Although technically described as dissecting forceps, Kelly forceps can also be used to carefully grasp and move tissues such as the proper ligament during laparoscopic ovariectomy. Grasping forceps are usually placed on locking handles to facilitate a more secure grip of tissues during surgery.

The most commonly used dissecting forceps include Kelly dissectors and Maryland dissectors (which resemble Crile hemostatic forceps) (Figure 4-5B). They are available with straight or curved jaws, but most surgeons find that curved instruments improve tissue visualization during dissection. Needle-nosed, tapered, bullet-nose, and micro-dissectors are also available. For dissection around ducts and vessels, right-angled dissectors (see Figure 4-5B) and Mixter spreader-dissectors are very useful. The Mixter dissector has a longer jaw and more acute angle at the tip than does the right-angle dissector. Dissecting forceps may be on either ratcheted or non-ratcheted handles. Using ratcheted handles allows some versatility when using the same instrument for both grasping and dissecting, as the locking mechanism allows for a more stable grasp. On the other hand, nonratcheted handles allow for a smoother motion when placing and spreading the instrument jaws during dissection and avoid accidental ratcheting of the handles. When dissecting around vessels, ducts, and other fragile tissue, it is best, however, to use a nonratcheted handle.

Biopsy forceps are available as cup biopsy forceps and as punch biopsy forceps (Figure 4-6). Punch biopsy forceps will cut tissue as one jaw "punches" through the fenestration in the opposite jaw. On the other hand, cup biopsy forceps provide some hemostasis by crushing and tearing tissues at the edges of the biopsy sample as the cup is closed and then gently twisted to obtain the specimen. Some cup biopsy instruments have a fine spike in one or both jaws to better secure tissue; however, this spike is not necessary to obtain adequate tissue samples for histologic analysis. In our practice, cup biopsy forceps are the most commonly used biopsy instrument for obtaining liver, splenic, pancreatic, adrenal, lymph node, and other soft tissue mass biopsies. Because punch biopsy forceps cut rather than tear, they may be more appropriate for use in tissues such as the pancreas, where tearing may incite inflammation and pancreatitis. Biopsy forceps can also be on either a ratcheted or nonratcheted handle; however, ratcheted handles allow for a better, more consistent grip on tissues while obtaining a biopsy sample.

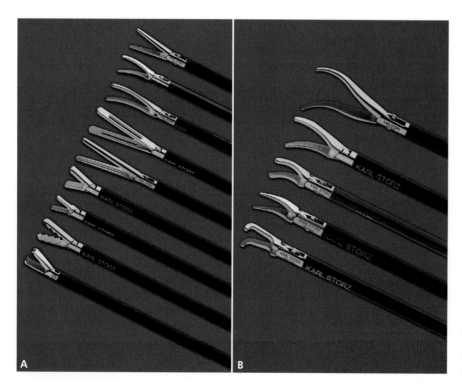

Figure 4-5 A. Grasping forceps (from top to bottom): straight dissecting and grasping forceps, curved dissecting and grasping forceps, DeBakey grasping forceps, bowel grasper with longitudinal fenestration, bowel forceps, robust Reddick-Olsen forceps, regular Reddick-Olsen forceps, alligator jaw forceps, and toothed grasping forceps ("Tiger Jaws"). **B.** Dissecting forceps (from top to bottom): 10-mm, long Kelly forceps (not shown to scale); 5-mm, long Kelly forceps; Kelly forceps; Noshiro forceps (for fine dissection); and right-angled forceps. (© 2014 Photos courtesy of KARL STORZ GmbH & Co. KG.)

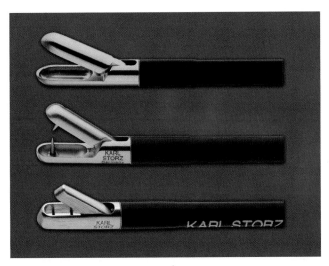

Figure 4-6 Biopsy forceps (from top to bottom): biopsy forceps without teeth, biopsy forceps with two teeth, and biopsy punch. (© 2014 Photo courtesy of KARL STORZ GmbH & Co. KG.)

Scissors

In veterinary surgery, endoscopic scissors are used for more advanced procedures, such as for transection of the common bile duct in laparoscopic cholecystectomy, transection of the pulmonary ligament of a caudal lung lobe in thoracoscopic lung lobectomy, thoracoscopic subtotal pericardiectomy, or cutting intracorporeal sutures (Figure 4-7). Curved Metzenbaum scissors are the most versatile for tissue transection and dissection. When used with a handle–shaft assembly with a connector for monopolar electrocoagulation, hemostasis may be achieved while cutting. Metzenbaum scissors are also available with straight blades and with long, fine blades (curved or straight) for finer dissection. Other dissecting scissor types include operating scissors with serrated blades, blunt-tipped scissors, sharp-tipped scissors, and micro-dissection scissors. Blades can be fine or robust, long or short, and straight or curved for most scissor sizes and shapes. Hook scissors have a wider, single-action blade that engages a thinner, stationary blade. Both blades are hooked toward each other. Hook scissors are used to cut suture intracorporeally, and the hook design hinders suture slippage during transection of the suture. All scissors are used with nonlocking handles.

Tissue Retractors

Palpation probes are very useful instruments and should be included in every laparoscopy pack (Figure 4-8A). Palpation probes are single-piece instruments with straight handles that come in 3- and 5-mm-diameter sizes to fit through 3- and 5-mm cannulas. They can also be used with a 10-mm cannula if a reducer cap is used. They have long, thin shafts that are marked in centimeter intervals to help with measurement of lesions within the body cavity. Whereas 3-mm palpation probes are available in 20- and 30-cm lengths, 5-mm probes are available in a 36-cm length. Probes can serve many different functions, starting with the obvious palpation of organs and structures within a body cavity. They can also be used in a sweeping motion to move and retract organs such as the intestines, omentum, or spleen out of the viewing field, such as during laparoscopic ovariectomy or gastropexy, and they can be used to help stabilize organs during tissue dissection or ligation.

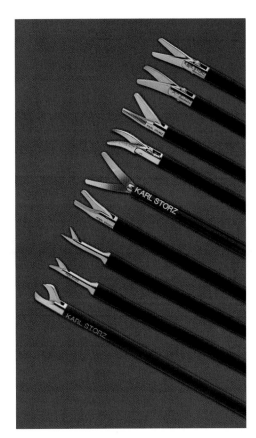

Figure 4-7 Endoscopic scissors (from top to bottom): straight scissors; curved Metzenbaum scissors; serrated Manhes scissors; scissors with curved, conical, serrated blades; scissors with spoon-shaped blades; Manhes micro scissors; straight micro-dissecting scissors; curved micro-dissecting scissors; and hook scissors. (© 2014 Photo courtesy of KARL STORZ GmbH & Co. KG.)

Several different kinds of retractors are available for human MIS. Of these, only the fan retractor is regularly used in veterinary surgery (Figure 4-8B). The fan retractor consists of a straight shaft with a series of flat blades at the end that distend in the shape of a paper fan when the outer sheath of the shaft is rotated. The completely opened retractor is sturdy and is used to retract organs with large surface areas, such as the liver or intestines. It is often used for advanced procedures such as laparoscopic cholecystectomy or adrenalectomy. Fan retractors are available in both 5- and 10-mm-diameter sizes.

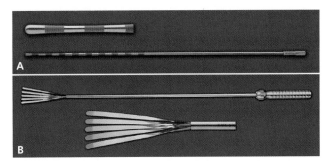

Figure 4-8 **A.** Palpation probe with centimeter markings. Inset shows detail of the instrument tip. **B.** Fan retractor. Inset shows detail of the collapsible fan blades at the working end. (© 2014 Photo courtesy of KARL STORZ GmbH & Co. KG.)

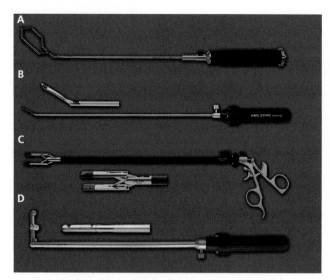

Figure 4-9 Retractors used in human minimally invasive surgery (from top to bottom): Cuschieri retractor with end deployed (**A**); retractor for gastric banding, with close-up of working end (inset) (**B**); Leroy H-retractor, with close-up of working end (inset) (**C**); and Leroy T-retractor with end deployed, with inset showing the closed end (**D**). (© 2014 Photo courtesy of KARL STORZ GmbH & Co. KG.)

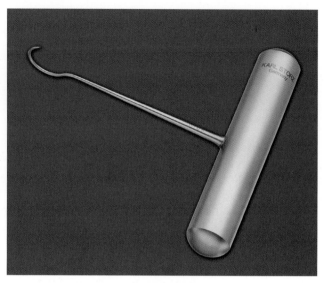

Figure 4-10 An ovariectomy hook with a T-shaped handle. (© 2014 Photo courtesy of KARL STORZ GmbH & Co. KG.)

Other types of retractors that are widely used in human laparoscopic surgery include the Cuschieri Retractor, gastric banding retractors, and Leroy Retractors (Figure 4-9). The Cuschieri Retractor was designed as safe retractor of the liver for extended periods of time during laparoscopic surgeries. When activated, the distal end roughly resembles a hexagon, allowing for support of a larger surface area. When closed, the retractor can also be used to move and retract other abdominal structures, such as the intestinal tract. A similar principle is used and advanced upon in newer designs based on the Cushieri articulating retractor. A variety of retractor shapes is available, including curved, triangular, circular, and pretzel shapes. Gastric banding retractors have a flat, angled distal end that is used to bluntly retract the stomach and intestines. A fenestration at the end of the instrument is used to secure a gastric band for passage around the esophagus. Leroy retractors come in a variety of configurations and are used in human colorectal surgery. These retractors may become more widely used as surgeons begin to perform more advanced procedures.

Ovariectomy hooks are used during laparoscopic ovariectomy and ovariohysterectomy to suspend the ovary against the body wall to facilitate ligation and transection of the ovarian pedicle (Figure 4-10). Ovariectomy hooks are placed percutaneously to capture the ovary and proper ligament within the curve of the hook. They have a heavy, T-shaped handle to facilitate retraction and to prevent rotation of the hook after being placed. The heavy handle allows positioning of the instrument without an assistant, and the small puncture that is created does not need to be closed. Both small and large ovariectomy hooks are available to accommodate patient size. A straight-handled hook may be used in some clinics but is no longer manufactured. When ovariectomy hooks are not available, a large-diameter suture on a large needle (i.e., 0 polypropylene on a CT-26 or CT-40 swaged needle) can be used to capture and retract the ovary in the same manner.

Needle Holders and Suturing Devices

Different methods of suturing for advanced laparoscopic and thoracoscopic procedures include extracorporeal knot tying, intracorporeal knot tying, and intracorporeal suturing. A variety of needle holders and suture assist devices are available for this purpose. The most common diameter needle holders used are 5 mm, although 3-mm-diameter instruments are available for smaller patients. Endoscopic needle holders most commonly come with straight handles (Figure 4-11) rather than ring handles to provide a more ergonomic motion while manipulating suture and needle. The handles lock via a ratchet mechanism.

The traditional endoscopic needle holder (see Figure 4-11) has straight jaws with tungsten carbide inserts to prevent needle slippage. It is used in combination with grasping forceps to pass the needle from one side of an incision to the other and to tie knots. Needle holders with right-handed and left-handed curved jaws (Figure 4-12) are used as a pair to pass the needle and tie knots. The curved configuration helps with loop formation and grasping of the suture end while tying knots.

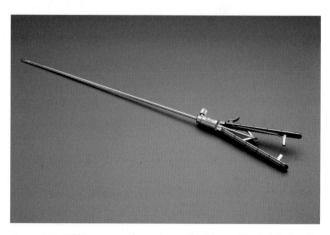

Figure 4-11 KOH macro-endoscopic needle driver with straight handle. Used with a wide range of suture and needle sizes; from 0/0 to 7/0. (© 2014 Photo courtesy of KARL STORZ GmbH & Co. KG.)

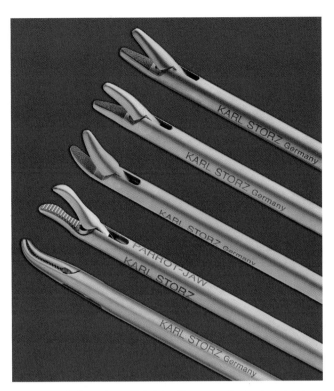

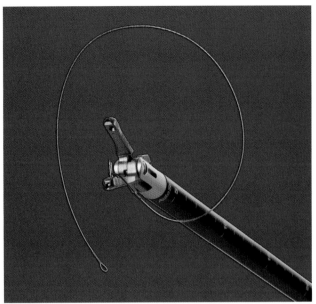

Figure 4-13 Endo Stitch Device with suture loaded into jaws. (Copyright © 2013 Covidien. All rights reserved. Used with the permission of Covidien.)

Figure 4-12 Endoscopic needle holders (from top to bottom): straight jaws, jaws curved to the left, jaws curved to the right, Szabo-Berci needle holder ("Parrot Jaw"), and Szabo-Berci assistant needle holder ("Flamingo Jaw"). (© 2014 Photo courtesy of KARL STORZ GmbH & Co. KG.)

Although marketed for human and large animal endoscopic surgery, the Szabo-Berci needle holder pair (see Figure 4-12) is also designed to facilitate easier needle passage, loop formation, knot tying, and grasping of tissues. The Szabo-Berci needle holder "Parrot Jaw" has a broad, flat jaw with a downward curve and blunt tips. Its counterpart, the Szabo-Berci Assistant needle holder "Flamingo Jaw," has a narrower, tapered jaw with pointed tips for grasping of suture ends through a loop. These needle drivers are designed to accommodate a fairly limited range of needle and suture sizes.

A self-righting needle holder is available that automatically places a curved needle in the correct vertical position for suturing. The needle holder has a single-action mechanism with a fixed, broad jaw with cut-outs that fit with the convex surface of a curved needle. The opposing jaw is narrow and meets with the concave surface of the needle when the jaws are closed to rotate the needle against the fixed jaw and hold it perpendicular to the axis of the instrument. Self-righting needle holders negate the need for a second instrument to position the needle and thereby facilitate more efficient needle handling during suturing. They also prevent needles from twisting within the grasp of the instrument during passage through tissues. However, the suture is easily damaged if grasped with the jaws of self-righting needle drivers, which is an important limitation.

The Endo Stitch device (Covidien, Mansfield, MA) (Figure 4-13) was designed to avoid needle handling during intracorporeal suturing. A double-pointed needle with centrally swaged suture is passed from one jaw to the other. This device will pass the suture through tissue, as well as through suture loops, to tie knots without the need to reload and reposition the needle. It comes in a 10-mm-diameter size only.

A needle must be passed carefully through the instrument cannula to prevent damage to the gaskets within. One way to avoid damage is by the use of an introducer sleeve, a valveless cannula that fits within a regular port cannula but is still wide enough to allow passage of a needle, suture, and other knot-tying equipment (Figure 4-14). However, in small animals with small cannula sizes, it is often more practical to simply remove the cannula from the body wall, thread it onto the needle driver, grasp the needle and suture, introduce them through the incision, and thereafter replace the cannula into the incision. Suture knots can be tied intracorporeally or extracorporeally. Intracorporeal knot tying using needle holders and graspers requires some practice for a surgeon to become proficient at this skill. The Suture Assistant (Ethicon Endo-Surgery, Somerville, NJ) is a 5-mm-diameter device that deploys pretied suture intracorporeally for simple interrupted suture patterns. Cartridges are available with different sizes and types of suture most commonly used for soft tissue closure. After the suture is loaded onto the Suture Assistant, it is passed into the body cavity. The needle is driven through the tissues with needle holders and then is passed through a pretied loop at the end of the device. Deployment of the device produces a secure intracorporeal knot.

It is often easier for an endoscopic surgeon who is starting to place endoscopic sutures to tie knots extracorporeally. Extracorporeal knot tying can be performed using standard suture material or using pretied loop sutures, such as the Endo-Loop Ligature. With standard suture, a single half-hitch, double half-hitch (i.e. surgeon's throw), or modified Roeder knot (for details, see Chapter 2) is created outside of the body and then is pushed through the cannula using a knot pusher. A knot pusher (Ethicon Endo-Surgery) is a plastic tube with a conical end through which the suture ends pass. The knot pusher then is used to slide the knot into the body cavity by pushing down on the knot while simultaneously pulling up on the suture ends. After placement, a half-hitch knot can be corrected to an overhand throw. Koeckerling Knot Tiers (Karl Storz GmbH, Tuttlingen, Germany) (see Figure 4-14) are 5-mm instruments on long shafts with a notch and hole at the end; they serve the same purpose as a knot pusher. Endoscopic Babcock forceps can also be used to advance and secure an extracorporeal knot.

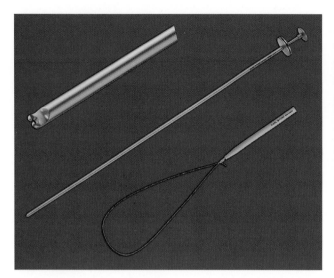

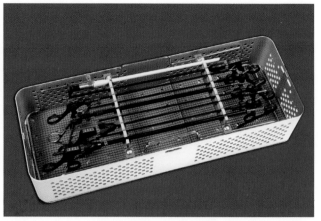

Figure 4-15 An example of a laparoscopic instrument pack in its tray for sterilization and storage. (Photo courtesy of Dr. Philipp Mayhew.)

Figure 4-14 Suture assist devices (from top left to bottom right): Koeckerling knot tier, introducer sleeve, and EndoLoop ligature. (© 2014 Photo courtesy of KARL STORZ GmbH & Co. KG.)

The Endo-Loop Ligature (Karl Storz GmbH) (see Figure 4-14) was developed for use over free vascular pedicles. It consists of a pretied loop of suture with a Roeder knot loaded into a single-use plastic cannula. After the loop is placed around the desired tissue, the cannula is snapped at a prescored line. The most distal end is used as a handle to tension the suture while the rest of the cannula serves as a knot pusher to close the ligature around the pedicle. After it is tightened, the suture can be cut and the remaining suture, and cannulas are removed.

Laparoscopy Packs

All instrument packs for MIS should include traditional open surgical instruments for the securing of drapes and initial port entry. Additionally, it is wise to always be prepared to convert to an open procedure when warranted. To that end, a general surgery pack containing at least drapes large enough to cover the patient and operating table; sufficient towel clamps to secure the drapes to the patient; a #3 scalpel handle; a pair each of Brown-Adson and DeBakey thumb forceps; several curved mosquito and either Crile or Kelly hemostatic forceps; Metzenbaum, Mayo, and suture scissors; needle holders; a saline bowl; and 4 × 4 x-ray detectable gauzes are needed.

A basic starting laparoscopic instrument pack for a beginning endoscopic surgeon using multiple-port approach should include a 5-mm, 0-degree telescope or a 10-mm, 0-degree telescope; a light cable; insufflator tubing; an endoscopic video camera; a Veress needle (if desired entry technique); three 5-mm cannulas with two sharp-tipped trocars and one blunt-tipped trocar; one to two 10-mm cannulas with one sharp and one blunt trocar (to accommodate a 10-mm telescope, instruments, or energy devices); two reducer caps; 10-mm double-action Babcock or Duval grasping forceps; a 5-mm double-or single-action Babcock forceps; two 5-mm curved Kelly or Maryland grasping-dissecting forceps; 5-mm Metzenbaum dissecting scissors; 5-mm cup biopsy forceps with or without spikes; 5-mm punch biopsy forceps; a-5 mm palpation probe; and an ovariectomy hook.

For more advanced surgeons, this basic pack may be expanded to include right-angle dissecting forceps; additional graspers such as atraumatic tissue graspers, bullet-nosed graspers, or bowel graspers; needle holders (straight or curved); additional suturing equipment such as a knot pusher or Suture Assistant; hook scissors; a suction and lavage device; a fan retractor; a 5-mm, 30-degree telescope; bipolar electrosurgical instrumentation; mini-laparoscopic telescopes and instrumentation; and single-port access cannulas with either articulating or roticulating instruments.

Instruments may be equipped with insulation and a connection for a monopolar electrosurgical device at the surgeon's preference. If modular instruments are chosen, at least one ratcheted and one nonratcheted handle should be included. Trays designed specifically for sterilization and safe storage of delicate endoscopic instruments are available and highly recommended (Figure 4-15). Often, the camera, telescopes, light cable, and insufflation tubing are packaged separately from the rest of the instruments.

4.2 Trocars and Cannulas

Nicole J. Buote

Key Points

- Trocar assembly includes a cannula, seal, and obturator.
- Veress needle use for insufflation requires blind insertion of a specially designed needle for CO_2 insufflation before trocar placement.
- In the direct insertion technique, the primary trocar is placed without preinsufflation with either a bladed trocar or an optical trocar.
- The Hasson technique requires a mini-laparotomy with visualization of intraabdominal structures before placement of the trocar.
- Reported complications of trocar placement include laceration to intraabdominal organs, hemorrhage from intraabdominal vessels, and subcutaneous emphysema.

The Trocar, Cannula, and Sheath

In its simplest configuration, a trocar is a pen-shaped instrument with a sharp triangular point at one end, typically used inside a hollow cylinder, known as a cannula or sleeve, which provides an access port into a cavity during surgery. Rigid telescopes must be placed through a cannula in order to gain access to the body cavity. The literature shows a notable inconsistency of terminology; often *trocar* is used to describe the assembly of a cannula with its associated obturator. A cannula–trocar assembly is made up of three components: a cannula, seal and obturator.

Cannula

A cannula is a tube-shaped metal or plastic shaft placed in the patient to allow access into the abdominal cavity during a laparoscopic procedure. Cannulas are sometimes sutured in place to the body wall or thoracic wall to ensure they do not migrate; they can also be screwed in place or held in place by inflatable balls and plastic flanges. Sheaths are protective shafts that are usually locked in place on the telescope, such as used with cystoscopes and arthroscopes.[1]

Seal

A seal is located at the top of the cannula, which allows instruments to pass through the cannula while preventing carbon dioxide (CO_2) from escaping from the abdominal cavity. A gas-tight valve is located at the top of the cannula to allow instruments to be inserted and removed during a procedure without permitting the insufflated carbon dioxide escape. Various types of valves are available (spring loaded, magnetic trap door, trumpet, silicone, and so on), offering different characteristics in terms of leakage, mode of operation, and

location on the cannula. More recently, a valveless cannula has been designed that makes use of a pressurized curtain of gas at the top of the instrument, eliminating the need for a valve altogether. This approach has the dual benefit of significantly reducing carbon dioxide leakage and smudging of the laparoscope lens, which is problem commonly associated with traditional valve types.[2]

Obturator

An obturator is the tool (either sharp or blunt) that allows the cannula to penetrate the abdomen for initial placement. Although it once was used to refer solely to the piercing tool (obturator), as mentioned earlier, the term *trocar* is now often used to refer to the whole assembly. The pointed pyramidal tip from which the trocar gained its name is now one of several different types available, with outer diameters ranging from around 2 to 15 mm.[3] Other designs include flat double-edged blades and pointed conical tips. Bladed trocars reduce the amount of force needed for the instrument to pass through the abdominal wall. For increased safety, some designs now include a spring-loaded plastic shield that automatically covers the blade as it enters the abdominal cavity. Conical tips can be either metal or plastic and require a small initial incision to be made using a scalpel. They pass through the tissues of the abdominal wall by stretching rather than cutting them. This leads to improved sleeve retention because it is surrounded by intact tissue layers that help hold it in place.[3]

Today, a very wide range of precision-engineered laparoscopic trocars exists, which has revolutionized patient care as we know it. Surgical trocars in human medicine are most commonly a single-patient use instrument and have graduated from the "three–point" design that gave them their name to either a flat bladed

---

Small Animal Laparoscopy and Thoracoscopy, First Edition. Edited by Boel A. Fransson and Philipp D. Mayhew.
© 2015 by ACVS Foundation. Published 2015 by John Wiley & Sons, Inc.
Companion website: www.wiley.com/go/fransson/laparoscopy

"dilating tip" product, or something that is entirely blade free. In veterinary medicine, the most commonly used trocar assemblies are reusable, reautoclavable configurations made of stainless steel or plastic or silicone materials.

Trocar–Cannula Placement

Laparoscopic entry is covered in detail in Chapter 8. However, a brief description as it relates to instrumentation follows here.

Initial trocar placement can be done after insufflation of the peritoneum or preceding it depending on the method chosen. Creating a pneumoperitoneum, or insufflation of the abdomen, allows for separation between the body wall and internal organs and allows for increased internal working space for manipulation of organs by surgical instruments. Cannula placement can be done by one of three methods: Veress needle, direct trocar insertion, or the open Hasson method. Insufflation can be performed using a Veress needle before placement of the primary trocar or via the trocar itself through a gas intake port, typically located on the side of the outer cannula. After the laparoscope has been introduced, secondary trocars can be placed under direct laparoscopic observation to minimize the risk of injury.

Veress Needle Technique

The Veress needle technique is the oldest and most traditional technique. One large retrospective study revealed that 81% of 155,987 gynecologic laparoscopic procedures used the Veress needle technique, but only 48% of 17,216 general surgical laparoscopic procedures used this method of insufflation.[4] The Veress needle is a specially designed instrument with an outer diameter of approximately 2 mm (Figure 4-16). The outer cannula consists of a beveled needle point for cutting through tissue and an inner spring-loaded dull-tipped stylet (Figure 4-17). After the sharp outer needle passes through the abdominal wall, the spring-loaded stylet springs forward to protect the inner organs. The needle can then be attached to insufflation tubing and CO_2 used to inflate the cavity. Blind placement of a Veress needle remains an important risk factor for complications. There are multiple reported safety tests to confirm that the Veress needle is properly placed before insufflation, including the "double click sound," "aspiration test," "hiss sound test," "waggle test," and "hanging drop test." Unfortunately, most of these tests have been shown to be unreliable.[5] In fact, waggling the Veress needle from side to side was considered contraindicated in clinical guidelines for MD surgeons because of the risk of organ laceration.[6] Two recent studies have looked at the diagnostic accuracy of tissue impedance measurement interpretation for correct Veress needle placement in cats and dogs.[7,8] In dogs, the impedance measurement had a 89.7% sensitivity, 100% specificity, and 90% accuracy.[7] In cats, tissue impedance measurement resulted in 94.7% sensitivity, 20% specificity, and 79.2% accuracy.[8] The differences between cats and dogs were thought to be due to the overdeveloped retroperitoneal fat pad in cats as well as their small size.

After an adequate volume of gas has been insufflated, the Veress needle is removed. In the blind technique for initial trocar insertion, a bladed trocar or trocar with a sharp obturator is inserted through an adequately sized incision. Trocar assemblies with sharp obturators are most commonly used in veterinary medicine; laparoscopic surgeons in human medicine tend to use bladed trocars. Bladed trocars

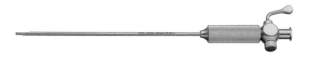

Figure 4-16 Veress needle. (© 2014 Photo courtesy of KARL STORZ GmbH & Co. KG.)

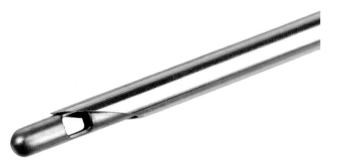

Figure 4-17 Close up photograph of the specialized tip to a Veress needle. (© 2014 Photo courtesy of KARL STORZ GmbH & Co. KG.)

are equipped with a spring-loaded safety shield that retracts when passed through the abdominal wall. This is often accompanied by an audible click as the blade retracts. Advancement of the trocar assembly is stopped at this point, and the bladed trocar or sharp obturator is removed from its outer cannula. The laparoscope can then be inserted to confirm the successful placement of the cannula in the peritoneal cavity and to rule out intraabdominal injury from either Veress needle or trocar insertion. If the cannula is appropriately located, the insufflation tubing is connected to the gas port of the cannula, and insufflation to the predetermined pressure occurs. The remaining cannulas are then placed under direct visualization.

Direct Insertion Technique

In the direct insertion technique, the primary cannula–trocar assembly is placed without preinsufflation. This technique is not regularly performed in veterinary medicine but can be performed with either a bladed trocar and a blind technique or an optical trocar under some measure of direct visualization. Theoretical advantages include decreased time to establish abdominal laparoscopic access, but potential disadvantages may include a higher rate of trocar-related intraabdominal injuries. Several published series evaluating the direct trocar placement technique have demonstrated that very low rates of injury are possible.[9] For inexperienced surgeons, the direct access technique is likely associated with unnecessary increased risk compared with alternative techniques.[4,10]

Optical trocar assemblies can also be placed with a direct technique. A gradual twisting motion is used, and distinct layers of the abdominal wall can be seen during entry.

Hasson Technique

In an effort to decrease the incidence of injuries associated with the blind penetration of the abdominal cavity during laparoscopy, Hasson[11] proposed a mini-laparotomy technique. He developed a reusable device similar to a standard laparoscopic port with a cork-shaped sleeve on the outside. The sleeve could be slid up or down on the cannula shaft depending on the thickness of the patient's abdominal wall.[10] Sutures in the fascia were used to anchor the outer sleeve and to create an airtight seal. Hasson-type cannulas that are fixed to the abdominal wall between a balloon and a dense foam cuff are also now commercially available.

In the open technique, the peritoneal cavity is entered under direct visualization. Theoretical advantages to the open technique may include a decreased likelihood of injury to adherent bowel or major vascular injuries during initial trocar insertion. Potential disadvantages may include increased operative time (especially in obese patients) and an increased risk of late port-related complications such as hematoma, wound infection, or hernia.[12] Leakage of gas around the cannula is occasionally a problem. If resulting in a loss of pneumoperitoneum, sutures may be placed around the cannulas to act as a purse string.

Alternatively, a balloon-tipped fixation trocar or a dilating "Olive" can be added to the trocar can be placed to seal the leak.[1,13]

Types of Trocar Assemblies

Multiple types of cannula–trocar assemblies are available in human and veterinary medicine. They can be divided into reusable or single use, rigid or flexible, and by the various fixation methods they used. Various designs of each type are available. Although the initial cost of a reusable trocar assembly is high, the per-use cost is significantly less than that of disposable types. However, reusable trocars can be difficult to sterilize because of the number of small parts that comprise the valve and gas inlet assemblies. Additionally, over time, the tips can become blunt and the valves leaky and stiff. Some manufacturers now offer a combination type using a reusable sleeve and piercing stylus in conjunction with a single-use valve assembly.

Disposable Trocar Assemblies

Disposable cannulas are very common in human medicine, but their cost limits their use in veterinary medicine. There are multiple different types of disposable trocars, including bladeless trocars with safety shields (Figure 4-18), inflatable flanges to help with retention, and optical trocars (Figure 4-19). Optical trocars have a transparent plastic sleeve, into which the laparoscope may be fitted before insertion of the trocar, enabling the surgeon to monitor the passage of the instrument through the layers of the abdominal wall. The internal surface of the sleeve must be nonreflective to avoid light from the laparoscope interfering with the surgeon's view.

Nondisposable Trocar Assemblies

Reusable trocar assemblies are the most common type used in veterinary medicine. These include smooth and threaded, a.k.a. Ternamian, stainless steel trocars (Figures 4-20 and 4-21). These have the advantages of being easy to clean and sterilize with a long shelf life. The plastic valves that attach to these trocars are also autoclavable, but they eventually wear or crack over time. The threaded cannulas can be used without an obturator as the distal end is shaped to penetrate the body wall and screw into place, avoiding the need for retention sutures. These may be difficult to place through very thick tissue planes without appropriate insufflation pressures or without an appropriately sized skin incision.

Flexible ports or plastic cannulas have been used to gain access to the abdomen or chest (Figure 4-22). Specialized Thoracoports (Covidien, Mansfield, MA) are plastic cannulas with plastic blunt trocars used for atraumatic entrance into the thoracic cavity to decrease the chance of iatrogenic damage to intercostal vessels or underlying structures (e.g., heart, esophagus, trachea) (Figure 4-23). There are also many multiport systems available to veterinary surgeons today, which allow for a telescope and up to three instruments to be passed

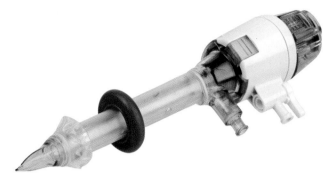

Figure 4-19 Disposable optical view cannula–trocar with an internal flange and balloon for improved retention.

into a body cavity simultaneously through one incision. These ports are discussed elsewhere in detail. They have different advantages and disadvantages, including cost, resterilization ability, flexibility of instrument handling after the cannulas are engaged, and so on.

Trocar Assembly-Related Complications

Most insertional complications can be avoided with special attention to detail and do not usually require the need for conversion to an open procedure. Complications associated with trocar placement and insufflation include damage to intraabdominal organs, vascular injury, subcutaneous insufflation (emphysema), fatal air embolism, and insufflation of falciform fat.[14] Insertion of the Veress needle via the intercostal technique in one article was associated with 35% grade 1 complications (subcutaneous emphysema, omental or falciform injuries), 10.7% grade 2 complications (liver of splenic injuries), and 1.7%

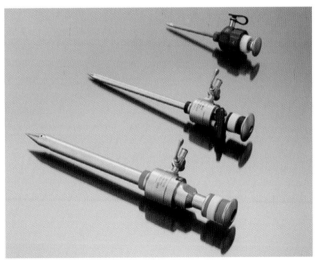

Figure 4-20 Different sizes of smooth stainless steel reusable cannulas. (© 2014 Photo courtesy of KARL STORZ GmbH & Co. KG.)

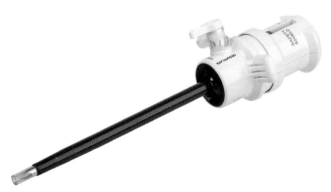

Figure 4-18 Disposable bladeless cannula with a safety shield.

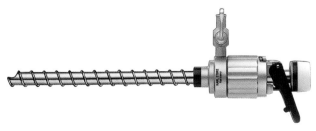

Figure 4-21 A Ternamian (i.e., threaded) EndoTIP stainless steel reusable cannula. (© 2014 Photo courtesy of KARL STORZ GmbH & Co. KG.)

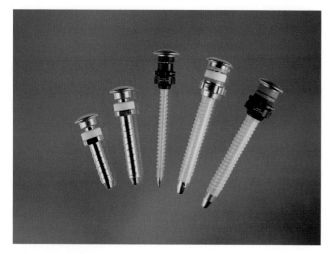

Figure 4-22 Multiple types of plastic re-usable thoracic ports. (© 2014 Photo courtesy of KARL STORZ GmbH & Co. KG.)

grade 3 complications (pneumothorax).[15] Insertion of the Veress needle and primary trocar for initial entry remains the most hazardous part of laparoscopy, accounting for 40% of all laparoscopic complications and the majority of the fatalities.[16] Despite decades of research and development to find safer methods for initial laparoscopic entry, major vessel injuries have been reported using virtually all types of trocar insertion methods. The overall morbidity and mortality rates related to laparoscopic access are low. The life-threatening complications include injury to the bowel, bladder, and major abdominal vessels. A recent Cochrane review included 17 randomized controlled trials concerning 3040 individuals undergoing laparoscopy. Overall, there was no evidence of advantage using any single abdominal access technique in terms of preventing major complications.[17]

Vascular Injury

Vascular injury can occur regardless of the method of access, and most vascular injuries (up to 80%) occur at the initial access. Recent studies have suggested that the incidence of major vascular injury is slightly higher with the closed technique (Veress and direct trocar insertion) as opposed to the open (Hasson) technique. Molloy *et al.*[4] suggests that the open technique decreased the rate of vascular injury to 0.01% compared with a rate of 0.04% associated with closed techniques using a Veress needle. Although the incidence of major vascular injuries is low, the mortality rate arising from these lesions reportedly ranges between 8% and 17%. Vessel

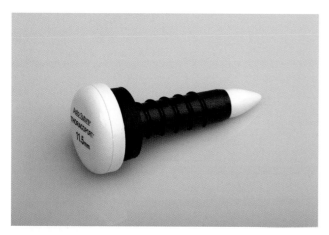

Figure 4-23 Reusable Thoracoport. (Photo courtesy of Dr. Philipp Mayhew.)

injuries attributable to trocars are usually more obvious and catastrophic than injuries related to Veress needle insertion. An expanding retroperitoneal hematoma, hemodynamic instability in the face of active bleeding, and active intraabdominal hemorrhage that cannot be managed laparoscopically are all indications for conversion to laparotomy and exploration or vascular repair.

Visceral Injury

Although studies have suggested that the open technique of initial trocar placement may be associated with a lower incidence of major vascular injuries, the same cannot be said for visceral injuries.[13] The incidence of this complication is about 0.05% of all open access procedures.[18] The main difference between bowel injuries occurring during the open technique compared with the closed technique is that with the open procedure, it is more likely that the injury will be immediately obvious and repaired without delay. Veress needle injuries to the large and small bowel may be associated with a higher incidence of peritonitis and other complications than injuries to the stomach, which can often be managed conservatively.

References

1 Rawlings, C.A. (2011) Laparoscopy. In: Tams, T.R., Rawlings, C.A. (eds.) Small Animal Endoscopy, 3rd edn. Elsevier Mosby, St. Louis.

2 Herati, A.S., Atalla, M.A., Rais-Bahrami, S., Andonian, S., Vira, M.A., Kavoussi, L.R. (2009) A new valve-less trocar for urologic laparoscopy: initial evaluation. J Endourol 23 (9), 1535-1539.

3 Laparoscopic MD. (n.d.) Laparoscopic trocars. [8/5/2014]; Available from: http://www.laparoscopic.md/instruments/trocar

4 Molloy, D., Kaloo, P.D., Cooper, M., Nguyen, T.V. (2002) Laparoscopic entry: a literature review and analysis of techniques and complications of primary port entry. Aust N Z J Obstet Gynaecol 42 (3), 246-254.

5 Teoh, B., Sen, R., Abbott, J. (2005) An evaluation of four tests used to ascertain Veress needle placement at closed laparoscopy. J Minim Invasive Gynecol 12 (2), 153-158.

6 Vilos, G.A., Ternamian, A., Dempster, J., Laberge, P.Y., The Society of Obstetricians and Gynaecologists of Canada. (2007) Laparoscopic entry: a review of techniques, technologies, and complications. J Obstet Gynaecol Can 29 (5), 433-465.

7 Whittemore, J.C., Mitchell, A., Hyink, S., Reed, A. (2013) Diagnostic accuracy of tissue impedance measurement interpretation for correct Veress needle placement in canine cadavers. Vet Surg 42 (5), 613-622.

8 Hyink, S., Whittemore, J.C., Mitchell, A., Reed, A. (2013) Diagnostic accuracy of tissue impedance measurement interpretation for correct Veress needle placement in feline cadavers. Vet Surg 42 (5), 623-638.

9 Mlyncek, M., Truska, A., Garay, J. (1994) Laparoscopy without use of the Veress needle: results in a series of 1,600 procedures. Mayo Clin Proc 69 (12), 1146-1148.

10 Woolcott, R. (1997) The safety of laparoscopy performed by direct trocar insertion and carbon dioxide insufflation under vision. Aust N Z J Obstet Gynaecol 37 (2), 216-219.

11 Hasson, H.M. (1971) A modified instrument and method for laparoscopy. Am J Obstet Gynecol. 110 (6), 886-887.

12 Giannios, N.M., Gulani, V., Rohlck, K., Flyckt, R.L., Weil, S.J., Hurd, W.W. (2009) Left upper quadrant laparoscopic placement: effects of insertion angle and body mass index on distance to posterior peritoneum by magnetic resonance imaging. Am J Obstet Gynecol. 201 (5), 522 e1-5.

13 Gould, J.C., Philip, A. (2011) Principles and techniques of abdominal access and physiology of pneumoperitoneum. In: ACS Surgery: Principles and Practice. PA Decker Intellectual Properties, Philadelphia.

14 Surgeons SfL. (2010) Prevention and Management of Laparoendoscopic Surgical Complications: Laparoscopic Trocar complications. [cited 2014 March]; Available from: http://laparoscopy.blogs.com/prevention_management_3/2010/11/laparoscopic-trocar-complications.html

15 Fiorbianco, V., Skalicky, M., Doerner, J., Findik, M., Dupre, G. (2012) Right intercostal insertion of a Veress needle for laparoscopy in dogs. Vet Surg 41 (3), 367-373.

16 Fuller, J., Ashar, B.S., Carey-Corrado, J. (2005) Trocar-associated injuries and fatalities: an analysis of 1399 reports to the FDA. J Minim Invasive Gynecol 12 (4), 302-307.

17 Ahmad, G., Duffy, J.M., Phillips, K., Watson, A. (2008) Laparoscopic entry techniques. Cochrane Database Syst Rev (2), CD006583.

18 McMahon, A.J., Baxter, J.N., O'Dwyer, P.J. (1993) Preventing complications of laparoscopy. Br J Surg 80 (12), 1593-1594.

4.3 Miscellaneous Surgical Instrumentation

Jessica K. Baron and Jeffrey J. Runge

Key Points
- Specimen retrieval bags allow for extraction of tissue with reduced risk of spilling and port contamination.
- Single-use integrated suction and irrigation devices are commercially available, but separate and resterilizable options are also available.
- Wound protector and retractor devices are very useful for increased surgical exposure and port protection.

Specimen Retrieval Bags

Numerous tissue extraction devices are available for laparoscopy and thoracoscopy, and many of these are pouchlike and preloaded within a delivery system (Figure 4-24). They are typically made from strong synthetic materials, which can withstand aggressive handling, and have a low incidence of tearing or rupture, which prevents escape of the removed tissue. Before development of retrieval bags, surgeons were required to remove diseased or contaminated tissue through unprotected port sites and mini incisions. The use of a retrieval bag allows extraction of tissue confined within a durable closed pouch, thus reducing the risk of content spillage during extraction. Retrieval bags also prevent contamination of the port or incision site from infected or malignant tissue.[1-4] Examples of homemade cost-effective specimen retrieval bags include fingers of powderless latex gloves, zip-close bags, and condoms[1,2,4] (Figure 4-25A and 4-25B). Most commercially available specimen retrieval bags require 10- to 12-mm cannulas for introduction into the body cavity, but small retrieval bags used with 5-mm cannulas are also available. Typically, the opening of commercially available bags have a rigid expandable rim (Figure 4-24C), which greatly facilitates tissue insertion into the bag. Many of the commercially available bags are deployed from a hollow instrument shaft[1,2,4] (Video Clip 4-1).

For proper removal of a retrieval bag from a body cavity, it is paramount that the tissue to be extracted has settled to the bottom of the bag. Lifting the bag and allowing the specimen to fall to the bottom can accomplish this but at times may not be sufficient. Alternatively, the tissue can be pushed with a grasper to the bottom of the bag. Some commercially available products allow for intracorporeal bag closure using an embedded purse string (see Figure 4-24B). The opening of the bag is then guided to the desired exit site (typically a cannula). When the opening of the bag is inside the cannula, the bag and cannula can be pulled from the site together. Smaller bags with less tissue can at time be removed through a larger cannula (12 mm). Bags filled with tissue can be slowly pulled through the incision after the cannula is removed, often without the need to extend the size of the incision. Homemade retrieval bags are often somewhat fragile, and one should be cautious to not tear these bags during extraction from the abdomen.[1,2,4] For larger specimens that cannot fit through the cannula site, either manual or power tissue morcellation or enlargement of the port incision may be performed to facilitate bag and specimen removal. Manual morcellation can be achieved by bringing the bag opening to the enlarged cannula incision and inserting a blunt instrument, such as ring forceps, which is used to disrupt the contained structure. Firmer tissue can be clamped, partially exposed, and circumferentially cored with a scalpel. With manual morcellation, one has to take precaution to not disrupt the integrity of the bag or to contaminate the cannula site. Fluid-filled structures, such as an excised gallbladder, can have their contents removed or aspirated while inside a bag to facilitate extraction. Importantly, one should not attempt to deliberately force or overzealously pull a retrieval bag through a small incision. If there are any concerns about feasibility of extraction, the incision should be extended to enable safe removal of bag and contents.

Small Animal Laparoscopy and Thoracoscopy, First Edition. Edited by Boel A. Fransson and Philipp D. Mayhew.
© 2015 by ACVS Foundation. Published 2015 by John Wiley & Sons, Inc.
Companion website: www.wiley.com/go/fransson/laparoscopy

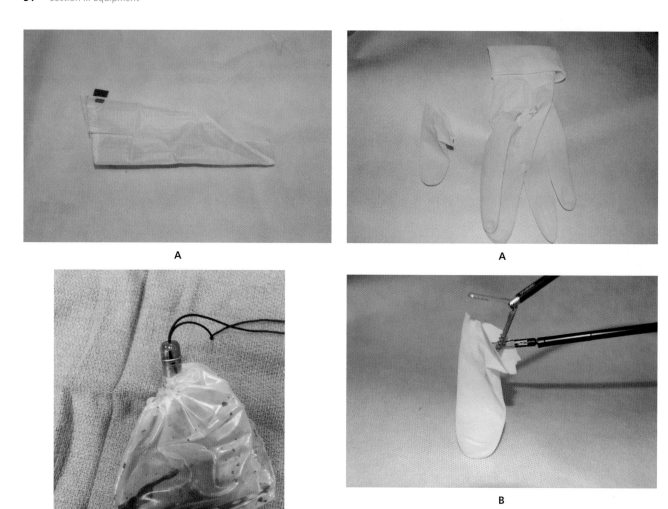

A

B

C

Figure 4-24 **A.** Homemade retrieval bags are cost effective. **B.** Commercially available retrieval bags have a purse string that closes the bag before exteriorizing it through a port site. **C.** Commercially available retrieval bags have a rigid rim that maintains a large opening of the bag, greatly facilitating insertion of tissue.

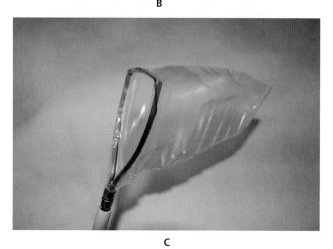

A

B

Figure 4-25 **A.** A homemade retrieval bag for small lesions can be made out of a surgical glove. **B.** Whereas a homemade retrieval bag requires a grasper to hold on to the bag, commercial bags often include a delivery system.

Suction and Irrigation Devices:

Suction and irrigation devices (Figure 4-26) are commonly used in both human and veterinary thoracoscopy and laparoscopy. Typically, suction and irrigation systems are combined into one device, but they can also be separate units; either type is available as disposable or resterilizable alternatives. The irrigation systems can be powered by a variety of mechanisms, including a pressure bag, compressed air pump, roller pump systems, or electrical motor system.[1-3] The irrigation function is typically used for lavage of debris and tissue, but a high-pressure water jet has also been used for hydrodissection.[1,2] Manufacturers provide a variety of suction tips, including single fenestration tips for more focal aspiration and multiple fenestration tips for aspiration of large fluid volumes (Video Clip 4-2). Aspiration of fluid and blood is important for visualization because blood can absorb light, leading to decreased overall laparoscopic illumination. However, the use of suction may affect visualization by loss of pneumoperitoneum if used excessively during laparoscopy.[1,2] To reduce this risk, a smaller probe, such as a 5-mm instrument should be used and the suction used only when the probe is inserted into the fluid to be aspirated.[1,2]

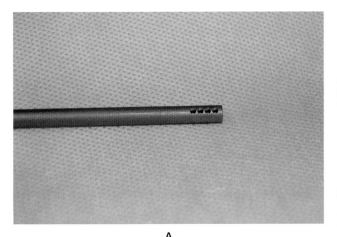

A

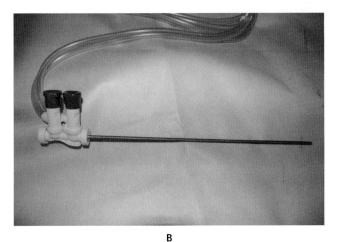

B

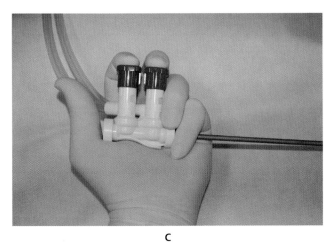

C

Figure 4-26 **A.** A suction irrigation device has many fenestrations in the tip for effective suctioning. **B.** Commercial units are surprisingly cost effective and include a pump, tubing, and a handpiece for regulation of suction and irrigation actions. **C.** Use of irrigation and suction.

Wound Protector and Retractor Devices:

Wound retraction devices (Figures 4-27 and 4-28) increase surgical exposure through reduced incision length while enabling a surgeon to insert at least one finger into the abdomen, allowing palpation with tactile sensation during exploration.[7] These retractors are available in

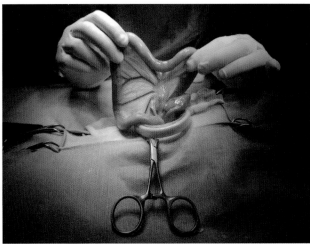

Figure 4-27 Use of a wound retractor in abdominal minimally invasive surgery.

a variety of size, corresponding to incision lengths from 2.5 to 25 cm, of which the smallest size is most frequently used in small animal MIS. Reports suggest that use of wound retraction devices significantly decreases the occurrence of surgical site infection in patients undergoing major intestinal surgery.[9,10] A wound retractor provides both a protective surgical wound barrier and 360-degree wound edge retraction. Its use in thoracic and abdominal surgeries has been well described in humans and has recently also been applied to companion animal surgery, including hand-assisted MIS (Figures 4-29 to 4-31). Previous studies have reported the use of a wound retractor in intestinal MIS, including resection and anastomosis in dogs and cats,[8] as well as in abdominal exploration and intestinal biopsy in cats.[11] More recently, its use was reported for thoracoscopic-assisted pulmonary surgery.[12] Benefits of using a wound retraction device include atraumatic circumferential wound retraction, direct barrier protection of the body wall and skin against contamination by intestinal bacteria and neoplastic cells, and improved extracorporeal intestine exposure without compromising vascular supply.[7,9,10]

Wound retractor placement is achieved by compressing the inner ring (internal ring) between the thumb and index finger creating

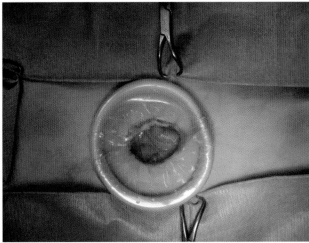

Figure 4-28 A wound retractor applies centrifugal force on the incision, greatly facilitating exteriorizing of intestines.

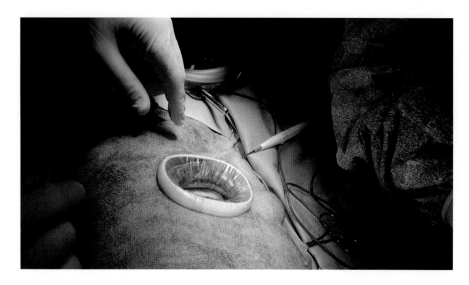

Figure 4-29 Wound retractor in the chest.

 an oval (Video Clip 4-3). The compressed ring is inserted into the incision until the entire ring is positioned within the cavity and compression released. A finger is used to palpate the inner ring's position within the cavity to ensure there is no entrapment of viscera. External traction is then applied to the outer ring (external ring) by the surgeon and assistant. The outer ring (external ring) is then rolled outward (similar to rolling down a tube sock), causing a shortening of the polyurethane sleeve relative to its original position. This rolling is completed when the outer ring (external ring) is in contact with patient's body wall, entrapping the body wall snugly between the inner (internal) and outer (external) rings (see Figure 4-31).

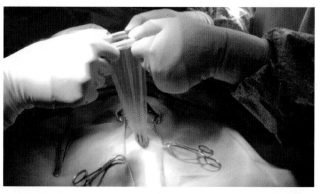

A

Morcellators

Morcellation entails division of bulky tissue into smaller pieces (typically strips), enabling extraction through a laparoscopic port or mini incision. Electromechanical morcellators (Figure 4-32)

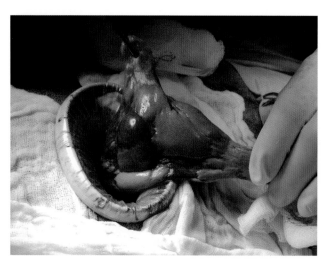

Figure 4-30 The wound retractor facilitates exteriorizing of organs while protecting the wound edges.

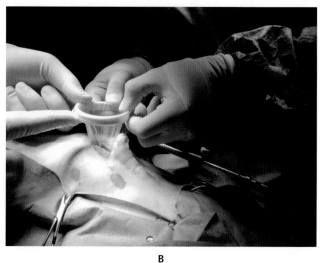

B

Figure 4-31 **A.** Application of a wound retractor. With the flexible ring positioned inside the body cavity, ventral tension is applied, and the stiffer ring is "rolled" in a dorsal direction, thus rolling the softer material and shortening the length of the retractor. **B.** With shortening of the retractor, 360-degree outward retraction force is applied to the edges of the incision.

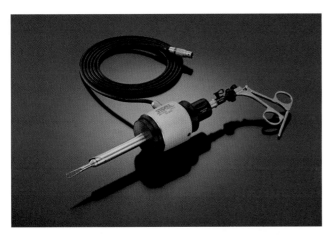

Figure 4-32 A morcellator. (©2014 Photo courtesy of KARL STORZ GmbH & Co. KG.)

are commercially available and commonly used in human laparoscopy for tissue extraction. Morcellators are considered to reduce operative time and decrease the risk of incision site hernia formation.[4] In humans, morcellation is most commonly performed during laparoscopic hysterectomies, myomectomies, and splenectomies.[1,2,4] Mechanical morcellators works through application of a sharp cylindrical blade to the specimen, which converts tissue into smaller strips that are exteriorized though a hollow tube or shaft inserted in a cannula.[1,2,4] Typically, forceps are used to grasp the tissue through the hollow tube; the tissue is then pulled externally toward the oscillating blade. This technique can also be used within a specimen retrieval bag, which may help prevent spillage of cells within a body cavity. Risks associated with use of power morcellation include iatrogenic tissue damage, seeding of cancerous tissues, and decreased ability to perform histopathologic cancer staging.[4-6] Recently, the Food and Drug Administration issued a recommendation to not use power morcellation in patients with suspected or confirmed cancer because of the risk for tumor cell seeding. A recent systematic review of laparoscopic morcellator-related complications underscored the need for surgeons' safe practices associated with its use.[5]

 All videos cited in this chapter can be found on the book's companion website at **www.wiley.com/go/fransson/ laparoscopy**

References

1 Mishra, R.K. (2013) Textbook of Practical Laparoscopic Surgery, 3rd edn. Jaypee Brothers Medical Publishers, New Delhi.

2 Palanivelu, C. (2007) Instrumentation and imaging system in laparoscopy. In: Parthasarathi, R (ed.) Art of Laparoscopic Surgery Textbook and Atlas, 1st edn. Jaypee Brothers Medical Publishers, New Delhi, pp 11-34.

3 Mencaglia, L., Minelli, L., Wattiez, A. (2013) Manual of Gynecological Laparoscopic Surgery, 11th edn. Endo Press, Tuttlingen, Germany.

4 Amer, N., Amer, M., Mishra, R.K. (2013) Different techniques of tissue retrieval from abdominal cavity during minimal access surgery. World J Lap Surg 6 (2), 63-68.

5 Milad, M.P., Milad, E.A. (2014) Laparoscopic morcellator-related complications. J Minim Invasive Gynecol 21 (3), 486-491.

6 Seidman, M.A., Oduyebo, T., Muto, M.G., Crum, C.P., Nucci, M.R., Quade, B.J. (2012) Peritoneal dissemination complicating morcellation of uterine mesenchymal neoplasms. PLoS One 7, e50058

7 Mayhew, P.D. (2009) Techniques for laparoscopic and laparoscopic-assisted biopsy of abdominal organs. Compend Contin Educ Pract Vet 31 (4), 170-176.

8 Gower, S.B., Mayhew, P.D. (2011) A wound retraction device for laparoscopic-assisted intestinal surgery in dogs and cats. Vet Surg 40 (4), 485-488.

9 Horiuchi, T., Tanishima, H., Tamagawa, K., et al. (2007) Randomized, controlled investigation of the anti-infective properties of the Alexis retractor/protector of incision sites. J Trauma 62 (2), 212-215.

10 Cheng, K.P., Roslani, A.C., Sehha, N., et al. (2012) Alexis O-Ring wound retractor vs conventional wound protection for the prevention of surgical site infections in colorectal resections. Colorectal Dis 14 (6), 346-351.

11 Baron, J.K., Giuffrida, M.A., Mayhew, P.D., Mayhew, K.N., Culp, W.T.N., Wormser, C., Holt, D.E., Singhal, S., Runge, J.J. (2014) Initial experience and clinical outcome of thoracoscopic assisted pulmonary surgery (TAPS) for complete and partial lung lobectomy in dogs and cats: 11 cases (2008-2013). In: Proceedings of the Veterinary Endoscopy Society Symposium, Florence, Italy, May 15-17.

12 Runge, J.J. (2014) Evaluation of minimally invasive abdominal exploration and intestinal biopsies. (MIAEB) using a Novel would retraction device in cats: 31 cases (2005-2013). In: Proceedings of the American College of Veterinary Surgeons Surgical Symposium, San Diego.

5 Energy Devices and Stapling Equipment

Sarah Marvel and Eric Monnet

Key Points

- A basic understanding of electrosurgical devices is required to allow for appropriate use and prevention of morbidity relating to their use.
- Three different type of coupling injuries can occur with monopolar devices: direct, indirect, and capacitive coupling.
- Indirect coupling results from defects in the insulating coating of the electrode (instrument), often leads to large current densities concentrated in small areas, and can result in high-morbidity injuries.
- Tissue fusion technology or vessel sealant devices measure tissue impedance and deliver the appropriate amount of energy to achieve a safe seal. They are approved for sealing vessels up to 7 mm in diameter.

Meticulous hemostasis, one of Halsted's seven principles, is important for any surgery but particularly for minimally invasive procedures in which a small amount of hemorrhage can compromise visualization. Numerous devices are available for hemostasis with laparoscopy and thoracoscopy, including hemostatic clips, endostapling equipment, and energy devices.

Energy has been used in surgery for thousands of years. The first form of energy used in surgery was thermal cautery, or the application of energy as heat to tissues. Although this was invaluable for controlling hemorrhage, lateral thermal damage to normal tissues was extensive. This technology evolved as William T. Bovie developed the first electrosurgical unit (ESU) that provided both cutting and coagulation settings. Rather than electrocautery, which relies on the transfer of heat directly to tissues, this new technology created an electrical current that was applied to the tissues and in turn created heat. Almost 100 years later, we are still using monopolar and bipolar electrosurgical devices similar to the "Bovie," but advances in technology have created safer units with more consistent tissue effects. More recently, vessel sealant technology has gained popularity in minimally invasive procedures. These bipolar electrosurgical devices have been used in numerous types of minimally invasive procedures, including surgeries of the reproductive tract, splenectomies, adrenalectomies, nephrectomies, lung biopsies, and pericardial surgery.

All surgeons should have a basic understanding of electrosurgical devices to allow for appropriate use of this equipment and to prevent unnecessary injury related to their use. Energy devices have their advantages and disadvantages for a given procedure, and it is up to the surgeon to understand the shortcomings of a particular device and decide which is most appropriate for a given situation.

Electrosurgical Theory

Electricity is the movement or flow of electrically charged particles from one electrode to another. Electrosurgery tools apply an electrical current to tissue, enabling cutting, coagulating, desiccating, or fulgurating by generating heat. There are three properties of electricity that affect the rise in temperature of the tissue: voltage, current, and resistance or impedance. The interaction of these three properties is explained by Ohm's law, which describes the flow of electricity along a circuit:

Voltage (V) = Current (I) × Resistance (R)

Whereas current is a measure of electron movement through tissue in a given time, voltage is the driving force that moves the electrons against the tissue resistance or impedance within the circuit. Tissue resistance or impedance is a function of both the composition of the tissues and blood supply. As voltage drives electrons through the circuit against impedance, heat is generated. This tissue resistance or impedance produces heat rather than the active electrode. Therefore, tissues with greater impedance will result in the generation of more heat. Tissue impedance constantly changes as an electrical

---

Small Animal Laparoscopy and Thoracoscopy, First Edition. Edited by Boel A. Fransson and Philipp D. Mayhew.
© 2015 by ACVS Foundation. Published 2015 by John Wiley & Sons, Inc.
Companion website: www.wiley.com/go/fransson/laparoscopy

Table 5-1 Tissue Effect in Relation to Temperature

Temperature (°C)	Tissue Effect
250	Tissue carbonized from dehydration
100	Cell wall rupture
90	Tissue desiccation
70	Protein denaturing
50	Enzymatic activity inactivated
40	Inflammation and edema

Modified from Dubiel, B., Shires, P.K., Korvick, D., Chekan, E.G. (2010) Electromagnetic energy sources in surgery. Vet Surg 39 (8), 910.

current is applied and the tissues become desiccated. The degree of heat leads to varying tissue effects (Table 5-1).

Another important concept in understanding electrosurgery is the concept of power. Power is a measure of work per unit time. It is a function of voltage and current and is measured in watts. Power tells you the rate at which the energy works. Power rises exponentially with increases in voltage and decreases inversely with increases in resistance or impedance. However, voltage is the main determinant of tissue effect and is a function of the waveform that the generator delivers (see waveform section below).

An ESU is composed of four basic components: a generator, an active electrode, the patient, and the return electrode. The ESU uses low-frequency alternating current (AC) from a wall outlet and converts it to a higher voltage radiofrequency (RF) output. The current can be used to induce diathermy but also stimulates muscle and nerve cells. Stimulation of muscle and nerve cells can lead to pain, muscle spasm, and even cardiac arrest. The sensitivity of nerves and muscles cells to electrical stimulation decreases and the excitability threshold increases with increasing frequency, meaning that nerve and muscle cell stimulation is refractory to electrical stimulation above 100 kHz.[1] Therefore, electrosurgical devices use frequencies in the range of 350 to 500 kHz. This range is referred to as the medium RF electromagnetic spectrum (Figure 5-1).

Waveforms

There are three basic types of waveforms generated in electrosurgery: cutting waveform, coagulation waveform, and blended waveforms (Figure 5-2). Cutting waveforms are continuous waveforms, and coagulation and blend are intermittent waveforms.

The continuous cutting waveform uses less peak voltage at a similar power setting to the intermittent waveform, resulting in less lateral thermal tissue damage. With pure cut, the amplitude of the continuous waveform is the same. This induces a localized effect on

the tissues, creating high tissue temperatures (>100°C), vaporization of the interstitial fluid, and tissue separation with little hemostasis. Heat is absorbed by water released from the cells, which minimizes thermal damage and provides minimal coagulation. Power settings for the cut waveform are often between 50 and 80 W.[2]

The intermittent waveform of the coagulation waveform produces a high current density delivered in pulses. This waveform has higher voltage than the continuous waveforms and delivers the electrical charge deeper into the tissues. The pauses between the pulses lead to decreased tissue heating, resulting in coagulation rather than cutting. Coagulation is achieved with a power setting between 30 and 50 W.[2] Coagulation can either be performed using desiccation or fulguration. Whereas fulguration uses a noncontact technique to control diffuse hemorrhage, desiccation is a contact technique used for local bleeding. Fulguration uses an intermittent waveform, which allows for proteins to melt and recongeal, forming a coagulum. Some ESUs also contain a spray mode, which is useful for oozing capillary beds. Spray mode does not penetrate as deeply into tissues and can be used in more delicate tissues. Desiccation or a contact technique leads to less heat production than fulguration. A coagulum is formed by tissues drying out and proteins melting.

A blended waveform results in simultaneous coagulation and cutting. Whereas blend 1 is more effective at cutting with minimal hemostasis, blend 3 results in better hemostasis and decreased cutting (see Figure 5-2). Many surgeons prefer to use the blend waveform because it provides a trade-off between thermal tissue damage and hemostasis.

Despite its name, the cutting waveform can be used for coagulation, and in some scenarios, it is recommended over the coagulation waveform. An example is when applying electrosurgery to the hemostat or forceps in what is referred to as *coaptive coagulation*. In this scenario, cutting energy is recommended because this produces deeper hemostasis and less thermal spread compared with coagulation energy. Coagulation results in rapid increase in impedance from char at the electrode. As impedance increases, more power is needed to penetrate deeper tissues. Instead, cutting energy heats up the tissue more quickly, minimizing char accumulation and allowing energy to penetrate deeper into the target tissues. With coaptive coagulation, the flattened vessel wall becomes fused as the current is applied to the instrument. Heat denatures the outer vessel wall and dehydrates the vessel, halting blood flow.

Monopolar Electrosurgery

The monopolar system is the most commonly used electrosurgical device. It consists of a generator; an electrosurgical pencil

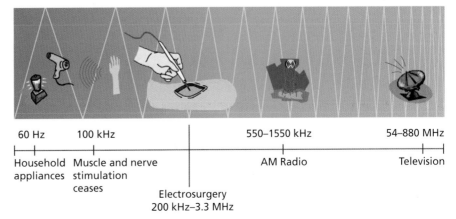

Figure 5-1 Most electrosurgery units operate within the medium radiofrequency electromagnetic spectrum. Some units operate at a higher radiofrequency (3–4 MHz) and are referred to as radio wave radiosurgery. (From Huhn, J.C. (2011) Stapling and energy devices for endoscopic surgery. In: Tams, T.R., Rawlings, C.A. (eds.) Small Animal Endoscopy, 3rd ed, Elsevier, St. Louis, p. 365.)

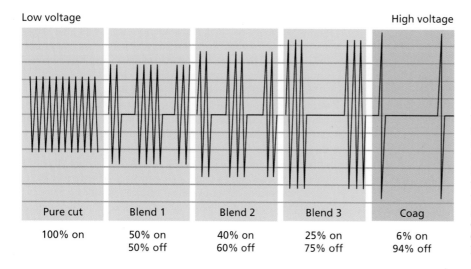

Figure 5-2 Pure cut is a continuous low-voltage waveform. Coagulation waveform is a high-voltage intermittent waveform that allows for cooling between energy pulses. Blended waveforms provide a continuum of intermittent waveforms of varying voltages, which allows for a tissue effect more geared toward cutting or coagulation. (From Huhn, J.C. (2011) Stapling and energy devices for endoscopic surgery. In: Tams, T.R., Rawlings, C.A. (eds.) Small Animal Endoscopy, 3rd ed, Elsevier, St. Louis, p. 366.)

(active electrode); and a return electrode, which is the grounding pad (passive electrode). The generator directs a current through the electrosurgical pencil, which contains the active electrode. The current then passes to the tissue through the patient's body to the grounding pad and back to the generator (Figure 5-3). The tissue effect is determined by the power setting, waveform, technique (contact, noncontact, and time), and electrode configuration. The passive electrode should maintain a wide contact area to minimize the chance of concentrating the current and patient burning. Previous rigid metal plates were associated with increased burns because of rigidity, which often led to decreased contact with the plate to the patient. Newer electrosurgery generators also come with return electrode monitoring (REM) in which a generator will cease operation if the return signal is outside programmed limits.

Monopolar electrosurgery provides hemostasis for vessels smaller than 2 mm in diameter, and collateral damage can occur up to 2 cm from the coagulation site.[3,4]

A multitude of electrodes are available for the electrosurgical pencil, with three basic shapes: needle tip, spatula, and J-hooks. The use of insulated electrode extensions has become popular for endoscopic surgery. These extensions enable the use of the standard electrosurgical pencil in endoscopic surgery (Figure 5-4). An L- or J-hook electrode is very commonly used during minimally invasive surgery (MIS) for dissection. These electrodes allow dissection of

tissue by hooking in the tip while the ESU is activated. This technique is used frequently during cholecystectomy. With the advent of the Triverse handpiece (Valley Lab, Boulder, CO), the surgeon can adjust the power level with the handpiece rather than relying on an assistant to adjust the power at the generator (Figure 5-5). Monopolar electrodes are available in a device that also allows for irrigation and suction at the surgical site. With the irrigation and suction present, the surgical field can be kept clean, and more precise and efficient dissection can be performed with the monopolar cautery tip. An insulated endoscopic instrument can be connected to an ESU and used as a monopolar electrosurgery device. Endoscopic grasping forceps may then be used to provide hemostasis. Insulated endoscopic scissors can also be used. A foot pedal is used to activate the electrocautery unit when the scissors are cutting tissue. Hand-activated switches are also available.

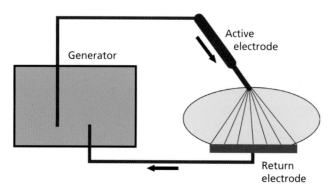

Figure 5-3 Alternating current flows from the generator to the handpiece. Electrical current then flows from the electrode (handpiece) to the patient and then to the return electrode. (From Taheri, A., Mansoori, P., Sandoval, L.F., Feldman, S.R., Pearce, D., Williford, P.M. (2014) Electrosurgery: part I. Basics and principles. J Am Acad Dermatol 70 (4), 591.)

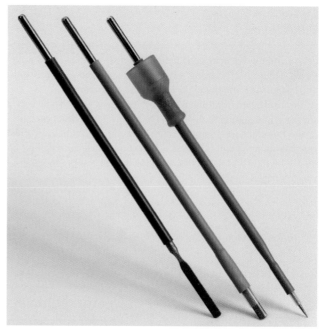

Figure 5-4 Electrode extensions are available in various tip configurations. (From Huhn, J.C. (2011) Stapling and energy devices for endoscopic surgery. In: Tams, T.R., Rawlings, C.A. (eds.) Small Animal Endoscopy, 3rd ed, Elsevier, St. Louis, p. 368.)

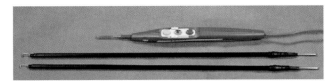

Figure 5-5 Both J- and L-shaped extensions are available for use with monopolar electrosurgery. Their extended lengths make them ideal for use in minimally invasive surgery. Also pictured is Valley Lab's Triverse handpiece, which has a sliding switch to allow for adjustment of power delivery at the handpiece in addition to the generator. (From Huhn, J.C. (2011) Stapling and energy devices for endoscopic surgery. In: Tams, T.R., Rawlings, C.A. (eds.) Small Animal Endoscopy, 3rd ed, Elsevier, St. Louis, p. 368.)

Safety of Monopolar Electrosurgery

Approximately 40,000 human patients sustain electrosurgical-related injuries each year. Up to 70% of electrosurgical burns go undetected at the time of laparoscopic surgery, often because the active electrode is outside of the surgeons field of view.[5] Three different types of coupling injuries can occur: direct coupling, indirect coupling, and capacitive coupling.[2,6-8] *Direct coupling* is the result of an electrically conductive object in close proximity to the target tissue. It occurs when the active electrode is activated before contact with the tissues resulting in energy transmission to the unwanted electrically conductive object, which can manifest as a burn (Figure 5-6). *Indirect coupling* results from a discontinuity in the insulating coating of the active electrode. If this occurs, current is drawn toward a neighboring electrically conductive object. Because of the lack of output on the target tissue, power settings are often increased, intensifying the misdirected current (Figure 5-7). These insulation breaks are often small and not visible to the naked eye. These small breaks in insulation are dangerous because large current densities are concentrated at these small discontinuities in insulation. *Capacitive coupling* results from a build-up of current between two conducting substances that are separated by an insulating substance. When the charge exceeds the insulating capacity, it can spark across the insulator to the other conducting substance, resulting in thermal injury. Capacitive coupling injuries occur most often with the use of "hybrid" cannula systems, or those that use both conductive (metal) and insulating (plastic) materials. All metal cannulas are less

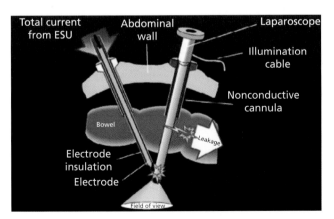

Figure 5-6 Direct coupling occurs when the active electrode is in close proximity to another metal instrument and activation of the electrosurgical device occurs, transmitting current to the metal instrument and ultimately the adjacent structures. ESU, electrosurgical unit. (From Dubiel, B., Shires, P.K., Korvick, D., Chekan, E.G. (2010) Electromagnetic energy sources in surgery. Vet Surg 39 (8), 913.)

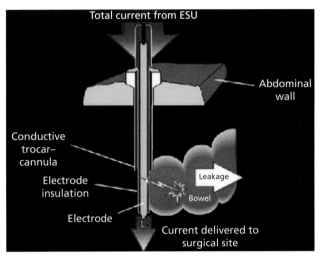

Figure 5-7 Indirect coupling or insulation failure occurs when there is damage to the insulation of the active electrode. This allows for stray current to be discharged and may result in injury to neighboring tissues. ESU, electrosurgical unit. (From Dubiel, B., Shires, P.K., Korvick, D., Chekan, E.G. (2010) Electromagnetic energy sources in surgery. Vet Surg 39 (8), 913.)

likely to result in this type of coupling injury because stray current is dispersed over a larger surface area. The extent of coupling injuries depends of the magnitude of the current applied.

Bipolar Electrosurgery

Bipolar electrosurgical devices differ from monopolar in that both the active and passive electrode are contained within the same electrosurgical device, meaning that the current does not pass through the patient. This achieves the desired hemostatic effect using less energy (30–50 W) while minimizing the risk to the patient as the current passes from one electrode to the tissue and then to the other electrode. Bipolar forceps requires more time to coagulate vessels and is more apt to stick to the vessel and carbonize tissues, which can lead to further hemorrhage upon removal. Bipolar forceps have minimal use in tissue dissection and are used for coagulation of tissue only and not cutting. Traditional bipolar electrosurgery devices use forceps with a foot pedal connected by a cord; thus, the current remains local. These traditional bipolar devices can coagulate vessels 3 mm or smaller in diameter.[9] Lateral thermal damage has been reported to occur up to 8 mm from the coagulation site.[10,11] Bipolar instruments used in MIS can coagulate and cut if a cutting blade is present in the instrument. Bipolar endoscopic scissors are available; however, these scissors may cut the tissue before sufficient coagulation. Additionally, the cutting blade on some instruments can push the tissue out of the jaws, which leads to incomplete cutting, and eventually these blades become dull. Bipolar endoscopic instruments are more expensive than monopolar instruments.

Tissue Fusion Device

Tissue fusion technology, or vessel sealant devices, are bipolar electrosurgery devices relying on tissue fusion for control of blood vessels and lymphatics. These devices measure tissue impedance and subsequently deliver the appropriate the amount of energy to achieve a safe seal. Vessel sealant devices have been approved for sealing vessels up to 7 mm in diameter.[12-14]

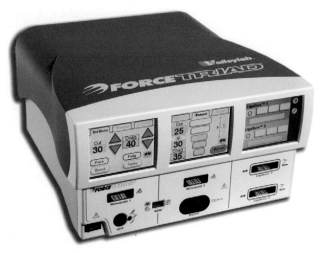

Figure 5-8 Valley Lab Force Triad generator, which combines monopolar, bipolar, and vessel sealant technology. It features three touchscreen modules. Handpieces are automatically recognized when they are plugged in. (From Huhn, J.C. (2011) Stapling and energy devices for endoscopic surgery. In: Tams, T.R., Rawlings, C.A. (eds.) Small Animal Endoscopy, 3rd ed, Elsevier, St. Louis, p. 370.)

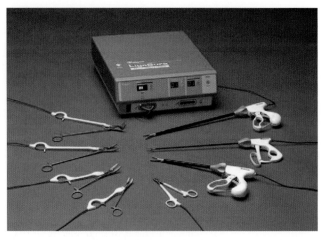

Figure 5-9 Valley Lab LigaSure generator with numerous bipolar handpieces for open and minimally invasive surgery. Some handpieces require foot-pedal activation; others are handswitch activated. (From Huhn, J.C. (2011) Stapling and energy devices for endoscopic surgery. In: Tams, T.R., Rawlings, C.A. (eds.) Small Animal Endoscopy, 3rd ed, Elsevier, St. Louis, p. 370.)

This system uses low voltage with high current. The generator senses tissue impedance (electrical resistance) and adjusts the energy to achieve hemostasis while minimizing heat and tissue carbonization (Figure 5-8). An acoustic signal is delivered to indicate that the sealing cycle has been completed. This system denatures elastin and collagen, and the strength of the seal is dependent on the ratio of elastin and collagen within the tissues.[15] The handpiece applies a certain amount of pressure on the tissue to fuse. This amount of pressure is characteristic of the device used. Vessel sealant devices can achieve hemostasis without dissection of the blood vessels. This is particularly valuable when blood vessels are surrounded by fat or other tissues (e.g., an ovarian pedicle). A 5-mm handpiece can also be used for blunt tissue dissection.

Bipolar vessel sealant devices have been used in several organ systems, including the reproductive tract, lung, liver, and other soft tissue structures.[16-19] There are numerous handpieces available for use in open surgery and MIS (Figure 5-9). Lateral thermal damage has been reported to occur between 1.5 and 6 mm from the coagulation site.[10,11,20] Bipolar vessel sealant technology has proven to be safe and effective for use in MIS with applications in numerous procedures, including reproductive surgery, adrenalectomy, splenectomy, nephrectomy, and pericardectomy. The resulting blood vessel seals have been tested to withstand pressure well above physiologic systolic pressures.[14,21] Although peripheral lung biopsies have been successfully obtained in experimental studies,[16] the variability of bronchus sealing makes this technique unreliable for larger biopsies.[22,23]

Ultrasonic Dissector

Ultrasound waves are sound waves with a frequency above the upper limit of human hearing (>20 kHz). Sound wave energy used in surgical devices typically occurs at frequencies of 23 to 55 kHz. Ultrasonic surgical devices are capable of cutting, desiccation, protein coagulation, and cavitation (hybrid form of vaporization facilitating dissection). The advantage of this form of energy is that no electrical circuit is required, which eliminates the risk of direct and indirect coupling injuries that may occur in laparoscopy, as well as neural stimulation, which can result in cardiac and respiratory arrest.

An ultrasonic generator delivers an alternating polarity electrical current that is modulated by the generator, directed through the transducer, and converted to sound energy. This conversion of current into sound energy occurs as the piezoelectric current is directed through a series of stacked ceramic plates within the transducer. The vibration of the ceramic plates at 55,500 times per second produces sound waves or *harmonic frequency,* which generates mechanical energy. Sound energy propagates down the shaft of the instrument to the tip, leading to axial displacement of the instrument tip. An increase in power on the generator leads to an increase in axial displacement of the instrument tip, leading to an increased cutting rate.

Ultrasonic energy devices generate minimal heat and therefore very little lateral thermal spread (<1.5 mm). Ultrasonic energy devices can seal vessels up to 3 mm in diameter. Table 5-2 lists various currently available ultrasonic dissectors as well as tissue fusion devices.

Table 5-2 Various Energy Devices and Their Capabilities

Energy Device (Manufacturer)	Monopolar	Bipolar	Tissue Sealing	Ultrasonic Dissector
Force Triad (Valley Lab, Boulder, CO)	✓	✓	✓	
Ethicon Endo-Surgery Generator (Ethicon, Cincinnati, OH)			✓	✓
Sonicision (Covidien, North Haven, CT)				✓
Altrus (Conmed, Utica NY)			✓	
Ultracision (Ethicon)				✓
Autosonix (Covidien North Haven, CT)				✓
Thunderbeat (Olympus, Center Valley, PA)			✓	✓

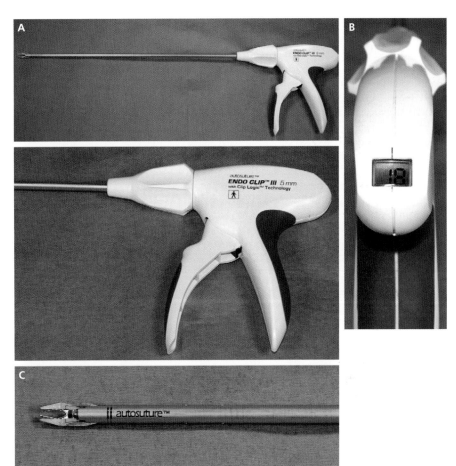

Figure 5-10 Endoclips come in different shaft diameters and clip sizes. They apply C-shaped clips that close from the tip first. (From Huhn, J.C. (2011) Stapling and energy devices for endoscopic surgery. In: Tams, T.R., Rawlings, C.A. (eds.) Small Animal Endoscopy, 3rd ed, Elsevier, St. Louis, p. 364.)

A recent study by Newcomb *et al.*[14] compared vessel sealing in a porcine model with electrosurgical and ultrasonic devices. They found that vessel sealant devices had the highest mean burst pressures compared with ultrasonic dissector. More seal failures were seen overall with the ultrasonic dissector than with the vessel sealant devices. However, for vessels 2 to 3 mm in diameter, the ultrasonic dissector did not have any seal failures, but the vessel sealant devices did. This study emphasizes that fact that ultrasonic dissectors consistently seal vessels less than 3 mm but perform inconsistently with larger vessel diameters.

Clips and Staple Applicators

Hemostatic clips have been adapted for endoscopic use. These are C-shaped clips, in which the tip of the clip closes first, preventing tissue from slipping out of the tip as the clip is closed. Endoclips (Covidien, New Haven, CT) are made in both a 5- and a 10-mm shaft diameter (Figure 5-10). The 10-mm clips have three sizes: medium, medium/large, and large. The 5-mm clip is available in medium/large sizes. Ethicon also manufactures hemostatic clips for endoscopic use (LigaMax; Ethicon Endo-Surgery, Blue Ash, OH), which are available in 5-, 10-, and 12-mm shaft diameters. Locking clip designs with the intent to provide superior clip stability are also available (Reflex ELC 530, Utica, NY). All devices have an indicator on the instrument that details the number of clips left in the device. Complications with clip application include placing too much tissue within the jaws of the clip and clip slippage. Impor-

tantly, clips should not be applied to tissue under tension because this can result in changes in diameter of the tissues and clip slippage when the tension is released.

Endoscopic staplers are commonly used in MIS. The most commonly used device is the Endo GIA stapler (Covidien), but the Endo TA (Covidien) stapler is also available. These are sold as multifire handpieces with disposable cartridges. The Endo GIA comes in three different lengths (30, 45, and 60 mm) and four different staple height sizes (2.0, 2.5, 3.5, and 4.8 mm) (Figure 5-11). This stapler fires six rows of staples and then cuts in between, leaving

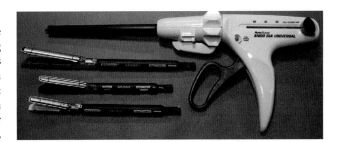

Figure 5-11 Endoscopic gastrointestinal anastomosis staplers have a 10-mm-diameter shaft that has three different length staplers with four different staple sizes. The largest staple leg length (4.8 mm, green) requires a 15-mm port because of the larger diameter of the stapler. (From Huhn, J.C. (2011) Stapling and energy devices for endoscopic surgery. In: Tams, T.R., Rawlings, C.A. (eds.) Small Animal Endoscopy, 3rd ed, Elsevier, St. Louis, p. 365.)

three rows of staples behind. The Endo TA stapler is available in a 30-mm length. It fires a triple staggered row of staples in either 2.5- or 3.5-mm leg length. These staples are composed of titanium and are B shaped when compressed, which allows for microvascular perfusion to the staple line, preventing necrosis, which could lead to delayed hemorrhage or leakage. The Endo GIA is also available reticulated, which allows a more precise placement of the cartridge of staples.

A study comparing two Endo GIA 30 vascular staple cartridges in a porcine model found both the 2.0- and the 2.5-mm staple height to be equivalent for hemostasis of large blood vessels (renal artery and vein, caudal vena cava, and aorta). Both achieved vessel sealing greater than 310 mm Hg and were able to seal arteries up to 17 mm and veins up to 22 mm.[24] Lansdowne et al.[25] reported thoracoscopic lung lobectomy in nine dogs. They recommended using the 3.5-mm staple height and longer staple cartridges because the 30-mm length alone often was not long enough to span the hilus of the lung lobe.

References

1 d'Arsonval, M.A. (1891) Action physiologique des courants alternatifs. CR Soc Biol 43, 283-286.

2 Wang, K., Advincula, A.P. (2007) "Current thoughts" in electrosurgery. Int J Gynaecol Obstet 97 (3), 245-250.

3 Hanrath, M., Rodgerson, D.H. (2002) Laparoscopic cryptorchidectomy using electrosurgical instrumentation in standing horses. Vet Surg 31 (2), 117-124.

4 Toombs, J.P., Crowe, D.T. (1985) Operative techniques. In: Slatter, D. (ed.) Textbook of Small Animal Surgery, 1st edn. WB Saunders, Philadelphia, pp 310-334.

5 Lee, J. (2002) Update on electrosurgery. Outpatient Surg 2 (2), 44-53.

6 Feldman, L.S., Fuchshuber, P.R., Jones, D.B. (2012) The SAGES Manual on the Fundamental Use of Surgical Energy (FUSE). Springer, New York.

7 Thompson, S.E., Potter, L. (1999) Electrosurgery, lasers, and ultrasonic energy. In: Freeman, L.J. (ed.) Veterinary Endosurgery. Mosby, St. Louis, pp. 61-72.

8 Massarweh, N.N., Cosgriff, N., Slakey, D.P. (2006) Electrosurgery: history, principles, and current and future uses. J Am Coll Surg 202 (3), 520-530.

9 Spivak, H., Richardson, W.S., Hunter, J.G. (1998) The use of bipolar cautery, laparosonic coagulating shears, and vascular clips for hemostasis of small and medium-sized vessels. Surg Endosc 12 (2), 183-185.

10 Phillips, C.K., Hruby, G.W., Durak, E., et al. (2008) Tissue response to surgical energy devices. Urology 71 (4), 744-748.

11 Hruby, G.W., Marruffo, F.C., Durak, E., et al. (2007) Evaluation of surgical energy devices for vessel sealing and peripheral energy spread in a porcine model. J Urol 178 (6), 2689-2693.

12 Carbonell, A.M., Joels, C.S., Kercher, K.W., Matthews, B.D., Sing, R.F., Heniford, B.T. (2003) A comparison of laparoscopic bipolar vessel sealing devices in the hemostasis of small-, medium-, and large-sized arteries. J Laparoendosc Adv Surg Tech A 13 (6), 3773-80.

13 Harold, K.L., Pollinger, H., Matthews, B.D., Kercher, K.W., Sing, R.F., Heniford, B.T. (2003) Comparison of ultrasonic energy, bipolar thermal energy, and vascular clips for the hemostasis of small-, medium-, and large-sized arteries. Surg Endosc 17 (8), 1228-1230.

14 Newcomb, W.L., Hope, W.W., Schmelzer, T.M., et al. (2009) Comparison of blood vessel sealing among new electrosurgical and ultrasonic devices. Surg Endosc 23 (1), 90-96.

15 Sindram, D., Martin, K., Meadows, J.P., et al. (2011) Collagen-elastin ratio predicts burst pressure of arterial seals created using a bipolar vessel sealing device in a porcine model. Surg Endosc 25 (8), 2604-2612.

16 Mayhew, P.D., Culp, W.T., Pascoe, P.J., Arzi, N.V. (2012) Use of the Ligasure vessel-sealing device for thoracoscopic peripheral lung biopsy in healthy dogs. Vet Surg 41 (4), 523-528.

17 Barrera, J.S., Monnet, E. (2012) Effectiveness of a bipolar vessel sealant device for sealing uterine horns and bodies from dogs. Am J Vet Res 73 (2), 302-305.

18 Risselada, M., Ellison, G.W., Bacon, N.J., et al. (2010) Comparison of 5 surgical techniques for partial liver lobectomy in the dog for intraoperative blood loss and surgical time. Vet Surg 39 (7), 856-862.

19 Brdecka, D.J., Rawlings, C.A., Perry, A.C., Anderson, J.R. (2008) Use of an electro-thermal, feedback-controlled, bipolar sealing device for resection of the elongated portion of the soft palate in dogs with obstructive upper airway disease. J Am Vet Med Assoc 233 (8), 1265-1269.

20 Landman, J., Kerbl, K., Rehman, J., et al. (2003) Evaluation of a vessel sealing system, bipolar electrosurgery, harmonic scalpel, titanium clips, endoscopic gastrointestinal anastomosis vascular staples and sutures for arterial and venous ligation in a porcine model. J Urol 169 (2), 697-700.

21 Lamberton, G.R., Hsi, R.S., Jin, D.H., Lindler, T.U., Jellison, F.C., Baldwin, DD. (2008) Prospective comparison of four laparoscopic vessel ligation devices. J Endourol 22 (10), 2307-2312.

22 Santini, M., Vicidomini, G., Baldi, A., et al. (2006) Use of an electrothermal bipolar tissue sealing system in lung surgery. Eur J Cardiothorac Surg 29 (2), 226-230.

23 Marvel, S., Monnet, E. (2013) Ex vivo evaluation of canine lung biopsy techniques. Vet Surg 42 (4), 473-477.

24 El-Hakim, A., Cai, Y., Marcovich, R., Pinto, P., Lee, B.R. (2004) Effect of Endo-GIA vascular staple size on laparoscopic vessel sealing in a porcine model. Surg Endosc 18 (6), 961-963.

25 Lansdowne, J.L., Monnet, E., Twedt, D.C., Dernell, W.S. (2005) Thoracoscopic lung lobectomy for treatment of lung tumors in dogs. Vet Surg 34 (5), 530-535.

6

Single-Incision Laparoscopic Surgery

Jeffrey J. Runge

Key Points

- Single-port surgery provides a natural progression to a less invasive approach compared with the multiport platform.
- Single-port surgery can be achieved using an operating laparoscope but is more commonly performed using a variety of commercially available single-port devices.
- Articulating instruments can be used to offset the limitations on triangulation that are inherent to the single-port approach although the use of rigid instrumentation is also possible.
- Single-port ovariectomy, gastropexy, intestinal biopsy, and cryptorchidectomy have been described in the veterinary literature, and many other procedures will be described using this approach in the future.

Surgery is forever evolving. As new evidence emerges on how to treat disease, the methods by which we apply this new knowledge to daily patient care are constantly refined. Within the past century, arguably one of the most important advancements to occur within surgery is the development of laparoscopy. This approach has completely revolutionized modern surgical practices, significantly changing the surgical way of thinking, operative techniques, and all other aspects of modern surgical care.[1] Laparoscopy gained acceptance among surgeons and patients alike because of its unquestionable advantages, which include smaller incisions, reduced postoperative pain, shorter hospital stays, and faster return to everyday living compared with the traditional open approach.[2] After the laparoscopic revolution occurred in humans during the 1980s, it was not long before diseases once commonly addressed through open surgery began to be performed by laparoscopic means. The tremendous advantages and benefits of laparoscopy witnessed in human health care impacted companion animal health as well, eventually changing the way many common operative procedures could be performed in veterinary surgery. To date, veterinary surgeons now have the ability to use a minimally invasive approach for almost every type of intrathoracic and intraabdominal procedure offered in canine and feline surgery.

Over the past decade, a second revolution in the field of laparoscopic surgery has occurred with striking technical advancements leading to the development of even less invasive operative procedures in both humans and animals. The journey to make minimally invasive techniques even less invasive has generated a drive within the surgical community to explore novel ways of achieving this paradigm.[3] New approaches to minimally invasive abdominal entry have included decreasing the overall number of trocar–cannula assemblies placed through the abdominal wall and attempting to eliminate them completely by using a natural orifice. These concepts have led to the birth of several new minimally invasive access platforms with the most notable being single-port surgery and natural orifice transluminal endoscopic surgery (NOTES). Because NOTES is still in its early experimental stages and continues to suffer from numerous hurdles preventing its broad implementation, single-port surgery has emerged as the more acceptable choice for most surgeons.[4] Unlike NOTES, single-port surgery remains within the comfort zone of most surgeons because the instrumentation and techniques are similar to those used in standard laparoscopy.[5]

Whereas conventional laparoscopy requires multiple, individually spaced incisions to accommodate ports ranging from 5 to 10 mm in length, the single-port platform differs from this by placing all instruments through one single (1.5–2 cm) incision into the abdomen. In humans, at present, procedures such as single-port cholecystectomy are gaining significant popularity, and with the aim of minimizing overall invasiveness, it is positioning itself to potentially replace conventional multiport

---

Small Animal Laparoscopy and Thoracoscopy, First Edition. Edited by Boel A. Fransson and Philipp D. Mayhew.
© 2015 by ACVS Foundation. Published 2015 by John Wiley & Sons, Inc.
Companion website: www.wiley.com/go/fransson/laparoscopy

laparoscopic cholecystectomy by achieving reduced postoperative pain and optimized cosmetic results compared with the multiport procedure.[6]

Development of a New Platform

The history of single-port surgery may date back to its early use in laparoscopic gynecologic surgery when Wheeless and Thompson described more than 1000 tubal ligations using a single puncture laparoscope with an offset eye piece.[7] However, purists within the contemporary single-port arena argue that operative laparoscopy differs significantly from modern day single-port surgery, and the origins of the single-port surgical revolution were developed more recently. The first use of separate instruments and ports through a single incision was initially described in 1997 by Navarra *et al.*, when they published their "one wound cholecystectomy" using two transumbilical trocars. At that time, single-port surgery seemed as if it was not ready to emerge as a viable access platform for the mainstream and even Navarra himself questioned the validity of that approach in terms of its safety, efficacy, and operative time.[8] It was not until 2007 when Curcillo revisited Navarra's work and described a stepwise approach for the reduction of port sites and consolidation of trocars, resulting in one umbilical incision for laparoscopic cholecystectomy named single-port access (SPA).[9] Since 2007, a massive emergence of single-port procedures has been successfully adapted to many common multiport laparoscopic abdominal procedures in both children and adults with the ultimate goal of reducing overall surgical invasiveness. The single-port platform evolved rapidly with the objectives of minimizing overall surgical trauma, reducing postoperative pain, shortening convalescence, and improving cosmesis.[9] In humans, it is speculated that the potential advantages that single-port surgery has over conventional multiport laparoscopy include superior cosmesis from a relatively hidden umbilical scar; a possible decrease in morbidity related to visceral and vascular injury during trocar placement; and risk reduction of postoperative wound infection, hernia formation, and elimination of multiple trocar site closures.[10] Although single-port surgery may seem to have potential benefits, comparative trials in humans have yet to find significant differences between single-port and conventional multiport laparoscopy in postoperative complications, postoperative pain, hospital stay, and cosmetic results.[11,12] It should also be noted that within the human literature, including both clinical case series and laboratory-based skill acquisition studies, evidence has demonstrated unique requirements of single-port surgery, with skill sets and ergonomic demands that cannot be directly adapted from existing laparoscopic experience, and the implementation of an evidence- and competency-based single-port training curriculum is necessary to ensure appropriate training of future single-port surgeons.[13]

Adoption into Veterinary Laparoscopy

Within veterinary laparoscopic surgery, reducing the number of portals of entry has been a concept embraced by many veterinarians for a number of common techniques. In 2009, Dupre *et al.* described the one portal operating laparoscopic ovariectomy (OVE) using a 10-mm telescope that incorporates a working channel that can accommodate 5-mm instruments.[14] An array of two-port laparoscopic-assisted techniques, including gastropexy,[15] cystopexy,[16] urinary calculi removal,[17] and

cryptorchidectomy,[18] have also been described. These two-port techniques enabled many common elective procedures to be done routinely by veterinary laparoscopic surgeons. It was only recently that many of the two-port procedures in veterinary laparoscopy took a leap toward the single-port platform in which multiple instruments as well as the telescope are consolidated to one point of entry for completion of the entire procedure. The earliest abstract reports on laparoscopic single-port veterinary techniques that did not use an operating laparoscope emerged in 2011.[19,20] The single-port platform gained rapid popularity among veterinary laparoscopic surgeons. Shortly after the initial single-port abstracts, a total laparoscopic ovariectomy using standard rigid instrumentation was described[21] using a commercially available single-port device (SILS [single-incision laparoscopic surgery] port, Covidien, Mansfield, MA). Shortly after, the SPA ovariectomy technique was reported.[22] Other single-port devices as well as novel bent and articulating instruments emerged as feasible instrumentation that could be used in veterinary single-port laparoscopy.[23] More recently, other techniques using the single-port approach were reported, including single-incision laparoscopic-assisted intestinal surgery (SILAIS) in dogs and cats using the EndoCone (Karl Storz Endoscopy, Goleta, CA) and the SILS port[24]; the single incision laparoscopic ovariectomy in cats[25]; the SPA gastropexy and ovariectomy (SPAGO) with the SILS port[26]; and the single-port laparoscopic cryptorchidectomy (SPLC), which was described using the EndoCone, SILS, and Triports (Olympus, Center Valley, PA).[27] An evaluation of the learning curve for the single-port ovariectomy using the SILS port has also been reported.[28] A study has also been published within the veterinary literature evaluating the effect of standard decontamination and sterilization methods on sterility after reuse of the SILS device.[29]

Access Methods for Single-Port Surgery

Operative Laparoscopy and Advanced Operative Laparoscopy

This uses a traditional simple operative laparoscope that incorporates a 5-mm working channel through which instruments can be passed (Figure 6-1). Advanced operating laparoscopes include a triangulating operating platform,[30] such as the SPIDER surgical system (TransEnterix Surgical Inc, Durham, NC), which gives a surgeon multiple independent flexible arms that can be extended through a rigid operating laparoscope shaft.

Single-Port Access

This uses a single skin incision (usually at the umbilicus) but separate individual facial incisions through which traditional

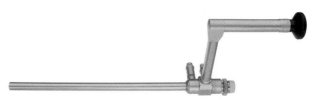

Figure 6-1 This operating laparoscope (Karl Storz Endoscopy, Goleta, CA) incorporates a 5-mm working channel through which 5-mm rigid instrumentation can be passed. (© 2014 Photo Courtesy of KARL STORZ GmbH & Co. KG.)

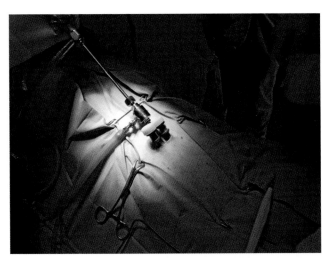

Figure 6-2 Single-port access laparoscopy is performed by the passage of three separate cannulae through one skin incision but separate fascial incisions.

trocar–cannula assemblies are passed through the abdominal wall (Figure 6-2).

Commercially Available Single-Port Devices

These devices have been specifically manufactured for single-port surgery and are intended to be inserted through a single full-thickness abdominal incision. These commercially available SPA devices can have multiple 5- to 12-mm access channels to enable an array of instrumentation to enter to the abdominal cavity (Figure 6-3).

Principles of Single-Port Surgery

The principles of single-port surgery are very similar to those of conventional multiport laparoscopy, although differences exist associated with the way triangulation is achieved. Having one point of entry inherently prevents the traditional principles of instrument triangulation. The close proximity of the instruments and optics both intraabdominally and extraabdominally causes the surgeon to perform the procedure without a lot of surgical working space intraabdominally. This ultimately causes increased tech-

nical complexity for any procedures because of inadequate triangulation, a compromised field of view, inadequate exposure, and frequent instrument collisions, which all occur as a result of the common entry point for the camera and instruments.[30] Single-port laparoscopy has been able to somewhat overcome this lack of triangulation by using angled optical telescopes, crossing instruments, or bent and articulating instruments. This novel arrangement of both the optics and instruments creates more internal and external working space, allowing for some triangulation which prevents instrument crowding. Although standard instruments can be used for single-port surgery, numerous instruments and devices have been developed to simplify and make single-port surgery more user friendly.

Access in Single-Port Surgery

The devices and equipment used for single-port surgery can be broadly classified as (1) specifically manufactured devices for single-port surgery, (2) standard instruments and trocar–cannula assemblies used for conventional laparoscopy inserted through one skin incision, or (3) innovative adoptions of existing equipment not primarily intended for laparoscopy.

Insertion Techniques for Specifically Manufactured Single-Port Devices

EndoCone Port (Karl Storz Endoscopy; Figure 6-4)

A 3-cm mini-laparotomy incision is created in advance of port insertion. To insert this single-port device, the bulkhead seal is removed, and a small amount of sterile lubricant is applied to the positive threads of the conical port (Video Clip 6-1). The flanged edge of the port is then inserted into the 3-cm incision and threaded 360 degrees in a clockwise direction. During port insertion, the abdominal viscera is observed through the port to ensure that no entrapment or inclusion of bowel or omentum occurs. When the threaded cannula is in place, the EndoCone is capped by snapping the bulkhead into position. The insufflation tubing is then connected to the gas valve on the port, and insufflation commenced. A major benefit for using this device is its ability to be steam sterilized in an autoclave. This is one of the only ports deliberately developed with reuse in mind. Another advantage is that this port has a ballast that can be removed repeatedly during

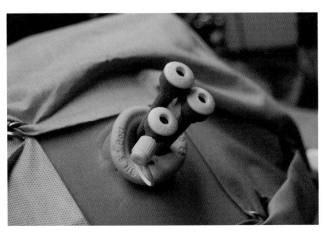

Figure 6-3 The SILS (single-incision laparoscopic surgery) port (Covidien, Mansfield, MA) allows the placement of three cannulae and has a separate CO_2 insufflation port.

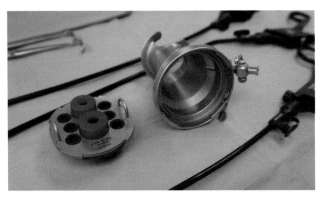

Figure 6-4 The EndoCone port (Karl Storz Endoscopy, Goleta, CA) has the advantage of being one of the only single-port devices that can be steam sterilized. (Image courtesy of J. Brad Case.)

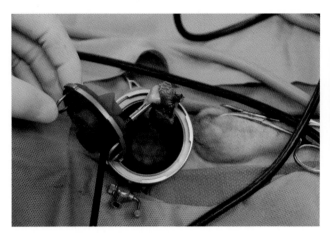

Figure 6-5 The EndoCone allows easy removal of tissue by removal of the bulkhead. (Image courtesy of J. Brad Case.)

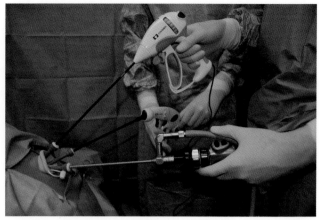

Figure 6-6 With some port devices, some triangulation can still be maintained, but this varies by device.

the procedure without compromising the ability to reinsufflate the abdomen. This can enable tissue removal at any time during the procedure (Figure 6-5).

GelPOINT Access System (Applied Medical Inc., Rancho Santa Margarita, CA)

A 2- to 7-cm mini-laparotomy incision is created in advance for insertion of the port (Video Clip 6-2). This single-port device consists of a wound retractor, GelSeal cap, and four 5- to 10-mm cannulae. The wound retractor portion of this port provides 360-degree atraumatic retraction of an abdominal incision 2 to 7 cm in length. The wound retractor portion is required to be inserted initially by passing the inner flexible ring through the abdominal incision. The outer ring is then rolled until it reaches the incision causing radial retraction. The cannulae are inserted through the GelSeal cap, and the GelSeal cap is then fitted to the outer ring of the wound retractor. The insufflator tubing is then attached, and the abdomen is insufflated to 8 to 10 mm Hg with carbon dioxide using a pressure-regulating mechanical insufflator. There are several advantages to using this device: the wound retractor sleeve is able to accommodate the widest range of body wall thicknesses compared with other single-port devices; the wound retractor portion can accommodate a 7-cm incision, which can enable large tissue removal; and the GelSeal cap can be removed and reattached repeatedly during the procedure without compromising the ability to reinsufflate the abdomen.

SILS Port (Covidien; Figures 6-3 and 6-6)

A 2- to 3-cm mini-laparotomy is created in advance for insertion of the port. To insert this single-port device, a small amount of sterile lubricant is applied to its soft base (Video Clip 6-3). The port is inserted into its 2- to 3-cm abdominal incision by clamping two curved Rochester carmalt forceps at the base in a staggered fashion. Varying techniques have been described for insertion into the incision: it can be performed without abdominal wall countertraction or with a form of countertraction such as grasping the facial edges with two large rat-toothed tissue forceps, Army-Navy retractors, or stay sutures. Regardless of traction, the tips of the Rochester carmalts are directed into the incision in a cranial direction toward the diaphragm or away from any underlying viscera. When the base is seeded within the incision, the clamps are then released to allow the bottom portion of the port

to expand and fit snugly within the incision. Three 5-mm cannulae (supplied with the port) are then inserted into the three inner cylinders with the aid of a 5-mm blunt obturator. The SILS port also is supplied with a 12- to 15-mm trocar–cannula assembly to allow for larger instruments to be inserted with two other 5-mm cannulae. The heights of the cannulae are staggered to minimize cannula contact (Figure 6-7). Insufflator tubing is then attached and the abdomen is insufflated to 8 to 10 mm Hg with carbon dioxide using a pressure-regulating mechanical insufflator. The multitrocar port can be positioned to have the three 5-mm cannulae at the 12, 4, and 8 o'clock positions relative to the surgical site, although any arrangement is possible. Advantages of this port include the relative ease of insertion and reinsertion during a procedure and its ability to fit snugly within the incision, preventing loss of pneumoperitoneum.

S-Port (Karl Storz Endoscopy; Figure 6-8)

A 2- to 4-cm mini-laparotomy incision is created in advance for insertion of the port. To insert this device, a 360-degree

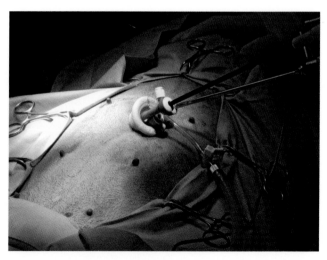

Figure 6-7 With the SILS (single-incision laparoscopic surgery) device (Karl Storz Endoscopy, Goleta, CA), it is recommended to stagger the cannulae to minimize interference.

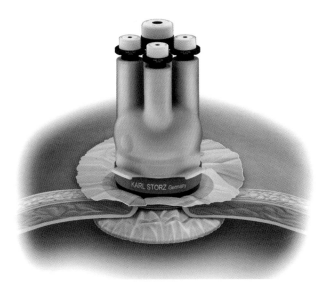

Figure 6-8 The S-port (Karl Storz Endoscopy, Goleta, CA) is shown in position across the body wall. (© 2014 Photo Courtesy of KARL STORZ GmbH & Co. KG.)

atraumatic wound retraction device is first inserted through the mini-laparotomy incision. The base adaptor ring of the S-Port is then fitted over the outer wound retractor ring. The outer ring of the wound retractor is then rolled until it reaches the adaptor ring directly over the incision causing the retractor to be pulled taut. Depending on what base ring adaptor is used, the appropriate seal (Figure 6-9; EndoCone ballast or X-Cone cap, Karl Storz Endoscopy) is fitted on to the adaptor ring with the wound retractor sheath evenly stretched over the ring (see Figure 6-9). The Luer-lock connector is inserted into one of the 5-mm port holes, the insufflator tubing is then attached, and the abdomen is insufflated to 8 to 10 mm Hg with carbon dioxide using a pressure-regulating mechanical insufflator. Advantages to using this device are that the wound retractor sleeve is able to accommodate a wide range of body wall thicknesses, and the soft outer cap can be removed and reattached repeatedly during the procedure to allow tissue extraction without compromising the ability to

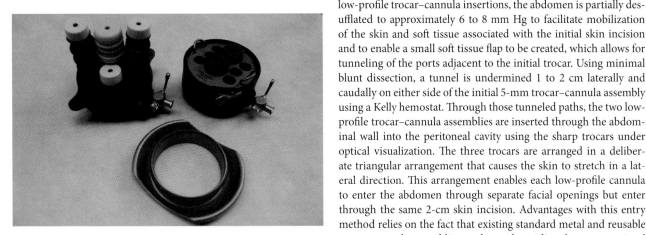

Figure 6-9 The components of the EndoCone or X-Cone (Karl Storz Endoscopy, Goleta, CA) are shown.

reinsufflate the abdomen. This device has also been designed with autoclave sterilization in mind.

Triport System (Olympus)

This single-port device is inserted into a 1.5- to 2-cm abdominal incision by directing the internal ring of the wound retractor through the incision (Video Clip 6-4). A small amount of sterile lubricant can be applied to the inner retractor ring to aid in insertion. The inner ring is released from the supplied introducer within the incision to the abdominal cavity. The ring is then adjusted to sit just on the inside of the incision. The transparent sleeve attached to this inner ring is pulled up and away from the patient while the outer ring is simultaneously pushed down toward the incision. The inner and outer rings of this entry system are firmly pushed together while the plastic sleeve is pulled to ensure the rings are tight against the abdominal wall. The excess transparent plastic sleeve is cut, allowing 1 to 2 cm of excess to be folded into the incision. The soft plastic trocar cap is then firmly fitted to the outer ring. The insufflator tubing is then attached, and the abdomen is insufflated to 8 to 10 mm Hg with carbon dioxide using a pressure-regulating mechanical insufflator. Advantages to using this device are similar to those of the other wound retractor devices: the wound retractor sleeve is able to accommodate a wide range of body wall thicknesses, and the soft outer cap can be removed and reattached repeatedly during the procedure to allow tissue extraction without compromising the ability to reinsufflate the abdomen.

Insertion Technique of Standard Trocars for Single-Port Entry

Single-Port Access Technique (see Figure 6-2, Video Clip 6-5)

A 1.5- to 2-cm skin incision is made on the ventral midline in the region of the umbilicus. Using the Hasson abdominal access technique, a 5-mm blunt laparoscopic low-profile trocar–cannula assembly is inserted into the abdomen. The abdomen is insufflated using a pressure-regulating mechanical insufflator to an intraabdominal pressure between 9 and 12 mm Hg. After brief abdominal exploration with a 30-degree telescope, two additional very-low-profile 5-mm trocar–cannula assemblies are then inserted in a triangular pattern adjacent to the initial port. For the second and third low-profile trocar–cannula insertions, the abdomen is partially desufflated to approximately 6 to 8 mm Hg to facilitate mobilization of the skin and soft tissue associated with the initial skin incision and to enable a small soft tissue flap to be created, which allows for tunneling of the ports adjacent to the initial trocar. Using minimal blunt dissection, a tunnel is undermined 1 to 2 cm laterally and caudally on either side of the initial 5-mm trocar–cannula assembly using a Kelly hemostat. Through those tunneled paths, the two low-profile trocar–cannula assemblies are inserted through the abdominal wall into the peritoneal cavity using the sharp trocars under optical visualization. The three trocars are arranged in a deliberate triangular arrangement that causes the skin to stretch in a lateral direction. This arrangement enables each low-profile cannula to enter the abdomen through separate facial openings but enter through the same 2-cm skin incision. Advantages with this entry method relies on the fact that existing standard metal and reusable trocar–cannula assemblies can be used, avoiding the cost associated with purchasing disposable equipment.

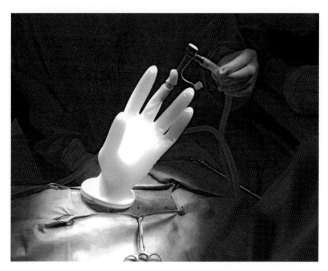

Figure 6-10 A wound retractor with latex glove and finger ports can be used as an inexpensive single-port device.

Innovative Adaptations of Existing Equipment

Wound Retractor with Latex Glove and Finger Ports (Figure 6-10)

A 2- to 3-cm mini-laparotomy incision is created in advance for insertion of the port. The inner ring of a 360-degree atraumatic wound retraction device (Alexis Wound Retractor; Applied Medical, or SurgiSleeve Wound Protector, Covidien) is first inserted through the mini-laparotomy incision (Figure 6-11). The outer ring of the wound retractor is then rolled until it reaches the level of the skin, causing the retractor sheath to be pulled taut. The tips of the fingers of a sterile latex glove are cut to just allow a 5- to 10-mm trocar–cannula assembly to be inserted. Suture is tied securely around the trocar–cannula assembly at the junction of the latex fingertip and the port. The wrist portion of the glove is then stretched over the external ring of the wound retractor. The insufflator tubing is then attached to any of the finger port Luer-lock fittings, and then insufflation of carbon dioxide to an

intraabdominal pressure of 8 to 10 mm Hg is delivered using a pressure-regulating mechanical insufflator. All five fingers can be used as ports of entry if necessary.[31]

Instrumentation

Conventional multiport laparoscopy is governed by the rule of triangulation such that a view is established in tandem with the simultaneously working extension of the human hand by means of the instruments.[3] Because the single-port platform follows the premise that all instruments enter the abdomen at the same site, one is forced to challenge the laws of traditional instrument triangulation. The single-port platform creates significant physical and ergonomic constraints that make traditional procedures more difficult to learn and perform compared with traditional laparoscopic surgery.[30] The proximity and parallel trajectory of the telescope and operating instruments placed through the single site lead to inevitable instrument and cannula collision, which ultimately interferes with smooth movements and makes the procedure more demanding than standard multiport laparoscopy.[30]

In trying to overcome some of the technical difficulties associated with single-port surgery, bent and articulating instruments have been developed to reproduce the triangulation that is experienced with conventional multiport laparoscopy and to limit some of the stated difficulties associated with using standard rigid instrumentation in single-port surgery.[27]

However, it should be noted that single-port surgery could successfully be performed using rigid instrumentation. An extensive body of literature exists describing single-port procedures completed by means of standard rigid laparoscopic instruments in both humans[32-35] and veterinary patients.[20,21,24] An array of articulating and double prebent laparoscopic instruments have been developed and marketed specifically for the single-port platform in an effort to correct the difficulties resulting from the loss of triangulation. Bent or coaxial deviating instruments are in a fixed position and were designed to be offset from the straight axis of a standard instrument, enabling the surgeon to have internal and external working space. The curved design provides acceptable intracorporeal triangulation and good ergonomic positioning for the hands (Figure 6-12). The articulating instruments have a design that mimics the movements of a surgeon's wrist and have a distal tip that can deflect relative to their shaft, offering seven degrees of freedom of movement.[3] Many of these instruments also offer axial 360-degree rotation for tip orientation similar to conventional rigid instruments. All of the articulating instruments can

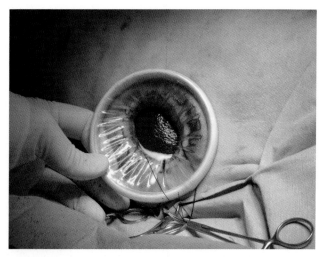

Figure 6-11 This wound retractor (Alexis; Applied Medical, Rancho Santa Margarita, CA) provides a protected retracted access incision through which organs can be exteriorized.

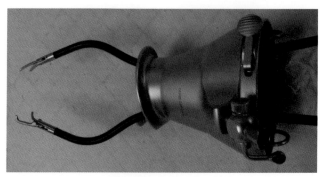

Figure 6-12 Coaxial instruments used through single-port devices can obviate some of the disadvantages encountered when the ability to triangulate is compromised. (Courtesy of J. Brad Case.)

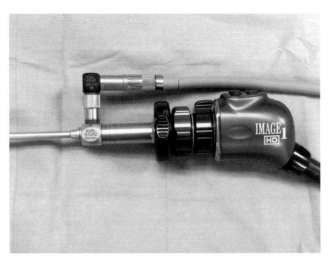

Figure 6-13 A right angle adaptor placed onto the connection between the light cable and telescope can reduce interference between the light cable and instruments during single-port surgery.

be introduced in both single-port devices and conventional rigid trocar–cannula assemblies. The double prebent instruments are intended to mimic triangulation through a curved design of both ends of the instrument shaft, which leads to antipodal directions of the tips and handles when the instruments are held in parallel.[36] The double-bent instruments can only be used with soft, flexible, or specifically designed entry devices for bent instruments because the bends in these instruments prevent their introduction into a rigid trocar–cannula assembly.

Optics

With the close proximity of the telescopes and instruments in single-port surgery, adjustments are required to create space both internally and externally to avoid instrument and optic interference. The easiest way to avoid optics and instrument clashing during the procedure is the use of an angled telescope. The most common telescope used for single-port laparoscopy in veterinary medicine is a telescope with a 30-degree angle. To further reduce the external clashing of instruments with the light cable, a right-angle adaptor for the light cable can be used (Figure 6-13). Recently, the development of advanced laparoscopes geared specifically for single-port surgery has emerged. A variety of deflectable telescopes with different mechanical design properties have recently been shown to be effective. One design involves a traditional fixed-rod design that contains a rotating lens at the distal end (EndoCAMeleon, Karl Storz Endoscopy), or alternatively a design that uses the "chip on the tip" concept by placing an image processor at the distal tip of an articulating laparoscope (EndoEye, Olympus; Idealeye Stryker, Kalamazoo, MI).[37] During veterinary single-port surgery, it has been shown that using either a 30-degree telescope[24,27] or an advanced deflecting optic[23] enables the telescope's camera head and tip to be directed away from the other instruments during the procedure, improving working space while simultaneously maintaining excellent visualization.

Conclusion

The single-port platform is a recent innovation in minimally invasive surgery. This platform may represent the next step forward in minimally invasive techniques. Early reports in the veterinary lit-

erature have shown this access method as a feasible and potentially more attractive approach for many common veterinary procedures. The focus of all new surgical techniques should be feasibility, safety, and efficacy, and they should provide a clinical advantage over other existing methods. Further studies are needed to determine if this platform of surgery can be considered a comparable alternative to multiport laparoscopy. Continually pursuing these types of research initiatives will help to drive emerging minimally invasive techniques and technology that ultimately benefits both human and veterinary patients alike.

 All videos cited in this chapter can be found on the book's companion website at **www.wiley.com/go/fransson/ laparoscopy**

References

1 Darzi ,A., Munz, Y. (2004) The impact of minimally invasive surgical techniques. Annu Rev Med 55, 223-237.

2 Keus, F., de Jong, J., Gooszen, H.G., et al. (2006) Laparoscopic versus open cholecystectomy for patients with symptomatic cholecystolithiasis. Cochrane Database Syst Rev 4, CD006229.

3 Kommu, S.S., Rane, A. (2009) Devices for laparoendoscopic single-site surgery in urology. Expert Rev Med Devices 6, 95-103.

4 Islam, A., Castellvi, A.O., Tesfay, S.T., et al. (2011) Early surgeon impressions and technical difficulty associated with laparoendoscopic single-site surgery: a Society of American Gastrointestinal and Endoscopic Surgeons learning center study. Surg Endosc 8, 2597-2603.

5 Galvao Neto, M., Ramos, A., Campos, J. (2009) Single port laparoscopic access surgery. Gastrointest Endosc 11, 84-93.

6 Qiu, J., Yuan, H., Chen, S., et al. (2013) Single-port versus conventional multiport laparoscopic cholecystectomy: a meta-analysis of randomized controlled trials and nonrandomized studies. J Laparoendosc Adv Surg Tech A 23, 815-831.

7 Wheeless, C.R. Jr, Thompson, B.H. (1973) Laparoscopic sterilization. Review of 3600 cases. Obstet Gynecol 42, 751-758.

8 Navarra, G., Pozza, E., Occhionorelli, S., et al. (1997) One-wound laparoscopic cholecystectomy. Br J Surg 84, 695.

9 Podolsky, E.R., Rottman, S.J., Pobete, H., et al. (2009) Single port access (SPA) cholecystectomy: a completely transumbilical approach. J Laparoendoscopic Adv Surg Tech A 19, 219-222.

10 Fader, A.N., Levinson, K.L., Gunderson, C.C., et al. (2011) Laparoendoscopic single-site surgery in gynaecology: a new frontier in minimally invasive surgery. J Minim Access Surg 7, 71-77.

11 Mencaglia, L., Mereu, L., Carri, G., et al. (2013) Single port entry—are there any advantages? Best Pract Res Clin Obstet Gynaecol 27, 441-455.

12 Antoniou, S.A., Koch, O.O., Antoniou, G. (2014) Meta-analysis of randomized trials on single-incision laparoscopic versus conventional laparoscopic appendectomy. Am J Surg 207, 613-622.

13 Pucher, P.H., Sodergren, M.H., Singh, P., et al. (2012) Have we learned from lessons of the past? A systematic review of training for single incision laparoscopic surgery. Surg Endosc 27, 1478-1484.

14 Dupré, G., Fiorbianco, V., Skalicky, M., et al. (2009) Laparoscopic ovariectomy in dogs: comparison between single portal and two-portal access. Vet Surg 38, 818-824.

15 Rawlings, C.A., Foutz, T.L., Mahaffey, M.B., et al. (2001) A rapid and strong laparoscopic-assisted gastropexy in dogs. Am J Vet Res 62, 871-875.

16 Rawlings, C.A., Howerth, E.W., Mahaffey, M.B., et al. (2002) Laparoscopic-assisted cystopexy in dogs. Am J Vet Res 63, 1226-1231.

17 Rawlings, C.A., Mahaffey, M.B., Barsanti, J.A., et al. (2003) Use of laparoscopic-assisted cystoscopy for removal of urinary calculi in dogs. J Am Vet Med Assoc 222, 759-761.

18 Miller, N.A., Van Lue, S.J., Rawlings, C.A. (2004) Use of laparoscopic-assisted cryptorchidectomy in dogs and cats. J Am Vet Med Assoc 224, 875-878.

19 Runge, J.J., Curcillo PG. (2011) Reduced port surgery: Single port access (SPA) technique for laparoscopic canine ovariectomy. In: Proceedings of the 8th Annual Meeting of the Veterinary Endoscopy Society, San Pedro, Belize, p. 13.

20 Wilson, D., Monnet, E. (2011) Utilization of SILS Port with standard instrumentation to perform laparoscopic procedures in dogs. In: Proceedings of the 8th Annual Meeting of the Veterinary Endoscopy Society, San Pedro, Belize, p. 12.

21 Manassero, M., Leperlier, D., Vallefuoco, R., et al. (2012) Laparoscopic ovariectomy in dogs using a single-port multiple-access device. Vet Rec 171, 69.

22 Runge, J.J., Curcillo, P.G. II, King, S.A., et al. (2012) Initial application of reduced port surgery using the single port access technique for laparoscopic canine ovariectomy. Vet Surg 41, 803-806.

23 Runge, J.J. (2012) The cutting edge: introducing reduced port laparoscopic surgery. Today's Vet Pract Jan/Feb, 14-20.

24 Case, J.B., Ellison, G. (2013) Single Incision laparoscopic-assisted intestinal surgery (SILAIS) in 7 dogs and 1 cat. Vet Surg 42, 629-634.

25 Coisman, J.G., Case, J.B., Shih, A., et al. (2013) Comparison of surgical variables in cats undergoing single-incision laparoscopic ovariectomy using a LigaSure or extracorporeal suture versus open ovariectomy. Vet Surg 43, 38-44.

26 Runge, J.J., Mayhew, P.D., Case, J.B., et al. (2014) Single-port cryptorchidectomy in dogs and cats: 25 cases (2009-2014). J Am Vet Med Assoc 245, 1258-65.

27 Runge, J.J., Mayhew, P.D. (2013) Evaluation of single port access gastropexy and ovariectomy using articulating instruments and angled telescopes in dogs. Vet Surg 42, 807-813.

28 Runge, J.J., Boston, R.C., Ross, S.B., et al. (2014) Evaluation of the learning curve for a board-certified surgeon performing laparoendoscopic single-site ovariectomy in dogs. J Am Vet Med Assoc 245, 828-835.

29 Coisman, J.G., Case, J.B., Clark, N.D., et al. (2013) Efficacy of decontamination and sterilization of a single-use single-incision laparoscopic surgery port. Am J Vet Res 74, 934-938.

30 Rieder, E., Martinec, D.V., Cassera, M.A., et al. (2011) A triangulating operating platform enhances bimanual performance and reduces surgical workload in single-incision laparoscopy. J Am Coll Surg 212, 378-384.

31 Shussman, N., Kedar, A., Elazary, R., et al. (2014) Reusable single-port access device shortens operative time and reduces operative costs. Surg Endosc 28, 1902-1907.

32 Podolsky, E.R., Curcillo, P.G. (2010b) Single port access (SPA) surgery—a 24-month experience. J Gastrointest Surg 14, 759-767.

33 Podolsky, E.R., Curcillo, P.G. (2010a) Reduced-port surgery: preservation of the critical view in single-port-access cholecystectomy. Surg Endosc 24, 3038-3043.

34 Tsai, Y.-C., Lin, V.C.-H., Chung, S.-D., et al. (2012) Ergonomic and geometric tricks of laparoendoscopic single-site surgery (LESS) by using conventional laparoscopic instruments. Surg Endosc 26, 2671-2677.

35 Yilmaz, H., Alptekin, H. (2013) Single-incision laparoscopic transabdominal preperitoneal herniorrhaphy for bilateral inguinal hernias using conventional instruments. Surg Laparosc Endosc Percutan Tech 23, 320-323.

36 Miernik, A., Schoenthaler, M., Lilienthal, K., et al. (2012) Pre-bent instruments used in single-port laparoscopic surgery versus conventional laparoscopic surgery: comparative study of performance in a dry lab. Surg Endosc 26, 1924-1930.

37 Goldsmith, Z.G., Astroza, G.M., Wang, A.J., et al. (2012) Optical performance comparison of deflectable laparoscopes for laparoendoscopic single-site surgery. J Endourol 26, 1340-1345.

SECTION III

Fundamental Techniques in Laparoscopy

7 Anesthesia Management of Dogs and Cats for Laparoscopy

Khursheed Mama and Marlis L. de Rezende

> **Key Points**
> - Anesthesia management requires an understanding of the physiological effects of capnoperitoneum.
> - The Trendelenburg (head-down) and Fowler (head-up) positions often used with laparoscopy can also influence venous return and cardiac output.
> - The physiological effects associated with laparoscopy lead to a requirement for attentive anesthesia monitoring and management.

Introduction

Laparoscopic-assisted interventions are gaining popularity in veterinary medicine[1] as in human medicine, in part because of the realized and potential reduction in tissue trauma when compared with laparotomy. A decrease in inflammatory mediators (e.g., C-reactive protein, interleukin-6) and cells (e.g., white blood cells) and a decrease in metabolic responses suggestive of stress (e.g., hyperglycemia) in patients undergoing laparoscopic versus open surgical intervention are taken as support of this.[2-5] Recent, albeit limited, direct and indirect evidence from animal studies[3,6,8] supports that as for human patients, there is less pain associated with a laparoscopic versus a traditional surgical approach for the same procedure. This in turn reduces the need for analgesic drugs and shortens hospital stays in human patients with that same potential in animals. Additional advantages include reduced adhesion formation[9] lower infection rates,[10] a shorter healing time, improved cosmetic results, and quicker return to function.[11-13] Because of these real and potential benefits to animals, laparoscopy is being used both as a diagnostic[14,15] and surgical tool[16-18] with increasing frequency in veterinary medicine.

Despite the many advantages associated with laparoscopic versus traditional approaches, there is the potential for complicating factors to adversely affect outcome that the anesthetist must consider. In addition to effects related to the disease state of the animal, the positioning for surgery, and the surgical procedure itself, there is the potential to significantly influence physiological functions when insufflating gas into the abdomen. These considerations are the focus of this chapter and are discussed in more detail in the subsequent text.

Anesthesia Considerations Related to Disease

In addition to routine procedures in healthy dogs and cats, animals with significant disease are increasingly presented for laparoscopy. The anesthetist must therefore be aware of the considerations related to the primary and any secondary disease processes in these patients. This information is available in broad-based anesthesia textbooks. As an example, consider a patient presenting for a liver biopsy. On the surface, this would seem a fairly straightforward procedure. However, if circulation is compromised because of hypoproteinemia and acid–base and electrolyte changes, insufflation of the abdomen can result in serious hypotension. If coagulation status is also compromised, significant blood loss from the biopsy site may exacerbate this, and the animal may require a transfusion. If lung metastases are present, respiratory complications are possible. The potential for side effects tends to increase with more complex procedures as in an animal with an adrenal pheochromocytoma in which manipulation can increase catecholamine release and result in hypertension and cardiac rhythm abnormalities. Timely intervention is facilitated if these potential complications are anticipated.

Anesthesia Considerations Related to Surgery

Surgical complications may be related specifically to the procedure or positioning for the procedure (discussed later) or may be of a more general nature. Again, prior preparation will facilitate rapid treatment if this occurs.

Hemorrhage from inadvertent puncture of organs or vessels during placement of the Veress needle or introduction of the trocars is

Small Animal Laparoscopy and Thoracoscopy, First Edition. Edited by Boel A. Fransson and Philipp D. Mayhew.
© 2015 by ACVS Foundation. Published 2015 by John Wiley & Sons, Inc.
Companion website: www.wiley.com/go/fransson/laparoscopy

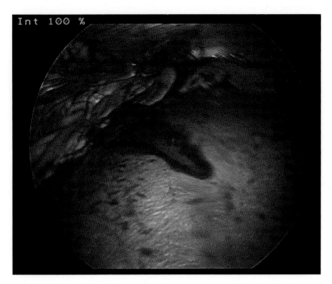

Figure 7-1 Inadvertent splenic puncture. (Courtesy of Eric Monnet.)

a reported complication in human and animal patients (Figure 7-1) even during entry into the abdomen for routine procedures and requires a quick response from the anesthetist.[19-23] Hemorrhage from either cause might also necessitate conversion from the laparoscopic to an open approach during which time the patient will need to continue to be supported aggressively until the surgeon can visualize and control the source of hemorrhage. A recent report in veterinary patients indicates excessive hemorrhage as one of the significant causes for conversion to celiotomy during diagnostic procedures.[24]

Hemorrhage has also been reported at the surgical site during routine procedures such as ovariectomy in dogs,[22,25] suggesting that vigilance on the part of the anesthetist for this complication is important.

Reported surgical complication rates for laparoscopy and laparotomy vary. Initial reports suggested that surgical complications occurred with a lower frequency for laparoscopy, but as the complexity of procedures performed using this approach has increased, the complication rate is now more comparable.[19,20]

In addition to vascular entry and organ puncture with subsequent hemorrhage as previously mentioned, surgical complications include bladder (Figure 7-2), bowel, or stomach puncture and gas

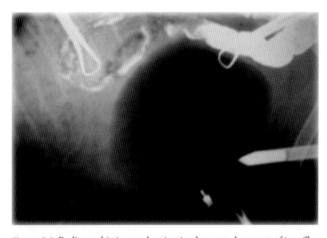

Figure 7-2 Radiographic image showing inadvertent placement of insufflation gas into the bladder. (Courtesy of David Twedt.)

distention; trauma to the bile duct; peritoneal detachment; and so on. A recent study in dogs and cats reports a 7.5% emergent conversion rate from laparoscopy to laparotomy because of surgical complications such as hemorrhage and biliary tract rupture.[24] Complication rates and surgical time, which can additionally contribute to morbidity, tend to decrease with surgeon experience.

Other causes of surgical complications are related to the unique equipment used for intervention. Just as it is important for the surgeon to have basal knowledge of anesthesia, it is important for the anesthetist to have at least a similar level of understanding of the surgical equipment used to facilitate laparoscopy. Complications associated with puncture of organs or vessels with the Veress needle have already been discussed. Additional complications may arise from use (intentional or accidental) of high insufflation pressures, intraabdominal use of cautery (especially if a potentially flammable gas is used), heat from the light source and cable, and so on.

Pathophysiology of Pneumoperitoneum

Hemodynamic Effects

Hemodynamic changes and complications result from many factors, including surgical intervention as previously mentioned, patient position, anesthesia, and variations in carbon dioxide (CO_2) tension. A body of literature indicates that peritoneal insufflation, regardless of the gas used, alters hemodynamics in both human beings and animals. Although variability is reported, the most consistent changes are those to cardiac output and vascular resistance. A decrease in cardiac output and concomitant increase in systemic vascular resistance are the most typical changes associated with increased abdominal pressure.[26-30] This occurs despite the frequently observed slight increase in heart rate with insufflation. The decrease in cardiac output has been measured using many different tools (e.g., pulmonary artery catheterization, esophageal Doppler echocardiography) and interestingly is seen in human and veterinary patients regardless of whether they are in a head-up or head-down position.[20,31,32] The decrease in cardiac output tends to parallel a decrease in venous return, which is believed to occur as a result of caval compression (with increasing insufflation pressure), pooling of blood in the caudal extremities, and changes in venous resistance.[26,27,33] It is interesting that despite a decrease in cardiac output, blood pressure changes are not consistent. In fact, blood pressure is often elevated in healthy patients with the increase in systemic vascular resistance offsetting the decrease in cardiac output.[19,27,28,30,33] This increase in resistance is thought at least in part to be the result of vasopressin release during peritoneal stretch resulting from insufflation.[27,34,35] The anesthetist is cautioned not to become complacent when recording normal blood pressure values because there is evidence that tissue perfusion to abdominal organs is progressively decreased with increases in abdominal insufflation pressures.

As insufflation pressures increase into the range of 10 to 15 mm Hg, hepatic, renal, and mesenteric blood flows are decreased. In studies with pigs, intraabdominal pressures greater than 10 mm Hg were associated with significant reductions in hepatic artery and splanchnic blood flow.[36,37] In dogs, intraabdominal pressures in the range of 16 to 20 mm Hg decreased portal venous and mesenteric arterial flow.[38,39] Impairment of blood flow in other vessels (e.g., celiac artery) and to the intestinal mucosa is also reported for both dogs and pigs in this similar pressure range.[27,37,40] Oliguria is reported with pressures in the 15 to 20 mm Hg range, and anuria may be seen when pressures exceed this ranges.[37,40,41] (In dogs, renal blood flow and glomerular filtration rate were decreased by more than 75% with intraabdominal pressures of 20 mm Hg, and anuria was observed when abdominal pressures reached 40 mm Hg.[27,41] Similar findings were reported in pigs, in which oliguria was observed with pressures over 15 mm Hg.[40] Interestingly, in a single study in healthy cats, pneumoperitoneum up to an intraabdominal pressure of 16 mm Hg with CO_2 as the insufflation gas did not significantly influence cardiovascular parameters; regional blood flow was not evaluated.[42]

Although healthy cats did not show changes in measured parameters during peritoneal insufflation, it is important to remember that cardiovascular function may be further influenced by the patient's health status, positioning during anesthesia and surgery, duration of the procedure, and type of insufflation gas.

For example, head-up (also known as Fowler or reverse Trendelenburg) (Figure 7-3) positioning can compromise venous return and cardiac output because of gravitational effects. This is of greater consequence during anesthesia because of the blunting of baroreceptor reflexes. During Trendelenburg positioning, cardiac output again decreases, but the reasons differ and include decreases in heart rate and vasomotor tone.[43,44] In anesthetized dogs, both body positions have further compromised cardiac output during pneumoperitoneum, with the Fowler position having the most significant impact.[32] There is also increasing concern regarding changes in intracranial pressure, which compound those seen with CO_2 pneumoperitoneum. A recent study has shown a correlation between laparoscopic insufflation pressures and intracranial pressure in human patients undergoing laparoscopic ventriculoperitoneal shunt placement.[45] Although unlikely to be serious in healthy patients, this could be of great significance in patients with intracranial disease.

Respiratory Effects

Respiratory function is also altered during laparoscopic intervention. The increase in abdominal pressure and volume limits diaphragmatic excursion and reduces pulmonary compliance, functional residual capacity, and vital capacity of the lung and may lead to ventilation/perfusion mismatch.[27,33,46-48] Hence, it is not surprising that the effects tend to be proportional to insufflation pressures

as is shown in young swine[49] and adult dogs.[33,50] In spontaneously breathing dogs, the respiratory rate remained unchanged with abdominal insufflation, but a significant reduction in tidal volume was reported.[50] With volume-controlled ventilation, maintenance of tidal volume results in an increase in peak inspiratory pressure,[33] and hypercapnia and hypoxemia might still occur. Similarly, when using pressure-controlled ventilation, the peak inspiratory pressure must be increased to overcome the decrease in lung compliance and avoid a reduction in tidal volume. The resulting positive pressure in the chest has an additional impact on reducing venous return, and thus cardiac output could be further compromised.

In spontaneously breathing animals, the decrease in tidal volume and increase in end-tidal CO_2 are proportional to increasing insufflation pressure, and the negative impact lasts longer in animals exposed to the higher pressures.[50] This reflects fatigue on the part of the patient and has led to the common recommendation for mechanical ventilation in patients when the procedure is anticipated to last longer than 15 to 30 minutes.

The inability for patients to compensate for the elevation in CO_2 by adjusting their ventilation is even more notable when CO_2 is used as the insufflation gas as is common practice. This is because CO_2 is highly diffusible and enters the bloodstream, contributing to a rise in arterial tension. Hence, the impact on ventilation is greater than insufflation with an inert gas such as helium or with other gases such as nitrous oxide (N_2O) or air (albeit those gases have other disadvantages).[51-53] An increase in arterial CO_2 tensions may initially be cardiovascularly supporting[26,51] but will ultimately result in a concurrent decrease in blood pH, which in turn has a potential to impact cellular metabolic processes. Elevated CO_2 tensions are also associated with increased cerebral blood flow,[54,55] but additional mechanisms may exist.[56] In compromised patients or those breathing a low inspired oxygen tension, excessive CO_2 levels may contribute to hypoxemia. In addition, CO_2 tensions greater than 90 mm Hg have anesthetic effects in their own right.[57]

As for the cardiovascular system, additional factors such as positioning may further impact respiratory effects.[19,46,47,58] Both the Trendelenburg and reverse Trendelenburg positions have a negative impact on lung expansion because of increased lung and chest wall impedance.[59] The observed decrease in lung compliance and volumes, such as functional residual capacity and total and vital lung capacity[46,47,60,61] lead to further increase in CO_2 tensions.[61-64] Therefore, the use of mechanical ventilation, with an increased peak inspiratory pressure, is important to maintain CO_2 levels within acceptable limits and to avoid decreases in arterial oxygen tensions.[62,65] In animals and humans, the Trendelenburg position is associated with greater respiratory depression, particularly regarding oxygenation.[47,59,62,66] These respiratory effects seem to be species dependent with dogs and cats less impacted than horses and sheep. In addition, horses with a higher body weight seem to be more affected, with higher arterial CO_2 and lower oxygen tensions.[66]

Complications Associated with Pneumoperitoneum

These are in addition to cardiovascular and respiratory changes expected with insufflation of a gas into the peritoneal space. They include retroperitoneal or subcutaneous emphysema, both of which are generally the result of insufflation of gas outside of the peritoneal cavity. The occurrence of subcutaneous emphysema has been reported in dogs after laparoscopic gastropexy, nephrectomy, and

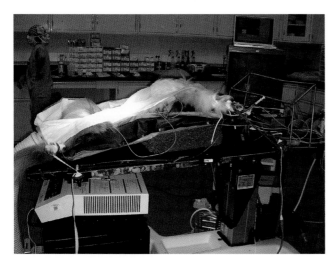

Figure 7-3 Dog prepared for laparoscopic intervention in the Fowler (reverse Trendelenburg) position.

ovariectomy.[22,67,68] A marked increase in CO_2 tension is typically observed in the face of extraperitoneal insufflation and should alert the anesthetist for this complication.[69] If the insufflation gas is CO_2, this tends to resolve fairly quickly after insufflation of gas is discontinued; one may also tap this virtual space and remove some gas to improve animal comfort. Additional analgesic therapy should be considered because pain is frequently observed in these animals. More serious complications include pneumomediastinum,[70] pneumothorax[71-73], and pneumopericardium,[74,75] which are all thought to be a result of insufflation gas (creating positive pressure) tracking through embryonic remnants or alternatively through potential diaphragmatic defects or weak points. Alveoli rupture, associated with the use of high peak inspiratory pressures to maintain minute ventilation, should also be considered as a possible cause. These complications may be life threatening, and the anesthetist should be ready to intervene rapidly if they occur. In a tension pneumothorax caused by alveoli rupture caused by high peak inspiratory pressures used during laparoscopy, cardiac output is compromised, and severe hypotension, oxygen desaturation, and a decrease in the partial pressure of end-tidal (but not arterial) CO_2 are commonly observed. In these animals, discontinuation of mechanical ventilation and thoracocentesis or chest tube placement should be performed quickly. On the other hand, when the pneumothorax is caused by migration of the CO_2 used for abdominal insufflation, similar cardiorespiratory depression is typically seen, except for the partial pressure of end-tidal CO_2, which might rise as the CO_2 is absorbed via the pleural surface.[19,73] In most of those cases, a chest drain may be avoided because the CO_2 can be removed from the chest via suction through the abdominal cavity.[71] CO_2 is absorbed much faster than air, and any residual pneumothorax is spontaneously absorbed. Mechanical ventilation with the addition of positive end-expiratory pressure has been advocated to minimize CO_2 accumulation in the chest and to maintain adequate ventilation and oxygenation.[19,71,73]

Perhaps the most concerning complication is the potential for gas embolism. This results when insufflation gas enters the vasculature and is transported to the heart and lungs. In small amounts, the gas is delivered to the lungs and usually cleared without much consequence to the patient. As volumes of gas increase, hypotension, tachycardia, arrhythmias, and a decrease in end-tidal CO_2 tension may be noted.[76,77] If a larger (patient size–dependent) volume of gas were to reach the heart, there is the potential for the gas to occupy one of the chambers of the heart and prevent blood flow that ultimately results in cardiac arrest.[77-80] Several studies using transesophageal echocardiography have demonstrated a very high incidence of subclinical gas emboli during different laparoscopic surgical procedures in both animals and humans.[81-84] The fact that no adverse effects were reported in those studies may be related to the use of CO_2 for abdominal insufflation. The potential for embolization exists with CO_2 but is lower than for air, nitrous oxide, or helium. This is why despite not being inert (and so contributing to a rise in arterial tensions more than caused by distention alone), CO_2 is still preferred as the insufflation gas for laparoscopic interventions.[19,81,82,85] Despite its relative safety, fatal embolism has been reported with CO_2 use in both humans and animals.[77,79] If gas embolism is suspected, abdominal insufflation should be immediately discontinued. When possible, the animal should be placed in left lateral recumbency and cardiac massage started in an attempt to dislodge the emboli from the heart. Placement of a central venous or pulmonary artery catheter may allow aspiration of the gas emboli.[19,58]

Anesthesia Management

Although there are some unique aspects to laparoscopic intervention, as noted in the preceding text, the basic principles of anesthesia must first be applied. General anesthesia should be a reversible event that provides amnesia, analgesia, unconsciousness, and muscle relaxation while supporting thermoregulation and cardiovascular, respiratory, neurologic, hepatic, and renal functions. To meet these basic principles, care should be individualized for the animal with consideration given to the reason for the presentation, the animal's signalment, general health status, and so on. Procedure-related risks should also be considered, and it may be warranted to consider the expertise of the surgical team when selecting anesthetic drugs and the support and monitoring plan. Additionally, one must factor in the pathophysiological implications of laparoscopic intervention as discussed earlier in this chapter.

A young healthy dog or cat presented for an elective procedure is unlikely to have restrictions when selecting anesthetic drugs. In our practice, an opioid would likely be used for premedication to provide analgesia and some sedation. The additional use of a tranquilizer or sedative might be warranted if the animal is excited or fractious. An anticholinergic could be considered to offset the bradycardia seen with many opioids and sometimes associated with peritoneal distention and visceral traction. Propofol (or another preferred induction agent) could be used for anesthesia induction and to facilitate intubation. Although many drugs, including ketamine and propofol, increase splenic size, thiopental, which is still available internationally, has been historically associated with the greatest potential to cause splenic enlargement. This may increase the potential for puncture of the spleen on entry into the abdomen and could compromise surgical visualization during cranial abdominal procedures, so its use should be weighed carefully. After intubation, the patient is commonly transitioned to maintenance with an inhaled anesthetic (isoflurane or sevoflurane). Local anesthetic infiltration at portal sites and a nonsteroidal antiinflammatory drug (when not contraindicated) are used in addition to postoperative opioids to provide additional analgesia. For debilitated or critically ill animals, the anesthetic plan is modified as appropriate.

In addition to the anesthetic drug plan, when considering the investment in time, training, and equipment for surgical aspects of laparoscopy, the veterinarian must consider whether the appropriate anesthesia equipment is available to support and monitor the patient during these procedures.

In addition to monitoring body temperature and providing external heat as appropriate, the heart rate and cardiac rhythm, which can vary during gas insufflation and organ manipulation (e.g., bradycardia with urinary bladder traction), should be monitored using an electrocardiogram. Blood pressure monitoring is essential and will alert the anesthetist to both anesthetic drug and insufflation related changes. Intravenous fluids (crystalloid or colloids as appropriate for the animal) are used to help maintain vascular volume and counteract the vasodilating effects of tranquilizers (e.g., acepromazine) and anesthetic drugs (e.g., propofol), as well as the additional influence of abdominal distention with insufflation gas and postural changes on venous return and subsequently cardiac output. Hypotension may be treated with rapid administration (bolus) of intravenous fluids, reducing the anesthetic dose, or decreasing insufflation pressure. When these interventions are not possible or not adequate, inotropes or vasoactive medications may be necessary.

Because of pneumoperitoneum and additional potential postural changes for surgery, access to a ventilator is highly desirable. As has been mentioned previously, pneumoperitoneum will increase

CO_2 tension. This occurs to a greater extent when the insufflation gas is CO_2 as is currently most common. If no adjustments are made to positive-pressure ventilation at the start of CO_2 insufflation, the arterial CO_2 tension ($PaCO_2$) rises. This increase tends to occur rapidly upon insufflation and generally plateaus in ventilated patients. Spontaneously breathing animals tend to fatigue and may not be able to maintain the plateau. Hence, for procedures in which insufflation will be sustained for more than 20 to 30 minutes, use of positive-pressure ventilation is recommended to minimize hypercapnia and a consequent reduction in pH and potential adverse effects on intracranial pressure and anesthesia depth. Typically, minute ventilation will need upward adjustment to compensate for the delivery of CO_2 with the insufflator. One should follow the basic principles of ventilation and consider the change in chest wall compliance when making these adjustments.

Because of the potential to cause barotrauma and compromise venous return (and so cardiac output) further with a significant increase in tidal volume, it is common to first increase respiratory rate and then if needed adjust the airway pressure or tidal or minute volume depending on the type of ventilator being used. Both pressure- and time-cycled (volume-limited) ventilators may be used, but the user should be familiar with the special considerations for each of these in the face of reduced pulmonary compliance caused by insufflation and potential postural changes. Although some elevation in arterial CO_2 tension is acceptable in a healthy patient, a general recommendation in patients without intracranial disease is to maintain this value at or below 60 mm Hg. In the absence of blood gas monitoring, the end-tidal CO_2, which may be up to 10 mm Hg (but is usually 0–5 mm Hg) lower than arterial CO_2 tensions, should be maintained below 55 mm Hg. Ventilation may also help prevent atelectasis of the lung resulting from cranial displacement of the diaphragm and so help maintain oxygenation.

Along with providing respiratory support, it is important to monitor respiratory function. CO_2 may be monitored in the airway with a capnograph or in the blood using a blood gas analyzer. The former has the benefit of being continuous and noninvasive. Additionally, the capnograph will alert the anesthetist to low cardiac output states as may occur for a number of reasons, including that resulting from an intravascular gas (CO_2) embolus.

A pulse oximeter similarly is easily applied and provides continuous measurement of oxygen saturation while also recording pulse rate. In most dogs and cats undergoing laparoscopic procedures, use of pulse oximetry is considered sufficient for monitoring of oxygenation because hypoxemia is not a likely complication even with insufflation in patients breathing a high fraction of inspired oxygen (FiO_2). However, in patients breathing a lower FiO_2, hypoxemia is possible and likely to occur more rapidly if a complication (e.g., pneumothorax) occurs. If nitrous oxide is used as part of the anesthetic protocol, oxygen saturation monitoring is especially important.

In a high-risk or critically ill animal, arterial blood gas analysis is useful and provides information about CO_2 and oxygen tensions. Blood pH and other parameters, including electrolytes, blood glucose, and lactate, are frequently included with blood gas results and provide additional information to facilitate appropriate management of the animal.

Summary

As laparoscopy increasingly gains popularity, it is important that the veterinary team is well versed in both surgical and anesthetic aspects of management to ensure a successful outcome.

References

1 Beedorn, J.A., Dykema, J.L., Hardie, R.J. (2013) Minimally invasive surgery in veterinary practice: a 2010 survey of diplomates and residents of the American College of Veterinary Surgeons. Vet Surg 42, 635-642.

2 Devitt, C.M., Cox, R.E., Hailey, J.J. (2005) Duration, complications, stress and pain of open ovariohysterectomy versus a simple method of laparoscopic-assisted ovariohysterectomy in dogs. J Am Vet Med Assoc 6, 921-927.

3 Jakeways, M.S., Mitchell, V., Hashim, I.A. (1994) Metabolic and inflammatory responses after open or laparoscopic cholecystectomy. Br J Surg 81, 127-131.

4 Joris, J., Cigarini, I., Legrand, M., et al. (1992) Metabolic and respiratory changes after cholecystectomy performed via laparotomy or laparoscopy. Br J Anaesth 69, 341-345.

5 Mealy, K., Gallagher, H., Barry, M., et al. (1992) Physiological and metabolic responses to open and laparoscopic cholecystectomy. Br J Surg 79, 1061-1064.

6 Gauthier, O., Holopherne-Doran, D., Gendarme, T., et al. (2014) Assessment of postoperative pain in cats after ovariectomy by laparoscopy, median celiotomy, or flank laparotomy. Vet Surg Jan 31. doi: 10.1111/j.1532-950X.2014.12150.x. [Epub ahead of print]

7 Davidson, E.B., Moll, H.D., Payton, M.E. (2004) Comparison of laparoscopic ovariohysterectomy and ovariohysterectomy in dogs. Vet Surg 33, 62-69.

8 Hancock, R.B., Lanz, O.I., Waldron, D.R., et al. (2005) Comparison of postoperative pain after ovariohysterectomy by harmonic scalpel-assisted laparoscopy compared with median celiotomy and ligation in dogs. Vet Surg 34, 273-282.

9 Schippers, E., Tittel, A., Ottinger, A., Schumpelick, V. (1988) Laparoscopy versus laparotomy: comparison of adhesion-formation after bowel resection in a canine model. Dig Surg 15, 145-147.

10 Barnett, J.C., Havrilesky, L.J., Bondurant, A.E., et al. (2011) Adverse events associated with laparoscopy vs laparotomy in the treatment of endometrial cancer. Am J Obstet Gynecol 205, 143.e1-6.

11 Gal, D., Lind, L., Lovecchio, J.L., Kohn, N. (1995) Comparative study of laparoscopy vs. laparotomy for adnexal surgery: efficacy, safety and cyst rupture. J Gynecol Surg 11, 153-158.

12 Grace, P.A., Quereshi, A., Coleman, J., et al. (1991) Reduced postoperative hospitalization after laparoscopic cholecystectomy. Br J Surg 78, 160-162.

13 Gerges, F.J., Kanazi, G.E., Jabbour-Khoury, S.I. (2006) Anesthesia for laparoscopy: a review. J Clin Anesth 18, 67-78.

14 Robertson, E., Twedt, D., Webb, C. (2014) Diagnostic laparoscopy in the cat: 1. Rationale and equipment. J Feline Med Surg 16, 5-16.

15 Radhakrishnan, A., Mayhew, P.D. (2013) Laparoscopic splenic biopsy in dogs and cats: 15 cases (2006-2008). J Am Anim Hosp Assoc 49, 41-45.

16 Smith, R.R., Mayhew, P.D., Berent, A.C. (2012) Laparoscopic adrenalectomy for management of a functional adrenal tumor in a cat. J Am Vet Med Assoc 241, 368-372.

17 Menendez, I.M., Fitch, G. (2012) Use of a laparoscopic retrieval device for urolith removal through a perineal urethrotomy. Vet Surg 41, 629-633.

18 Naan, E.C., Kirpensteijn, J., Dupre, G., et al. (2013) Innovative approach to laparoscopic adrenalectomy for treatment of unilateral adrenal gland tumors in dogs. Vet Surg 42, 710-715.

19 Joris, J.L. (2010) Anesthesia for laparoscopic surgery. In: Miller, R.D. (ed.) Millers Anesthesia, 7th edn. Churchill Livingstone/Elsevier, Philadelphia, pp. 2185-2202

20 Cunningham, A.J. (1998) Anesthetic implications of laparoscopic surgery. Yale J Biol Med 71, 551-578.

21 Strasberg, S.M., Sanabria, J.R., Clavien, P.A. (1992) Complications of laparoscopic cholecystectomy. Can J Surg 35, 275-280.

22 Case, J.B., Marvel, S.J., Boscan, P., et al. (2011) Surgical time and severity of postoperative pain in dogs undergoing laparoscopic ovariectomy with one, two or three instrument cannulas. J Am Vet Med Assoc 239, 203-208.

23 Desmaiziere, L.M., Martinot, S., Lepage, O.M., et al. (2003) Complications associated with cannula insertion techniques used for laparoscopy in standing horses. Vet Surg 32, 501-506.

24 Buote, N.J., Kovk-McClaran, J.R., Schold, J.D. (2011) Conversion from diagnostic laparoscopy to laparotomy: risk factors and occurrence. Vet Surg 40, 106-114.

25 Dupre, G., Fiorbianco, V., Skalicky, M., et al. (2009) Laparoscopic ovariectomy in dogs: comparison between single portal and two-portal access. Vet Surg 38, 818-824.

25 Solis-Herruzo, J.A., Moreno, D., Gonzalez, A., et al. (1991) Effect of intrathoracic pressure on plasma arginine vasopressin levels. Gastroenterology 101, 607-617.

26 Ivankovich, A.D., Miletich, D.J., Albrecht, R.F., et al. (1975) Cardiovascular effects of intraperitoneal insufflation with carbon dioxide and Nitrous oxide in the dog. Anesthesiology 42, 281-287.

27 Barnes, G.E., Laine, G.A., Giam, P.Y., et al. (1985) Cardiovascular responses to elevation of intra-abdominal hydrostatic pressure. Am J Physiol 248, R208-R213.

28 Joris, J.L., Noirot, D.P., Legrand, M.J., et al. (1993) Hemodynamic changes during laparoscopic cholecystectomy. Anesth Analg 76, 1067-1071.

29 Kashtan, J., Green, J.F., Parsons, E.Q., et al. (1981) Hemodynamic effects of increased abdominal pressure. J Surg Res 30, 249-255.

30 Johannsen, G., Andersen, M., Juhl, B. (1989) The effect of general anaesthesia on the haemodynamic events during laparoscopy with CO_2-insufflation. Acta Anaesthesiol Scand 33, 132-136.

31 Cunningham, A.J., Turner, J., Rosenbaum, S., et al. (1993) Transoesophageal echocardiographic assessment of haemodynamic function during laparoscopic cholecystectomy. Br J Anaesth 70, 621-625.

32 Williams, M.D., Murr, P.C. (1993) Laparoscopic insufflation of the abdomen depresses cardiopulmonary function. Surg Endosc 7, 12-16.

33 Richardson, J.D., Trinkle, J.K. (1976) Hemodynamic and respiratory alterations with increased intra-abdominal pressure. J Surg Res 20, 401-404.

34 Melville, R.J., Frizis, H.I., Forsling, M.L., et al. (1985) The stimulus for vasopressin release during laparoscopy. Surg Gynecol Obstet 161, 253-256.

36 Diebel, L.N., Wilson, R.F., Dulchavsky, S.A., et al. (1992) Effect of increased intra-abdominal pressure on hepatic arterial, portal venous, and hepatic microcirculatory blood flow. J Trauma 33, 279-283.

37 Diebel, L.N., Dulchavsky, S.A., Wilson, R.F., et al. (1992) Effect of increased intra-abdominal pressure on mesenteric arterial and intestinal mucosal blood flow. J Trauma 33, 45-48.

38 Ishizaki, Y., Bandai, Y., Shimomura, K., et al. (1993) Safe intraabdominal pressure of carbon dioxide pneumoperitoneum during laparoscopic surgery. Surgery 114, 549-554.

39 Ishizaki, Y., Bandai, Y., Shimomura, K., et al. (1993) Changes in splanchnic blood flow and cardiovascular effects following peritoneal insufflation of carbon dioxide. Surg Endosc 7, 420-423.

40 Bongard, F., Pianim, N., Dubecz, S., et al. (1995) Adverse consequences of increased intra-abdominal pressure on bowel tissue. J Trauma 39, 519-525.

41 Harman, P.K., Kron, I.L., Mclachlan, H.D., et al. (1982) Elevated intra-abdominal pressure and renal function. Ann Surg 196, 594-597.

42 Mayhew, P.D., Pascoe, P.J., Kass, P.H., et al. (2013) Effects of pneumoperitoneum induced at various pressures on cardiorespiratory function and working space during laparoscopy in cats. Am J Vet Res 74, 1340-1346.

43 Abel, F.L., Pierce, J.H., Guntheroth, W.G. (1963) Baroreceptor influence on postural changes in blood pressure and carotid blood flow. Am J Physiol 285, 360-364.

44 Slinker, B.K., Campbell, K.B., Alexander, J.E., et al. (1982) Arterial baroreflex control of the heart rate in the horse, pig, and calf. Am J Vet Res 43, 1926-1933.

45 Kamine, T.H., Papavassiliou, E., Schneider, B.E. (2014) Effect of abdominal insufflation for laparoscopy on intracranial pressure. JAMA Surg 149, 380-382.

46 Obeid, F., Saba, A., Fath, J., et al. (1995) Increases in intra-abdominal pressure affect pulmonary compliance. Arch Surg 130, 544-547.

47 Oikkonen, M., Tallgren, M. (1995) Changes in respiratory compliance at laparoscopy: measurements using side stream spirometry. Can J Anaesth 42, 495-497.

48 Duke, T., Steinacher, S.L., Remedios, A.M. (1996) Cardiopulmonary effects of using carbon dioxide for laparoscopic surgery in dogs. Vet Surg 25, 77-82.

49 Liem, T., Applebaum, H., Herzberger, B. (1994) Hemodynamic and ventilatory effects of abdominal CO_2 insufflation at various pressures in the young swine. J Pediatr Surg 29, 966-969.

50 Gross, M.E., Jones, B.D., Bergstresser, D.R., et al. (1993) Effects of abdominal insufflation with nitrous oxide on cardiorespiratory measurements in spontaneously breathing isoflurane-anesthetized dogs. Am J Vet Res 54, 1352-1358.

51 Rademaker, B.M.P., Odoom, J.A., de Wit, L., et al. (1994) Haemodynamic effects of pneumoperitoneum for laparoscopic surgery: a comparison of CO_2 with N_2O insufflation. Eur J Anaesthesiol 11, 301-306.

52 Rademaker, B.M.P., Bannenberg, J.J.G., Kalkman, C.J., et al. (1995) Effects of pneumoperitoneum with helium on hemodynamics and oxygen transport: a comparison with carbon dioxide. J Laparoendosc Surg 5, 15-20.

53 Rammohan, A., Manimaran, A.B., Manohar, R.R. et al. (2011) Nitrous oxide for pneumoperitoneum: no laughing matter this! A prospective single blind case controlled study. Int J Surg 9, 173-176.

54 Fujii, Y., Tanaka, H., Tsuruoka, S., et al. (1994) Middle cerebral artery blood flow velocity increases during laparoscopic cholecystectomy. Anesth Analg 78, 80-83.

55 Schob, O.M., Allen, D.C., Benzel, E., et al. (1996) A comparison of the pathophysiologic effects of carbon dioxide, nitrous oxide, and helium pneumoperitoneum on intracranial pressure. Am J Surg 172, 248-253.

56 Huettemann, E., Terborg, C., Sakka, S.G., et al. (2002) Preserved CO(2) reactivity and increase in middle cerebral arterial blood flow velocity during laparoscopy surgery in children. Anesth Analg 94, 255-258.

57 Clowes, G.H.A. Jr, Kretchmer, H.E., McBurney, R.W., et al. (1953) The electroencephalogram in the evaluation of the effects of anesthetic agents and carbon dioxide accumulation during surgery. Ann Surg 138, 558-568.

58 Bailey, J.E., Pablo, L.S. (1999) Anesthetic and physiologic considerations for veterinary endosurgery. In: Freeman, L.J. (ed.) Veterinary Endosurgery. Mosby, St Louis, pp. 24-43.

59 Fahy, B.G., Barnas, G.M., Flowers, J.L., et al. (1995) The effects of increased abdominal pressure on lung and chest wall mechanics during laparoscopy surgery. Anesth Analg 81, 744-750.

60 Mutoh, T., Lamm, W.J.E., Embree, L.J., et al. (1991) Abdominal distension alters regional pleural pressures and chest wall mechanics in pigs in vivo. J Appl Physiol 70, 2611-2618.

61 Pelosi, P., Foti, G., Cereda, M., et al. (1996) Effects of carbon dioxide insufflation for laparoscopic cholecystectomy on the respiratory system. Anaesthesia 51, 744-749.

62 Peroni, J., Fischer, A.T. Jr. (1995) Effects of carbon dioxide insufflation and body position on blood gas values and cardiovascular parameters in the anesthetized horse undergoing laparoscopy. ACVS Veterinary Symposium 30, Chicago, Oct 29-Nov 1.

63 Kadono, Y., Yaegashi, H., Machioka, K., et al. (2013) Cardiovascular and respiratory effects of the degree of head-down angle during robot assisted laparoscopic radical prostatectomy. Int J Med Robotics Comput Assist Surg 9, 17-22.

64 Salihoglu, Z., Demiroluk, S., Cakmakkaya, S., et al. (2002) Influence of the patient positioning on respiratory mechanics during pneumoperitoneum. Middle East J Anesthesiol 16, 521-528.

65 Wahba, R.W., Mamazza, J. (1993) Ventilatory requirements during laparoscopic cholecystectomy. Can J Anaesth 40, 206-210.

66 Hofmeister, E., Peroni, J.F., Fisher, A. T. Jr. (2008) Effects of carbon dioxide insufflation and body position on blood gas values in horses anesthetized for laparoscopy. J Equine Vet Sci 28, 549-553.

67 Hardie, R.J., Flanders, J.A., Schmidt, P., et al. (1996) Biomechanical and histological evaluation of a laparoscopic stapled gastropexy technique in dogs. Vet Surg 25, 127-133.

68 Kim, Y.K., Park, S.J., Lee, S.Y., et al. (2013) Laparoscopic nephrectomy in dogs: an initial experience of 16 experimental procedures. Vet J 198, 513-517.

69 Mullet, C.E., Viale, J.P., Sagnard, P.E., et al. (1993) Pulmonary CO_2 elimination during surgical procedures using intra- or extraperitoneal CO_2 insufflation. Anesth Analg 76, 622-626.

70 Dehours, E., Valle, B., Bournes, V., et al. (2013) A pneumomediastinum with diffuse subcutaneous emphysema. J Emerg Med 44, e81-e82.

71 Philips, S., Falk, G.L. (2011) Surgical tension pneumothorax during laparoscopic repair of massive hiatus hernia: a different situation requiring different management. Anesth Intensive Care 39, 1120-1123.

72 Y, V.S., Suresh, Y.A., Sequeira, T.F. (2014) Laparoscopy-pneumothorax and ocular emphysema, a rare complication—a case report. J Clin Diagn Res 8, GD01-GD02.

73 Joris, J.L., Chiche, J.D., Lamy, M.L. (1995) Pneumothorax during laparoscopic fundoplication: diagnosis and treatment with positive end-expiratory pressure. Anesth Analg 81, 993-1000.

74 Ko, M.L. (2010) Pneumopericardium and severe subcutaneous emphysema after laparoscopic surgery. J Minim Invasive Gynecol 17, 531-533.

75 Knos, G.B., Sung, Y.F., Toledo, A. (1991) Pneumopericardium associated with laparoscopy. J Clin Anesth 3, 56-59.

76 Couture, P., Boudreault, D., Derouin, M., et al. (1994) Venous carbon dioxide embolism in pigs: an evaluation of end-tidal carbon dioxide, transesophageal echocardiography, pulmonary artery pressure, and precordial auscultation as monitoring modalities. Anesth Analg 79, 867-873.

77 Staffieri, F., Lacitignola, L., De Siena, R., et al. (2007) A case of spontaneous venous embolism with carbon dioxide during laparoscopic surgery in a pig. Vet Anesth Analg 34, 63-66.

78 Gilroy, B.A., Anson, L.W. (1987) Fatal air embolism during anesthesia for laparoscopy in a dog. J Am Vet Med Assoc 190, 552-554.

79 Lantz, P.E., Smith, J.D. (1994) Fatal carbon dioxide embolism complicating attempted laparoscopic cholecystectomy—case report and literature review. J Forensic Sci 39, 1468-1480.

80 Haroun-Bizri, S., ElRassi, T. (2001) Successful resuscitation after catastrophic carbon dioxide embolism during laparoscopic Cholecystectomy. Eur J Anaesthesiol 18, 118-121.

81 Hong, J.Y., Kim, W.O., Kil, H.K. (2010) Detection of subclinical CO_2 embolism by transesophageal echocardiography during laparoscopic radical prostatectomy. Urology 75, 581-584.

82 Kim, C.S., Kim, J.Y., Kwon, J.Y., et al. (2009) Venous air embolism during total laparoscopic hysterectomy. Anesthesiology 111, 50-54.

83 Schmandra, T.C., Mierdl, S., Bauer, H., et al. (2002) Transesophageal echocardiography shows high risk of gas embolism during laparoscopic hepatic resection under carbon dioxide pneumoperitoneum. Br J Surg 89, 870-876.

84 Derouin, M., Couture, P., Boudreault, D., et al. (1996) Detection of gas embolism by transesophageal echocardiography during laparoscopic cholecystectomy. Anesth Analg 82, 119-124.

85 Self-Education and Evaluation Program. (2010) ASA Safety Bulletin 74, 44.

8 Laparoscopic Access Techniques

Gilles Dupre

Key Points

- Single-port surgery provides a natural progression to a less invasive approach compared with the multiport platform.
- Single-port surgery can be achieved using an operating laparoscope but is more commonly performed using a variety of commercially available single-port devices.
- Articulating instruments can be used to offset the limitations on triangulation that are inherent to the single-port approach, although the use of rigid instrumentation is also possible.
- Single-port ovariectomy, gastropexy, intestinal biopsy, and cryptorchidectomy have been described in the veterinary literature, and many other procedures will be described using this approach in the future.

The first step in laparoscopic procedures is establishment of a working space. This is usually accomplished by insufflating carbon dioxide (CO_2) into the abdominal cavity to create capnoperitoneum. The first entry into the abdominal cavity is associated with higher risk than subsequent entries. Despite considerable progress in the performance of laparoscopic procedures in humans, major complications occur in about 1 of every 1000 patients during the first entry,[1] and half of these complications involve the colon. After the first entry has been achieved, additional instrument portals can be safely introduced under laparoscopic visualization.

Laparoscopic access can be described as open (following the performance of a mini-laparotomy), closed (no surgical access to the abdominal cavity), blind (no view of the abdominal cavity during entry), or visual (with the help of a telescope inserted through the port). Additionally, the first port can be inserted into an insufflated or noninsufflated abdomen.

Several techniques, instruments, and approaches have been introduced during the past few decades to minimize entry-related injuries in both human and veterinary surgery.[2,3] Nevertheless, meta-analyses and evidence-based reviews have failed to document systematic advantages of one technique over any other. Moreover, the results of such studies should be interpreted with caution because not all complications are reported, particularly minor complications, and the surgeon's preferences and expertise influence the results. In veterinary medicine, entry-related injuries

during either establishment of pneumoperitoneum or portal placement are very well described in textbooks,[4,5] but are relatively rare in clinical trials. We are aware of one clinical trial in the field of large animal medicine that examined the safety of various trocar placement techniques and identified problems with insufflation or cannula insertion in 12 of 40 horses.[6] Complications during access to the abdominal cavity have also been reported in a few clinical studies within the field of small animal medicine and include: subcutaneous emphysema,[3,7] fatal gas embolism,[8] and splenic injury.[3,9-11]

Because of the increase in the size of the canine spleen during general anesthesia, splenic injury is one of the most commonly encountered serious access injuries that may warrant conversion. Therefore, caution is required when using human data for small animal patients because abdominal anatomy, body size, and abdominal wall elasticity and resistance differ greatly between small animals and humans. This is also true when comparing a 3-kg cat with an 80-kg Great Dane.

Finally, most currently available abdominal access devices are designed for use in human patients, in whom an intraabdominal free space is known to exist. This fact should also be taken into account when using these devices in small animals, in which such a free space is sometimes almost nonexistent.

For the above-mentioned reasons, it is necessary to (1) describe the most commonly used abdominal access techniques in both

---

Small Animal Laparoscopy and Thoracoscopy, First Edition. Edited by Boel A. Fransson and Philipp D. Mayhew.
© 2015 by ACVS Foundation. Published 2015 by John Wiley & Sons, Inc.
Companion website: www.wiley.com/go/fransson/laparoscopy

veterinary and human surgery and (2) discuss the most clinically important aspects of laparoscopic access in small animal surgery based on both current studies and personal experience.

Necessary Considerations Before Laparoscopic Access

Physics of Entry

The various aspects of different laparoscopic access techniques can be grouped under the acronym MIS: M, method (blind vs. open); I, access instrument (push vs. pull trocar); and S, access site (umbilical, retrocostal, or other). Regardless of the method, instrument, and site used for abdominal access, the surgeon must carefully consider the tissue layers to be traversed, the instrument design, and the penetration force.[12] Most surgeons hold a conventional trocar and cannula assembly with the dominant hand and apply significant linear force generated by the shoulder and trunk muscles toward the body part being accessed. This linear propulsion dictates that the instrument design involves a pointed or sharp end to decrease the entry force necessary to transect the different tissue layers during port placement.[13] Additionally, when the peritoneal layer has been transfixed, a sudden loss of resistance is registered. A more sudden and uncontrolled loss of resistance induces a greater extent of trocar overshoot and hence a greater likelihood of inadvertent injury.

Peritoneal Tenting and Curtain Effect

The trocar type, trocar or Veress needle (VN) handling technique, and local anatomic characteristics of the patient can contribute to displacement of the peritoneum during abdominal entry. This effect, known as peritoneal tenting or the curtain effect, can have deleterious consequences if the trocar or VN is inadvertently advanced to a deep subperitoneal location without reaching the intraabdominal cavity.

Relevant Anatomic Knowledge

The first access, whether blind or open, should be performed in an area with low tissue resistance to limit the linear force necessary for entry into the abdominal cavity. Thus, in both human and small animal laparoscopic techniques, the first entry is generally performed along the linea alba in the periumbilical region. Use of this location also guarantees that abdominal wall vessels will not be encountered during penetration. Although the placement of ports for various instruments is considered to be essential, no consensus on trocar–cannula assembly placement, even for the same procedures, has been reached. The explanations of port location among various studies are often vague and leave substantial room for error, especially in the hands of novice surgeons. This was illustrated in one study in which the performance of two different trocar placement techniques described in the veterinary literature was tested among 64 students in their final year of veterinary medical school. Correct placement was achieved by only 40.8% of the students. In contrast, after introducing a mapping system (a coordinate system of the abdominal wall), correct placement was achieved by 95% of the students. These findings support the need for development of an accurate system with which to adequately locate the ports.[14]

Trocar and Cannula Design

A trocar is a pen-shaped instrument with a sharp triangular point at one end. This pointed end is typically located within a hollow tube, known as a cannula, and is used to create an opening into the body through which the cannula may be introduced. This process provides a surgical access port. Such devices have been in use for thousands of years. A gas-tight valve is usually located at the top of the trocar to allow for insertion and removal of instruments during a procedure without permitting escape of the insufflated CO_2. The appearance of the pointed pyramidal tip can differ; the outer diameter typically ranges from approximately 2 to 15 mm but may even reach several centimeters for placement of specialized instruments such as staplers or tissue morcellators. The trocar may also have either a blunt or cutting tip (bladed trocar). Bladed trocars reduce the amount of force needed to pass the instrument through the abdominal wall. For increased safety, some designs include a spring-loaded plastic shield that automatically covers the blade as it enters the abdominal cavity. The use of these spring-loaded safety shields is generally recommended in veterinary medicine because the distance between the abdominal wall and the spleen, aorta, or other large vessels is relatively small in veterinary patients. Conical tips can be either metal or plastic and require the creation of a small initial incision using a scalpel. They pass through the tissues of the abdominal wall by stretching rather than cutting the tissues. This leads to improved sleeve retention. However, both blunt and conical tips require a higher linear force to enter the abdomen.

Trocar–cannula assemblies may be for single-patient-use, reusable, or a hybrid. Reusable trocars and cannulae, or those with reusable components, may be the most economical choice for veterinary clinical practice. However, many veterinary practitioners who perform minimally invasive procedures currently reprocess and sterilize laparoscopic instruments, including trocars and cannulae, for reuse.[15]

Closed-Entry Techniques (Blind)

Capnoperitoneum can be achieved for subsequent abdominal entry in several different ways. In blind-entry techniques, the structures located behind the peritoneum cannot be visualized. Such techniques are performed by first inserting either a VN or trocar (direct trocar insertion [DTI]) to establish pneumoperitoneum. Among the 35 clinical studies published in veterinary medicine, Fiorbianco *et al.* identified 17 blind entries (VN insertion, $n = 15$; DTI, $n = 2$) and 19 open methods (most of which were not precisely described).[3]

Blind Abdominal Access Using a Veress Needle Followed by Blind Trocar Insertion

Use of a Veress Needle to Establish Pneumoperitoneum

The VN was developed by Janos Veress in 1938 to achieve safer access during establishment of therapeutic pneumothorax in the treatment of tuberculosis. In 1947, Raoul Palmer popularized the use of the VN using CO_2 to induce pneumoperitoneum for laparoscopy; he subsequently published a report on its safety in the first 250 patients in which it was used.[16] The VN is a long needle with a blunt, hollow, spring-loaded trocar in its center. The blunt trocar springs back through the resistance of the abdominal wall and springs out again when the resistance disappears, thus protecting the viscera from the sharp tip of the needle (Figure 8-1). Gas flows through the hollow trocar to create the initial pneumoperitoneum. VNs may be reusable or disposable. A recent study compared 13 different VNs and found significant differences in the spring constant (compressive force of the spring), final force (force required to depress the stylet to release the cutting envelope), and axis intercept (preload of the spring) (P.J. Schramel, A. Kindslehner, G. Dupré, unpublished data). In addition to the bevel

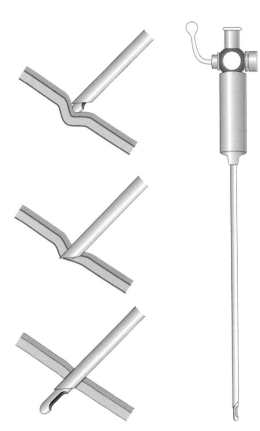

Figure 8-1 When the Veress needle (VN) is used to achieve abdominal access, the blunt trocar springs back through the resistance of the abdominal wall and springs out again when the resistance disappears, thus protecting the viscera from the sharp tip of the needle. The double-click test is one of the most important VN placement tests. It ensures that the needle adequately passed through the peritoneal layer.

sharpness, these three parameters have a significant influence on peritoneal displacement when the needle passes through the abdominal wall. Therefore, further studies are required to document which type of needle induces the least amount of peritoneal tenting (Figure 8-2).

Holding and Manipulating the Veress Needle
The VN is grasped by the hub during its insertion, thus allowing for retraction of the blunt inner stylet. Several placement techniques have been described (see later discussion); regardless of the technique used,

A
B

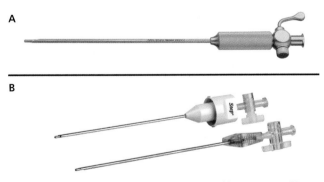

Figure 8-2 Veress needles (VNs) come in a variety of forms. **A**, Reusable VN (Karl Storz Veterinary Endoscopy, Goleta, CA). **B**, Single-use VN (Covidien Inc., Mansfield, MA). Many factors influence the amount of peritoneal tenting generated by VNs. Among them, the sharpness of the trocar and the spring resistance are of upmost importance.

the tip of the needle should be maintained at a safe distance from any underlying abdominal organs. Additionally, depending on the resistance of the spring, different forces may be needed to penetrate the thick muscular layer of the abdominal wall. Uncontrolled and deep penetration must be avoided. A 1-mm skin incision is performed at the selected site, and forceps are used to lift and tent the abdominal wall. The VN is then inserted in a caudal direction at an angle to the skin, thus avoiding the spleen and falciform ligament. Other measures directed at minimizing the risk of iatrogenic organ damage include placing the animal with its head slightly lower than the hind legs (Trendelenburg position) and resting the heel of the surgeon's nondominant hand on the patient's abdominal wall to control the needle entry. After insertion of the VN and conduction of placement tests (see later), the needle is gently swept in a circular pattern against the abdominal wall, freeing it from any adhesions or omentum.

Veress Needle Entrance Location
In humans, the VN is usually inserted into the periumbilical area with or without elevation of the anterior abdominal wall.[17,18] Insertion into the left upper quadrant (Palmer's point) has been suggested as an alternative to the periumbilical approach to reduce the risk of penetrating injuries in patients with periumbilical adhesions.[16] In small animals, on the other hand, several sites have been reported and are largely based on the surgeon's preference. However, the VN is usually inserted either caudal or caudolateral to the umbilicus, where the abdominal wall is consistently thin.[4,17] In an effort to reduce the risk of injuries during blind access, some authors have evaluated the regions of the body with the least contact with the underlying abdominal organs when the patient is placed in dorsal recumbency.[17] In one canine cadaver study, intercostal placement of the VN has been evaluated, and the right ninth intercostal space was associated with the lowest number of organ penetrations after VN insertion.[17] Another study performed on canine patients[3] suggested that VN insertion through the last palpable intercostal space with the dog positioned in dorsal recumbency is safe and likely to result in less frequent falciform ligament penetration than other locations. This insertion point offers the advantages of resistance of the rib cage during insertion and being located a safe distance from the spleen and intestines, thus minimizing the risk of damage. This is the author's method of choice whenever the abdominal cavity is blindly accessed using a VN (Fig-

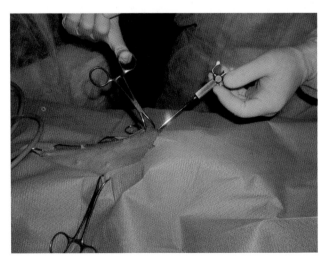

Figure 8-3 Intercostal placement of a Veress needle.

ure 8-3). In humans, pneumoperitoneum has also been established by inserting a long VN through the fundus of the uterus.[2]

After correct placement of the needle has been confirmed, pneumoperitoneum is established by slowly insufflating the abdominal cavity. The author recommends the use of an intraabdominal pressure of 12 mm Hg in dogs and 8 to 10 mm Hg in cats before insertion of the first port; after the first port has been placed, the pressure can be reduced to 8 to 10 mm Hg in dogs and 6 to 8 mm Hg in cats. Overdistension should be avoided because it leads to decreased venous return and impaired ventilation.

Verification of Appropriate Intraabdominal Veress Needle Placement

Correct placement of the VN is extremely important because placement into an organ, vessel, or mass may cause hemorrhage, which may interfere with visualization or result in fatal embolism or peritonitis. Several tests can be conducted to ensure appropriate placement of the VN.

Double-Click Test

Passage of the VN through the different layers of the abdominal wall creates an audible double click. The first click occurs as the VN passes through the rectus abdominis, and the second occurs as it passes through the peritoneum (see Figure 8-1).

Aspiration Test

In the aspiration test, a 2- to 5-mL syringe is attached to the hub of the VN, and the plunger of the syringe is pulled back. If the needle is correctly positioned, no fluid or other material should be aspirated. Aspiration of blood or bowel contents warrants repositioning of the needle.

Injection Test

This test involves injection of saline into the peritoneal cavity. Injection of saline without resistance indicates that the VN is correctly positioned. Obtaining saline on aspiration indicates that fluid has been trapped in an inappropriate location and warrants repositioning of the VN.

Hanging-Drop Test

In the hanging-drop test, a drop of saline is placed into the hub of the needle, and the abdominal wall is tented. If the needle is properly positioned within the peritoneal cavity, the negative pressure within the abdominal cavity aspirates the drop into the needle hub.

Intraabdominal Pressure Test

If the intraabdominal pressure (measured on the mechanical insufflator) increases dramatically or if the flow rate is close to zero, the needle tip is likely to be occluded because of placement against a viscus, within the omentum, or in a subcutaneous location. In such cases, the needle should be gently manipulated in and out of the abdomen to dislodge the occlusion, avoiding lateral movements to prevent injury to nearby structures. If the pressure remains elevated, the needle must be replaced.

Misplacement of the Veress Needle

The needle can be incorrectly placed into the subcutaneous tissue, omentum, falciform ligament, liver, or spleen (Video Clip 8-1). Subcutaneous placement results in subcutaneous emphysema, which greatly increases the difficulty of the procedure.

Subcutaneous emphysema resolves in approximately 48 hours. Similarly, insufflation of CO_2 below the omentum or within the falciform ligament causes expansion of these structures and consequent obstruction of the field of view. In one human study, the VN was adequately placed in the peritoneal cavity in 85% to 86% of cases.[18] In a prospective study involving intercostal placement of the VN in dogs, pneumoperitoneum was successfully established by VN insertion in 49 (88%) dogs after one (45 dogs) or two attempts (4 dogs).[3]

Blind Trocar Insertion After Establishment of Pneumoperitoneum

After insufflation of the abdominal cavity, the laparoscopic access site is chosen. The optimal site in small animals is usually on the midline or in the subumbilical region. A skin and subcutaneous tissue incision of adequate size for trocar insertion is then created. Whereas an excessively large incision will result in gas leakage and dislodgement of the cannula, an excessively small incision increases the force required to penetrate the abdominal wall, thus causing the trocar tip to get too close to the viscera. A hemostat can be used to bluntly separate the muscle layers. The trocar–cannula assembly is passed through the abdominal wall with a controlled thrusting–twisting motion of the hand and wrist while directing it caudally and to the right to avoid the spleen. The upper end of the cannula is held firmly against the heel of the hand. After abdominal penetration, the trocar is removed, the scope is introduced, and the abdominal viscera are evaluated for trauma. The CO_2 hose from the insufflator is connected to the Luer-lock stopcock of the cannula, and the VN is removed.

Access Through Direct Trocar Insertion

Dingfelder was the first to describe the use of a trocar for direct entry into the abdominal cavity.[19] The suggested advantage of this method of entry is the avoidance of VN-related complications, including failed pneumoperitoneum, preperitoneal insufflation, intestinal insufflation, and the more serious CO_2 embolism. Laparoscopic entry is initiated with only one blind step (trocar) instead of three (VN, insufflation, trocar). Direct entry is a more rapid technique than any other method of entry; however, it is reportedly one of the least frequently performed laparoscopic techniques in clinical practice today.[20]

The technique begins with the creation of a skin incision wide enough to accommodate the diameter of a sharp-tipped trocar–cannula assembly. In humans, the anterior abdominal wall must be adequately elevated by hand; the trocar is then inserted directly into the cavity, aiming toward the pelvic hollow. Alternatively, the abdominal wall is elevated by pulling on two towel clips placed 3 cm from each side of the umbilicus, and the trocar is then inserted at a 90-degree angle. Upon removal of the sharp trocar, the laparoscope is inserted to confirm the presence of omentum or bowel within the field of view. The following factors are considered to be critical for safe performance of DTI in humans: complete relaxation, a sharp trocar, a skin incision large enough to avoid undue skin resistance, and adequate elevation of the abdominal wall.

Several points must be considered before extrapolating human data to the performance of DTI in small animals. The distance between the abdominal wall and underlying organs or vessels is dependent on the patient's body size, but may be very small. In commercially available trocar–cannula assemblies, the distance between the extremity of the cannula and the tip of the bevel of the

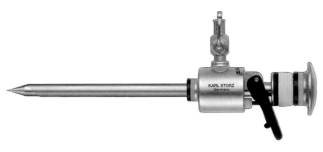

Figure 8-4 In some commercially available ports, the distance between the extremity of the trocar and the bevel of the cannula might be too long to ensure a safe entry in small animals with shallow abdomens. (© 2014 Photo Courtesy of KARL STORZ GmbH & Co. KG.)

trocar can be so long that the sharp end of the trocar may come into contact with the spleen, intestine, or large vessels even though the cannula has not yet entered the abdomen (Figure 8-4). Lifting the abdominal wall along with the peritoneum may be difficult, especially in small patients.

For the above-mentioned reasons, DTI should only be performed in small animals with an adequately large body size and only when the abdominal wall can be lifted either by hand or stay sutures. Ports with retractable trocar blades, plastic blades, and very short bevels are generally preferred (Figure 8-5). Because of the potential risks associated with closed entry. open access is often preferred in small animals.

Open-Entry Techniques

Open Laparoscopic Entry (Hasson Technique)

The open technique to establish pneumoperitoneum was first devised by Hasson in 1971.[21] This technique is suggested to prevent gas embolism, preperitoneal insufflation, and possibly visceral and major vascular injury. The technique involves the use of a cannula fitted with a cone-shaped sleeve, a blunt-tipped trocar, and sometimes a second sleeve to which stay sutures can be attached (Figure 8-6). Abdominal entry is essentially accomplished by performing a mini-laparotomy. In small animals, a small transverse or longitudinal incision is made at the umbilicus or in the subumbilical region. This incision should be long enough to allow for dissection down to the fascia, incision of the fascia, dissection of the rectus abdominis fibers, identification of the peritoneum, and entrance into the peritoneal cavity under

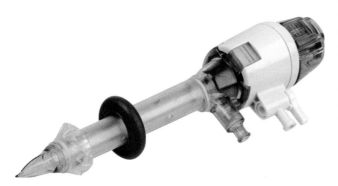

Figure 8-5 Cannula design compatible with use in small patients. A very short bevel or a very short distance between the tip of the trocar and the bevel of the cannula ensures a safer placement of the trocar.

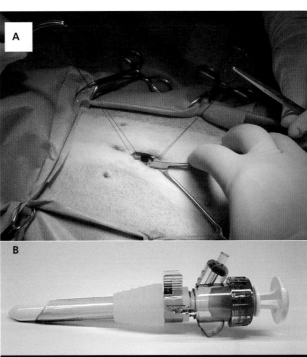

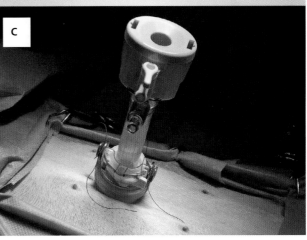

Figure 8-6 Open placement with the Hasson technique. **A,** Dissection of the abdominal wall. **B,** The Hasson cannula. **C,** The Hasson cannula in place fixed with stay sutures.

direct visualization. The cannula is inserted into the peritoneal cavity with the blunt trocar in place. Sutures are placed in the fascia on either side of the cannula and attached to the cannula to seal the abdominal wall incision to the cone-shaped sleeve. The laparoscope is then introduced, and insufflation is commenced.

The modified Hasson technique is an open technique in which a normal trocar is inserted. The absence of a cone-shaped sleeve increases the risk of CO_2 leakage around the cannula and subsequent subcutaneous emphysema due to gas leaking through the relatively large incision.

Visual Entry Techniques

Optical-access trocars were introduced in 1994 to limit the risk of inadvertent organ injury.[2] Several disposable visual entry systems that retain the use of a conventional but translucent trocar and cannula push-through design are available, including the Endopath

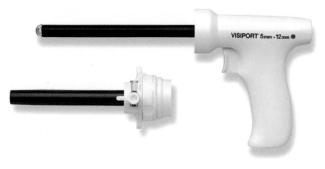

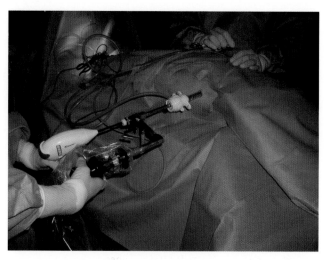

Figure 8-8 Single-port-single Instrument surgery. In this technique (here a laparoscopic ovariectomy), the instrument is introduced into the working channel of the operating laparoscope (Karl STORZ Endoscopy, Tuttlingen, Germany).

Optiview optical trocar (Ethicon Endo-Surgery, Cincinnati, OH), the VisiPort optical trocar, (Figure 8-7, Covidien/Medtronic, Salem, CT), and the Kii Balloon and Kii access system (Applied Medical, Rancho Santa Margarita, CA). A zero-degree laparoscope is loaded into these single-use visual trocars and transmits real-time monitor images while transecting the tissue layers of the abdominal wall. Application of these systems recruits significant axial thrust through the surgeon's dominant upper body muscles to transect the myofascial layers of the abdominal wall.

In contrast, the endoscopic threaded imaging port EndoTIP (Karl Storz Veterinary Endoscopy, Goleta, CA) is a reusable visual cannula system that allows for push-force reduction (see Chapter 4, Figure 4-21).[12] It comprises a stainless steel threaded cannula and is designed for use without a trocar. In the technique originally described by Ternamian, the EndoTIP is inserted after capnoperitoneum has been established with a VN. A skin and fascial incision is made under direct visualization. The surgeon rotates the cannula clockwise while the notched tip of the cannula engages the fascial window and stretches it radially. Downward axial pressure during rotation is minimized. The rectus abdominis fascia, rectus muscle, and transparent grayish peritoneal membrane are all observed sequentially.[1] One other advantage of the EndoTIP system is the lack of vertical displacement of the trocar because of its screw threads. Some veterinarians use EndoTIP cannulas without first performing insufflation and either with or without the laparoscope placed within the cannula to perform the first entry into the abdominal cavity. Data on the safety and efficacy of this access technique are lacking.

Closed Access, Open Access, and Direct Trocar Insertion: Evidence of Efficacy

A group of authors performed a meta-analysis of 28 randomized controlled trials involving 4860 individuals undergoing laparoscopy and evaluated 14 different parameters to compare the different laparoscopic entry techniques.[22] No single technique exhibited any advantages in terms of preventing major vascular or visceral complications. However, lower rates of failed entry, extraperitoneal insufflation, and omental injury were seen with DTI than with VN entry. Fewer failed entries and no increase in the complication rate were seen when the abdominal wall was not lifted before VN insertion than when it was lifted. These findings are supported by another meta-analysis suggesting that the commonly used VN entry technique is associated with a substantial risk of minor com-

plications[23] as well as by a previous study of intercostal VN insertion in small animals.[17] The lack of statistically significant differences in the incidence of major vascular and visceral injury among different entry techniques may be explained by the low rate of reported complications associated with laparoscopic entry and the small number of participants within the included studies.

In veterinary medicine, the results of these various studies should be interpreted with caution because outcomes of human studies cannot necessarily be applied to small animals. In addition, clinicians must also remember that splenic dilation in small animals under general anesthesia is specific to the veterinary setting and does not seem to be clinically relevant in humans.

Single-Access Surgery

Transition from multiple- to single-port surgery is the next step after completion of the initial transition from open to laparoscopic surgery because studies in humans have shown that single-port approaches minimize soft tissue trauma and improve the cosmetic outcome.[24]

Single-port surgery can be performed using either an operating laparoscope or commercially available single-port devices. The operating laparoscope is generally a 10-mm device and is therefore placed through a regular cannula capable of accepting 10-mm instrumentation (Figure 8-8). Single-port devices allow several instruments and the laparoscope to enter the abdominal cavity through a single port that is generally placed through a 2- to 3-cm open laparotomy incision. Thus, obtaining abdominal access using these devices is usually simpler than when access is performed using a VN or open technique. Greater discussion of single-port laparoscopic surgery can be found in Chapter 6.

Natural orifice transluminal endoscopic surgery was recently introduced as a method of reaching the peritoneal cavity through the wall of the stomach. However, the term *natural orifice surgery* is now more widely used because it encompasses transvaginal, transgastric, and even transanal approaches. In small animals, the learning curve for laparoscopic ovariectomy performed by natural orifice transluminal endoscopic surgery has been evaluated[25] and warrants further work before being routinely applied in practice. Further discussion of natural orifice surgery can be found in Chapter 28.

As procedures become more advanced, additional innovative features are incorporated into trocar and instrument designs.[15] For instance, intelligent visual trocars in which the length adapts to the size of the abdominal wall have recently been developed (AnchorPort; SurgiQuest, Orange, CT).

On the other hand, because of the costs of single-port platforms and single-use instruments, alternative innovative techniques that combine medical and "hand-made" devices are currently being investigated in developing countries[26] and could become interesting for the veterinary market.

Conclusion

Abdominal access is the first and among the most important steps in laparoscopic surgery. Although misplacement of a VN might prolong the duration of surgery or lead to minor complications, erroneous DTI can have disastrous consequences and requires prompt conversion. No rational guidelines regarding where to place the additional ports have been published; thus, placement is often extrapolated from expert opinions. Although the morbidity associated with laparoscopic access is relatively low, there is a need for adequate, evidence-based descriptions of abdominal access in laparoscopic surgery that will be applicable in all animals from 2-kg cats to 80-kg Great Danes. This step is necessary for further development of laparoscopic surgery in small animals.

 All videos cited in this chapter can be found on the book's companion website at **www.wiley.com/go/fransson/ laparoscopy**

References

1 Ternamian, A.M. (2001) How to improve laparoscopic access safety: ENDOTIP. Minim Invasive Ther Allied Technol 10, 31-39.
2 Merdan, I. (2013) Laparoscopic entry: a review of techniques, technologies, and complications. Bas J Surg 19;10-23.
3 Fiorbianco, V., Skalicky, M., Doerner, J., et al. (2012) Right intercostal insertion of a Veress needle for laparoscopy in dogs. Vet Surg 41, 367-373.
4 Freeman, L.J. (1999) Veterinary Endosurgery. Mosby, St. Louis.
5 Bonath, K.H., Kramer, M. (2014) Kleintierkrankheiten 2: Minimal-invasive Chirurgie. In: Bonath, KH [Hrsg.]: Kleintierkrankheiten: Chirurgie der Weichteile, 2nd edn. Ulmer, Stuttgart, pp. 552-580.
6 Desmaizières, L.-M., Martinot, S., Lepage, O.M., et al. (2003) Complications associated with cannula insertion techniques used for laparoscopy in standing horses. Vet Surg 32, 501.
7 Nickel, R., Stürtzbecher, N., Kilian, H., et al. (2007) Postoperative Rekonvaleszenz nach laparoskopischer und konventioneller Ovariektomie: eine vergleichende Studie. Kleintierpraxis 52, 413-424.
8 Gilroy, B.A., Anson, L.W. (1987) Fatal air embolism during anesthesia for laparoscopy in a dog. J Am Vet Med Assoc 190, 552-554.
9 Dupré, G., Fiorbianco, V., Skalicky, M., et al. (2009) Laparoscopic ovariectomy in dogs: comparison between single portal and two-portal access. Vet Surg 38, 818-824.
10 Mayhew, P.D., Brown, D.C. (2007) Comparison of three techniques for ovarian pedicle hemostasis during laparoscopic-assisted ovariohysterectomy. Vet Surg 36, 541-547.
11 Davidson, E.B., Moll, H.D., Payton, M.E. (2004) Comparison of laparoscopic ovariohysterectomy and ovariohysterectomy in dogs. Vet Surg 33, 62-69.
12 Ternamian, A.M. (1997) Laparoscopy without trocars. Surg Endosc 11, 81581-8.
13 Corson, S.L., Batzer, F.R., Gocial, B., et al. (1989) Measurement of the force necessary for laparoscopic trocar entry. J Reprod Med 34, 282-284.
14 Katic, N., Katic, C., Dupre, G.P. (2014, May) Development and preclinical application of a mapping system (LAPMAP) for portal placement in laparoscopic surgery. Proceedings of the 11th Veterinary Endoscopy Society meeting, Florence, Italy.
15 Van Lue, S.J., Van Lue, A.P. (2009) Equipment and Instrumentation in veterinary endoscopy. Vet Clin North Am Small Animal Pract 39, 817-837.
16 Palmer, R. (1974) Safety in laparoscopy. J Reprod Med 13, 1-5.
17 Doerner, J., Fiorbianco, V., Dupré, G. (2012) Intercostal insertion of Veress needle for canine laparoscopic procedures: a cadaver study. Vet Surg 41, 362-366.
18 Hudelist, G., Keckstein, J. (2011) Surgical technique of traditional laparoscopic access. In: Tinelli, A. (ed.). Laparoscopic Entry. Springer, London, pp. 19-32.
19 Dingfelder, J.R. (1978) Direct laparoscope trocar insertion without prior pneumoperitoneum. J Reprod Med 21, 45-47.
20 Molloy, D., Kaloo, P.D., Cooper, M., et al. (2002) Laparoscopic entry: a literature review and analysis of techniques and complications of primary port entry. Aust NZ J Obstet Gynaecol 42, 246-254.
21 Hasson, H.M. (1971) A modified instrument and method for laparoscopy. Am J Obstet Gynecol 110, 886-887.
22 Ahmad, G., O'Flynn, H., Duffy, J.M.N., et al. (2012) Laparoscopic entry techniques. Cochrane Database Syst Rev 2, CD006583.
23 Jiang, X., Anderson, C., Schnatz, P.F. (2012) The safety of direct trocar versus Veress needle for laparoscopic entry: a meta-analysis of randomized clinical trials. J Laparoendosc Adv Surg Tech A 22, 362-370.
24 Kommu, S.S., Rané, A. (2009) Devices for laparoendoscopic single-site surgery in urology. Expert Rev Med Devices 6, 95-103.
25 Freeman, L., Rahmani, E.Y., Burgess, R.C.F., et al. (2011) Evaluation of the learning curve for natural orifice transluminal endoscopic surgery: bilateral ovariectomy in dogs. Vet Surg 40, 140-150.
26 Khiangte, E., Newme, I., Phukan, P., et al. (2011) Improvised transumbilical glove port: a cost effective method for single port laparoscopic surgery. Indian J Surg 73, 142-145.

9 The Laparoscopic Working Space: Pneumoperitoneum Techniques and Patient Positioning

Boel A. Fransson

Key Points

- Carbon dioxide (CO_2) is the most commonly used gas for pneumoperitoneum and is considered safe compared with other gases, such as nitrous oxide, nitrogen, helium, and argon, but CO_2 gets systemically absorbed.
- Gasless laparoscopy by abdominal wall lift devices circumvent the physiological changes of capnoperitoneum but provide a smaller working field.
- Patient positioning entails gravitational effect of organs in order to increase intraabdominal visualization and is imperative for surgical success.

The first steps in laparoscopic surgery are to enter the abdominal cavity and to create a working space for visualization and instrument manipulation. Most commonly, the latter is accomplished by gas insufflation at positive pressures, creating a pneumoperitoneum. These initial steps in the surgical procedure are imperative for the success of the surgery, and both carry a significant risk for morbidity and even mortality. Fortunately, serious complications to laparoscopic surgery are uncommon in humans[1] and animals.[2] However, entry of the abdomen has been recognized as the most common cause of serious laparoscopic complications in humans, including bowel and abdominal vessel perforation.[3] The fatal outcome from an entry-related splenic puncture with resulting air embolism was reported in a dog.[4] The complication rate of laparoscopic entry has not been prospectively studied in small animals. A review of the veterinary literature noted that of 36 reports in dogs and cats, only 7 had entry technique complications, for a total of 30 of 749 procedures (4%) entry technique complication rate.[5] The retrospective nature of the included reports was noted to likely severely underestimate the true rate of entry technique complications. In horses, 30% were shown to experience insufflation or cannula insertion problems,[6] including peritoneal detachment, splenic puncture, and bowel perforation. The complication rates relating to the pneumoperitoneum are unknown in small animal surgery.

In addition, even with uncomplicated abdominal entry, gas insufflation is associated with morbidity, which the veterinary laparoscopic surgeon needs to be aware of and take in consideration in the case selection for laparoscopic procedures.

The Pneumoperitoneum

After successful entry into the abdominal cavity (see Chapter 8), the pneumoperitoneum provides the visual field. The pneumoperitoneum can be hyperbaric (higher than atmospheric pressure); resulting from gas insufflation (Figure 9-1). Pneumoperitoneum can also consist of isobaric room air. The latter is a result of gasless, or lift, laparoscopy (Figure 9-2). The physiological effects on the patients vary with the gas type and pressure of the pneumoperitoneum.

Gas Types for Hyperbaric Pneumoperitoneum

Carbon dioxide (CO_2) is by far the most commonly used gas for pneumoperitoneum because it is safe and inexpensive, but it is not the perfect gas. The absorption of CO_2 causes hypercapnia and acidosis, which have to be avoided by hyperventilation.[7] Various cardiopulmonary complications (i.e., tachycardia, cardiac arrhythmias, and pulmonary edema) and postoperative pain from peritoneal irritation are among the adverse effects of capnoperitoneum.[7] Other gases such as helium (He), argon (Ar), nitrogen (N_2), and nitrous oxide (N_2O, or laughing gas) have been introduced as alternatives to capnoperitoneum. Helium and argon are inert gases but are less soluble than CO_2 and may increase the risk for venous gas embolism. Although helium pneumoperitoneum has been reported

Small Animal Laparoscopy and Thoracoscopy, First Edition. Edited by Boel A. Fransson and Philipp D. Mayhew.

© 2015 by ACVS Foundation. Published 2015 by John Wiley & Sons, Inc.

Companion website: www.wiley.com/go/fransson/laparoscopy

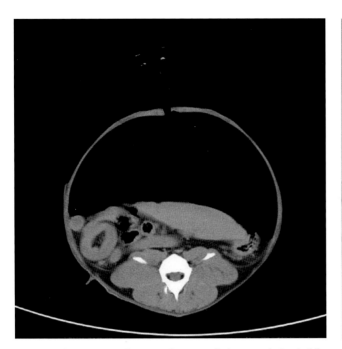

Figure 9-1 A transsectional computed tomography image at the level of the umbilical cannula (radiolucent) of a dog with a 12–mm Hg capnoperitoneum. The abdomen assumes a dome-like shape with a large field for laparoscopic visualization. However, the intraabdominal pressure is affecting organ perfusion and pulmonary compliance.

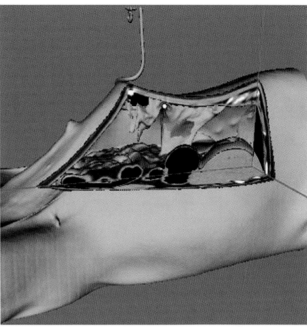

Figure 9-2 Lift laparoscopy in a computed tomography reconstructed image of a dog. A lift device is applied at the umbilicus and tents up the body wall to provide an isobaric pneumoperitoneum, formed by room air gaining entrance into the abdomen. The visual field is smaller compared with capnoperitoneum, but the avoidance of pressurized capnoperitoneum, requiring an airtight seal, may be advantageous in select cases.

to decrease cardiopulmonary effects compared with capnoperitoneum, the safety of its use has not been established.[7] N_2O is a mild anesthetic and was shown to reduce postoperative pain, but N_2O is flammable and have caused explosions associated with electrocautery during laparoscopy.[7] Gases other than helium and N_2O have not been compared with capnoperitoneum in clinical trials in humans.

Early in the history of small animal laparoscopy, N_2O was the preferred gas for diagnostic laparoscopy,[8] and it was noted that this gas enabled laparoscopy under local anesthesia, in contrast to CO_2, which was associated with peritoneal irritation. Capnoperitoneum in dogs leads to decreased peritoneal fluid pH,[9] which has been suggested as one of the reasons for irritation.[10] Attempts to improve removal of residual CO_2 by aspiration, abdominal compression, and other maneuvers have been demonstrated to decrease postoperative pain in humans.[11-13]

Pressure Effects of Pneumoperitoneum

Regardless of the gas used for pneumoperitoneum, the pressurized pneumoperitoneum will exert effects on physiological parameters. Increased heart rate, increased systemic vascular resistance, increased arterial and central venous pressures, and decreased pulmonary compliance have been reported in humans, dogs, and horses with pressurized pneumoperitoneum.[14-17] These effects can be severe in dogs, especially when the intraabdominal pressures exceeds 15 mm Hg.[16] These negative effects are most pronounced during induction, and healthy dogs compensate well,[18] but patients with cardiopulmonary compromise may not be able to compensate to the same extent.

In addition to cardiopulmonary effects, pressures of 12 to 14 mm Hg may have clinically relevant negative effects on intraabdominal organ perfusion, especially the renal flow in patients with already impaired perfusion.[19] In healthy dogs, hepatic and intestinal perfusion changes associated with high intraabdominal pressures (15–16 mm Hg) lead to increased blood levels of hepatic enzymes and evidence of bacterial translocation.[20,21]

The intracranial pressure (ICP) increases by elevations in intraabdominal pressure and by the Trendelenburg position.[19] The hypercapnia associated with capnoperitoneum may further exacerbate ICP elevation. Therefore, standard or high-pressure capnoperitoneum should likely be avoided in small animals with head injury or neurological disorders.

A Cochrane systematic review evaluated the effects of low pneumoperitoneum pressure (<12 mm Hg) compared to standard pressure (12–16 mm Hg) in humans, with the main finding of decreased postoperative pain in the low-pressure group.[22] Previous clinical guidelines have stated that gasless or low-pressure laparoscopy should be considered in patients with limited cardiac function and that in general, the lowest possible pressure allowing adequate exposure should be used rather than a routine pressure.[19]

A decade ago, capnoperitoneum pressures of 12 mm Hg were generally recommended in small animals, but more recent work appears to advocate pressures of 8 to 10 mm Hg. Evidence-based recommendations are lacking. The practical clinical guideline to use the lowest possible pressure allowing adequate exposure[19] seems appropriate also in small animals.

Gasless Laparoscopy

Abdominal wall lift laparoscopy was developed to circumvent the physiological changes of capnoperitoneum. During abdominal wall lift laparoscopy, the abdominal cavity is not pressurized, but air gains entrance through the ports and creates an isobaric pneumoperitoneum, which allows working space for the laparoscopic instrumentation. The advantages of gasless laparoscopy include absence of adverse cardiovascular hemodynamic changes, hypercapnia, and adrenergic response associated with pressurized capnoperitoneum in humans.[17] These advantages have made gasless lift laparoscopy indicated for surgery in compromised patients,[19] including abdominal trauma victims.[23]

Disadvantages include that the lifting creates a tenting effect, in contrast to the dome shape of the pressurized abdomen, which is associated with a reduction in the working space in the abdomen.[24] A device for lift laparoscopy, the LapLift (Figure 9-3), has been developed by our research group, and a report of its feasible use in seven dogs and five cats was presented.[25] Lift laparoscopy was noted to have some significant practical advantages, particularly for laparoscopic-assisted procedures. The lift device is easy to use and is very atraumatic in its design. Through its use for several years at our institution, it has not been associated with entry complications such as splenic perforations, which are common with conventional entry, especially when performed by inexperienced surgeons. The most common adverse effect with lift laparoscopy is that omentum is caught with the lift, in which case the surgeon simply derotates the device, releases the omentum, and reinserts the lift. Without the need for air-tight seals on ports, the surgeon has the freedom to use instruments of different size, and the work space is also maintained during laparoscopic-assisted incisions. The device is also amendable for use in a single-incision laparoscopic surgery/laparoendoscopic single-site surgery fashion (Figure 9-4), which will be reported on in the future. Despite the suboptimal tenting effect, we have noted similar surgery times and the advantage of less pain response in a

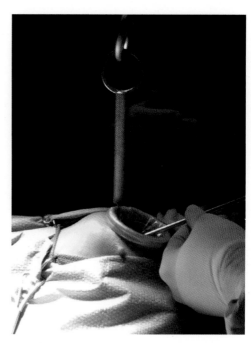

Figure 9-4 A lift device used in a laparoendoscopic single-site surgery fashion.

randomized, controlled, blinded study of ovariohysterectomy performed with lift laparoscopy compared with capnoperitoneum.[18] Currently, we find lift laparoscopy indicated in patients for diagnostic procedures, multiple laparoscopic-assisted procedures in the same patient, and especially if the patient is systemically ill or otherwise compromised. It is important to note that the benefit of avoiding the capnoperitoneum in a systemically ill animal may be offset by longer anesthesia times caused by laparoscopy under suboptimal visualization. Therefore, lift laparoscopy should not be used when a large field of visualization is necessary, such as if intracorporeal electrocautery is used, associated with risks of unobserved trauma, or with intracorporeal suturing. Lift laparoscopy is also most effective in the cranial abdomen, where the rib cage is adding to the tenting effect. The pelvic inlet is not well visualized,[26] and in our experience, lateral lifting of the abdominal wall is not as effective as ventral lifting.

Patient Positioning

The body position of the patient is of great importance for visualization of target areas during laparoscopy. Several organs' positions are heavily influenced by gravity, and changes in position during the surgery can greatly improve the surgeon's ability to visualize the abdomen.

Laparoscopy is often performed with the patient in the Trendelenburg position (i.e., with the head lower than the abdomen). This moves the organs cranially, which may improve the working space but adds to reduction in pulmonary compliance. Therefore, the general recommendation is to not use a steeper angle than 15 degrees to the horizontal plane. In this author's experience, a 10-degree Trendelenburg position is usually sufficient. A reversed Trendelenburg position may affect venous return, exacerbating negative effects of the intraabdominal pressure, and the animal need to be appropriately monitored for cardiovascular changes if maintained in this position.

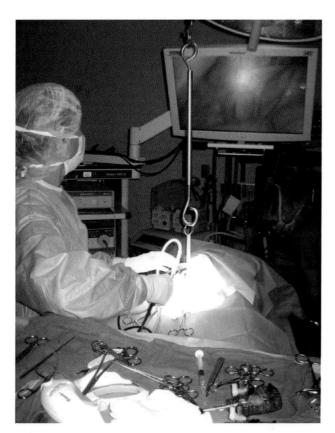

Figure 9-3 Lift laparoscopy in a clinical case. In this particular patient, the lift device is suspended from a custom made hook.

Ideal body positions for surgery will be outlined together with the specific surgical technique in this text. Very little evidence-based information is available on body position during small animal minimally invasive surgery. Sternal recumbency without abdominal support (a "hanging belly") was recently described as advantageous for canine laparoscopic adrenalectomy.[27] An experimental computed tomography investigation of body position's effects on exposure of the canine abdomen before and during capnoperitoneum was performed, and the following conclusions were drawn:[28]

- Dorsal recumbency provides best exposure to the liver (all lobes), gallbladder, and pancreas.
- The dorsal Trendelenburg position provides the best exposure to the stomach, pancreas, pylorus, bladder, and cervix and good exposure to the liver.
- The right lobes of the liver are best exposed by left lateral recumbency together with the cystic duct, duodenum, right kidney, right ovary, and uterine horn.
- The right lateral recumbency provides best exposure of left liver lobes, spleen, left kidney, left ovary, and uterine horn.
- Interestingly, the body and left limb of the pancreas were better exposed during the noninsufflated condition, but this finding may be of limited clinical relevance.
- Gastroesophageal reflux (GER) was noted in almost all scans after insufflation, but before insufflation, only 3 of 24 scans, from 6 anesthetized dogs, showed GER. The clinical significance of GER in association with laparoscopy is not known.[28]

In general, the body position may need to change once or several times during a surgical procedure. In a study assessing the safety of gasless laparoscopy for exploratory laparoscopy after blunt or penetrating abdominal trauma in humans, the exploration was started in reverse Trendelenburg position to assess the liver, pancreas, spleen, diaphragm, transverse colon, and stomach. The body position was changed to dorsal recumbency for midabdomen exploration, and finally the Trendelenburg position was used for pelvic cavity examination.[23] In contrast to humans, dogs' abdomens are flattened side to side, such that lateral tilting provides additional opportunity for excellent visualization. Therefore, an electrical table with a lateral tilt feature, in addition to Trendelenburg or reversed Trendelenburg position, is extremely advantageous for procedures requiring access to both sides of an animal abdomen. The lateral tilt on different type of tables often ranges between ±10 and 30 degrees, and the upper range is preferable. Electrically adjustable operating tables are fairly costly. However, simple and fairly inexpensive tilt tables are also commercially available, including the VetOvation tilt table (VetOvation, Raleigh, NC) and TT tilt positioner (Karl Storz Veterinary Endoscopy, Goleta, CA) (Figure 9-5).

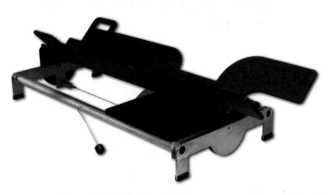

Figure 9-5 A lateral tilt device intended for use on top of a conventional operating table. (© 2014 Photo courtesy of Apexx Veterinary Equipment.)

Retroperitoneal Laparoscopy

Most, if not all, laparoscopic techniques in small animals to date have been performed with a transperitoneal technique. An alternative to pneumoperitoneum does, however, exist. In humans, retroperitoneal laparoscopy for renal, proximal ureteral, and adrenal surgery has been systematically reviewed compared with a transperitoneal approach. Advantages associated with retroperitoneoscopy are a more direct access to the posterior kidney and renal hilus, without the need to retract intraabdominal organs.[28] Also, if abdominal adhesions exist, a retroperitoneal approach may be advantageous. Disadvantages include spatial limitations, loss of anatomic landmarks, and the lack of view. Despite these, retroperitoneoscopy for partial nephrectomy was shown to be safe, was faster than transperitoneal surgery, and led to faster patient recovery.[28,29] Retroperitoneal adrenalectomy was found to have similar outcomes as transperitoneal adrenalectomy.[30] In contrast, for ureteropelvic junction obstruction, transperitoneal surgery was shown to be faster and had lower conversion rate compared with retroperitoneal access.[31]

Retroperitoneal laparoscopic surgery has not yet been reported in dogs, to this author's knowledge.

References

1 Ahmad, G., O'Flynn, H., Duffy, J.M., et al. (2012) Laparoscopic entry techniques. Cochrane Database Syst Rev 2, CD006583.
2 Buote, N.J., Kovak-McClaran, J.R., Schold, J.D. (2011) Conversion from diagnostic laparoscopy to laparotomy: risk factors and occurrence. Vet Surg 40 (1), 106-214.
3 Compeau, C., McLeod, N.T., Ternamian, A. (2011) Laparoscopic entry: a review of Canadian general surgical practice. Can J Surg 54 (5), 315-320.
4 Gilroy, B.A., Anson, L.W. (1987) Fatal air embolism during anesthesia for laparoscopy in a dog. J Am Vet Med Assoc 190 (5), 552-554.
5 Whittemore, J.C., Mitchell, A., Hyink, S., Reed, A. (2013) Diagnostic accuracy of tissue impedance measurement interpretation for correct Veress needle placement in canine cadavers. Vet Surg 42 (5), 613-622.
6 Desmaizieres, L.M., Martinot, S., Lepage, O.M., et al. (2003) Complications associated with cannula insertion techniques used for laparoscopy in standing horses. Vet Surg 32 (6), 501-506.
7 Cheng, Y., Lu, J., Xiong, X., et al. (2013) Gases for establishing pneumoperitoneum during laparoscopic abdominal surgery. Cochrane Database Syst Rev 1, CD009569.
8 Johnson, G.F., Twedt, D.C. (1977) Endoscopy and laparoscopy in the diagnosis and management of neoplasia in small animals. Vet Clin North Am 7 (1), 77-92.
9 Duerr, F.M., Twedt, D.C., Monnet, E. (2008) Changes in pH of peritoneal fluid associated with carbon dioxide insufflation during laparoscopic surgery in dogs. Am J Vet Res 69 (2), 298-301.
10 Lunardi, A.C., Paisani Dde, M., Tanaka, C., Carvalho, C.R. (2013) Impact of laparoscopic surgery on thoracoabdominal mechanics and inspiratory muscular activity. Respir Physiol Neurobiol 186 (1), 40-44.
11 Fredman, B., Jedeikin, R., Olsfanger, D., et al. (1994) Residual pneumoperitoneum: a cause of postoperative pain after laparoscopic cholecystectomy. Anesth Analg 79 (1), 152-154.
12 Phelps, P., Cakmakkaya, O.S., Apfel, C.C., Radke, O.C. (2008) A simple clinical maneuver to reduce laparoscopy-induced shoulder pain: a randomized controlled trial. Obstet Gynecol 111 (5), 1155-1160.
13 Radosa, J.C., Radosa, M.P., Mavrova, R., et al. (2013) Five minutes of extended assisted ventilation with an open umbilical trocar valve significantly reduces postoperative abdominal and shoulder pain in patients undergoing laparoscopic hysterectomy. Eur J Obstet Gynecol Reprod Biol 171 (1), 122-1227.
14 Donaldson, L.L., Trostle, S.S., White, N.A. (1998) Cardiopulmonary changes associated with abdominal insufflation of carbon dioxide in mechanically ventilated, dorsally recumbent, halothane anaesthetised horses. Equine Vet J 30 (2), 144-151.
15 Casati, A., Valentini, G., Ferrari, S., et al. (1997) Cardiorespiratory changes during gynaecological laparoscopy by abdominal wall elevation: comparison with carbon dioxide pneumoperitoneum. Br J Anaesth 78 (1), 51-54.
16 Gross, M.E., Jones, B.D., Bergstresser, D.R., Rosenbauer, R.R. (1993) Effects of abdominal insufflation with nitrous oxide on cardiorespiratory measurements in spontaneously breathing isoflurane-anesthetized dogs. Am J Vet Res 54 (8), 1352-1358.
17 Gurusamy, K.S., Samraj, K., Davidson, B.R. (2008) Abdominal lift for laparoscopic cholecystectomy. Cochrane Database Syst Rev 2, CD006574.

18 Fransson, B.A., Grubb, T.L., Perez, T.E., et al. (2014) Cardiorespiratory changes and pain response of lift laparoscopy compared to capnoperitoneum laparoscopy in dogs. Vet Surg May 7. doi: 10.1111/j.1532-950X.2014.12198.x. [Epub ahead of print].

19 Neudecker, J., Sauerland, S., Neugebauer, E., et al. (2002) The European Association for Endoscopic Surgery clinical practice guideline on the pneumoperitoneum for laparoscopic surgery. Surg Endosc 16 (7), 1121-1143.

20 Nesek-Adam, V., Rasic, Z., Kos, J., Vnuk, D. (2004) Aminotransferases after experimental pneumoperitoneum in dogs. Acta Anaesthesiol Scand 48 (7), 862-866.

21 Tug, T., Ozbas, S., Tekeli, A., et al. (1998) Does pneumoperitoneum cause bacterial translocation? J Laparoendosc Adv Surg Tech A 8 (6), 401-407.

22 Gurusamy, K.S., Samraj, K., Davidson, B.R. (2009) Low pressure versus standard pressure pneumoperitoneum in laparoscopic cholecystectomy. Cochrane Database Syst Rev 2, CD006930.

23 Liao, C.H., Kuo, I.M., Fu, C.Y., et al. (2014) Gasless laparoscopic assisted surgery for abdominal trauma. Injury 45 (5), 850-854.

24 Watkins, C., Fransson, B.A., Ragle, C.A., et al. (2013) Comparison of thoracic and abdominal cavity volumes during abdominal CO_2 insufflation and abdominal wall lift. Vet Surg 42 (5), 607-612.

25 Fransson, B.A., Ragle, C.A. (2011) Lift laparoscopy in dogs and cats: 12 cases (2008-2009). J Am Vet Med Assoc 239 (12), 1574-1579.

26 Kennedy, K., Fransson, B.A., Gay, J. M., Roberts, G. (2013) Comparison of abdominal pneumoperitoneum volumes in lift laparoscopy with variable lift location and tensile force. Veterinary Endoscopy Society, May 2-4, Key Largo, FL, p. 33.

27 Naan, E.C., Kirpensteijn, J., Dupre, G.P., et al. (2013) Innovative approach to laparoscopic adrenalectomy for treatment of unilateral adrenal gland tumors in dogs. Vet Surg 42 (6), 710-715.

28 Ren, T., Liu, Y., Zhao, X., et al. (2014) Transperitoneal approach versus retroperitoneal approach: a meta-analysis of laparoscopic partial nephrectomy for renal cell carcinoma. PLoS One 9 (3), e91978.

29 Fan, X., Xu, K., Lin, T., et al. (2013) Comparison of transperitoneal and retroperitoneal laparoscopic nephrectomy for renal cell carcinoma: a systematic review and meta-analysis. BJU Int 111 (4), 611-621.

30 Nigri, G., Rosman, A.S., Petrucciani, N., et al. (2013) Meta-analysis of trials comparing laparoscopic transperitoneal and retroperitoneal adrenalectomy. Surgery 153 (1), 111-119.

31 Wu, Y., Dong, Q., Han, P., et al. (2012) Meta-analysis of transperitoneal versus retroperitoneal approaches of laparoscopic pyeloplasty for ureteropelvic junction obstruction. J Laparoendosc Adv Surg Tech A 22 (7), 658-662.

10 Laparoscopic Contraindications, Complications, and Conversion

Nicole J. Buote and Janet Kovak McClaran

Anatomic and Physiologic Contraindications to Laparoscopy: Relative and Definitive

Before a laparoscopic procedure is considered, the surgeon should have specific knowledge regarding any preexisting contraindications in the patient. Contraindications to laparoscopy can be divided into relative or definitive and anatomic or physiologic. Definitive or absolute contraindications are those that eliminate a patient from a laparoscopic procedure completely. Relative contraindications are those in which exceptions can and are made when taking into account varying factors related to the patient. Anatomic contraindications can include difficulty accessing the cavity, obliteration of the peritoneal or thoracic space, organomegaly, intestinal distension, congenital abnormalities, and potential for dissemination of cancer.[1] The major physiologic considerations regarding safety of these procedures include pregnancy, increased intracranial pressure, abnormal cardiac output and gas exchange in the lung, chronic liver disease and coagulopathy.[1] One of the most important limitations that should also be considered is the surgeon's own boundaries to his or her laparoscopic skills. Although this may be difficult to discuss, inadequate training or experience may lead to serious injuries during more advanced procedures. Outdated or poorly maintained equipment and inadequately trained assistants can also be contraindications for some laparoscopic procedures. This discussion should focus on patient variables commonly used to determine eligibility for minimally invasive procedures, but surgical judgment should also be mentioned.

Anatomic Limitations (Box 10-1)
Port Access and Adhesions

The ability to place ports in the appropriate locations for specific procedures is the first step in successfully performing minimally invasive surgery (MIS). If there are anatomic reasons why ports cannot be placed safely in the required location, such as previous adhesion to the body wall from other procedures (stomach, urinary bladder), the procedure should be performed open. In humans, any type of previous abdominal or thoracic surgery may be a relative contraindication because up to 30% of reoperative patients have bowel or other organs that are directly adherent to the abdominal scar,[2-7] and in autopsy studies, 75% to 90% of patients with previous abdominal surgery had adhesions.[8] Care must be taken to develop a thorough anamnesis to ensure no previous surgeries may interfere with proposed port placements. In the reoperative abdomen, several early prospective human studies illustrated fewer injuries when the Hasson or open "cut-down" method was used compared with the blind "Veress" needle (VN) port insertion method.[9-11] However, the risk is quite low with either technique as long as the first port is placed distant to the previous abdominal incisions. Failure to produce a pneumoperitoneum after two or three passes of the VN is considered sufficient cause to switch to the Hasson technique. New optical trocars, discussed in detail elsewhere, are another option that allows the surgeon to view the layers of tissue as they are traversed.

Even after the first port has been established, the formation of adhesions from previous surgeries must be contended with and may be cause to convert to an open procedure if sufficient progress cannot be made. Adhesions decrease the peritoneal working space and hinder visibility; many times, adhesiolysis is extremely time consuming. Although not a common problem reported in veterinary medicine, adhesions do occur in our patient population (Figure 10-1) and can lead to all of the same difficulties in maneuverability.[12,13] Although not encountered commonly in veterinary medicine, adhesion of organs to peritoneal mesh is a specific consideration in human medicine. These adhesions are extremely difficult to break down, and this is an absolute contraindication for laparoscopy in the region surrounding the mesh placement. There have been studies showing that laparoscopy is associated with less adhesion formation compared with open procedures, which is beneficial for patients.[14]

Small Animal Laparoscopy and Thoracoscopy, First Edition. Edited by Boel A. Fransson and Philipp D. Mayhew.
© 2015 by ACVS Foundation. Published 2015 by John Wiley & Sons, Inc.
Companion website: www.wiley.com/go/fransson/laparoscopy

Box 10-1 Relative Anatomic Contraindications for Minimally Invasive Surgery

Obesity
Reoperative abdomen or thorax (adhesions)
Aberrant anatomy
Cirrhosis, portal hypertension (varicosities)
Small bowel obstruction
Septic peritonitis
Disseminated abdominal cancer

Cirrhosis and Portal Hypertension

Liver disease increases the risk of morbidity and mortality with any type of surgical procedure because of malnutrition, coagulopathies, ascites, and renal dysfunction.[15] Initially, the major concern with laparoscopic procedures in this patient population centered on the meshwork of abdominal wall varicosities (Figure 10-2) that can be formed, which makes port placement exceedingly dangerous. More recent concerns include the effects of carbon dioxide (CO_2) insufflation on liver physiology (decreased portal venous return); therefore, gasless and low-pressure techniques have been advocated.[16] Recommendations are to perform an open Hasson technique for port placement for laparoscopic procedures in these patients to

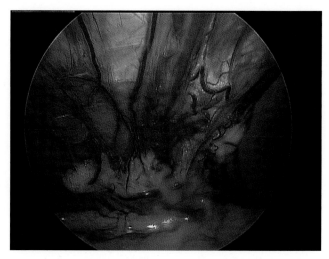

Figure 10-2 Intraoperative view of abdominal wall varicosities in a canine patient with advanced liver disease.

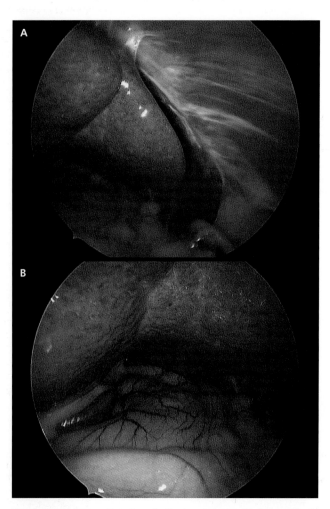

Figure 10-1 Intraoperative view of adhesions between the liver and body wall and liver and linea alba (**A**). Note how the dorsal surface of the liver is completely elevated off the underlying structures and the stomach is more cranial than normal (**B**).

decrease the chance of iatrogenic laceration to varicosities.[15,16] Although we do not see advanced cirrhosis as commonly in veterinary medicine, the author has encountered cirrhosis and varicose vessels during diagnostic laparoscopic liver biopsy. Special care is always taken to avoid these fragile vessels and stay in the periphery of the liver lobes because the larger intrahepatic vessels are closer to the surface in a cirrhotic liver.

Many times in veterinary medicine, we have not diagnosed portal hypertension before surgery, so caution should be taken in any patient with suspected cirrhosis. In patients with ascites but no portal hypertension, a VN may be used, but the patient should be placed in a Trendelenburg (head-down) position to move any air-filled bowel that may be floating in abdominal fluid away from the needle. Depending on the amount of fluid present, removal of the ascites may be warranted before the procedure starts. If a large amount of ascites is present, insufflation can lead to frothy bubbly fluid (caused by the albumin present in the fluid), markedly decreasing visualization. Patients with ascites may also have an increased risk of wound complications because leakage of fluid decreases healing of the port incisions.[1]

Septic Peritonitis

Preexisting septic peritonitis was once thought to be a contraindication to laparoscopic procedures because of the potential for abscess formation at the port sites. There have been multiple studies looking at laparoscopic appendectomy and closure of peptic ulcers that have illustrated no greater incisional complication rate compared with open procedures, so this is a relative contraindication and left up to the surgeon's discretion.[18-21] Most veterinary cases of septic peritonitis do not have a localized diagnosis before surgery, and many patients are quite unstable. Although the presence of sepsis in and of itself is not a contraindication, the surgeon would have to determine the best way to effectively and efficiently explore the abdomen and treat the problem after it is found in these critically ill patients. Bedside diagnostic laparoscopy[22] for critically ill patients suspected of having intraabdominal sepsis has been performed in humans and holds the benefit of a highly accurate diagnosis with decreased morbidity. An important point to consider is the well-documented effect of pneumoperitoneum on translocation of bacteria into the circulation at certain intraabdominal pressures,[23,24] but much controversy exists over the effect of CO_2 insufflation on the innate immune system of the peritoneum (morphology of peritoneal mesothelium and macrophages).[25-28]

Small Bowel Obstruction

Another relative anatomic contraindication is mechanical bowel obstruction, which leads to a decrease in the available working space and increased risk of bowel injury (serosal tearing or enterotomy). This topic is again controversial with some authors feeling strongly that laparoscopy should not be used in these cases and others reporting decreased healing times and improved gastrointestinal (GI) function postoperatively.[29-32] Baiocchi et al. report specific standards that should be followed if laparoscopic treatment for small bowel obstruction is to be considered, although no such guidelines exist in veterinary medicine.[33] These factors include proximal obstruction, small bowel dilation less than 4 cm, single adhesion band, mild abdominal distention, partial obstruction, and previous appendectomy. Reported success rates range from 46% to 84%,[34,35] with an overall rate of intestinal damage during the procedure of 5.8%.[24] The threshold for conversion should be very low in these cases, especially during the first few cases, and if possible, the GI tract should be decompressed preoperatively (orogastric tube placement after induction).

Abdominal Malignancy

Planning or staging laparoscopy has been successfully used in cases of abdominal malignancy in humans and in the authors' practices[36-38] when visualization of the disease could cause a significant change in patient management to nonoperative treatment. This spares the patient recovery from a major surgical procedure, and in combination with laparoscopic ultrasonography or peritoneal cytology, specifically tailored treatments can be provided.[39] Laparoscopic staging has become the standard of care in human medicine before resection of any upper intestinal tumors (Figure 10-3).[40] In human medicine, many definitive treatments for intraabdominal cancer can be performed laparoscopically or laparoscopically assisted, so conversion is unnecessary. It is, however, generally considered that any locally invasive (involving the body wall, adjacent organs, or retroperitoneum) tumor of the abdomen (GI or other intraabdominal organ) may be better suited to open resection.

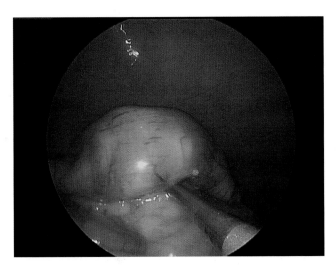

Figure 10-3 Intraoperative view of solitary small intestinal mass with no evidence of metastatic peritoneal lesions.

Staging laparoscopy helps identify metastatic disease that may not be evident on computed tomography or ultrasonography (peritoneal carcinomatosis) as well as gives information as to resectability (location and mobility of the organ of interest).

Port-site recurrences have been linked mostly to technical error with no convincing evidence of an increased incidence of port-site metastasis or acceleration of disease with laparoscopy.[39] In veterinary medicine, to the authors' knowledge, there have been no large-scale studies reporting the overall incidence of port site metastasis, and currently port-site metastasis has only been reported after thoracoscopic procedures. Another important factor is the varied biologic activity of some tumors. In human medicine, mucinous cystadenocarcinoma of the ovary and signet cell or mucinous GI adenocarcinomas may exhibit a higher implantation rate onto the peritoneal surface after laparoscopic procedures.[1] It may be that as laparoscopy is used more commonly in veterinary surgical oncology that such tumor-specific differences in complication rates also become apparent.

Physiologic Limitations (Box 10-2)
Pneumoperitoneum

The cardiopulmonary effects of CO_2 insufflation for establishment of a pneumoperitoneum have been established. Insufflation with CO_2 is associated with two potential problems: (1) absorption of CO_2 across the peritoneal surface may cause hypercarbia, leading to respiratory acidosis, and (2) transmission of increased intraabdominal pressure through the diaphragm raises intrathoracic pressures by 5 to 15 mm Hg, depending on diaphragmatic compliance. Absorption of CO_2 and the ensuing hypercarbic acidosis require intraoperative compensation by the anesthetist. Increasing the minute ventilation, usually by hyperventilation, lowers the $PaCO_2$ and raises the pH. In patients with marginal pulmonary reserve (e.g., obese patients) or those who require positive end-expiratory pressure for adequate oxygenation, adequate compensation may not be possible; in these cases, refractory respiratory acidosis may develop. End-tidal CO_2 monitoring is essential in the management of the ventilation of patients undergoing laparoscopy but may underestimate the true arterial $paCO_2$ by as much as 10 mm Hg in an individual with chronic lung disease.[1] Therefore, arterial monitoring is recommended in these patients. In children and in patients who cannot be adequately ventilated during laparoscopic surgery, lower peak insufflation pressures should be used. If this fails, alternative measures, including the use of an abdominal wall-lifting device (gasless technique), administration of an alternative insufflation gas such as nitrous oxide or helium, or conversion to an open technique should be considered.[41-43]

Venous return to the heart is decreased in response to peritoneal insufflation. This is most often seen in hypovolemic patients because insufflation compresses the low-pressure caudal vena cava and other large veins. In a well-hydrated patient, return is near normal. Cardiac output will be decreased if venous return is decreased,

Box 10-2 Relative Physiologic Contraindications to Minimally Invasive Surgery

Pulmonary disease
Cardiovascular disease
Intracranial disease
Coagulopathy
Pregnancy
Shock

which can then lead to metabolic acidosis because of decreased visceral perfusion. This is why laparoscopic procedures were once thought to be contraindicated in elderly humans, but with improved anesthetic techniques and monitoring, this is no longer true, and there have actually been studies showing improved outcomes.[44] Patients with severe cardiac disease or hypovolemic shock may not compensate well and may manifest a dramatic drop in cardiac output during peritoneal insufflation. Although laparoscopy has been used as a diagnostic tool in some intensive care unit patients,[45] it should not be recommended in patients with acute hemorrhagic shock.

Intracranial Disease

Any intracranial pressure concerns should be taken into account before laparoscopic procedures are chosen. A combination of the Trendelenburg (head-down) position and peritoneal insufflation can cause increased intracranial pressure, and with an accompanying metabolic acidosis, this can be severe; therefore, these procedures should be avoided in patients with acute brain injury. There have been reports of ventriculoperitoneal shunt failure after laparoscopic procedures as well as a theoretical risk of intracranial insufflation if the one-way valve fails. Some surgeons recommend exteriorizing the shunt before insufflation and then replacing it.[45,46]

Pregnancy

There have been many studies on laparoscopic procedures during pregnancy and the effects on the mother and fetus. Although the need for surgery during pregnancy may be rare in veterinary medicine, it is not impossible to think there may be certain necessary situations. In experimental studies, peritoneal insufflation has been found to increase intrauterine pressure, decrease uterine blood flow, and cause maternal and fetal acidosis.[47] There have been clinical studies showing that adverse outcomes were rare when laparoscopy was performed in the second trimester, but these do not illustrate long-term effects on the development of the child.[48-51] In human medicine, any elective procedures are recommended during the second trimester to avoid the teratogenic effects of anesthetics and the obliteration of peritoneal space by a gravid uterus.

Coagulopathy

A preexisting coagulopathy was once thought to be a definitive contraindication for laparoscopic surgery in human medicine, but this is rarely the case now because of improved operative techniques and recombinant coagulation factors. Any congenital coagulopathy should be corrected before any surgery, laparoscopic or open, because an uncorrected coagulopathy holds the same risk of uncontrolled hemorrhage with both procedure types. There are some specific diseases of the hemolymphatic system, such as medically refractory immune thrombocytopenia purpura, that are almost exclusively treated with laparoscopic splenectomy in humans.[1,52]

Preventing and Preparing for Complications

Preventing complications during laparoscopic procedures requires the same thoughtfulness and planning as used with traditional open procedures. Although every specific procedure may require specific planning and each patient may have individual needs, these are discussed in detail in different chapters. However, a few important tenants specific to minimally invasive procedures and surgery in general will be discussed in this chapter (Box 10-3).

Box 10-3 Steps to Prevent Complications in Minimally Invasive Surgery

> Have blood products available.
> Ensure appropriate venous or arterial access.
> Have mechanical ventilation available.
> Ensure appropriate staffing.
> Check all equipment preoperatively.
> Plan for conversion.
> Have appropriate postoperative care available.
> Do not place pride over patient care; convert when necessary.

Blood Products and Venous Access

The benefit to many minimally invasive procedures includes very small incisions from which samples from various organs can be removed. Even in cases in which incisions are enlarged to remove intact organs in sterile specimen retrieval bags, these incisions do not allow for the same type of hemostatic control that an open approach may provide. Therefore, with regards to biopsies of the liver, spleen, and kidney, blood products should be available in the hospital for patients during and after the procedure if necessary. Obviously, the surgeon's best judgment will need to be used to determine whether blood products alone will be sufficient or if conversion is necessary to control hemorrhage. Along with available blood products, venous and/or arterial access should be established before any patient is taken into the operating suite. Debilitated patients may need vasopressor support or blood; therefore, a second venous catheter should be considered. An arterial line placed before the procedure begins will allow invasive blood pressure monitoring to be performed.

Mechanical Ventilation and Appropriate Equipment

Many patients undergoing laparoscopic procedures need mechanical ventilation because of their inability to adapt to the CO_2 insufflation or because of positioning for the procedure. Without this availability, the patient may be at risk for dangerous physiologic consequences. Along with a ventilator, it behooves the surgeon to ensure before every MIS procedure that he or she has all of the required instrumentation necessary for the procedure and that it is in working order. As discussed in other parts of this chapter, elective conversions have been reported in human medicine because of failure of one or more pieces of equipment. Although some malfunctions (camera, light source, telescope damage) cannot be detected until the equipment is all in place during the procedure, a simple checklist of necessary instruments, ports, specimen bags, electrosurgical units, and so on should be created and viewed before each MIS procedure to ensure a seamless and consistent experience.

Surgical Judgment

In human and veterinary medicine, surgical judgment is born from training and experience. It should be noted that in human medicine, much controversy exists over the training of laparoscopists, and building the foundation for appropriate training, which is occurring in veterinary medicine, is ongoing in human medicine also.[53] Many veterinary facilities offer weekend courses in basic and advanced laparoscopic techniques currently, and the advent of human MIS began in that fashion also. Laparoscopic cholecystectomy was the first to be taught and discussed in a seminar or workshop manner, but in the beginning, complication rates were found to be greater compared with open procedures. The research illustrated that this was because of the steep learning curve associated with this procedure[54-56] as well as the fact that there appears to be limited transfer of training from one procedure to another.[57,58] Although results revealed that attending workshops or seminars did not enable surgeons to safely perform laparoscopic procedures,[59,60] the need is so great that residency or fellowship training alone may simply not be enough to fulfill this requirement. The laparoscopic ability and experience of the surgeon must be taken into account every time the feasibility of a particular surgery is considered. Therefore, inexperience in the surgeon or assistants should be considered a relative contraindication for advanced minimally invasive procedures.

Appropriate Staffing

Making sure that the anesthesia staff is prepared for the specific physiologic changes that occur during MIS when patient positioning is changed (e.g., Trendelenburg, reverse Trendelenburg, lateral), and changes associated with insufflation and desufflation are critical to the safety of the patient as well as the timeliness of the surgery. The surgeon should also have available surgical assistants, whether they are other doctors or scrub nurses who are able to appropriately help during these procedures, because many times multiple hands are needed to hold the telescope, instruments, vessel sealing devices, retrieval bags, and other equipment. Being sure to have enough help at the table and well-trained anesthesia technicians is a simple yet vital factor in preventing and preparing for surgical complications.

Always Prepare for Conversion

Although no surgeon likes to contemplate defeat, the need for elective or emergent conversions should always be prepared for ahead of time with every MIS case. The abdomen should be aseptically prepared for a traditional open approach or other appropriate approach (e.g., paracostal, flank) for every laparoscopic procedure in case a complication arises requiring a rapid response.

Intraoperative Complications Associated with Laparoscopy

Complications associated with laparoscopy may be anticipated in a small number of patients. Overall rates of complications in human medicine vary widely depending on procedures performed. Cited major complications associated with laparoscopic procedures in animals include anesthetic-related events, such as air embolism,[61] as well as operative issues such as bleeding, organ penetration, or incisional complications.[62] The rate of previously reported complications with laparoscopic surgery in animals ranges from 2% to 35%.[63,64] Of reported complications, the most common is minor bleeding.[65-67] Complications may be associated with anesthesia and maintenance of a pneumoperitoneum, equipment malfunction, or trocar insertion, as well as during organ manipulation and biopsy. Box 10-4 outlines potential complications that may be encountered with laparoscopy.

Anesthetic Complications

Reported anesthetic complications associated with laparoscopy may involve patients' inability to tolerate pneumoperitoneum as well as equipment malfunction. Hypercarbia and hypoxia are generally encountered in patients with a history of preexisting pulmonary or cardiac disease.[69] Abdominal insufflation using CO_2 to a pressure of 15 mm Hg for 180 minutes resulted in significant increases in heart rate, minute ventilation, and saphenous vein pressure, as

Box 10-4 Intraoperative Complications

Anesthesia-related complications (hypotension, cardiovascular compromise)

Veress needle or trocar insertion (injury to abdominal wall vasculature, penetration of hollow viscus, penetration of organ)

Pulmonary complication (air embolus, pneumothorax)

Loss of insufflation or inappropriate insufflation (subcutaneous emphysema)

Equipment malfunction

Inability to remove sample

Excessive hemorrhage

Adhesions

Failure to progress; inexperience

well as decreases in pH and PaO_2. These changes, however, were found to be acceptable in healthy, well-ventilated dogs.[70] In a study of the cardiopulmonary effects of CO_2 for laparoscopic surgery in cats, insufflation produced increases in heart rate, mean blood pressure, and diastolic arterial pressure.[71] These changes were found to be well tolerated and within physiologically acceptable limits. In another study of healthy cats, cardiopulmonary parameters were minimally changed by induction of intraabdominal pressure up to 8 mm Hg, and no increase in working space or visualization was found by increasing intraabdominal pressure to 15 mm Hg, suggesting that maintenance of lower pressures in feline patients may be advisable.[72] To date, no specific criteria have been made to predict ventilatory failure during laparoscopic procedures. It is also important to remember that there can be effects of patient positioning on pulmonary compliance with a greater decrease in compliance seen in Trendelenburg position (head down by 15–30 degrees) compared with the reverse Trendelenburg position.[73]

Minor anesthetic complications, such as transient hypotension, are commonly encountered in laparoscopic procedures and were reported in 54% of veterinary patients undergoing laparoscopic procedures.[64] However, serious anesthetic complications, including death and air or CO_2 embolism, are rare.[61,74] Careful monitoring of CO_2 tension and ventilation minute volume is required to identify patients that develop CO_2 embolism, which occurs by direct injection of CO_2 into the venous system via a VN. Patients become profoundly hypotensive, cyanotic, or bradycardic or develop asystole. Treatment includes cessation of insufflation, delivery of 100% oxygen, placement of the patient in steep left lateral Trendelenburg position, and placement of a central line to aspirate gas from the venous system.[75] Tension pneumothorax has been reported in patients with a congenital or iatrogenic diaphragmatic defect.[76] Other reported complications after CO_2 pneumoperitoneum include signs of reperfusion injury and peritoneal acidosis, which may lead to attenuation of the inflammatory response after laparoscopic surgery.[77,78]

Operative Complications

Operative complications are considered unintentional intraoperative events that require additional management to correct or reduce the risk of a poor outcome.[69] The most common complications are encountered with trocar and portal placement.[79] The closed technique uses a VN for insufflation followed by blind insertion of a sharp trocar and cannula (Figure 10-4). Damage may include minimal hemorrhage, but major complications, including large vessel rupture, urinary bladder damage, GI tract perforation, and splenic laceration, may be encountered. In a review of laparoscopic

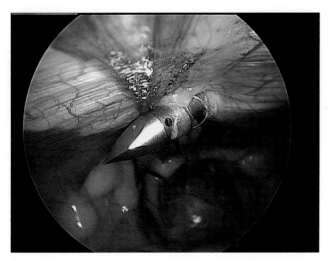

Figure 10-4 Intraoperative view of a sharp trocar and cannula.

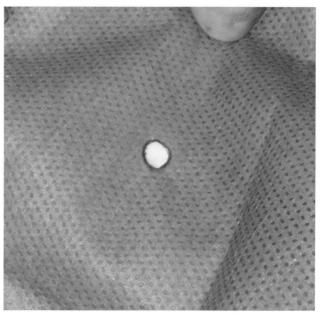

Figure 10-5 Photograph of a burn through surgical drape material from the telescope with the light source turned on. This burn was produced in a matter of seconds.

complications in a study of 2324 operative laparoscopic gynecologic procedures in women, the overall rate of complications was low (0.22%), but there were more complications (n = 15) from VN and trocar insertion than from actual operative procedures (n = 3).[79] Various needle safety tests or checks have been proposed to avoid VN damage such as the double-click test, the aspiration test, the hanging drop test, the "hiss" sound test, and serial intraabdominal gas pressure tests. These tests have been shown to have limited accuracy in humans.[80] Furthermore, certain tests, such as wiggling of the VN, should be avoided because they can enlarge a 1.6-mm puncture injury to an injury of up to 1 cm in viscera or blood vessels.[81] The use of tissue impedance measurements has been studied in canine and feline cadavers[82,83] and may have a high diagnostic accuracy for identifying incorrect VN placement. If VN placement is to be used for an intercostal approach in dogs, it appears that placement in the right ninth intercostal space at the mid distance between the xiphoid cartilage and the most caudal extent of the costal arch resulted in the fewest complications.[84,85]

An alternative approach to trocar placement is the open, or Hasson, technique, which involves making a small subumbilical incision under direct visualization followed by insertion of a blunt trocar and cannula. Although minor lacerations may be successfully repaired with intracorporeal suturing, most cases of perforation require conversion to an open laparotomy. A serious complication may occur if injuries to bowel or vasculature are not recognized at the time of trocar insertion and hemoabdomen, peritonitis, or abscessation occurs.[76] Box 10-5 outlines measures that may be taken to decrease risks associated with trocar and cannula placement. As discussed earlier, newer, self-dilating optical

Box 10-5 Steps to Avoid Iatrogenic Trocar Insertion Complications

Empty the patient's bladder before the procedure.
Place the animal in a slight Trendelenburg (head-down) position.
Use the Hasson technique.
Ensure adequate insufflation.
Aim the first trocar toward the right cranial quadrant.
Plan subsequent portal sites with transillumination.
Place instrument portals under direct visualization.
Fully inspect the abdomen before closure.

trocars allow direct visualization through each abdominal layer and have been associated with fewer reported complications.[75] A prospective study of 14,243 laparoscopic procedures performed on human patients documented an incidence of trocar-related vascular and visceral injury in 0.18% of patients. These injuries were repaired laparoscopically in 21.7% of patients and via laparotomy in 78.2% of individuals. Only one death was reported related to trocar injury.[75]

Equipment malfunction is often cited as a potential cause of complications in human patients undergoing laparoscopic procedures[86-88] but is rarely reported in the veterinary literature.[64] Malfunctions have been categorized as those affecting imaging, transmission of fluids and light, the electric circuit, and surgical instruments.[86] A study of 116 gynecologic surgeries in women noted equipment failure was encountered in 38.8% of operative procedures, although the mean delay in procedures was only 5.6 ± 4 minutes, and no reported morbidity or mortality resulted as a consequence of the malfunctions.[86] Another study evaluated the incidence of stapler malfunction in laparoscopic procedures by survey of 124 minimally invasive surgeons and found that 86% reported experience with linear staple malfunction and 25% had to significantly alter the planned operative procedure because of the malfunction.[87] A simple complication to avoid is burns though draping material when the telescope light source is kept on while sitting on the patient or instrument table (Figure 10-5). It is unclear if the lack of cited equipment malfunction in veterinary medicine is due to fewer complex procedures being attempted or if underreporting of adverse events occurs.

Other major complications that may occur during laparoscopic procedures include damage to viscera during organ manipulation as well as hemorrhage after organ biopsy (Figure 10-6). Specific complications vary widely depending on the procedure type. Overall, the complications in therapeutic laparoscopy are higher than those encountered during diagnostic laparoscopy.[79] Hemorrhage after diagnostic liver biopsies in human medicine is rare and has

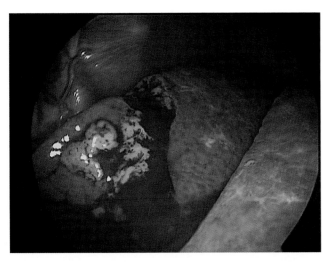

Figure 10-6 Intraoperative view of excessive arterial bleeding from a liver biopsy site.

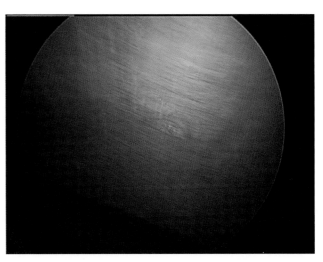

Figure 10-7 Intraoperative view of peritoneal burns when the telescope is gently cleaned off on the peritoneum.

been reported to be 1.3% in a study of 603 patients that underwent diagnostic laparoscopy.[89] In a study of 80 small animal patients undergoing laparoscopic liver biopsy, no fatalities were reported, and although 4% of animals required blood transfusion, all had been anemic before surgery.[68] Laparoscopic ovariectomy has been performed with increasing frequency in dogs and cats, with a low rate of reported complications, including hemorrhage from ovaries or from inadvertent splenic laceration.[89-93] This is in contrast to human gynecologic laparoscopic surgery in which ureteral injury, bladder injury, intestinal injury, and major vascular injuries have all been reported.[94,95]

Thermal bowel injury may also occur after use of electrosurgical or electrocautery devices. Occurrence of this complication has been reported to be 0.2%.[75] The true incidence of this and other complications is difficult to assess because of underreporting. For example, a survey at an American College of Surgeons meeting reported that 18% of respondents had had an inadvertent laparoscopic electrosurgical injury occur in their practice, but 54% of these individuals knew of at least one other surgeon who had such an event.[75] Peritoneal burns from the telescope also can occur and are usually mild and therefore not reported either (Figure 10-7).

Conversion from Minimally Invasive Surgery to Open Surgery

In human surgery, conversion from laparoscopy to laparotomy (celiotomy) is defined as either an *elective* (conversion to laparotomy in the absence of a complication) or *emergent* (conversion because of development of a complication that cannot be adequately managed using laparoscopy) conversion.[69] Elective conversions are cases that are converted because of factors that preclude safe and timely laparoscopic completion of procedures. Failure to progress occurs because of factors that include adhesions from prior procedures, poor exposure (for reasons such as patient obesity or aberrant or unclear anatomy), or surgeon inexperience. Emergent conversions require immediate conversion to an open laparotomy and include cases of uncontrollable bleeding or rupture of a hollow viscus. In a veterinary study, 20 of 94 animals (21%) that had diagnostic laparoscopic procedures had conversion (65% elective, 35% emergent) to a celiotomy, with an overall rate of 7.5% when considering emergent

conversions alone.[64] A preoperative finding of a solitary liver tumor, low total solids, and a diagnosis of malignancy were all significant risk factors for conversion from laparoscopy to laparotomy (Figures 10-8 and 10-9, Video Clip 10-1). In human studies, rates of conversions vary depending on procedure type and conversion risk factors include patient age, sex, obesity, and preoperative comorbidity.[95] Many human studies highlight that there is no expected increase in postoperative complications or hospitalization stay for patients who had a laparoscopic procedure converted to an open laparotomy.[96,97]

Postoperative Complications

After the completion of laparoscopic procedures, reported complications documented in the human literature include postoperative hemorrhage; anastomotic leakage; subcutaneous emphysema; persistent pneumoperitoneum; and portal site inflammation, infection, or herniation.[76,89] Major complications are generally classified as those requiring additional surgery or transfusion. These generally vary depending on the surgical procedure and organ system

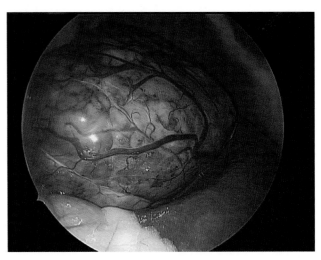

Figure 10-8 Intraoperative view of large hepatic mass.

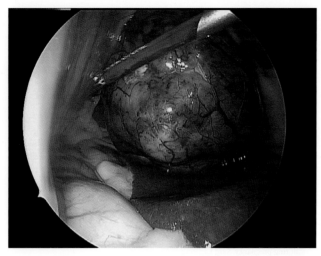

Figure 10-9 Intraoperative view of large hepatic mass being manipulated by a blunt probe. It was pedunculated and easily moveable, and no other metastatic disease was found, so the decision to convert for a liver lobectomy was made.

involved. Many major postoperative complications may be avoided by thorough inspection of the abdominal cavity after completion of every laparoscopic procedure to evaluate for bleeding or any organ damage. In a prospective study of 603 human patients undergoing diagnostic laparoscopic procedures, minor complications occurred in 5.1% of patients and included port site leakage of ascites, cellulitis, hematoma, and wound dehiscence.[89]

Late complications reported in human medicine related to portal sites include herniation, infection, and port site metastasis.[97-99] Herniation of omentum through 5-mm laparoscopic port sites in dogs has been reported.[100] It is important to ensure that all abdominal organs and fat are adequately within the abdomen as ports are removed, and the fascial layer should be closed under direct visualization. To reduce wound complications after laparoscopic procedures, as with open laparotomy, animals should be adequately exercise restricted with Elizabethan collars, and their owners should be instructed to monitor incision sites daily. Many theories exist for the formation of port site metastasis and include direct implantation during sample retrieval, exfoliation of cells during tumor manipulation, and dispersion after CO_2 insufflation or via hematogenous spread.[101,102] Controversy exists as to whether or not higher rates occur after laparoscopy or laparotomy. A study surveying 607 human surgeons who reported on a total of 117,840 total patients undergoing laparoscopic procedures reported an overall rate of tumor reoccurrence in 0.09% of cases regardless of whether specimen retrieval bags were used.[103] A study comparing laparoscopy to laparotomy found there was no evidence of an increase in circulating tumor cells after laparoscopy, but use of specimen retrieval bags for exteriorization of tumor samples is still recommended.[104]

In a veterinary study of 94 patients undergoing diagnostic laparoscopic procedures, 33 (35%) had a documented postoperative complication. Of these 26 (78%) with hypotension and 18 (54%) with anemia (not present preoperatively), 14 (42%) required a transfusion of some type of blood product, and 4 (12%) had other complications, including seroma (3), subcutaneous emphysema (3), and regurgitation (1).[64] In general, many human studies document a shorter length of hospitalization and lower rate of postoperative complications after laparoscopic procedures compared with open surgery.[105-107]

Effects on Hospital Discharge of Complications and Conversions

The effects of complications and conversion on outcome and time to discharge have been extensively studied in human medicine.[108-111] The effects of conversion vary depending on the procedure being performed with no evidence of increased morbidity in one study[110] of colorectal disease. An increase in medical complication rate after conversion from laparoscopic adrenalectomy was appreciated in a different study.[111] In veterinary medicine, only one retrospective study has specifically looked at complications and conversions in diagnostic laparoscopic procedures with regards to outcome.[64] The presence of complications did not affect survival to discharge because most were minor and treatable, but there was an increase in hospitalization from 2 to 3 days. Conversion did not increase the time to discharge or affect survival rates.[64]

Conclusion

Although relative contraindications do exist for laparoscopic procedures, appropriate case selection, surgical experience, and postoperative care allow us to perform a wide variety of procedures on patients that were historically considered contraindicated. Complications can occur in laparoscopic procedures, and surgeons must always be prepared to manage these intraoperatively with conversion if necessary.

 All videos cited in this chapter can be found on the book's companion website at **www.wiley.com/go/fransson/laparoscopy**

References

1 Bowers, S.P., Hunter, J.G. (2006) Contraindications to laparoscopy. In: Whelan, R.L., Fleshman, J.W., Fowler, D.L. (eds.) The SAGES Manual Perioperative Care in Minimally Invasive Surgery. Springer, New York, pp. 25-32.

2 Miller, K., Holbling, N., Hutter, J., et al. (1993) Laparoscopic cholecystectomy for patients who have had previous abdominal surgery. Surg Endosc 7, 400-403.

3 Halpern, N.B. (1996) The difficult laparoscopy. Surg Clin North Am 76, 603-613.

4 Halpern, N.B. (1998a) Access problems in laparoscopic cholecystectomy: postoperative adhesions, obesity, and liver disorders. Semin Laparosc Surg 5, 92-106.

5 Gersin, K.S., Heniford, B.T., Arca, M.J., et al. (1998) Alternative site entry for laparoscopy in patients with previous abdominal surgery. J Laparoendosc Adv Surg Tech A 8, 125-130.

6 Kumar, S.S. (1998) Laparoscopic cholecystectomy in the densely scarred abdomen. Am Surg 64, 1094-1096.

7 Audebert, A.J., Gomel, V. (2000) Role of microlaparoscopy in the diagnosis of peritoneal and visceral adhesions and in the prevention of bowel injury associated with blind trocar insertion. Fertil Steril 73, 631-635.

8 Weibel, M.A., Majno, G. (1973) Peritoneal adhesions and their relation to abdominal surgery. A postmortem study. Am J Surg 126, 345-353.

9 Sigman, H.H., Fried, G.M., Garzon, J., et al. (1993) Risks of blind versus open approach to celiotomy for laparoscopic surgery. Surg Laparosc Endosc 3, 296-299.

10 McKernan, J.B., Champion, J.K. (1995) Access techniques: Veress needle-initial blind trocar insertion versus open laparoscopy with the Hasson trocar. Endosc Surg Allied Technol 3, 35-38.

11 Mayol, J., Garcia-Aguilar, J., Ortiz-Oshiro, E., et al. (1997) Risks of the minimal access approach for laparoscopic surgery: multivariate analysis of morbidity related to umbilical trocar insertion. World J Surg 21, 529-533.

12 el Ghoul, W. (2005) The effects of combined liquid and membrane barriers in prevention of postoperative intra-abdominal adhesions after experimental jejunal anastomosis in dogs. Deutsch Tierarztl Wochenschr 112, 3-10.

13 Di Cicco, M.F., Bennett, R.A., Ragetly, C., et al. (2011) Segmental jejunal entrapment, volvulus, and strangulation secondary to intra-abdominal adhesions in a dog. J Am Anim Hosp Assoc 47, e31-e35.

14 Gutt, C.N., Oniu, T., Schemmer, P., et al. (2004) Fewer adhesions induced by laparoscopic surgery? Surg Endosc 18, 898-906.

15 Massaband, P., Curet, M.J. (2010) Laparoscopy in special conditions: previous abdominal surgery, pregnancy and liver disease. In: Assalia, A., Gagner, M., Schein, M. (eds.) Controversies in Laparoscopic Surgery. Springer, Berlin, pp. 55-76.

16 Giraudo, G., Brachet Contul, R., Caccetta, M., et al. (2001) Gasless laparoscopy could avoid alterations in hepatic function. Surg Endosc 15, 741-746.

17 Abdel-Atty, M.Y., Farges, O., Jagot, P., et al. (1999) Laparoscopy extends the indications for liver resection in patients with cirrhosis. Br J Surg 86, 1397-1400.

18 Navez, B., Tassetti, V., Scohy, J.J., et al. (1998b) Laparoscopic management of acute peritonitis. Br J Surg 85, 32-36.

19 Khalili, T.M., Hiatt, J.R., Savar, A., et al. (1999) Perforated appendicitis is not a contraindication to laparoscopy. Am Surg 65, 965-967.

20 Faranda, C., Barrat, C., Catheline, J.M., et al. (2000) Two-stage laparoscopic management of generalized peritonitis due to perforated sigmoid diverticula: eighteen cases. Surg Laparosc Endosc Percutan Tech 10, 135-138.

21 Navez, B., Delgadillo, X., Cambier, E., et al. (2001) Laparoscopic approach for acute appendicular peritonitis: efficacy and safety: a report of 96 consecutive cases. Surg Laparosc Endosc Percutan Tech 11, 313-316.

22 Ceribelli, C., Adami, E.A., Mattia, S., et al. (2012) Bedside diagnostic laparoscopy for critically ill patients, a retrospective study of 62 patients. Surg Endosc 26, 3612-3615.

23 Polat, C., Aktepe, O.C., Akbulut, G., et al. (2003) The effects of increased intra-abdominal pressure on bacterial translocation. Yonsei Med J 44, 259-264.

24 Fowler, D.L. (2010) Laparoscopy in the acute abdomen. In: Assalia, A., Gagner, M., Schein, M. (eds.) Controversies in Laparoscopic Surgery. Springer, Berlin, pp. 45-53.

25 Bloechle, C., Emmerman, A., Achilles, E., et al. (1995) The role of laparoscopy in patients with suspected peritonitis: experience of a single institution. J Laparoendosc Adv Surg Tech 9, 898-900.

26 West, M.A., Baker, J., Bellingham, J., et al. (1996) Kinetics of decreased LPS-stimulated cytokine release by macrophages exposed to CO_2. J Surg Res 63, 269-274.

27 West, M.A., Hackam, D.J., Baker, J., et al. (1997) Mechanism of decreased in vitro murine macrophage cytokine release after exposure to carbon dioxide: relevance to laparoscopic surgery. Ann Surg 226, 179-182.

28 Bloechle, C., Emmerman, A., Strate, T., et al. (1998) Laproscopic vs open repair of gastric perforation and abdominal lavage of associated peritonitis in pigs. Surg Endosc 12, 212-218.

29 Bloechle, C., Kluth, D., Holstein, A.F., et al. (1999) A pneumoperitoneum perpetuates severe damage to the ultrastructural integrity of parietal peritoneum in gastric perforation-induced peritonitis in rats. Surg Endosc 13, 683-688.

30 Leon EL, Metzger A, Tsiotos GG, et al. (1998) Laparoscopic management of small bowel obstruction: indications and outcome. J Gastrointest Surg 2, 132-140.

31 Strickland, P., Lourie, D.J., Suddleson, E.A., et al. (1999) Is laparoscopy safe and effective for treatment of acute small-bowel obstruction? Surg Endosc 13, 695-698.

32 Fazio, V.W., Lopez-Kostner, F. (2000) Role of laparoscopic surgery for treatment of early colorectal carcinoma. World J Surg 24, 1056-1060.

33 Baiocchi, G.L., Vettoretto, N., Zago, M., et al. (2014) A common case with common problems, laparoscopic treatment of small bowel obstruction (SBO). Ann Ital Chir Apr 7;85(ePub). pii: S2239253X14021525.

34 Navez, B., Arimont, J.M., Guiot, P. (1998a) Laparoscopic approach in acute small bowel obstruction. A review of 68 patients. Hepatogastroenterology 45, 132-140.

35 Chosidow, D., Johanet, H., Montariol, T., et al. (2000) Laparoscopy for acute small bowel obstruction secondary to adhesions. J Laparoendosc Adv Surg Tech 10, 155-159.

36 Rumstadt, B., Schwab, M., Schuster, K., et al. (1997) The role of laparoscopy in the preoperative staging of pancreatic carcinoma. J Gastrointest Surg 1, 245-250.

37 Bhalla, R., Formella, L., Kerrigan, D.D. (2000) Need for staging laparoscopy in patients with gastric cancer. Br J Surg 87, 362-373.

38 Lavonius, M.I., Laine, S., Salo, S., et al. (2001) Role of laparoscopy and laparoscopic ultrasound in staging of pancreatic tumors. Ann Chir Gynaecol 90, 252-255.

39 Wayman, J., Jamieson, G.G. (2010) Laparoscopy in abdominal malignancy. In: Assalia, A., Gagner, M., Schein, M. (eds.) Controversies in Laparoscopic Surgery. Springer, Berlin, pp. 87-100.

40 O'Brien, M.G., Fitzgerald, E.F., Lee, G., et al. (1995) A prospective comparison of laparoscopy and imaging in the staging of esophogastric cancer before surgery. Am J Gastroenterol 90, 2191-2194.

41 Hunter, J.G., Staheli, J., Oddsdottir, M., et al. (1995) Nitrous oxide pneumoperitoneum revisited. Is there a risk of combustion? Surg Endosc 9, 501-504.

42 Neuberger, T.J., Andrus, C.H., Wittgen, C.M., et al. (1996) Prospective comparison of helium versus carbon dioxide pneumoperitoneum. Gastrointest Endosc 43, 38-41.

43 Fleming, R.Y., Dougherty, T.B., Feig, B.W. (1997) The safety of helium for abdominal insufflation. Surg Endosc 11, 230-234.

44 Schwandner, O., Schiedeck, T.H., Bruch, H.P. (1999a) Advanced age: indication or contraindication for laparoscopic colorectal surgery? Dis Colon Rectum 42, 356-362.

45 Orlando, R. III, Crowell, K.L. (1997) Laparoscopy in the critically ill. Surg Endosc 11, 1072-1074.

46 Baskin, J.J., Vishteh, A.G., Wesche, D.E., et al. (1998) Ventriculoperitoneal shunt failure as a complication of laparoscopic surgery. J Soc Laparoendosc Surg 2, 177-180.

47 Curet, M.J., Vogt, D.A., Schob, O., et al. (1996) Effects of CO_2 pneumoperitoneum in pregnant ewes. J Surg Res 63, 339-344.

48 Halpern, N.B. (1998a) Laparoscopic cholecystectomy in pregnancy: a review of published experiences and clinical considerations. Semin Laparosc Surg 5, 129-134.

49 Conron, R.W. Jr, Abruzzi, K., Cochrane, S.O., et al. (1999) Laparoscopic procedures in pregnancy. Am Surg 65, 259-263.

50 Holthausen, U.H., Mettler, L, Troidl, H. (1999) Pregnancy: a contraindication? World J Surg 23, 856-862.

51 de Perrot, M., Jenny, A., Morales, M., et al. (2000) Laparoscopic appendectomy during pregnancy. Surg Laparosc Endosc Percutaneous Tech 10, 368-371.

52 Ray, U., Gupta, S., Chatterjee, S., et al. (2012) Laparoscopic versus open splenectomy in the treatment of idiopathic thrombocytopenic purpura: an Indian experience. J Indian Med Assoc 110, 889-893.

53 Park, A., Witzke, D. Education and training. (2010) In: Assalia, A., Gagner, M., Schein, M. (eds.) Controversies in Laparoscopic Surgery. Springer, Berlin, pp. 1-13.

54 Cagir, B., Rangraj, M., Maffuci, L., et al. (1994) The learning curve for laparoscopic cholecystectomy. J Laparoendosc Surg 4, 419-427.

55 Hunter, J.G., Sackier, J.M., Berci, G. (1994) Training in laparoscopic cholecystectomy: quantifying the learning curve. Surg Endosc 8, 28-31.

56 Voitk, A.J., Tsao, S.G.S., Ignatius, S. (2001) The tail of the learning curve for laparoscopic cholecystectomy. Am J Surg 182, 250-253.

57 See, W.A., Cooper, C.S., Fisher, R.J. (1993) Predictors of laparoscopic complications after formal training in laparoscopic surgery. JAMA 270, 2689-2692.

58 Morino, M., Festa, V., Garrone, C. (1995) Survey on Torino courses. The impact of a two-day practical course on apprenticeship and diffusion of laparoscopic cholecystectomy in Italy. Surg Laparosc Endosc 9, 46-48.

59 Cuschieri, A. (1993) Reflections on surgical training [editorial]. Surg Endosc 7, 73-74.

60 Rogers, D.A., Elstein, A.S., Bordage, G. (2001) Improving continuing medical education for surgical techniques: applying the lessons learned in the first decade of minimal access surgery. Ann Surg 233, 159-166.

61 Gilroy, B.A., Anson, L.W. (1987) Fatal air embolism during anesthesia for laparoscopy in a dog. J Am Vet Med Assoc 190, 552-554.

62 Monnet, E., Twedt, D.C. (2003) Laparoscopy. Vet Clin North Am Sm Anim Pract 33, 1147-1163.

63 Twedt, D.C., Monnet, E. (2005) Laparoscopy: technique and clinical experience. In: McCarthy, T.C. (ed.) Veterinary Endoscopy for the Small Animal Practitioner. Elsevier, Philadelphia, pp. 357-386.

64 Buote, N.J., Kovak-McClaran, J.R., Schold, J.D. (2011) Conversion from diagnostic laparoscopy to laparotomy, risk factors and occurrence. Vet Surg 40, 106-114.

65 Davidson, E.B., Moll, H.D., Payton, M.E. (2004) Comparison of laparoscopic ovariohysterectomy and ovariohysterectomy in dogs. Vet Surg 33, 62-69.

66 Devitt, C.M., Cox, R.E., Hailey, J.J. (2005) Duration, complications, stress, and pain of open ovariohysterectomy versus a simple method of laparoscopic-assisted ovariohysterectomy in dogs. J Am Vet Med Assoc 227, 921-927.

67 Mayhew, P.D., Mehler, S.J., Radhakrishnan, A. (2008) Laparoscopic cholecystectomy for management of uncomplicated gall bladder mucocele in six dogs. Vet Surg 37, 625-630.

68 Petre, S.L., McClaran, J.K., Bergman, P.J., et al. (2012) Safety and efficacy of laparoscopic hepatic biopsy in dogs: 80 cases (2004-2009). J Am Vet Med Assoc 240, 181-185.

69 Halpin, V.J., Soper, N.J. (2006) Decision to convert to open methods. In: Whelan, R.L., Fleshman, J.W., Fowler, D.L. (eds.) The SAGES Manual Perioperative Care in Minimally Invasive Surgery. New York, Springer, pp. 296-306.

70 Duke, T., Steinacher, S.L., Remedios, A.M. (1996) Cardiopulmonary effects of using carbon dioxide for laparoscopic surgery in dogs. Vet Surg 25, 77-82.

71 Beazley, S.G., Cosford, K., Duke-Novakovski, T. (2011) Cardiopulmonary effects of using carbon dioxide for laparoscopic surgery in cats. Can Vet J 52, 973-978.

72 Mayhew, P.D., Pascoe, P.J., Kass, P.H., et al. (2013) Effects of pneumoperitoneum induced at various pressures on cardiorespiratory function and working space during laparoscopy in cats. Am J Vet Res 74, 1340-1346.

73 Rizvi, A.Z., Hunter, J.G. (2010) Establishing pneumoperitoneum: the ideal gas and physiologic consequences. In: Assalia, A., Gagner, M., Schein, M. (eds.) Controversies in Laparoscopic Surgery. Springer, Berlin, pp. 27-44.

74 Staffieri, F., Lacitignola, L., De Siena, R., et al. (2007) A case of spontaneous venous embolism with carbon dioxide during laparoscopic surgery in a pig. Vet Anaesth Analg 34, 63-66.

75 LeBlanc, K.A. (2004) General laparoscopic surgical complications. In: LeBlanc, K.A. (ed.) Management of Laparoscopic Surgical Complications. Marcel Dekker, New York, pp. 43-62.

76 McMahon, A.J., Baxter, J.N., O'Dwyer, P.J. (1993) Preventing complications of laparoscopy. Br J Surg 80, 1593-1594.

77 Hanly, E.J., Aurora, A.A., Shih, S.P., et al. (2007) Peritoneal acidosis mediates immunoprotection in laparoscopic surgery. Surgery 142, 357-364.

78 Nickkholgh, A., Barro-Bejarano, M., Liang, R., et al. (2008) Signs of reperfusion injury following CO_2 pneumoperitoneum: an in vivo microscopy study. Surg Endosc 22, 122-128.

79 Bateman, B.G., Kolp, L.A., Hoeger, K. (1996) Complications of laparoscopy—operative and diagnostic. Fertil Steril 66, 30-35.

80 Teoh, B., Sen, R., Abbott, J. (2005) An evaluation of four tests used to ascertain Veress needle placement at closed laparoscopy. J Minim Invasive Gynecol 12, 153-158.

81 Vilos, G.A., Ternamian, A., Dempster, J., et al. (2007) Laparoscopic entry: a review of techniques, technologies, and complications. J Obstet Gynaecol Can 29, 433-465.

82 Whittemore, J.C., Mitchell, A., Hyink, S., et al. (2013) Diagnostic accuracy of tissue impedance measurement interpretation for correct Veress needle placement in canine cadavers. Vet Surg 42, 613-622.

83 Hyink, S., Whittemore, J.C., Mitchell, A., et al. (2013) Diagnostic accuracy of tissue impedance measurement interpretation for correct Veress needle placement in feline cadavers. Vet Surg 42, 623-628.

84 Doerner, J., Fiorbianco, V., Dupré, G. (2012) Intercostal insertion of Veress needle for canine laparoscopic procedures: a cadaver study. Vet Surg 41, 362-366.

85 Fiorbianco, V., Skalicky, M., Doerner, J., et al. (2012) Right intercostal insertion of a Veress needle for laparoscopy in dogs. Vet Surg 41, 367-373.

86 Courdier, S., Garbin, O., Hummel, M., et al. (2009) Equipment failure: causes and consequences in endoscopic gynecologic surgery. J Minim Invasive Gynecol 16, 28-33.

87 Kwazneski, D. 2nd, Six, C., Stahlfeld, K. (2013) The unacknowledged incidence of laparoscopic stapler malfunction. Surg Endosc 27, 86-89.

88 Ahmed, S., Ali, A.A., Hasan, M., et al. (2013) Problems leading to conversion in laparoscopic cholecystectomy. Mymensingh Med J 22, 53-58.

89 Kane, M.G,. Krejs, G.J. (1984) Complications of diagnostic laparoscopy in Dallas: a 7-year prospective study. Gastrointest Endosc 30, 237-240.

90 Mayhew, P.D., Brown, D.C. (2007) Comparison of three techniques for ovarian pedicle hemostasis during laparoscopic-assisted ovariohysterectomy. Vet Surg 36, 541-547.

91 Culp, W.T.N., Mayhew, P.D., Brown, D.C. (2009) The effect of laparoscopic versus open ovariectomy on postsurgical activity in small dogs. Vet Surg 38, 811-817.

92 Coisman, J.G., Case, J.B., Shih, A., et al. (2014) Comparison of surgical variables in cats undergoing single-incision laparoscopic ovariectomy using a LigaSure or extracorporeal suture versus open ovariectomy. Vet Surg 43, 38-44.

93 Härkki, P., Kurki, T., Sjöberg, J., et al. (2001) Safety aspects of laparoscopic hysterectomy. Acta Obstet Gynecol Scand 0, 383-391.

94 Miranda, C.S., Carvajal, A.R. (2003) Complications of operative gynecological laparoscopy. JSLS 7, 53-58.

95 Papandria, D., Lardaro, T., Rhee, D., et al. (2013) Risk factors for conversion from laparoscopic to open surgery: analysis of 2138 converted operations in the American College of Surgeons National Surgical Quality Improvement Program. Am Surg 79, 914-921.

96 Heijnsdijk, E.A., de Visser, H., Dankelman, J., et al. (2004) Slip and damage properties of jaws of laparoscopic graspers. Surg Endosc 18, 974-979.

97 Bianchi, P.P., Rosati, R., Bona, S., et al. (2007) Laparoscopic surgery in rectal cancer, a prospective analysis of patient survival and outcomes. Dis Colon Rectum 50, 2047-2053.

98 Feingold, D.L., Widmann W.D., Calhoun, S.K., et al. (2003) Persistent post-laparoscopy pneumoperitoneum. Surg Endosc 17, 296-299.

99 Kirchhoff, P., Dincler, S., Buchmann, P. (2008) A multivariate analysis of potential risk factors for intra- and postoperative complications in 1316 elective laparoscopic colorectal procedures. Ann Surg 248, 259-265.

100 Freeman, L.J. (1999) Complications. In: Freeman, L.J. (ed.) Veterinary Endosurgery. Mosby, St. Louis, pp. 92-102.

101 Martinez, J., Targarona, E.M., Balagué, C., et al. (1995) Port site metastasis. An unresolved problem in laparoscopic surgery. A review. Int Surg 80, 315-321.

102 Brundell, S., Ellis, T., Dodd, T., et al. (2002) Hematogenous spread as a mechanism for the generation of abdominal wound metastases following laparoscopy. Surg Endosc 16, 292-295.

103 Paolucci, V., Schaeff, B., Schneider, M., et al. (1999) Tumor seeding following laparoscopy: international survey. World J Surg. 23, 989-995; discussion 996-997.

104 Lelievre, L., Paterlini-Brechot, P., Camatte, S., et al. (2004) Effect of laparoscopy versus laparotomy on circulating tumor cells using isolation by size of epithelial tumor cells. Int J Gynecol Cancer 14, 229-233.

105 Wilson, M.Z., Hollenbeak, C.S., Stewart, D.B. (2013) Laparoscopic colectomy is associated with a lower incidence of postoperative complications compared with open colectomy: a propensity score-matched cohort analysis. Colorectal Dis Dec 21 (Epub ahead of print).

106 Park, J.Y., Kim, D.Y., Kim, J.H., et al. (2013) Laparoscopic versus open radical hysterectomy in patients with stage IB2 and IIA2 cervical cancer. J Surg Oncol 108, 63-69.

107 Kelly, K.N., Iannuzzi, J.C., Rickles, A.S., et al. (2014) Laparotomy for small-bowel obstruction: first choice or last resort for adhesiolysis? A laparoscopic approach for small-bowel obstruction reduces 30-day complications. Surg Endosc 28, 65-73.

108 Schwandner, O., Schiedeck, T.H.K., Bruch, H.P. (1999b) The role of conversion in laparoscopic colorectal surgery: do predictive factors exist? Surg Endosc 13, 151-156.

109 Rotholtz, N.A., Laporte, M., Pereyra, L., et al. (2008) Predictive factors for conversion in laparoscopic colorectal surgery. Tech Coloprotocol 12, 27-31.

110 Gaujoux, S., Bonnet, S., Leconte, M., et al. (2011) Risk factors for conversion and complications after unilateral laparoscopic adrenalectomy. Br J Surg 98, 1392-1399.

111 Van der Steeg, H.J., Alexander, S., Houterman, S., et al. (2011) Risk factors for conversion during laparoscopic cholecystectomy—experiences from a general teaching hospital. Scand J Surg 100, 169-173.

Laparoscopic Surgical Procedures

11 Diagnostic Laparoscopy of the Gastrointestinal Tract

J. Brad Case

> **Key Points**
>
> - Gastrointestinal (GI) exploratory laparoscopy can be performed safely in dogs and cats provided that the minimally invasive surgeon is thorough and possesses good decision-making ability.
> - A complete understanding of GI anatomy and physiology is a mandatory prerequisite before considering a laparoscopic approach to GI disease.
> - Accurate preoperative diagnostic evaluation is critical in patient selection for laparoscopic GI surgery.
> - Intraoperative alteration of patient position is often necessary for complete evaluation of the GI tract.
> - The minimally invasive GI surgeon must be ready and willing to convert to traditional laparotomy if the procedure can not be completed safely and effectively.

Preoperative Considerations

Gastroenteric Pathophysiology

A myriad of gastrointestinal (GI) diseases affect dogs and cats, with the most common being obstructive and nonobstructive foreign bodies, infectious, inflammatory, and neoplastic conditions. GI disease disrupts normal physiologic mechanisms and can lead to significant debilitation in dogs and cats, including hypovolemia, hypoproteinemia, electrolyte and acid–base imbalance, inflammation, perforation, and sepsis.[1-6] In the case of obstructive GI disease, acute vomiting can result in fluid and electrolyte losses, but the relative significance to overall fluid and electrolyte balance may be minimal with lower intestinal obstruction.[7,8] Clinically, however, hypochloremia, metabolic alkalosis, hypokalemia, and hyponatremia appear to be common in both upper and lower GI obstruction.[4] Vomiting is a common sequela to GI obstruction that puts the patient at risk for aspiration pneumonia and further debilitation.[8] Obstructed bowel becomes distended, hypersecretory, malabsorptive, hyper- or hypomotile, and ischemic, which can lead to microbial translocation and eventual perforation.[1,2,9-11] Intraluminal fluid accumulation appears to be significant in the upper GI tract in contrast to the lower intestinal tract, where minimal to no fluid accumulation occurs after acute obstruction for up to 72 hours.[2] Acute small intestinal obstruction also affects electromotor activity of the bowel.[10] A pattern of orad hypermotility results initially, which progresses in an orad direction to the level of the proximal duodenum. Simultaneously, aborad to the obstruction, hypomotility results, which progresses aborad to the level of the terminal ileum.[9] As chronicity develops, eventual diffuse intestinal ileus ensues.[10] A significant and immediate reduction of intestinal blood flow occurs with intestinal obstruction at intraluminal pressures of 30 mm Hg. As intraluminal pressure increases beyond 30 mm Hg, a corresponding worsening of intestinal blood flow results until a residual 20% to 35% of original flow remains.[11] Oxygen extraction by the small intestine also declines as intraluminal pressure increases.[11]

Nonobstructive or partially obstructive GI disease in dogs and cats may be associated with a more chronic and subtle onset of signs, including intermittent vomiting, gradual weight loss, mild hypoproteinemia, and hypokalemia.[12] Appropriate recognition and resuscitation of compromised patients before anesthesia and surgery is important regardless of whether or not laparoscopy is to be performed. A laparoscopic approach to GI surgery, when performed safely, should not present any significant additional risks versus a traditional laparotomy. Accordingly, the surgeon and support staff must be trained, experienced, and ready to convert to exploratory laparotomy in both elective and emergent situations if indicated.[13-15] GI laparoscopy is beneficial in staging and determining operability in certain cancers[16] and is associated with minimal morbidity and improved patient recovery compared with more

Small Animal Laparoscopy and Thoracoscopy, First Edition. Edited by Boel A. Fransson and Philipp D. Mayhew.

© 2015 by ACVS Foundation. Published 2015 by John Wiley & Sons, Inc.

Companion website: www.wiley.com/go/fransson/laparoscopy

invasive methods in humans.[17] Similar benefits likely exist with veterinary patients, but comparative studies have not been performed.

Relevant Anatomy

The GI tract in dogs and cats occupies most of the peritoneal cavity and extends from the esophageal hiatus of the diaphragm to the rectum in the pelvic canal. Therefore, complete gastroenteric exploration requires abundant working space and visibility within the majority of the peritoneal cavity. The stomach is divided into four major anatomic regions: the cardia, fundus, body, and pylorus. It is supported in position by surrounding soft tissues, including the esophagus and diaphragm; hepatogastric, hepatoduodenal, and gastrosplenic ligaments; and the liver and mesentery. In diagnostic GI laparoscopy, the ventral parietal gastric surface is readily visible, which facilitates evaluation. In contrast, the dorsal visceral surface is obscured by gravity and the surrounding adjoining soft tissues and thus requires alteration of patient position or gastric manipulation for evaluation in most cases. The pylorus is continuous with the descending duodenum at the cranial duodenal flexure, which is anchored in place by the hepatoduodenal ligament and the mesoduodenum. The descending duodenum originates in the right hypochondriac region and is anchored at the caudal duodenal flexure to the mesocolon.[18] Consequently, laparoscopic evaluation of the stomach and descending duodenum is performed intracorporeally in most cases. The ascending duodenum continues craniosinistrally from the caudal duodenal flexure, where it dives dorsally to the mesentery of the remaining small intestine and transitions into the jejunum. The ascending duodenum and jejunum are only loosely tethered dorsally by a relatively long mesenteric root, which facilitates extracorporeal laparoscopic-assisted evaluation. At the ileocecocolic junction (ICJ), the mesenteric attachments become shorter and therefore anchor the ICJ and colon more dorsally and caudally in the abdominal cavity. As a consequence, exteriorization and extracorporeal evaluation is more difficult but accomplishable in most cases with a laparoscopic-assisted approach.

The major arterial blood supply to the GI tract originates from the abdominal aorta via either the celiac or the cranial mesenteric artery (Figure 11-1). The stomach and proximal duodenum are supplied primarily by the major celiac branches: splenic, gastroepiploic, left and right gastric, gastroduodenal, hepatic, and cranial pancreaticoduodenal. The intestine, in contrast, is supplied almost exclusively by the caudal pancreaticoduodenal and jejunal branches of the cranial mesenteric artery, the major exception being the descending colon, which is derived from the left colic branch of the caudal mesenteric artery (see Figure 11-1). The venous drainage of the GI tract is ultimately via the portal vein, which is derived by four major veins: the cranial and caudal mesenteric, splenic, and gastroduodenal (see Figure 11-1). The caudal rectal vein, however, drains directly to the caudal vena cava. The main portal vein is enveloped by the mesoduodenum and is therefore visualized intracorporeally (Figure 11-2) along with the right limb of the pancreas and descending duodenum.

Diagnostic Workup

The preoperative diagnostic workup is typical of dogs and cats presenting with clinical signs of GI disease and is not usually different compared with patients undergoing laparotomy. In general, patients with GI disease should undergo preoperative complete blood count, serum biochemistry, urinalysis, coagulation testing, and appropriate diagnostic imaging. Dogs with GI hemorrhage may have a chronic nonregenerative anemia and associated azotemia. An inflamma-

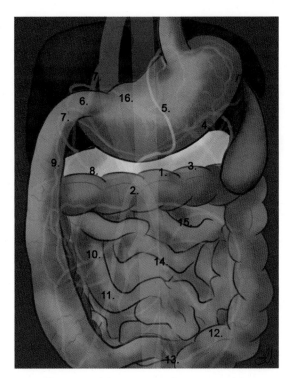

Figure 11-1 Illustration of the major vascular anatomy of the gastrointestinal tract in dogs and cats. Celiac artery (1), cranial mesenteric artery (2), splenic artery (3), gastroepiploic artery (4), left and right gastric artery (5 and 6), gastroduodenal artery (7), hepatic artery (8), cranial pancreaticoduodenal artery (9), caudal pancreaticoduodenal artery (10), jejunal arteries (11), left colic artery (12), caudal mesenteric artery (13), portal vein (14), mesenteric vein (15), splenic vein (16), and gastroduodenal vein (17).

tory leukogram is common with many GI diseases. A degenerative, left-shifted leukogram with evidence of sepsis (e.g., hypoglycemia, hyperbilirubinemia) should raise the suspicion of septic peritonitis, currently a contraindication to laparoscopic-assisted GI exploration. Serum biochemistry and urinalysis allow for assessment of hepatic and renal function and fluid and electrolyte status and are helpful in targeted therapy and resuscitation. Although uncommon

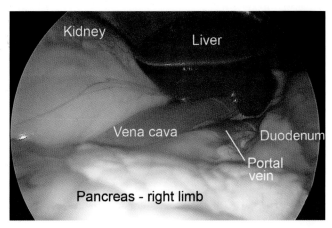

Figure 11-2 Intracorporeal view of the right cranial abdomen of a dog in left lateral recumbency during laparoscopic-assisted exploration. Notice that the parietal surface of the right pancreatic limb, duodenum, portal vein, vena cava, right lateral and caudate liver lobes, and right kidney are well visualized in this recumbency.

in an experienced minimally invasive surgeon's hands, intraoperative hemorrhage was responsible for 85% of emergent diagnostic laparoscopic conversions in one study.[13] Preoperative coagulation testing should therefore be considered in patients undergoing laparoscopic GI exploratory surgery, especially if biopsy of a vascular organ or mass is anticipated.

Depending on the nature of the disease, abdominal radiography may be sufficient for diagnosis, as is the case with the majority of simple intestinal obstructions.[19] Proximal duodenal and gastric outflow obstructions typically demonstrate a fluid distended duodenum and stomach, but more distal small intestinal obstructions typically reveal gas distention orad to the obstruction. Free peritoneal fluid creating loss of serosal detail and pneumoperitoneum, usually apparent as a thin gas lucency along the diaphragmatic margin, are consistent with hollow viscous rupture and potential septic peritonitis. In contrast, patients with nonobstructive GI disease may require abdominal ultrasonography (AUS) or computed tomography (CT) for preoperative evaluation.[19,20] AUS allows for accurate assessment of bowel diameter and wall thickness.[21] AUS is also useful in documenting small volumes of peritoneal fluid and gas, loss of wall layering, and hyperechoic mesentery, which are findings consistent with peritonitis.[22] However, AUS evaluation can be limited by operator experience; by the presence of large amounts of GI gas; and by the length of the examination, particularly in compromised patients.[23,24] Preoperative CT is used commonly for evaluation of humans with abdominal and GI disease and is becoming more popular in veterinary patients.[20,23-25] Contrast-enhanced CT has been found to be more accurate at lesion measurement versus AUS and is reported to be 100% accurate in differentiating surgical from nonsurgical acute abdominal conditions in dogs.[24] CT may possess unique benefits related to differentiating dogs and cats amenable to laparoscopic versus traditional GI exploration via laparotomy. In the author's experience, noncontrast CT has been effective at facilitating lesion measurement and localization within the specific segment of the GI tract (Figure 11-3) as well as at defining lesion association with adjacent structures. Thus, CT has helped to screen for patients less ideal for laparoscopic-assisted GI exploratory in some cases. However, compared with AUS, CT is likely more expensive and may be less accurate in regards to spatial and temporal resolution of certain structures.

Patient Selection

Selection criteria for diagnostic laparoscopic GI exploration have not been determined for dogs and cats. However, a recent study looking at conversion rates from diagnostic laparoscopy to laparotomy found that a low preoperative total solids, presence of a solitary liver tumor, and diagnosis of neoplasia were associated with an increased risk of conversion to laparotomy.[13] In the same study, a total conversion rate of 21% was determined. There are currently only two clinical reports describing the use of diagnostic and therapeutic GI laparoscopy in dogs and cats.[14,15] Both of these studies used a laparoscopic-assisted technique to explore the GI tract and reported excellent outcomes with few complications. However, conversions were reported in both case series, and a number of limitations and potential contraindications were suggested. For example, lesion diameter appears to be important, and the author of this chapter considers an intestinal lesion diameter of approximately 5 cm to be a reasonable upper limit when considering a laparoscopic-assisted approach in most dogs and cats.[15] Similar lesion sizes have been proposed in human laparoscopic-assisted GI surgery,[17] but there are conflicting recommendations.[26,27] Large-diameter lesions require significant enlargement of the port incision and may obviate some of the benefits of a minimal approach. Because the bowel is tubular, the length of the lesion is not as important in regard to exclusion as long as the affected bowel can be exteriorized safely. GI lesion lengths of up to 9 cm have been reported to be amenable to a laparoscopic-assisted exploratory approach.[14] The specific region of the affected bowel also appears to be important when considering patients as candidates for laparoscopic-assisted GI exploration. Dogs and cats with GI lesions affecting the stomach, orad duodenum, or bowel aborad to the ICJ may not be ideal candidates for a laparoscopic-assisted approach if significant exteriorization is required for complete evaluation and treatment.[14,15] Adhesions of the GI tract appear to be a contraindication to laparoscopic-assisted GI exploration in dogs and cats as well. Adhesions tether bowel to the mesentery and to other bowel segments, which results in the inability to safely exteriorize bowel from the peritoneal cavity without significant lengthening of port incisions.[15] Dense GI adhesions are associated with an increased risk of conversion from laparoscopic-assisted to traditional GI surgery in humans for management of small bowel obstruction,[28] and caution should be exercised when considering a laparoscopic approach in veterinary patients with known adhesions.[14,15] Other potential contraindications for GI laparoscopy in dogs and cats include GI perforation, septic peritonitis, linear foreign bodies, association with adjacent structures such as the common bile duct or pancreas, and inexperience of the surgery team. The stability of the patient needs to also be considered, and effort should be made to correct metabolic and cardiovascular disturbances before anesthesia and surgery regardless of whether or not a laparoscopic approach is performed. The operating surgeon should, however, elect for the most rapid and efficacious approach if patient stability is at all in question. As time progresses and minimally invasive GI surgeons gain experience, improved guidelines and specific recommendations will evolve to improve patient selection.

Patient Preparation

Patients undergoing laparoscopic-assisted GI surgery are prepared similarly to dogs undergoing traditional exploratory laparotomy because conversion to laparotomy is necessary in some cases. Aspiration is a known risk after anesthesia, especially in dogs and cats with GI disease. Efforts should therefore be made to reduce gastric content and volume as much as possible before induction of anesthesia. The presence of gastric material and inflammation

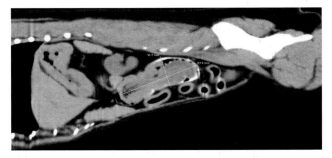

Figure 11-3 Preoperative sagittal abdominal computed tomography (CT) image of a dog with an ileocecocolic intussusception. Abdominal CT is accurate in lesion localization within the specific region of the gastrointestinal tract and at measuring lesion diameter and length. This dog would not be a good candidate for a laparoscopic-assisted approach because of the excessively large nature of the mass.

and the use of opioid medications delay gastric emptying,[29] possibly increasing the chance of reflux and aspiration of gastric fluid. If oropharyngeal reflux is observed during induction of anesthesia, the endotracheal tube cuff should be checked for an adequate seal and the oropharynx well evacuated using a suction system. Fasting supports gastric emptying and decreases gastric pH.[30] Proton pump inhibitors (PPIs) and prokinetic medications may reduce not only the risk for gastric acid–associated esophageal erosion or ulceration but also gastric emptying time, respectively, and should be considered in patients with GI pathology undergoing laparoscopic-assisted exploration. Compared with histamine-2 blockers, PPIs increase the duration that gastric pH remains above 3 to 4 and are more potent.[30,31] Whereas metoclopramide has been found to have a dose-related efficacy curve in experimental situations,[32] a lack of significant improvement in gastric myoelectric activity has been documented in certain pathologic conditions such as gastric dilatation and volvulus.[33] Because prokinetic medications are contraindicated in obstructive disease, use of these medications should be considered after the obstruction has been relieved. A recommended protocol is to start pantoprazole at 1 mg/kg IV every 24 hours before anesthesia and metoclopramide at 2 mg/kg/24 hr as an intravenous constant-rate infusion after the obstruction (if present) has been resolved. In nonobstructive and/or pseudo-obstructive gastric disease, prokinetics can be started before surgery. Fluid deficits as well as electrolyte and acid–base abnormalities are corrected before anesthesia. The urinary bladder is completely expressed or a retrograde urinary catheter is placed to maintain an empty bladder during the procedure. This is especially important for laparoscopic examination of the colon and caudal abdomen.

The patient is clipped widely from the inguinal region to approximately 5 cm cranial to the xyphoid process and laterally at least halfway along the abdominal wall in a dorsoventral orientation. Because conversion from diagnostic GI laparoscopy to exploratory laparotomy is necessary in some cases, the preparation must be adequate for emergent or elective conversion if the indication arises.

The decision to administer perioperative antibiotics is surgeon and case dependent. However, in the author's experience, most procedures will require at least 90 minutes of surgery time and ultimately lead to either gastrotomy or enterotomy; thus, perioperative antibiotics are usually indicated. Either first- (cefazolin) or second- (cefoxitin) generation cephalosporins are good options and can be administered at 22 mg/kg intravenously. Perioperative antibiotics should be delivered within 30 minutes of the skin incision being made and continued every 120 minutes until skin closure is complete to maintain antibiotic presence at the surgical site. Continuation of antibiotic prophylaxis beyond this time is rarely indicated.

Patient Position

Patients are positioned in dorsal recumbency and prepared using a standard aseptic technique. An operating table with the capacity for Trendelenburg and reverse Trendelenburg positions is very helpful. Alternatively or in addition to a motorized tilt table, a TT Endoscopic positioner (Apexx Veterinary Equipment, Englewood, CO) (Figure 11-4) is recommended when performing exploratory GI laparoscopy because alteration of the patient's position is often necessary. In small patients (cats and dogs <10 kg), however, the mechanical tilt table can be cumbersome, and its use is not necessary. Rather, the patient's position can be altered intermittently by the operating room (OR) technician, and the dog or cat can be stabilized in lateral recumbency using sand bags. The surgeon and assistant should stand on the left or right of the patient toward the *foot of the table*. If multiple video monitors are available, they are positioned at the *head of the table* on the right and left side. A single monitor is acceptable as long as it can easily be moved to the opposite side of the surgeon performing the exploration (Figure 11-5). Ceiling or boom-mounted monitors are preferable because movement of laparoscopy towers around the anesthetist and surgery table is cumbersome. The surgeon performing laparoscopic GI exploration will need to work from both the left and right of the patient. Thus, enough room should exist in the OR to allow the surgeon to move safely between the right and left sides of the patient. The instrument table is best placed at the *foot of the table,* leaving enough room for the surgeon and assistant to move around the back of the instrument table, thus avoiding collisions with the anesthetist or anesthesiologist. An extra large patient drape is recommended to prevent exposure of the patient and operating table during tilting of the patient.

Port Type and Position

Port type and position depend on the technique to be performed (single vs. multiple cannula) and the anticipated location of the lesion within the abdominal cavity. The multiport technique is performed with the laparoscope cannula placed subumbilically and the instrument cannula either midway between the umbilicus and xyphoid or between the umbilicus and pubis (Figure 11-6). Paramedian instrument port placement is helpful if laparoscopic-assisted feeding tube placement is to be performed.[34] Threaded cannulae are recommended for multiport procedures to prevent slippage of the cannula from within the peritoneum. With single-port procedures, a 20- to 30-mm skin incision is made 1 to 2 cm caudal to the umbilicus on midline (Figure 11-7). If the lesion is suspected to involve the ileocecocolic region, the port can be placed in a more caudal location. However, the port should not be placed farther caudal than midway between the umbilicus and pubis because doing so will restrict extracorporeal evaluation of the small intestine. For single-port placement, an index finger is used to palpate the peritoneal surface to ensure that no adhesions of abdominal viscera are present. If using the SILS port (SILSl Covidien, Mansfield, MA), it is grasped with two Carmalt forceps, the first engaging the cranial two thirds and the second engaging the caudal third. Sterile lubricant is applied to the surface of the port. The port is then placed by advancing the tips of the Carmalt forceps into the peritoneal cavity.

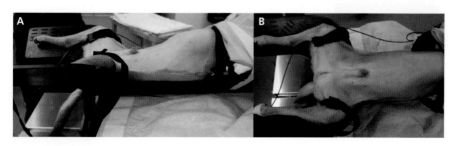

Figure 11-4 Preoperative images (**A** and **B**) of a dog with a small intestinal foreign body properly prepared and positioned on the mechanical tilt table. The tilt table allows for alteration between dorsal and both right and left lateral recumbency. The operating table facilitates both Trendelenburg and reverse Trendelenburg positioning.

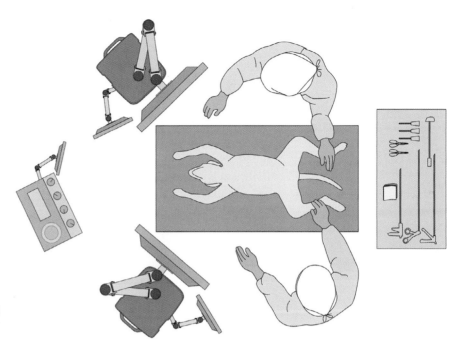

Figure 11-5 Illustration of the operating room set up for laparoscopic-assisted gastrointestinal surgery.

The Carmalt forceps are removed starting with the cranial forceps.[15] The EndoCone (Karl Storz, Veterinary Endoscopy, Goleta, CA) is inserted by engaging the abdominal wound with the leading edge (flange) of the threaded portion and twisting one revolution in a clockwise direction. The EndoCone is placed with the steel cap (bulkhead) detached to visualize the viscera during port insertion.[15] Three 5-mm inner cannulas are used with the SILS port. Although the EndoCone accommodates two 15-mm instruments, a 5-mm laparoscope and 5-mm instruments are recommended to minimize instrument interference, which is compounded with larger diameter instruments in the narrow base of the cone.

Working Space and Exposure

The peritoneal cavity is insufflated to a pressure of 8 to 10 mm Hg using CO_2 gas. Although insufflation up to 15 mm Hg in dogs is safe in most instances,[35] there is little clinical improvement in working space with additional pressure in cats,[36,37] and increased pressure may lead to additional pain or potentially time-dependent adverse sequelae.[38] A 5-mm, 30-degree, 29-cm laparoscope is used to examine the abdominal cavity. A 30-degree laparoscope is recommended for improved visualization of visceral surfaces, especially along the diaphragm and abdominal gutters. A number of positional maneuvers are helpful and necessary for thorough evaluation of the GI viscera. For example, examination of the gastric fundus and visceral surface of the stomach is facilitated by right lateral and reverse Trendelenburg positioning of the patient with concurrent retraction of the spleen and gastrosplenic ligament medially (Video Clip 11-1). A blunt probe or fan retractor can also be used to elevate the gastric body (Figure 11-8). The parietal surface of the stomach (especially the antral and pyloric regions) is evaluated in dorsal recumbency (Video Clip 11-2) with concurrent retraction of the liver lobes ventrally using a blunt probe or fan retractor (Figure 11-9). Expo-

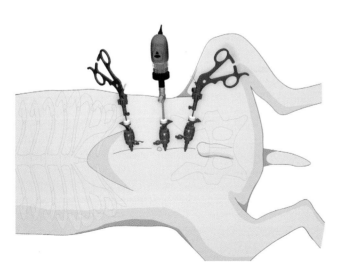

Figure 11-6 Illustration for correct port location for a multiport laparoscopic-assisted gastrointestinal exploratory procedure.

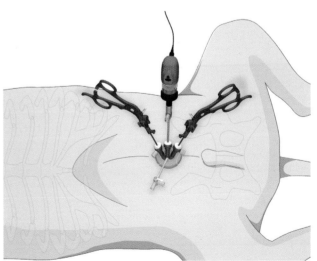

Figure 11-7 Illustration of correct location for a single incision port for laparoscopic-assisted gastrointestinal exploratory procedure.

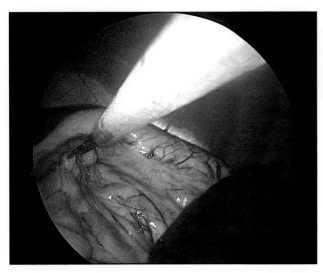

Figure 11-8 Intracorporeal view of the visceral gastric surface during retraction using a laparoscopic fan retractor.

sure cranially can be improved with caudal retraction of the gastric body using laparoscopic Babcock forceps. These maneuvers are also useful in observing the gallbladder, cystic duct, and common bile duct. The distal tip of the left limb of the pancreas can be evaluated and biopsied with the patient in right lateral recumbency with concurrent medial retraction of the gastrosplenic region (Video Clip 11-3). The left kidney and adrenal gland can also be evaluated in this position. For extracorporeal examination of the small intestine, a commercial wound retractor device or baby Gelpi forceps (Figure 11-10) can be used to distract the body wall and provide unrestricted access to the majority of the intestinal tract.

Instrumentation

Instruments needed include a SILS or EndoCone port (required for single-port procedures), straight laparoscopic Babcock forceps (required), straight or articulating laparoscopic DeBakey forceps (recommended), coaxial deviating laparoscopic Babcock forceps (optional if used with EndoCone), 5-mm 30-degree laparoscope (required), blunt palpation probe (required) or fan retractor (recommended), threaded or smooth 5.5-mm cannulae (required for multiport techniques), wound retractor (facilitative), small Gelpi retractor (facilitative), biopsy instruments (required), and basic surgical pack (required).

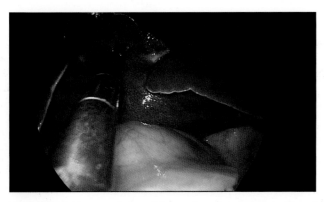

Figure 11-9 Intracorporeal view of the gastric antrum during elevation of the liver using a blunt palpation probe. Notice the primary peristaltic contraction.

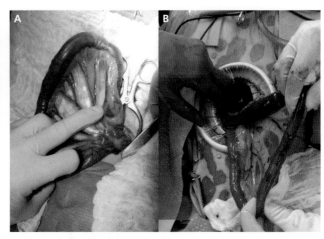

Figure 11-10 Intraoperative view of extracorporealized bowel using a Gelpi retractor (**A**) or a wound retractor (**B**). The ileocecocolic junction and lymph nodes are visible in A, and a segment of jejunum after enterotomy is demonstrated in B. (Part B courtesy of Dr. Ameet Singh.)

Surgical Techniques

Laparoscopic-Assisted Gastrointestinal Exploration

The GI tract can be challenging to explore completely and accurately using laparoscopy because of its length as well as its variation in size and location within the peritoneal cavity. For example, the stomach and orad duodenum are relatively deep and fixed within the cranial abdomen, which makes extracorporeal evaluation impossible. In contrast, the small intestine just aborad to the duodenocolic ligament through the ICJ is ideal for extracorporeal evaluation and is easily accomplished with a minimal *extraction* or *assist incision* (see Figure 11-10). Because GI disease often affects the upper and lower GI tract of dogs and cats, the operating surgeon must pay careful attention to technique when performing laparoscopic-assisted GI exploratory and ensure that all regions are adequately examined. Otherwise, GI lesions will be missed, and an unacceptable level of morbidity may result.

At the present time, three methods of GI exploration have been described in the primary veterinary literature. In an experimental report, Rawlings *et al.* described evaluation of the small intestine from the caudal duodenal flexure to the ileum using a *hand-over-hand* technique, but no description of gastric or colonic evaluation was included.[34] The *hand-over-hand* method is a previously reported method of intracorporeal intestinal evaluation in human laparoscopic surgery.[39,40] This method is time consuming and requires frequent grasping and repositioning of bowel within the laparoscopic forceps, which may increase the risk of iatrogenic bowel injury (Figure 11-11). Consequently, it has largely been replaced with an extracorporeal *hand-assisted* method of small bowel exploration. Gower and Mayhew described a laparoscopic-assisted intestinal exploration technique using a wound retractor.[14] In 2013, a single-incision laparoscopic-assisted method of exploration of the abdominal GI tract was described.[14] In this study, novel single-incision ports were used to explore the stomach, descending duodenum, ICJ, and colon intracorporeally while the remaining intestinal tract was explored extracorporeally in a *hand-assisted* fashion, similar to the method described by Gower and Mayhew. Conversion to exploratory laparotomy was required in only one out of eight animals because of an inability to complete the diagnostic GI exploration in that study.

Although a standardized technique has not been described, diagnostic GI laparoscopy should be performed systematically and in the

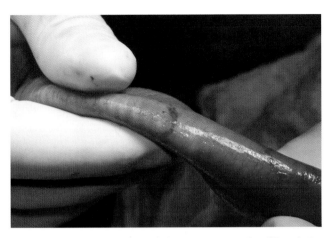

Figure 11-11 Intraoperative view of a hyperemic region of small bowel after grasping using 5-mm laparoscopic Babcock forceps.

same manner between patients. A *cranial-to-caudal* and *side-to-side* approach has been most useful in the author's experience. Initially, the stomach is evaluated using a blunt palpation probe while the parietal surface is imaged (see Video Clip 11-2). Aborad gastric contractions and peristaltic waves are easily observed. Ventral retraction of the hepatic lobes using a blunt probe (see Figure 11-9) or fan retractor is required for complete evaluation of the antrum and cardia. Caudal retraction of the gastric body using laparoscopic Babcock or DeBakey forceps facilitates visualization of the craniad stomach. The gastric fundus can be evaluated by positioning of the patient in right lateral and reverse Trendelenburg recumbency with concurrent caudal and medial retraction of the gastrosplenic region using a blunt probe or fan retractor (see Video Clip 11-1). Evaluation of the visceral gastric surface is accomplished by displacing the greater omentum and gastric body medially while in the same recumbency, although this is often difficult. The patient is positioned in left lateral recumbency for evaluation of the pylorus and descending duodenum (Video Clip 11-4). The blunt probe is used to elevate the bowel segment ventrally for visceral evaluation and medially for parietal visualization (see Figure 11-2). The right limb of the pancreas, main portal vein, vena cava, right kidney, and adrenal gland are easily observed at this time (Video Clip 11-5). The descending duodenum is then explored aborad to the level of the caudal duodenal flexure. The duodenocolic ligament and associated duodenum are difficult to visualize completely intracorporeally. This region can be digitally palpated using the *assist incision* after the port has been removed. For exploration of the remaining small intestine, the patient is positioned in dorsal recumbency, and a convenient loop of jejunum is grasped using the laparoscopic DeBakey or Babcock forceps then is brought ventrally to the port. The abdomen is then evacuated of CO_2, followed by removal of the port while maintaining a grasp of the jejunum using the atraumatic forceps. Conversely, a finger can be inserted through the *extraction incision* to grasp a convenient loop of small intestine after port removal. The margins of the celiotomy are then retracted and protected using a wound retractor[14] or baby Gelpi forceps (see Figure 11-10) and laparotomy sponges.[15] The jejunum is then exteriorized and grasped by the surgeon's fingers. Alternatively, with multiport exploration, individual port incisions are enlarged or connected, and a wound retractor is placed.[14] After it is exteriorized, the bowel is examined in an orad direction to the level of the caudal duodenal flexure and then aborally to the ICJ. Ileocecocolic lymph nodes are typically easy to examine with this approach. Depending

on the intestinal diameter and thickness, minimal enlargement of the port incision may be needed to prevent vascular occlusion of the mesentery during extracorporeal exploratory. The bowel is *run*, with the surgeon being sure to replace the bowel within the abdominal cavity before exteriorizing further bowel segments. Exteriorization of excessive bowel can create vascular occlusion and bowel ischemia if the *extraction incision* is not large enough. Because of the short and caudal mesenteric attachments of the colon, extracorporeal evaluation is difficult without creating a relatively long *extraction incision*. However, intracorporeal examination of the colon is relatively simple and is facilitated by right lateral recumbency (Video Clip 11-6). The colon is retracted ventrally similar to the duodenum using a blunt probe or laparoscopic Babcock forceps. The author minimizes direct grasping of bowel and instead uses blunt instruments to palpate and elevate by levering. The risk of iatrogenic bowel injury is most likely reduced using this approach. Exploration of the colon should be performed along with the gastric fundus to avoid repeat changes in recumbency and permanent loss of pneumoperitoneum associated with incisional enlargement. It is important to make sure that the urinary bladder is relatively empty during evaluation of the descending colon and pelvic canal.

Challenges

The main difficulties associated with laparoscopic-assisted diagnostic GI exploration are adequate visualization and palpation of all visceral anatomy and achieving unrestricted exteriorization of intestine. Adequate examination of the GI tract requires appropriate positioning and repositioning of the patient, intracorporeal manipulation and retraction of viscera, and consistency of methodology. Safe exteriorization of intestine requires recognition of potential contraindications such as *adhesion* formation or the presence of a *linear* foreign body. Additionally, adequacy of the incision length to avoid vascular constriction during intestinal evaluation is critical. The author has found an *extraction incision* length of 4 to 5 cm in large breed dogs and 3 cm in small breed dogs and cats to allow unrestricted exteriorization of intestine in most cases. Careful digital palpation of the caudal duodenal flexure and accurate examination of the pylorus and cranial duodenal flexure are critical to avoid missed obstructive or mass lesions. If intracorporeal GI exploration is performed, care must be taken to avoid dropping the bowel segment in between instrument grasps because it may be difficult to reidentify the same bowel segment being explored. In this case, the intracorporeal intestinal exploration will need to be reinitiated to ensure that all bowel segments are examined.

Complications

Reported complications associated with laparoscopic diagnostic GI exploration in veterinary surgery are limited to inability to evaluate specific regions of the intestinal tract and necessity for conversion to laparotomy (13%)[14,15] or minor incisional alteration (38%).[15] Although the efficacy of laparoscopic-assisted exploration has not been evaluated in a controlled manner, preliminary results are excellent assuming appropriate case selection and decision making by the operating surgeon. Complications reported in human laparoscopic GI surgery include perforation of viscera with laparoscopic instrumentation and hemorrhage[41] and wound infection.[27,41]

 All videos cited in this chapter can be found on the book's companion website at **www.wiley.com/go/fransson/ laparoscopy**

References

1 Enquist, I.F., Baumann, F.G., Rehder, E. (1968) Changes in body fluid spaces in dogs with intestinal obstruction. Surg Gynecol Obstet 127, 17-22.

2 Mishra, N.K., Appert, H.E., Howard, J.M. (1974) The effects of distention and obstruction on the accumulation of fluid in the lumen of small bowel of dogs. Ann Surg 180, 791-795.

3 Allen, D. Jr, Kvietys, P.R., Granger, D.N. (1986) Crystalloids versus colloids: implications in fluid therapy of dogs with intestinal obstruction. Am J Vet Res 47, 1751-1755.

4 Boag, A.K., Coe, R.J., Martinez, T.A., et al. (2005) Acid-base and electrolyte abnormalities in dogs with gastrointestinal foreign bodies. J Vet Intern Med 19, 816-821.

5 Ralphs, S.C., Jessen, C.R., Lipowitz, A.J. (2003) Risk factors for leakage following intestinal anastomosis in dogs and cats: 115 cases (1991-2000). J Am Vet Med Assoc 223, 73-77.

6 Grimes, J.A., Schmiedt, C.W., Cornell, K.K., et al. (2011) Identification of risk factors for septic peritonitis and failure to survive following gastrointestinal surgery in dogs. J Am Vet Med Assoc 238, 486-494.

7 Shields, R. (1965) The absorption and secretion of fluid and electrolytes by the obstructed bowel. Br J Surg 52, 774-779.

8 Kogan, D.A., Johnson, L.R., Sturges, B.K., et al. (2008) Etiology and clinical outcome in dogs with aspiration pneumonia: 88 cases (2004-2006). J Am Vet Med Assoc 233, 1748-1755.

9 Prihoda, M., Flatt, A., Summers, R.W. (1984) Mechanisms of motility changes during acute intestinal obstruction in the dog. Am J Physiol 247, G37-G42.

10 Summers, R.W., Yanda, R., Prihoda, M., et al. (1983) Acute intestinal obstruction: an electromyographic study in dogs. Gastroenterology 85, 1301-1306.

11 Boley, S.J., Agrawal, G.P., Warren, A.R., et al. (1969) Pathophysiologic effects of bowel distention on intestinal blood flow. Am J Surg 117, 228-234.

12 Hayes, G. (2009) Gastrointestinal foreign bodies in dogs and cats: a retrospective study of 208 cases. J Small Anim Pract 50, 576-583.

13 Buote, N.J., Kovak-McClaran, J.R., Schold, J.D. (2011) Conversion from diagnostic laparoscopy to laparotomy: risk factors and occurrence. Vet Surg 40, 106-114.

14 Gower, S.B., Mayhew, P.D. (2011) A wound retraction device for laparoscopic-assisted intestinal surgery in dogs and cats. Vet Surg 40, 485-488.

15 Case, J.B., Ellison, G. (2013) Single incision laparoscopic-assisted intestinal surgery (SILAIS) in 7 dogs and 1 cat. Vet Surg 42, 629-634.

16 Nair, C.K., Kothari, K.C. (2012) Role of diagnostic laparoscopy in assessing operability in borderline resectable gastrointestinal cancers. J Minim Access Surg 8, 45-49.

17 Cai, W., Wang, Z.T., Wu, L., et al. (2011) Laparoscopically assisted resections of small bowel stromal tumors are safe and effective. J Dig Dis 12, 443-447.

18 Evans, H.E. (1993) The digestive apparatus and abdomen: the small intestine. In: Miller's Anatomy of the Dog, 3rd edn. Saunders, Philadelphia, pp. 441-444.

19 Sharma, A., Thompson, M.S., Scrivani, P.V., et al. (2011) Comparison of radiography and ultrasonography for diagnosing small-intestinal mechanical obstruction in vomiting dogs. Vet Radiol Ultrasound 52, 248-255.

20 Fields, E.L., Robertson, I.D., Brown, J.C. Jr. (2012) Optimization of contrast-enhanced multidetector abdominal computed tomography in sedated canine patients. Vet Radiol Ultrasound 53, 507-512.

21 Delaney, F., O'Brien, R.T., Waller, K. (2003) Ultrasound evaluation of small bowel thickness compared to weight in normal dogs. Vet Radiol Ultrasound 44, 577-580.

22 Boysen, S.R., Tidwell, A.S., Penninck, D.G. (2003) Ultrasonographic findings in dogs and cats with gastrointestinal perforation. Vet Radiol Ultrasound 44, 556-564.

23 Shanaman, M.M., Hartman, S.K., O'Brien, R.T. (2012) Feasibility for using dual-phase contrast-enhanced multi-detector helical computed tomography to evaluate awake and sedated dogs with acute abdominal signs. Vet Radiol Ultrasound 53, 605-612.

24 Shanaman, M.M., Schwarz, T., Gal, A., et al. (2013) Comparison between survey radiography, B-mode ultrasonography, contrast-enhanced ultrasonography and contrast-enhanced multi-detector computed tomography findings in dogs with acute abdominal signs. Vet Radiol Ultrasound 54, 591-604.

25 Hryhorczuk, A.L., Lee, E.Y. (2012) Imaging evaluation of bowel obstruction in children: updates in imaging techniques and review of imaging findings. Semin Roentgenol 47, 159-170.

26 Karakousis, G.C., Singer, S., Zheng, J., et al. (2011) Laparoscopic versus open gastric resections for primary gastrointestinal stromal tumors (GISTs): a size-matched comparison. Ann Surg Oncol 18, 1599-1605.

27 De Vogelaere, K., Van Loo, I., Peters, O., et al. (2011) Laparoscopic resection of gastric gastrointestinal stromal tumors (GIST) is safe and effective, irrespective of tumor size. Surg Endosc 26, 2339-2345.

28 O'Connor, D.B., Winter, D.C. (2011) The role of laparoscopy in the management of acute small-bowel obstruction: a review of over 2,000 cases. Surg Endosc 26, 12-17.

29 Daniel, E.E. (1965) The electrical and contractile activity of the pyloric region in dogs and the effects of drugs. Gastroenterology 49, 403-418.

30 Bersenas, A.M., Mathews, K.A., Allen, D.G., et al. (2005) Effects of ranitidine, famotidine, pantoprazole, and omeprazole on intragastric pH in dogs. Am J Vet Res 66, 425-431.

31 Tolbert, K., Bissett, S., King, A., et al. (2011) Efficacy of oral famotidine and 2 omeprazole formulations for the control of intragastric pH in dogs. J Vet Intern Med 25, 47-54.

32 Burger, D.M., Wiestner, T., Hubler, M., et al. (2006) Effect of anticholinergics (atropine, glycopyrrolate) and prokinetics (metoclopramide, cisapride) on gastric motility in beagles and Labrador retrievers. J Vet Med A Physiol Pathol Clin Med 53, 97-107.

33 Hall, J.A., Solie, T.N., Seim, H.B., et al. (1996) Effect of metoclopramide on fed-state gastric myoelectric and motor activity in dogs. Am J Vet Res 57, 1616-1622.

34 Rawlings, C.A., Howerth, E.W., Bement, S., et al. (2002) Laparoscopic-assisted enterostomy tube placement and full-thickness biopsy of the jejunum with serosal patching in dogs. Am J Vet Res 63, 1313-1319.

35 Duke, T., Steinacher, S.L., Remedios, A.M. (1996) Cardiopulmonary effects of using carbon dioxide for laparoscopic surgery in dogs. Vet Surg 25, 77-82.

36 van Nimwegen, S.A., Kirpensteijn, J. (2007) Laparoscopic ovariectomy in cats: comparison of laser and bipolar electrocoagulation. J Feline Med Surg 9, 397-403.

37 Mayhew, P.D., Pascoe, P.J., Kass, P.H., et al. (2013) Effects of pneumoperitoneum induced at various pressures on cardiorespiratory function and working space during laparoscopy in cats. Am J Vet Res 74, 1340-1346.

38 Case, J.B., Marvel, S.J., Boscan, P., et al. (2011) Surgical time and severity of postoperative pain in dogs undergoing laparoscopic ovariectomy with one, two, or three instrument cannulas. J Am Vet Med Assoc 239, 203-208.

39 Young-Fadok, T.M. (2005) Laparoscopic surgery of the small bowel. In: Mastery of endoscopic and laparoscopic surgery, 2nd edn. Philadelphia, Lippincott, Williams & Wilkins, pp. 421-428.

40 Kawahara, H., Kobayashi, T., Watanabe, K., et al. (2009) Where is the best surgical incision for laparoscopic anterior resection? Hepatogastroenterology 56, 1629-1632.

41 Vestweber, B., Galetin, T., Lammerting, K., et al. (2013) Single-incision laparoscopic surgery: outcomes from 224 colonic resections performed at a single center using SILS. Surg Endosc 27, 434-442.

12

Laparoscopic-Assisted Gastrotomy, Enterotomy, Enterectomy, and Anastomosis

J. Brad Case and Gary W. Ellison

Key Points

- Laparoscopic-assisted gastrointestinal (GI) surgery is ideal for a subset of dogs and cats suspected of IBD or alimentary neoplasia and for dogs and cats with jejunal segment obstruction caused by a foreign body.
- Contraindications to laparoscopic-assisted GI exploratory include linear foreign bodies, septic peritonitis, and the presence of adhesions.
- Accurate patient and port positioning are critical to ensure successful evaluation of the GI tract.
- Adequate experience and accurate application of traditional GI surgical principles is critical to success.
- The minimally invasive GI surgeon must be ready and willing to convert to traditional laparotomy if the procedure cannot be completed safely and effectively.

Preoperative Considerations

Gastrointestinal Wound Healing

The gastrointestinal (GI) tract follows the same basic healing curve as the skin but has accelerated healing properties. The lag or inflammatory phase of healing lasts 3 to 4 days. Immediately after wounding, contraction of blood vessels occurs, platelets aggregate, the coagulation mechanism is activated, and fibrin clots are deposited to control hemorrhage. The fibrin clot offers some minimal wound strength on the first postoperative day, but the main wound support during the lag phase of healing comes from the sutures.[1] Enterocyte regeneration begins almost immediately after wounding; however, the epithelium offers little biomechanical support.[1] The lag phase is the most critical period during visceral wound healing because most dehiscences take place within 72 to 96 hours after the wound has been created. Wound dehiscence of an intestinal wound (Figure 12-1) often leads to generalized bacterial peritonitis and subsequent death. Therefore, factors that negatively affect visceral healing are potentially of great clinical significance to the surgeon. Factors that cause intestinal wounds to leak include failure to adequately identify ischemic tissue; improper suturing or stapling technique; and factors that negatively affect wound healing such as sepsis, malnutrition, and antineoplastic therapy. The GI submucosa

is composed primarily of dense type 1 collagen,[2] which provides the majority of the tensile strength of the GI tract and is responsible for holding sutures after gastrotomy or enterotomy.[1] Submucosal appositional closure of gastrotomy and enterotomy is preferred because inaccurate apposition causes eversion of mucosa, resulting in secondary healing, which is significantly delayed and increases the risk of leakage when compared to direct GI healing.[1,3]

For a discussion of the important anatomic concerns with regard to GI laparoscopic procedures, please see Chapter 11.

Diagnostic Workup

The general preoperative evaluation of dogs and cats undergoing laparoscopic-assisted GI surgery is similar to that of patients to be treated via laparotomy and is discussed in Chapter 11. However, it is important to consider advances in diagnostic imaging and specific characteristics of GI disease in patients being considered for a laparoscopic approach to better predict surgical success and to minimize frequency of conversion. In the past decade, significant improvements in diagnostic imaging have been made. For example, ultrasound and three-dimensional imaging modalities have become readily available in most referral institutions. Abdominal ultrasonography (AUS) allows for accurate assessment of bowel diameter and wall thickness[4] and is also useful in documenting small

Small Animal Laparoscopy and Thoracoscopy, First Edition. Edited by Boel A. Fransson and Philipp D. Mayhew.

© 2015 by ACVS Foundation. Published 2015 by John Wiley & Sons, Inc.

Companion website: www.wiley.com/go/fransson/laparoscopy

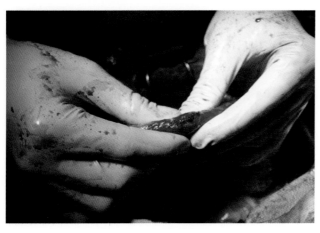

Figure 12-1 Intraoperative image of an intestinal dehiscence in a dog with septic peritonitis 4 days after enterotomy for a linear foreign body.

volumes of peritoneal fluid and gas, loss of wall layering, and hyperechoic mesentery, which are findings consistent with peritonitis.[5] However, given the limitations of AUS (e.g., inadequate operator experience, presence of large amounts of GI gas, and length of the exam),[6,7] advanced diagnostics may be particularly useful in preoperative evaluation of patients being considered for laparoscopic-assisted GI surgery. Preoperative abdominal computed tomography (CT) is used commonly for evaluation of humans with abdominal and GI disease and is becoming more popular in veterinary patients.[7-9] Contrast-enhanced CT is more accurate at lesion measurement versus AUS (Video Clip 12-1) and is reported to be 100% accurate in differentiating surgical from nonsurgical acute abdominal conditions in dogs.[7] The authors of this chapter have found preoperative CT helpful in dogs and cats before laparoscopic-assisted GI surgery for a few reasons, including evaluation and measurement of intestinal lesions, location of lesions within the specific region of the GI tract, association with other abdominal structures, identification of adhesions, and exploration of the abdominal cavity before surgery (Figure 12-2). Accurate information regarding these parameters is helpful in predicting dogs and cats more likely to be amenable to a laparoscopic-assisted surgical approach. Abdominal CT may also be a useful diagnostic test for staging dogs and cats with alimentary neoplasia.[10]

Patient Selection

Careful consideration of the patient and the particular condition is required before performing laparoscopic GI surgery. The general considerations are discussed in Chapter 11. Although not defined specifically in veterinary surgery, the authors believe linear foreign bodies, septic peritonitis or previous peritonitis, intestinal adhesions (Figures 12-3 and 12-4), and large-diameter lesions to be potential contraindications to a laparoscopic approach.[11] Linear foreign bodies cause plication and tethering of the bowel, which limit bowel exteriorization and may increase the risk of iatrogenic mesenteric perforation. Furthermore, linear foreign bodies are associated with a high rate (31%) of perforation and preexisting septic peritonitis,[12] requiring careful exploration of the entire GI tract, and the accuracy of laparoscopic-assisted GI exploration is currently unknown. Adhesions have been noted to be a contraindication for laparoscopic GI surgery in humans.[13,14] Large lesion diameter may also be a contraindication because exteriorization of affected bowel would require significant enlargement of the *extraction incision*, which might negate the benefits of the laparoscopic approach. A wide range of lesion diameters have been suggested by human GI laparoscopists, but more current guidelines suggest a maximal diameter of approximately 5 cm, although larger lesions are reported.[15-17] Conversely, laparoscopic-assisted GI biopsy is an excellent alternative to an open approach in obtaining GI biopsies in conditions such as inflammatory bowel disease (IBD) and alimentary lymphoma in dogs and cats and is routinely performed in many centers.

Prognostic Factors

Aside from the systemic health of the patient, a number of prognostic factors should be considered when performing laparoscopic-assisted enterotomy or enterectomy. Linear foreign bodies are associated with increased morbidity and mortality in dogs undergoing open enterotomy and enterectomy.[17-19] Because a laparoscopic approach is more limited, identification of a linear foreign body should prompt the surgeon to perform or convert to an exploratory laparotomy. Nonlinear GI foreign bodies have recently been shown to be protective for postoperative dehiscence and septic peritonitis after open enterotomy and enterectomy.[20] Clinically, dogs with nonlinear foreign bodies and intestinal mass lesions appear to have an excellent prognosis with laparoscopic-assisted enterotomy and enterectomy,[11,21] although large-scale studies have not been performed. Preoperative septic peritonitis is associated with a greater risk of intestinal dehiscence after GI surgery.[20,22,23] Furthermore, septic peritonitis results in cardiovascular and metabolic compromise of the patient, which may increase the risks of anesthesia. Increased length of anesthetic and surgical time may have deleterious consequences in some cases; thus, a laparoscopic approach may not be advisable. The clinical use of laparoscopic-

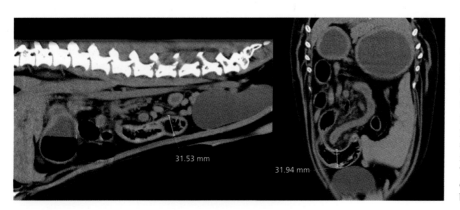

Figure 12-2 Sagittal and frontal plane computed tomography (CT) images from a dog with an orad jejunal cloth foreign body. The exact location within the gastrointestinal tract and lesion size are easily assessed with preoperative CT. Abdominal ultrasonography was also performed in this patient, but acoustic shadowing complicated lesion localization and measurement (Video Clip 12-1). This dog was considered an excellent candidate for a laparoscopic-assisted approach based on the CT.

31.53 mm

31.94 mm

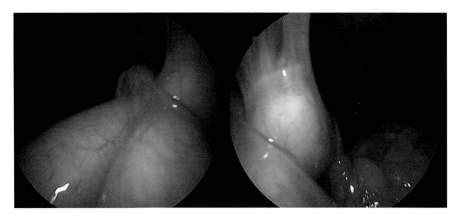

Figure 12-3 Intracorporeal view of a dog with small intestinal obstruction and multiple small intestinal adhesions. The laparoscopic-assisted approach was converted to an exploratory laparotomy after identification of the adhesions.

assisted enterectomy or enterotomy in dogs and cats with preoperative septic peritonitis has not been reported. In human surgery, laparoscopy was found to be less accurate than exploratory celiotomy for penetrating abdominal injuries involving the stomach and small intestine, missing up to 19% of injuries in one study.[24] Conversely, appendicular peritonitis is associated with an excellent prognosis when treated laparoscopically.[25]

Patient Preparation

Patient Positioning, Port Positions, and Working Space

For laparoscopic or laparoscopic-assisted gastrotomy, enterotomy, and enterectomy, the patient is positioned in a similar manner to when diagnostic procedures of the GI tract are performed; these are described in detail in Chapter 11. After establishment of a pneumoperitoneum, intracorporeal examination of the viscera is performed. Thereafter, pneumoperitoneum is discontinued, and either the stomach or intestine is exteriorized for gastrotomy, enterotomy, or enterectomy and anastomosis as indicated.

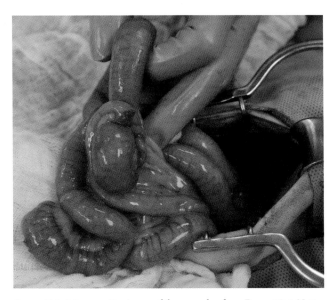

Figure 12-4 Intraoperative image of the same dog from Figure 12-3. Notice the multiple adhesions and bunching of the bowel, which would have precluded extracorporealization via the extraction incision.

Surgical Techniques

Instrumentation

Instruments needed include a straight laparoscopic Babcock forceps (required); straight or articulating DeBakey forceps (recommended); coaxial deviating laparoscopic Babcock forceps (optional if used with EndoCone; Karl Storz Endoscopy, Goleta, CA); a 5-mm, 30-degree laparoscope (required); blunt palpation probe (required) or fan retractor (facilitative); two threaded or smooth 5.5-mm cannulas (required for multiport technique); SILS (Covidien, Mansfield, MA) or EndoCone (required for a single-port approach); wound retractor (facilitative); baby Gelpi retractor (facilitative); biopsy instruments (required); basic surgical pack (required); and Thoraco-abdominal (e.g., TA, Covidien), Gastrointestinal Anastomotic (e.g., GIA, Covidien), or Endo-Gastrointestinal Anastomotic (e.g., EndoGIA, Covidien) staplers (required for stapled anastomosis).

Laparoscopic and Laparoscopic-Assisted Gastrotomy

Laparoscopic gastrotomy for removal of gastric foreign bodies has been described in 20 clinical dogs.[26] In this report, a midline, three-port technique was used, and the gastrotomy was closed in a single inverted pattern or with an endoscopic surgical stapler. Foreign bodies were removed using an endoscopic retrieval bag, and contamination was minimal. The clinical outcome was good in all dogs with no complications reported.

Flexible endoscopy is successful for the removal of gastric foreign bodies in 90% of cases and is an ideal method for gastric foreign body removal in dogs.[27] However, in some cases, flexible endoscopy has been ineffective, and a laparoscopic-assisted method can be used for *rescue gastrotomy*. Although not reported in the primary veterinary literature, the procedure is simple. A two- or single-port technique can be used. The authors' preference is to perform a single-port procedure. The port is placed on midline, approximately midway between the umbilicus and caudal xyphoid. After the peritoneum is insufflated, the endoscope is positioned in the most caudal 5-mm inner cannula and the abdomen explored. A 5-mm laparoscopic Babcock forceps is inserted via one of the remaining 5-mm inner cannulas and is used to grasp the parietal body of the stomach, which is then elevated ventrally. The endoscope and inner cannulae (SILS port) or the bulkhead of the EndoCone is carefully removed while a stable gentle grasp of the gastric body is maintained. This results in rapid desufflation of the peritoneal cavity. The port is removed, and the laparoscopic DeBakey or Babcock forceps are used to minimally extracorporealize the stomach. Two

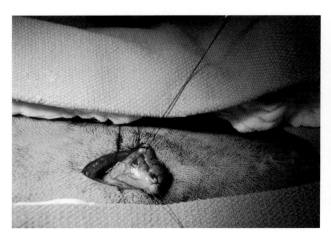

Figure 12-5 Intraoperative image of a dog after laparoscopic-assisted gastrotomy and gastroscopy. The gastrotomy has been closed in two layers.

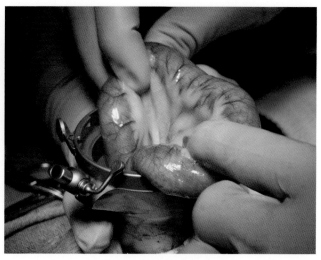

Figure 12-6 Intraoperative view of a dog undergoing extracorporeal small intestinal exploration via a conical single-incision laparoscopic surgery port (EndoCone; Karl Storz Endoscopy, Goleta, CA). The bulkhead of this port has been removed, and the intestine is evaluated in segments.

stay sutures are placed in the stomach approximately 4 cm apart (Figure 12-5). The abdominal wound can be retracted using baby Gelpi retractors or a wound retractor (see Figure 12-10). Laparotomy sponges are used to pack off the stomach, and an extracorporeal gastrotomy is performed. Minimal enlargement of the celiotomy is usually required depending on the size of the patient and the foreign material to be removed. The gastrotomy is performed using standard technique. Briefly, a stab incision is made in the body and extended 3 to 5 cm using Metzenbaum scissors. Five- or 10-mm endoscopic Babcock forceps can be used to retrieve foreign bodies from the gastric lumen. The endoscope is used as a *gastroscope* to guide and ensure complete removal of the gastric foreign material, but it should not be used again for laparoscopy because of contamination of the endoscope. After removal of all foreign material has been accomplished, a single-layer, simple-continuous closure of the gastrotomy is performed.[28] Alternatively, a two-layer closure may be performed (Figure 12-5). Monofilament absorbable suture is preferred for closure of the gastrotomy. Knotless suture can also be used to close the gastrotomy and is associated with a faster closure time and similar tensile properties as standard suture.[29]

Enterotomy and Intestinal Biopsy

Laparoscopic-assisted enterotomy has been described using a two-port[21] and single-port[11] technique with or without a wound retractor device. After the intracorporeal exploratory is completed, a segment of jejunum is exteriorized from the peritoneum, and the small intestine is *run* (Figure 12-6), eventually leading to extracorporeal isolation of the affected segment of bowel. The *extraction incision* may need to be minimally enlarged to facilitate exteriorization and to prevent strangulation of the mesenteric vasculature. A baby Gelpi or polyurethane wound retractor (Alexis; Applied Medical, Rancho Santa Margarita, CA) is used to maintain retraction of the abdominal wound during the extracorporeal enterotomy, and the affected bowel is isolated and packed off using laparotomy sponges. Use of a polyurethane wound retractor is preferable in cases of suspected or documented GI neoplasia to minimize the risk of port site metastasis.[21,30]

Antimesenteric enterotomy is performed aborad to the site of an intestinal foreign body to avoid incising compromised intestinal tissue. For intestinal biopsy, the enterotomy is made in an elliptical fashion using a scalpel blade or in a circular manner using a 4- to 5-mm biopsy punch (Video Clip 12-2). The enterotomy is closed in either a transverse or longitudinal (Figure 12-7) orienta-

tion depending on the concern for luminal compromise, which can be significant, especially in small animals. The enterotomy is closed in a single-layer appositional pattern to minimize tissue eversion and mucosal necrosis.[3] Either a continuous or interrupted pattern can be used.[28] Knotless suture can be used as well for enterotomy closure and is faster with no difference in bursting strength than comparable absorbable suture.[29,31]

Enterectomy and Anastomosis

Laparoscopic-assisted intestinal resection and anastomosis is performed in humans for small bowel obstruction of various causes, including small bowel tumors,[15,32] IBD,[33] and postoperative adhesion formation.[32,34] In most instances, resection and anastomosis is performed extracorporeally using standard techniques after the affected bowel has been exteriorized via the *extraction incision*. In veterinary surgery, laparoscopic-assisted enterectomy and anastomosis has been performed for small intestinal intussusception[11] and neoplasia.[21] This approach appears to minimize tissue

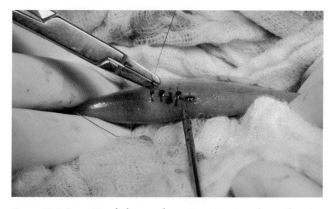

Figure 12-7 Appositional closure of an enterotomy in a dog undergoing single-incision laparoscopic-assisted exploratory and biopsy. Notice the lack of eversion and careful attention to good apposition during the closure. This enterotomy was created using a circular punch biopsy instrument (Video Clip 12-2).

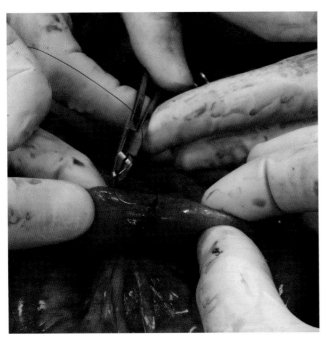

Figure 12-8 Appositional, simple interrupted, small intestinal anastomosis after single-incision laparoscopic-assisted enterectomy in a dog.

trauma, visceral manipulation, and peritoneal contamination. If a hand-sewn anastomosis is to be performed, either an interrupted (Figure 12-8) or continuous appositional pattern (Figure 12-9) is preferable to minimize mucosal eversion and promote primary intestinal healing.[28,35] Lack of submucosal apposition or tissue eversion is associated with prolonged inflammation and mucosal necrosis, increasing the risk of subsequent dehiscence.[3] Crushing suture patterns are also associated with prolonged inflammation and mucosal eversion; thus, they are not recommended.[36] Alternatively, a stapled side-to-side *functional end-to-end* anastomosis is appropriate[37] and is associated with higher bursting strength at 3 days after surgery.[38]

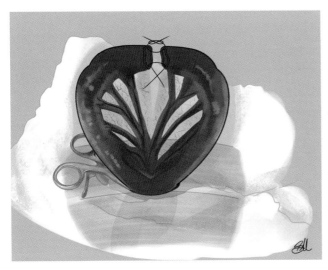

Figure 12-9 Illustration of a simple continuous, small intestinal anastomosis after single-incision laparoscopic-assisted enterectomy. Each of the two suture lines is continued 180 degrees on the respective side of the anastomosis before being tied off.

Omentalization

Both intracorporeal and extracorporeal GI omentalization can be performed with a laparoscopic-assisted approach. In most cases, the greater omentum is easily exteriorized along with the enterotomy or anastomosis site. The omentum can then be wrapped around the circumference of the bowel and tacked in place with one or two seromuscular sutures. Conversely, intracorporeal omentalization can be performed in dogs in which the original *extraction incision* has not been enlarged too much to prevent reinsertion of the port. The port is reinserted and the peritoneum examined to identify the affected intestine. The greater omentum is grasped using laparoscopic Babcock forceps (Figure 12-10) and is wrapped around the enterotomy or enterectomy site.[11] The benefits of omentalization include the addition of efferent and afferent blood and lymphatic supply as well as serosal sealing of the enterotomy site.[39]

Challenges

Potential challenges include an inability to exteriorize the affected viscera for extracorporeal procedures and an inability to adequately evaluate the GI tract and other organs of interest. These challenges are minimized by careful patient selection and appropriate clinical decision making. The GI laparoscopist must be ready and willing to convert to traditional laparotomy if the procedure cannot be completed safely and effectively or if emergent (e.g., significant hemorrhage) circumstances dictate.

Complications and Prognosis

Complications after laparoscopic-assisted GI surgery include dehiscence, septic peritonitis, pneumonia, and GI ileus. The prognosis after laparoscopic gastrotomy appears to be excellent with no leaking or dehiscence reported in 20 dogs undergoing either sutured or stapled gastric closure.[26] Laparoscopic-assisted gastrotomy is likely associated with a similar minor risk of dehiscence as traditional gastrotomy and total laparoscopic gastrotomy, but this has not been studied in veterinary surgery. In two recent clinical studies, no cases of gastrotomy dehiscence were reported.[28,40]

Dehiscence after laparoscopic-assisted enterotomy or enterectomy was not reported in any of nine dogs and seven cats in two recent reports.[11,21] The overall risk for dehiscence after GI surgery

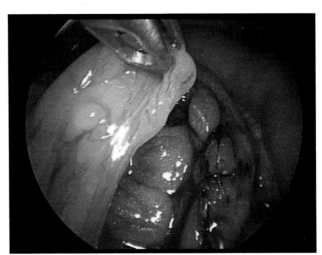

Figure 12-10 Intracorporeal omentalization of the enterectomy and anastomosis site in a dog that underwent single-incision laparoscopic-assisted surgery.

via traditional celiotomy typically ranges from 7% to 16%[20,22,23,41] and is affected by species and a variety of risk factors. Cats appear to develop intestinal leakage less frequently than dogs, and the following risk factors for intestinal leakage have been identified: presence of a foreign body, hypoalbuminemia (<2.5 g/dL), preexisting peritonitis, left shift, and use of blood products.[23] Any two of these findings together was 90% sensitive for predicting dehiscence.[23] However, enteric biopsy in hypoalbuminemic dogs was not associated with an increased risk of dehiscence in another study.[42] Another study identified preoperative septic peritonitis, hypoalbuminemia, hypoproteinemia, and hypotension as risk factors for dehiscence.[20] The mortality rate after intestinal dehiscence is reported to be as high as 74%.[22] The number of procedures, dehiscence, and peritonitis have also been associated with a significantly reduced survival rate.[41] Thus, the operating surgeon must be exact in his or her technique regardless of whether or not a laparoscopic-assisted technique is used.

Obstructive GI foreign bodies in particular are associated with an excellent (>90% survival) outcome when performed via traditional celiotomy.[18,40] Although large-scale studies have not been performed examining the outcome associated with laparoscopic-assisted enterotomy or enterectomy, reported prognoses appear to be excellent with no reported deaths in two recent case series.[11,21] In the authors' experience, uncomplicated jejunal foreign bodies are an excellent indication for a laparoscopic-assisted GI approach in dogs and cats. Likewise, suspected inflammatory or neoplastic conditions in which diagnostic GI biopsy is the goal of surgery are also excellent indications for a minimally invasive approach.

Postoperative Care

Pain Control

Pain control is easily accomplished in most dogs and cats after laparoscopic GI surgery; however, there is a paucity of controlled studies on the subject.[43] Numerous controlled studies, however, have evaluated pain after laparoscopic versus open sterilization and have demonstrated significant reductions in pain indices with laparoscopic techniques.[44-47] Reduced pain indices[48] and requirement for injectable analgesics[49] have also been demonstrated clinically with laparoscopic gastropexy and laparoscopic-assisted cystotomy, respectively.

Because of the possibility of delayed tissue healing,[50,51] the authors do not use nonsteroidal medications in dogs and cats undergoing GI procedures. Nonsteroidal drugs interfere with cyclooxygenase-2 (COX-2) and prostaglandin eicosanoid 1 functions, which are important for normal collagen deposition and gain in GI wound strength during healing.[51,52] COX-2 inhibition has been associated with an increased risk of dehiscence even at therapeutic levels.[52] Although nonsteroidal drugs are effective analgesics, the absence of their use has not appeared to adversely affect patient comfort after laparoscopic GI surgery. In general, dogs and cats undergoing laparoscopic-assisted GI surgery are treated with local incisional analgesics and injectable opioids until they are eating and drinking. When the patient is eating and drinking, tramadol hydrochloride is offered at 2 to 4 mg/kg per os every 8 hours. Most dogs and cats do not require oral analgesics within 3 days of surgery and do not demonstrate signs of pain or discomfort after that time.

Prophylactic Measures

Continuation of antacid and other GI-modifying medications after laparoscopic GI surgery is based on the underlying pathophysiology of the disease and surgeon preference. In the case of acute GI obstruction, the use of these medications is rarely indicated longer than 24 hours after surgery. In dogs and cats with inflammatory or possibly neoplastic (e.g., lymphoma) GI disease, continued use of GI protectants and antiemetics may be indicated to palliate clinical signs until definitive treatment (e.g., immunosuppressive therapy) can be instituted.

Postoperative ileus, if present, may lead to persistent vomiting, inappetence, and abdominal discomfort. In these patients, metoclopramide administered at 2 mg/kg/24 hr intravenously as a constant-rate infusion may be helpful in hastening bowel recovery. Maropitant administered at 1.0 mg/kg subcutaneously is effective at reducing nausea associated with opioid medications.[53,54]

Early enteral feeding has been shown to hasten healing of intestinal anastomosis in dogs. Bursting pressures and collagen deposition of ileal and colorectal anastomosis were compared in beagles fed elemental diets versus those fed only electrolyte and water for 4 days. The dogs fed elemental diets had nearly twice the bursting strength and nearly double the amount of collagen at the surgical site as the control dogs.[55] Human studies have demonstrated reduced septic complications, quicker bowel recovery, and shorter hospitalization time in patients fed enterally within 8 to 24 hours after GI surgery.[56] The authors typically feed patients within 8 hours of surgery if there is no evidence of nausea, vomiting, or regurgitation.

Hospitalization Time

Hospitalization time for most dogs and cats undergoing laparoscopic-assisted GI surgery appears to be relatively short. In two recent studies, eight of eight dogs and six of eight cats were discharged no later than the day after surgery,[11,21] and all animals had good postoperative outcomes. No comparisons of hospitalization time have been made with traditional laparotomy in veterinary medicine. However, in multiple human studies, reduced hospitalization has been documented.[15,57] Reduced hospitalization time has been attributed to less postoperative pain, improved bowel recovery, and fewer complications associated with the surgical procedure.[15,57]

 All videos cited in this chapter can be found on the book's companion website at **www.wiley.com/go/fransson/laparoscopy**

References

1 Ellison, G.W. (1989) Wound healing in the gastrointestinal tract. Semin Vet Med Surg Sm Anim 4, 287-293.

2 Graham, M.F., Diegelmann, R.F., Elson, C.O., et al. (1988) Collagen content and types in the intestinal strictures of Crohn's disease. Gastroenterology 94, 257-265.

3 Jansen, A., Becker, A.E., Brummelkamp, W.H., et al. (1981) The importance of the apposition of the submucosal intestinal layers for primary wound healing of intestinal anastomosis. Surg Gynecol Obstet 152, 51-58.

4 Delaney, F., O'Brien, R.T., Waller, K. (2003) Ultrasound evaluation of small bowel thickness compared to weight in normal dogs. Vet Radiol Ultrasound 44, 577-580.

5 Boysen, S.R., Tidwell, A.S., Penninck, D.G. (2003) Ultrasonographic findings in dogs and cats with gastrointestinal perforation. Vet Radiol Ultrasound 44, 556-564.

6 Shanaman, M.M., Hartman, S.K., O'Brien, R.T. (2012) Feasibility for using dual-phase contrast-enhanced multi-detector helical computed tomography to evaluate awake and sedated dogs with acute abdominal signs. Vet Radiol Ultrasound 53, 605-612.

7 Shanaman, M.M., Schwarz, T., Gal, A., et al. (2013) Comparison between survey radiography, B-mode ultrasonography, contrast-enhanced ultrasonography and contrast-enhanced multi-detector computed tomography findings in dogs with acute abdominal signs. Vet Radiol Ultrasound 54, 591-604.

8 Hryhorczuk, A.L., Lee, E.Y. (2012) Imaging evaluation of bowel obstruction in children: updates in imaging techniques and review of imaging findings. Semin Roentgenol 47, 159-170.

9 Fields, E.L., Robertson, I.D., Brown, J.C. Jr. (2012) Optimization of contrast-enhanced multidetector abdominal computed tomography in sedated canine patients. Vet Radiol Ultrasound 53, 507-512.

10 Hoey, S., Drees, R., Hetzel, S. (2013) Evaluation of the gastrointestinal tract in dogs using computed tomography. Vet Radiol Ultrasound 54, 25-30.

11 Case, J.B., Ellison, G. (2013) Single incision laparoscopic-assisted intestinal surgery (SILAIS) in 7 dogs and 1 cat. Vet Surg 42, 629-634.

12 Evans, K.L., Smeak, D.D., Biller, D.S. (1994) Gastrointestinal linear foreign bodies in 32 dogs: a retrospective evaluation and feline comparison. J Am Anim Hosp Assoc 30, 445-450.

13 Young-Fadok, T.M. (2005) Laparoscopic surgery of the small bowel. In: Mastery of Endoscopic and Laparoscopic Surgery, 2nd edn. Lippincott, Williams & Wilkins, Philadelphia, pp. 421-428.

14 O'Connor, D.B., Winter, D.C. (2012) The role of laparoscopy in the management of acute small-bowel obstruction: a review of over 2,000 cases. Surg Endosc 26, 12-17.

15 Cai, W., Wang, Z.T., Wu, L., et al. (2011) Laparoscopically assisted resections of small bowel stromal tumors are safe and effective. J Dig Dis 12, 443-447.

16 Karakousis, G.C., Singer, S., Zheng, J., et al. (2011) Laparoscopic versus open gastric resections for primary gastrointestinal stromal tumors (GISTs): a size-matched comparison. Ann Surg Oncol 18, 1599-1605.

17 Demetri, G.D., Benjamin, R.S., Blanke, C.D., et al. (2007) NCCN Task Force report: management of patients with gastrointestinal stromal tumor (GIST)–update of the NCCN clinical practice guidelines. J Natl Compr Canc Netw 5(suppl 2):S1-29; quiz S30.

18 Hayes, G. (2009) Gastrointestinal foreign bodies in dogs and cats: a retrospective study of 208 cases. J Small Anim Pract 50, 576-583.

19 Hosgood, G., Salisbury, S.K. (1988) Generalized peritonitis in dogs: 50 cases (1975-1986). J Am Vet Med Assoc 193, 1448-1450.

20 Grimes, J.A., Schmiedt, C.W., Cornell, K.K., et al. (2011) Identification of risk factors for septic peritonitis and failure to survive following gastrointestinal surgery in dogs. J Am Vet Med Assoc 238, 486-494.

21 Gower, S.B., Mayhew, P.D. (2011) A wound retraction device for laparoscopic-assisted intestinal surgery in dogs and cats. Vet Surg 40, 485-488.

22 Allen, D.A., Smeak, D.D., Schertel, E.R. (1992) Prevalence of small intestinal dehiscence and associated clinical factors: a retrospective study of 121 dogs. J Am Anim Hosp Assoc 28, 70-76.

23 Ralphs, S.C., Jessen, C.R., Lipowitz, A.J. (2003) Risk factors for leakage following intestinal anastomosis in dogs and cats: 115 cases (1991-2000). J Am Vet Med Assoc 223, 73-77.

24 Rossi, P., Mullins, D., Thal, E. (1993) Role of laparoscopy in the evaluation of abdominal trauma. Am J Surg 166, 707-710.

25 Navez, B., Delgadillo, X., Cambier, E., et al. (2001) Laparoscopic approach for acute appendicular peritonitis: efficacy and safety: a report of 96 consecutive cases. Surg Laparosc Endosc Percutan Tech 11, 313-316.

26 Lew, M., Jalynski, M., Brzeski, W. (2005) Laparoscopic removal of gastric foreign bodies in dogs—comparison of manual suturing and stapling viscerosynthesis. Pol J Vet Sci 8, 147-153.

27 Gianella, P., Pfammatter, N.S., Burgener, I.A. (2009) Oesophageal and gastric endoscopic foreign body removal: complications and follow-up of 102 dogs. J Small Anim Pract 50, 649-654.

28 Weisman, D.L., Smeak, D.D., Birchard, S.J., et al. (1999) Comparison of a continuous suture pattern with a simple interrupted pattern for enteric closure in dogs and cats: 83 cases (1991-1997). J Am Vet Med Assoc 214, 1507-1510.

29 Ehrhart, N.P., Kaminskaya, K., Miller, J.A., et al. (2013) In vivo assessment of absorbable knotless barbed suture for single layer gastrotomy and enterotomy closure. Vet Surg 42, 210-216.

30 Brisson, B.A., Reggeti, F., Bienzle, D. (2006) Portal site metastasis of invasive mesothelioma after diagnostic thoracoscopy in a dog. J Am Vet Med Assoc 229, 980-983.

31 Miller, J., Zaruby, J., Kaminskaya, K. (2012) Evaluation of a barbed suture device versus conventional suture in a canine enterotomy model. J Invest Surg 25, 107-111.

32 Tierris, I., Mavrantonis, C., Stratoulias, C., et al. (2011) Laparoscopy for acute small bowel obstruction: indication or contraindication? Surg Endosc 25, 531-535.

33 Canin-Endres, J., Salky, B., Gattorno, F., et al. (1999) Laparoscopically assisted intestinal resection in 88 patients with Crohn's disease. Surg Endosc 13, 595-599.

34 Liao, C.H., Liu, Y.Y., Chen, C.C., et al. (2012) Single-incision laparoscopic-assisted surgery for small bowel obstruction. J Laparoendosc Adv Surg Tech A 22, 957-961.

35 Ellison, G.W., Jokinen, M.P., Park, R.D. (1982) End-to-end approximating intestinal anastomosis in the dog: a comparative fluorescein dye, angiographic and histologic evaluation. J Am Anim Hosp Assoc 18, 729-736.

36 Bone, D.L., Duckett, K.E., Patton, C.S., et al. (1983) Evaluation of anastomoses of small intestine in dogs: crushing versus noncrushing suturing techniques. Am J Vet Res 44, 2043-2048.

37 Ullman, S.L., Pavletic, M.M., Clark, G.N. (1991) Open intestinal anastomosis with surgical stapling equipment in 24 dogs and cats. Vet Surg 20, 385-391.

38 Hess, J.L., McCurnin, D.M., Riley, M.G., et al. (1981) Pilot study for comparison of chromic catgut suture and mechanically applied staples in enteroanastomoses. J Am Anim Hosp Assoc 17, 409-414.

39 Heller, J., Hunt, G.B. (2002) Clinical applications of the omentum in dogs and cats. Aust Vet Pract 32, 66-73.

40 Boag, A.K., Coe, R.J., Martinez, T.A., et al. (2005) Acid-base and electrolyte abnormalities in dogs with gastrointestinal foreign bodies. J Vet Intern Med 19, 816-821.

41 Wylie, K.B., Hosgood, G. (1994) Mortality and morbidity of small and large intestinal surgery in dogs and cats, 74 cases (1980-1992). J Am Anim Hosp Assoc 30, 469-474.

42 Harvey, H.J. (1990) Complications of small intestinal biopsy in hypoalbuminemic dogs. Vet Surg 19, 289-292.

43 Hewitt, S.A., Brisson, B.A., Sinclair, M.D., et al. (2004) Evaluation of laparoscopic-assisted placement of jejunostomy feeding tubes in dogs. J Am Vet Med Assoc 225, 65-71.

44 Davidson, E.B., Moll, H.D., Payton, M.E. (2004) Comparison of laparoscopic ovariohysterectomy and ovariohysterectomy in dogs. Vet Surg 33, 62-69.

45 Hancock, R.B., Lanz, O.I., Waldron, D.R., et al. (2005) Comparison of postoperative pain after ovariohysterectomy by harmonic scalpel-assisted laparoscopy compared with median celiotomy and ligation in dogs. Vet Surg 34, 273-282.

46 Devitt, C.M., Cox, R.E., Hailey, J.J. (2005) Duration, complications, stress, and pain of open ovariohysterectomy versus a simple method of laparoscopic-assisted ovariohysterectomy in dogs. J Am Vet Med Assoc 227, 921-927.

47 Culp, W.T., Mayhew, P.D., Brown, D.C. (2009) The effect of laparoscopic versus open ovariectomy on postsurgical activity in small dogs. Vet Surg 38, 811-817.

48 Mayhew, P.D., Brown, D.C. (2009) Prospective evaluation of two intracorporeally sutured prophylactic laparoscopic gastropexy techniques compared with laparoscopic-assisted gastropexy in dogs. Vet Surg 38, 738-746.

49 Arulpragasam, S.P., Case, J.B., Ellison, G.W. (2013) Evaluation of costs and time required for laparoscopic-assisted versus open cystotomy for urinary cystolith removal in dogs: 43 cases (2009-2012). J Am Vet Med Assoc 243, 703-708.

50 Syk, I., Agren, M.S., Adawi, D., et al. (2001) Inhibition of matrix metalloproteinases enhances breaking strength of colonic anastomoses in an experimental model. Br J Surg 88, 228-234.

51 Terzioglu, T., Sonmez, Y.E., Eldegez, U. (1990) The effect of prostaglandin E1 on colonic anastomotic healing. A comparison study. Dis Colon Rectum 33, 44-48.

52 de Hingh, I.H., van Goor, H., de Man, B.M., et al. (2006) Selective cyclo-oxygenase 2 inhibition affects ileal but not colonic anastomotic healing in the early postoperative period. Br J Surg 93, 489-497.

53 Hay Kraus, B.L. (2013) Efficacy of maropitant in preventing vomiting in dogs premedicated with hydromorphone. Vet Anaesth Analg 40, 28-34.

54 Koh, R.B., Isaza, N., Xie, H., et al. (2014) Effects of maropitant, acepromazine, and electroacupuncture on vomiting associated with administration of morphine in dogs. J Am Vet Med Assoc 244:820-829.

55 Moss, G., Greenstein, A., Levy, S., et al. (1980) Maintenance of GI function after bowel surgery and immediate enteral full nutrition. I. Doubling of canine colorectal anastomotic bursting pressure and intestinal wound mature collagen content. J Parenter Enteral Nutr 4, 535-538.

56 Braga, M., Gianotti, L., Gentilini, O., et al. (2001) Early postoperative enteral nutrition improves gut oxygenation and reduces costs compared with total parenteral nutrition. Crit Care Med 29, 242-248.

57 Ding, J., Xia, Y., Liao, G.Q., et al. (2013) Hand-assisted laparoscopic surgery versus open surgery for colorectal disease: a systematic review and meta-analysis. Am J Surg 207, 109-119.

13 Laparoscopic-Assisted Feeding Tube Placement

J. Brad Case

Key Points

- Enteral nutrition is critical in patient recovery and uncomplicated gastrointestinal (GI) healing.
- Early enteral feeding may be preferable to delayed feeding in postoperative GI patients.
- Enteral feeding is associated with early hospital discharge in dogs after GI surgery.
- Accurate surgical technique in laparoscopic feeding tube placement is critical to minimize complications.
- Resting energy requirement (RER) kcal = Body weight$^{0.75}$ x 70.

Preoperative Considerations

Enteral nutrition is of critical importance to perioperative surgical patients. Enteral feeding maintains the health of the gastrointestinal (GI) tract and provides critical substances (e.g., amino acids and calories) integral for uncomplicated wound healing. In many instances, the dog or cat may have been clinically ill, resulting in prolonged periods of hypo- or anorexia or may develop anorexia as a postoperative complication. Ideally, caloric and nitrogen deficits are corrected before surgery, and maintenance of both is addressed after surgery. However, feeding can be challenging in many ill or refractory veterinary patients, and some dogs and cats may require a more emergent surgical procedure, putting them at increased risk for complications. This is especially true in dogs and cats with significant comorbidities such as pancreatitis. Recent experimental studies have examined the effects of enteral versus no feeding or parenteral feeding in acute pancreatitis models. These studies have demonstrated a number of deleterious effects associated with prolonged anorexia or parenteral feeding versus early enteral feeding in dogs. These include reduction of intestinal wall and mucosal thickness as well as villus atrophy.[1] A major adverse consequence of these pathologies is intestinal barrier compromise, which allows translocation of enteral microflora.[2] Increased levels of circulating endoxin and bacteria as well as greater bacterial volume at end tissues, such as the lungs and abdominal lymph nodes, also results when enteral nutrition is withheld or replaced by parenteral supplementation.[1] In human surgery, large meta-analyses examining the clinical outcomes in patients undergoing early enteral or oral feeding versus those withheld from feeding after GI surgery have demonstrated significant reductions in postsurgical infection and hospital stay.[3,4] In dogs, an experimental study found that early fed versus not fed beagles undergoing colorectal anastomosis had 55% more collagen deposition and two times the bursting strength of the anastomosis 4 days after surgery.[5] Clinically, dogs fed early (<24 hours) after surgery for septic peritonitis were discharged from the hospital 1.6 days before delayed fed dogs in one study.[6] A number of potential explanations, including mitigation of a hypercatabolic state, prevention of protein-caloric malnutrition, and preservation of GI barrier function, were speculated at.[6] Another retrospective study of 467 dogs and 55 cats found a significant association between caloric intake and hospital discharge. However, most of these dogs and cats had voluntary caloric intake, and the severity of disease was negatively associated with both caloric intake as well as outcome, making cause-and-effect deduction difficult.[7] Given the significant morbidity associated with perioperative malnutrition and the potential contraindications to upper GI feeding devices, minimally invasive, laparoscopic-assisted feeding tube placement is likely an important and useful procedure to maintain in the armamentarium of small animal veterinary surgeons.

Patient Selection

Any perioperative patient with inadequate voluntary nutritional intake is a candidate for supplemental enteral feeding. Enteral feeding is preferable to the parenteral route unless the GI tract is not functional. In general, enteral feeding should be performed in the

---

Small Animal Laparoscopy and Thoracoscopy, First Edition. Edited by Boel A. Fransson and Philipp D. Mayhew.
© 2015 by ACVS Foundation. Published 2015 by John Wiley & Sons, Inc.
Companion website: www.wiley.com/go/fransson/laparoscopy

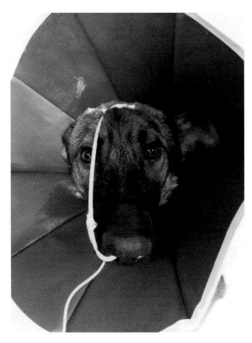

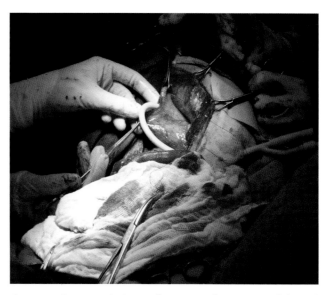

Figure 13-3 Intraoperative image of a patient undergoing open abdominal surgery for gastrostomy tube placement.

Figure 13-1 Postoperative image of a patient with a nasoesophageal feeding tube in place. The author prefers these devices for short-term enteral support in perioperative patients. (Courtesy of Dr. Justin Shmalberg.)

upper GI tract unless a patient's medical condition (e.g., persistent vomiting, esophageal or gastric neoplasia) contraindicates this. In this scenario, feeding aborad to the stomach or proximal duodenum may be indicated. The author has found nasoesophageal feeding tubes (Figure 13-1) to be most useful for temporary enteral support in patients with expected short-term (<48 hours) perioperative hypo- or anorexia. In dogs and cats with historical anorexia and malnutrition or in patients in which prolonged hyporexia is expected, a surgically placed feeding device may be indicated. Esophageal feeding tubes (Figure 13-2) are simple to place and to manage and are preferable to gastrostomy and enterostomy feeding devices, patient permitting. Dogs and cats who are not candidates for an esophageal feeding tube may require a gastrostomy or enterostomy device for nutritional support. Selecting a surgical approach (i.e., traditional

celiotomy vs. laparoscopy) for placement of these devices is largely up to the discretion of the operating surgeon and the medical condition of the patient. With a laparoscopic-assisted approach, the surgeon and technical staff should be comfortable with laparoscopy to facilitate timely and uncomplicated interventions. Because many patients being considered for enteral feeding device placement are sick or may require other surgical interventions, careful consideration and the potential limitations of a laparoscopic approach need to be considered. All patients are stabilized and prepared before anesthesia and surgery regardless of the surgical approach used. The most commonly indicated concomitant surgical indications in these patients are GI exploration and biopsy. Exploration of the GI tract can be performed using a combination of intracorporeal and extracorporeal maneuvers and can be performed in both multiple- and single-incision fashion as described in Chapter 11.[8-10] The author of this chapter prefers a laparoscopic-assisted approach for feeding tube placement in most cases when GI diagnostic exploration and biopsy is also indicated. When no other major abdominal procedure is indicated, a laparoscopic-assisted approach may be preferable to an open approach (Figure 13-3) because minimization of tissue trauma, systemic inflammation, and pain has been shown to improve patient recovery.[11] In dogs and cats, size limitations have not been established, and the author has not identified any limitations because of patient size with a laparoscopic-assisted approach to gastrostomy or enterostomy tube placement. However, patients with diaphragmatic defects or patients in which peritoneal insufflation will not be tolerated are not ideal candidates for a laparoscopic-assisted approach unless a lift laparoscopy system is available.[12]

Patient Preparation

Patient Position
Both dorsal and right lateral recumbency have been described for laparoscopic-assisted jejunostomy tube placement in dogs.[8,11] Because accurate exploration of the GI tract is often indicated, the author's preference is to position patients in dorsal recumbency and to then alter to right and left lateral recumbency to facilitate

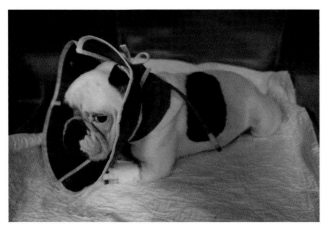

Figure 13-2 Image of a patient with an esophageal feeding tube in place. The author prefers an esophageal feeding device over a surgically placed enterostomy or gastrostomy tube for longer term enteral support in patients with no contraindications.

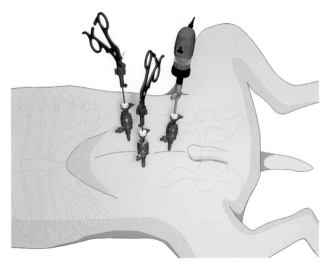

Figure 13-4 Recommended port locations for laparoscopic-assisted enterostomy tube placement.

intracorporeal evaluation of individual liver lobes, stomach, duodenum, pancreas, and colon. In large dogs (>10 kg), this is facilitated by use of a laparoscopic positioner table (see Figure 11-4). In small patients (cats and dogs <10 kg), however, the mechanical tilt table may be too large, and its use is not necessary. These patients' position can be altered intermittently by the operating room technician, and the dog or cat can be stabilized using sand bags.

Port Type and Position

The initial camera port is placed on ventral midline 2 to 3 cm caudal to the umbilicus. The second cannula is located just lateral to the rectus abdominis muscle and in the middle of the right flank region. If intracorporeal evaluation of the GI tract is chosen, a third cannula is placed to the left of the rectus abdominis approximately 1 to 2 cm cranial to the umbilical port (Figure 13-4). If a single-port device is to be used, the port is placed 1 to 2 cm caudal to the umbilicus on ventral midline. The procedure is modified by the addition of a second 5-mm port placed just lateral to the rectus abdominis muscle and in the middle of the right flank region (Figure 13-5).

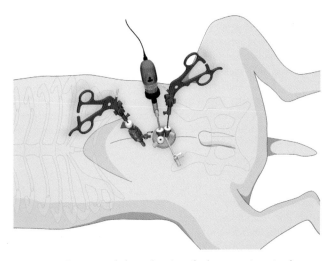

Figure 13-5 Recommended port locations for laparoscopic-assisted enterostomy tube placement if using a single-incision port.

Working Space and Exposure

The peritoneal cavity is insufflated to a pressure of 8 to 10 mm Hg using carbon dioxide. A 5-mm, 30-degree laparoscope is recommended for improved visualization of visceral surfaces especially along the diaphragm and abdominal gutters. Alternating patient position facilitates identification of specific anatomical regions of the GI tract. For example, the descending duodenum and right pancreatic limb are more easily accessed with the patient in left lateral recumbency, and the duodenostomy tube site is better presented to the operating surgeon.[8]

Surgical Techniques

Instrumentation

Two threaded or smooth 5.5-mm cannulae are required for a multiport technique. SILS (Covidien, Mansfield, MA) or EndoCone (Karl Storz Endoscopy, Goleta, CA) is required for a single-port approach. Other necessary instruments include straight laparoscopic Babcock forceps (required); straight or articulated laparoscopic DeBakey forceps (recommended); coaxial deviating laparoscopic Babcock forceps (optional if used with EndoCone); 5-mm, 30-degree laparoscope (required); blunt palpation probe (required) or fan retractor (facilitative); biopsy instruments (required); basic abdominal surgery pack (required); 5-French infant feeding tube (enterostomy); and 12- to 24-French Foley tube (gastrostomy).

Laparoscopic-Assisted Gastrostomy

Laparoscopic and laparoscopic-assisted gastrostomy tube placement has not been described clinically in dogs and cats. In contrast, a number of laparoscopic gastrostomy tube procedures have been described in humans.[13,14] In dogs and cats, percutaneous endoscopically placed gastrostomy and gastrojejunostomy tubes have been used successfully and are more common.[15,16] However, laparoscopic-assisted gastrostomy tube placement can be performed easily in most cases. The author of this chapter prefers to place these devices via a single incision in the left hypochondriac region. The patient is positioned in right lateral oblique recumbency, and a 3-cm skin incision is made 1 to 2 cm caudal to the 13th rib and midway between the umbilicus and the ventral margin of the 13th rib. The incision is continued through the subcutaneous tissues as well as the aponeurosis of the oblique abdominal muscles. The transversus abdominis muscle is incised, and a SILS or EndoCone port is placed as described in Chapter 11. A laparoscopic Babcock forceps is used to grasp the gastric fundus, which is then exteriorized via the 3-cm celiotomy after the port is removed. Two stay sutures are placed in the seromuscular layers of the stomach, and a stab incision using a #15 blade is created between them. A Foley-style gastrostomy tube is then placed into the gastric lumen, and the Foley tube is infused with saline. A purse-string suture is then placed, creating a tight seal around the gastrostomy tube. Four interrupted gastropexy sutures are then placed between the fundus and the transversus abdominis muscle. Caution is exercised to prevent needle puncture of the Foley balloon during the gastropexy. The surgical site is lavaged with sterile saline, and the wound is closed in three layers.

Laparoscopic-Assisted Enterostomy

Laparoscopic-assisted enterostomy tube placement should be performed after evaluation of the GI viscera when using the multiport technique because loss of pneumoperitoneum results with enlargement of the paramedian instrument incision. The procedure is

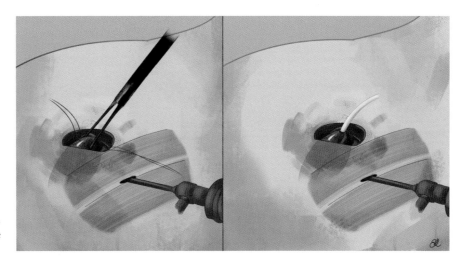

Figure 13-6 Illustration of a dog undergoing laparoscopic-assisted enterostomy tube placement.

straightforward and is performed with the dog in slight left lateral recumbency.[8] The 5-mm telescope is maneuvered from the caudal midline position, and the 5-mm laparoscopic Babcock forceps are introduced via the right paramedian cannula. Briefly, the descending duodenum (duodenostomy) or orad jejunum (jejunostomy) is grasped gently and elevated to the transversus abdominis muscle at the base of the instrument port. While maintaining intracorporeal visualization of the intestine, the port site is enlarged minimally to allow placement of four extracorporeal enteropexy sutures, one each at the orad, aborad, visceral, and parietal regions of the proposed enterostomy site. The intestine should be grasped and retracted away from the port site during incision enlargement to avoid iatrogenic injury of the bowel segment. After the intestine has been sutured to the transversus abdominis muscle, a loose purse-string suture is placed in the antimesenteric border of the bowel, and a #15 blade used to create an enterotomy in the middle of the purse string. Either a 3-0 or 4-0 monofilament absorbable suture on a tapered needle is ideal for the enteropexy and purse-string sutures. A 5-French feeding tube is then advanced in an aborad direction approximately 20 to 30 cm under laparoscopic visualization and the purse-string suture tightened to secure the enterostomy tube in place (Figure 13-6).[8] The surgical wound is lavaged with sterile saline and the subcutaneous tissues closed with monofilament absorbable suture. The skin is closed with nonabsorbable monofilament suture. A finger trap suture using 2-0 monofilament nonabsorbable suture is the preferred method of securing the enterostomy tube in place.[17]

Complications

Potential complications associated with laparoscopic-assisted enterostomy tube placement are likely similar to those encountered with traditional enterostomy tube procedures. Although clinical evaluation in compromised dogs and cats has not been performed, two experimental studies demonstrated negligible procedural complications; port site hemorrhage and jejunostomy tube kinking during insertion[11] and minor postoperative ostomy site inflammation.[8,11] Other reported complications of surgical enterostomy tube use in clinical patients include premature tube removal, septic peritonitis, vomiting, and diarrhea.[18,19] Regardless of whether or not a minimally invasive approach is used, careful attention to surgical technique is necessary to minimize the chance of complications associated with enterostomy tube implantation.

Postoperative Care

Pain Control

All surgery, including laparoscopic-assisted procedures, induces tissue trauma and discomfort, thus necessitating perioperative analgesia. With laparoscopic-assisted procedures including feeding tube placement, this is accomplished with local anesthetics and postoperative opioids without the use of nonsteroidal drugs.[11] Pain associated with laparoscopic-assisted enterostomy tube placement is minor and in one controlled study was found to be less than that of dogs undergoing jejunostomy tube placement via traditional midline celiotomy.[11] In this same study, rescue analgesia using an opioid medication was effective in all dogs, and no dogs developed severe pain scores (all <4 of 10) after surgery.

Prophylactic Measures

The use of antacids, antiemetics, and other GI-modifying medications after laparoscopic GI surgery is based on personal preference and the underlying pathophysiology of the disease. In dogs and cats with chronic vomiting or regurgitation, the use of antacids and antiemetics should be considered paramount to the medical management of their underlying disease. These medications not only reduce nausea but also reduce the caustic nature of gastric acid propelled into the esophagus. Exposure of the esophageal epithelium to gastric acid ultimately leads to erosion, ulceration, and subsequently stricture formation and is often associated with anesthesia and GI disease.[20,21] Because proton pump inhibitor drugs are more potent antacids than histamine blockers, their use may be preferable.[22,23]

Hospitalization Time

Hospitalization time in veterinary patients undergoing laparoscopic-assisted enterostomy tube placement depends on the physical status and concurrent illness of the patient. In dogs and cats, enterostomy tubes are best managed in the hospital because patients are often debilitated and require other supportive care and monitoring. In addition, constant-rate infusion feeding may be preferable to intermittent bolus feeding, and tube obstruction is commonly encountered with smaller diameter feeding tubes. In-hospital monitoring facilitates timely and effective remedy of these technical considerations. It is important to note that enterostomy tubes should be left in place for at least 7 days to allow for adhesion formation before removal is considered.

References

1 Qin, H.L., Su, Z.D., Hu, L.G., et al. (2002) Effect of early intrajejunal nutrition on pancreatic pathological features and gut barrier function in dogs with acute pancreatitis. Clin Nutr 21, 469-473.

2 Mohr, A.J., Leisewitz, A.L., Jacobson, L.S., et al. (2003) Effect of early enteral nutrition on intestinal permeability, intestinal protein loss, and outcome in dogs with severe parvoviral enteritis. J Vet Intern Med 17, 791-798.

3 Lewis, S.J., Egger, M., Sylvester, P.A., et al. (2001) Early enteral feeding versus "nil by mouth" after gastrointestinal surgery: systematic review and meta-analysis of controlled trials. BMJ 323, 773-776.

4 Braga, M., Gianotti, L., Gentilini, O., et al. (2001) Early postoperative enteral nutrition improves gut oxygenation and reduces costs compared with total parenteral nutrition. Crit Care Med 29, 242-248.

5 Moss, G., Greenstein, A., Levy, S., et al. (1980) Maintenance of GI function after bowel surgery and immediate enteral full nutrition. I. Doubling of canine colorectal anastomotic bursting pressure and intestinal wound mature collagen content. J Parenter Enteral Nutr 4, 535-538.

6 Liu, D.T., Brown, D.C., Silverstein, D.C. (2012) Early nutritional support is associated with decreased length of hospitalization in dogs with septic peritonitis: a retrospective study of 45 cases (2000-2009). J Vet Emerg Crit Care 22, 453-459.

7 Brunetto, M.A., Gomes, M.O., Andre, M.R., et al. (2010) Effects of nutritional support on hospital outcome in dogs and cats. J Vet Emerg Crit Care 20, 224-231.

8 Rawlings, C.A., Howerth, E.W., Bement, S., et al. (2002) Laparoscopic-assisted enterostomy tube placement and full-thickness biopsy of the jejunum with serosal patching in dogs. Am J Vet Res 63, 1313-1319.

9 Gower, S.B., Mayhew, P.D. (2011) A wound retraction device for laparoscopic-assisted intestinal surgery in dogs and cats. Vet Surg 40, 485-488.

10 Case, J.B., Ellison, G. (2013) Single incision laparoscopic-assisted intestinal surgery (SILAIS) in 7 dogs and 1 cat. Vet Surg 42, 629-634.

11 Hewitt, S.A., Brisson, B.A., Sinclair, M.D., et al. (2004) Evaluation of laparoscopic-assisted placement of jejunostomy feeding tubes in dogs. J Am Vet Med Assoc 225, 65-71.

12 Fransson, B.A., Ragle, C.A. (2011) Lift laparoscopy in dogs and cats: 12 cases (2008-2009). J Am Vet Med Assoc 239, 1574-1579.

13 Duh, Q.Y., Way, L.W. (1993) Laparoscopic gastrostomy using T-fasteners as retractors and anchors. Surg Endosc 7, 60-63.

14 Sampson, L.K., Georgeson, K.E., Winters, D.C. (1996) Laparoscopic gastrostomy as an adjunctive procedure to laparoscopic fundoplication in children. Surg Endosc 10, 1106-1110.

15 Salinardi, B.J., Harkin, K.R., Bulmer, B.J., et al. (2006) Comparison of complications of percutaneous endoscopic versus surgically placed gastrostomy tubes in 42 dogs and 52 cats. J Am Anim Hosp Assoc 42, 51-56.

16 Jergens, A.E., Morrison, J.A., Miles, K.G., et al. (2007) Percutaneous endoscopic gastrojejunostomy tube placement in healthy dogs and cats. J Vet Intern Med 21, 18-24.

17 Song, E.K., Mann, F.A., Wagner-Mann, C.C. (2008) Comparison of different tube materials and use of Chinese finger trap or four friction suture technique for securing gastrostomy, jejunostomy, and thoracostomy tubes in dogs. Vet Surg 37, 212-221.

18 Swann, H.M., Sweet, D.C., Michel, K. (1997) Complications associated with use of jejunostomy tubes in dogs and cats: 40 cases (1989-1994). J Am Vet Med Assoc 210, 1764-1767.

19 Crowe, D.T. Jr, Devey, J., Palmer, D.A., et al. (1997) The use of polymeric liquid enteral diets for nutritional support in seriously ill or injured small animals: clinical results in 200 patients. J Am Anim Hosp Assoc 33, 500-508.

20 Leib, M.S., Dinnel, H., Ward, D.L., et al. (2001) Endoscopic balloon dilation of benign esophageal strictures in dogs and cats. J Vet Intern Med 15, 547-552.

21 Wilson, D.V., Walshaw, R. (2004) Postanesthetic esophageal dysfunction in 13 dogs. J Am Anim Hosp Assoc 40, 455-460.

22 Bersenas, A.M., Mathews, K.A., Allen, D.G., et al. (2005) Effects of ranitidine, famotidine, pantoprazole, and omeprazole on intragastric pH in dogs. Am J Vet Res 66, 425-431.

23 Tolbert, K., Bissett, S., King, A., et al. (2011) Efficacy of oral famotidine and 2 omeprazole formulations for the control of intragastric pH in dogs. J Vet Intern Med 25, 47-54.

14 Laparoscopic and Laparoscopic-Assisted Gastropexy Techniques

Kayla M. Corriveau, Jeffrey J. Runge, and Clarence A. Rawlings

Key Points

- Laparoscopic gastropexy is the creation of a permanent adhesion of the stomach to the body wall to prevent gastric dilatation and volvulus syndrome.
- A variety of minimally invasive gastropexy techniques have been described, including laparoscopic assisted, total (or intracorporeally sutured) laparoscopic, and endoscopically assisted.
- Minimally invasive gastropexy techniques can be combined with other laparoscopic procedures and can be performed using multiport or single-port approaches.

Preoperative Considerations

A gastropexy is the creation of a permanent adhesion of the stomach to the body wall and is most commonly performed for prevention of gastric dilatation and volvulus (GDV) either in animals currently having an episode of GDV or prophylactically in those that have not had the syndrome yet. GDV is a life-threatening condition of uncertain etiology that affects approximately 60,000 dogs annually.[1] It is characterized by gastric dilatation, varying degrees of malpositioning of the stomach, compression of the portal, splanchnic, and caudal vena caval blood flow, hypotensive and cardiogenic shock, gastric necrosis, tissue acidosis, cardiac arrhythmias, disseminated intravascular coagulation, and possibly death.[2] Without surgical intervention, most GDV-affected dogs die, but only 1% or fewer die when the stomach is dilated (GD) but no torsion has occurred.[3] Even with aggressive management and surgical correction, the mortality rate for GDV-affected dogs remains high at 10% to 33%.[3-7] Mortality rates increase with need for splenectomy (32%), partial gastrectomy (35%), or both (55%).[8] Dogs treated surgically for GDV without a gastropexy have recurrence rates of more than 50%, but recurrence of GDV after gastropexy is less than 5%.[5] As a result, gastropexy is now considered a standard of care adjunctive procedure that should be performed at the time of surgical GDV correction.[5]

Because of the high morbidity and mortality rates associated with the development of GDV, prophylactic gastropexy should be considered in at-risk dogs. Unfortunately, few risk factors for GDV have been clearly identified, and the condition is assumed to be multifactorial.[9] Dog breed has consistently been found to be a predisposing factor with a 24% lifetime likelihood of GDV in large breed show dogs and 21.6% in giant breed show dogs.[10] Reported predisposed breeds include Great Danes, German shepherds, Gordon setters, Irish setters, Bassett hounds, Airedale terriers, Irish wolfhounds, Borzois, bloodhounds, Akitas, bull mastiffs, chow chows, and Weimaraners.[3,4,11] When evaluating Great Danes, Irish setters, Rottweilers, standard poodles, and Weimeraners, studies have shown that prophylactic gastropexy reduced lifetime mortality over a range of 2.2-fold for Rottweilers to 29.6-fold for Great Danes.[12] Other significant dog-related risk factors include increased age,[4,13,14] first-degree relative with GDV,[14] and increased thoracic depth-to-width ratio.[15,16] Less consistent dog-specific risk factors include an aggressive or fearful temperament,[9,14] being underweight,[9] and male gender.[9] Concurrent medical conditions have been noted in association with GDV, including histologic evidence of inflammatory bowel disease,[17] gastric foreign body,[18] and history of splenectomy,[19] but causal relationships have not been established. Environmental factors may also influence risk of GDV such as experiencing a stressful event within 8 hours prior.[4] Lastly, dietary management is considered a contributing factor with increased risk associated with small particle size (<30 mm diameter),[13] the presence of oil or fat among the first four ingredients in a dry food,[20] once-daily feeding,[9,21] feeding from an elevated bowl,[14]

Small Animal Laparoscopy and Thoracoscopy, First Edition. Edited by Boel A. Fransson and Philipp D. Mayhew.
© 2015 by ACVS Foundation. Published 2015 by John Wiley & Sons, Inc.
Companion website: www.wiley.com/go/fransson/laparoscopy

eating quickly,[9,14] and aerophagia.[21] Recent studies have brought into question the long-standing theory that pre- and postprandial exercise increases the risk of GDV. A large study of 1637 show dogs concluded no advantage to exercise restriction[14] around feeding time, but in a large cross-sectional study, moderate physical activity after a meal significantly decreased risk of GDV.[22] The only other factors found to be associated with a decreased incidence of GDV were owner-perceived personality trait of happiness[14] and supplements with fish or eggs.[22]

A variety of gastropexy techniques have been described, including incisional, belt loop,[23] circumcostal,[14] incorporating,[24] and fundic gastropexy.[25] Gastric fixation via gastrojejunostomy[26] and gastrocolopexy[27] have also been reported but are rarely used. Right-sided grid (mini-laparotomy),[28] endoscopically assisted,[29,30] totally laparoscopic,[31-34] and laparoscopic assisted[35-38] approaches have been described as minimally invasive options to perform prophylactic gastropexy. Right-sided percutaneous endoscopic gastrostomy (PEG) is another minimally invasive technique reported for permanent gastropexy but is not recommended because of inconsistent weak adhesion formation and greater procedure-related complications.[39]

Other than the PEG technique, biomechanical testing on a variety of the gastropexy techniques has been very comparable (Table 14-1). Unfortunately, the maximal tensile strength needed to prevent GDV is not known and may differ among individual dogs. Therefore, prevention of GDV recurrence and reliability of adhesion formation are arguably better clinical evaluation parameters for gastropexy techniques. Current published GDV recurrence rates after gastropexy are as follows: incisional, 0%[40]; belt loop, 0%[23]; circumcostal technique, 3.3% to 9%[41,42]; and gastrocolopexy, 15%.[42] Barium gastrography, ultrasonography, follow-up laparoscopy, and necropsy studies have been used to confirm formation of permanent gastropexy adhesions. Consistent formation of permanent adhesions has been confirmed by one or more of these methods with incisional gastropexy,[24,43] incorporating,[24] right-sided grid approach,[28] laparoscopic-assisted techniques,[35,37,44] totally laparoscopic stapled gastropexy,[32] and intracorporeally sutured gastropexy.[31,33]

With many of the commonly performed gastropexy techniques having comparable biomechanical values and clinical outcomes (i.e., GDV recurrence rate and consistency of adhesion formation), the type of gastropexy performed is largely up to surgeon preference

and the stability of the patient (see Table 14-1). Typically, an open laparotomy technique is used for GDV-affected dogs; however, there has been one report of laparoscopic correction of GDV in clinically affected dogs.[44] In this report, two dogs with confirmed GDV in which a stomach tube could be passed were successfully treated laparoscopically. The gastric contents from the tube in these cases did not indicate gross gastric hemorrhage, and the dogs were hemodynamically stable after fluid resuscitation. Although select patients may fall into this category, our current recommendation is to reserve minimally invasive gastropexy techniques for prophylaxis of GDV syndrome in noncritical patients with no signs of current GDV. Emergency open laparotomy, in the authors' opinion, remains the treatment of choice for GDV patients to allow rapid gastric decompression, derotation of the stomach, evaluation of gastric and splenic viability, and gastropexy. This chapter focuses on laparoscopic and laparoscopic-assisted prophylactic gastropexy techniques.

As stated earlier, indications for prophylactic gastropexy include clinically stable dogs at risk for GDV. Laparoscopic and laparoscopic-assisted gastropexy can also be easily performed concurrently with other elective laparoscopic procedures such as ovariectomy,[37,38] cryptorchidectomy,[45] and abdominal organ biopsy. Before prophylactic gastropexy, a routine preoperative biochemical panel and complete blood count are recommended. Screening thoracic radiographs are recommended in older patients (older than 8 years) or if clinical suspicion warrants thoracic investigation.

Patient Preparation

As with other elective abdominal surgeries, the dog should be fasted for at least 12 hours before anesthesia. The dog's abdomen should be clipped and aseptically prepared from the xiphoid to the pubic brim. For laparoscopic-assisted techniques that place the gastric antrum to the adjacent body wall; the right lateral abdominal wall may benefit from a wider clipping to a midlateral level to accommodate the creation of a right paramedian port (Figure 14-1). For an

Table 14-1 Biomechanical Testing of Gastropexy Techniques

Gastropexy Technique	Strength (Newtons)	Time of Testing (days postoperative)	References
Circumcostal	109	21	Fox et al.[46]
Incisional	60	21	Fox et al.[46]
Incisional	62	44	Waschak et al.[39]
Incisional	85	7	Hardie et al.[32]
	71	30	
Belt loop	53	Immediate, cadaver	Coolman et al.[47]
Belt loop	109	50	Wilson et al.[46]
Right-sided percutaneous endoscopic gastrostomy	22	44	Waschak et al.[39]
Laparoscopic assisted	77	50	Wilson et al.[48]
Laparoscopic assisted	107	30	Rawlings et al.[36]
Laparoscopic assisted	51	70	Mathon et al.[35]
Total laparoscopic stapled	45	7	Hardie et al.[32]
	72	30	

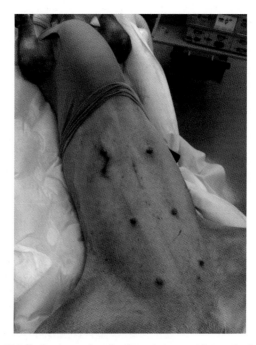

Figure 14-1 For laparoscopic-assisted gastropexy, a wide margin should be clipped around the planned site of the incision.

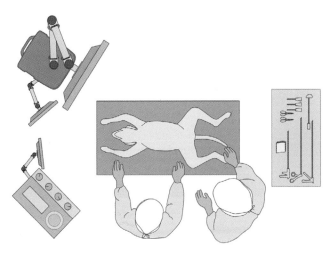

Figure 14-2 The operating room layout for a multiport or single-port laparoscopic-assisted gastropexy.

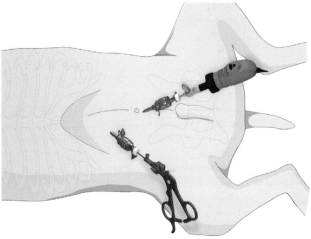

Figure 14-3 Port placement for two-port laparoscopic-assisted gastropexy.

intracorporeally sutured laparoscopic gastropexy, the dog is draped for a conventional open celiotomy in case conversion or additional port placement is required.

Prophylactic perioperative antibiotics are recommended (cefazolin, 22 mg/kg intravenously every 90 minutes) because during the early portions of the learning curve, surgical time may be significant with this procedure, especially when the intracorporeally sutured technique is used.[31]

For the single-port and multiport laparoscopic gastropexy techniques, the dog is placed in dorsal recumbency with the front and rear limbs secured for the procedure. The primary surgeon should be positioned on the dog's right side with the laparoscopic monitor on the opposite side of the patient (Figure 14-2). Abdominal access is obtained via either Veress needle or with the Hasson technique; the location of the initial port placement depends on the particular gastropexy technique used. Pneumoperitoneum is established with carbon dioxide (CO_2) using a mechanical insufflator to a pressure not exceeding 10 to 15 mm Hg. After the initial trocar–cannula assembly is placed (or single-port device is inserted), the insufflator pressure should be reduced to 6 to 10 mm Hg. Depending on which gastropexy technique is selected (or if additional laparoscopic procedures are performed), the number and location of laparoscopic ports can vary because the gastropexy can be performed using one, two, or three ports.

Surgical Techniques

Laparoscopic-Assisted Gastropexy (Multiport Technique)

The laparoscopic-assisted gastropexy was originally described by Rawlings *et al.* in 2001.[36] To perform a laparoscopic-assisted gastropexy, the dog is placed in dorsal recumbency. The abdomen is clipped and aseptically prepared from the xiphoid cartilage to the brim of the pubis. The telescope is initially placed through a submumbilical port, and the second port is inserted adjacent to the lateral margin of the rectus abdominis on the patients right side, approximately 3 to 5 cm caudal to the last rib depending on the patient's size (Figure 14-3). The second trocar–cannula assembly should be large enough to accommodate 10-mm instrumentation (Figure 14-4). After the telescope has been placed into the abdomen, transillumi-

nation of the body wall at the proposed location of the instrument portal can help identify a safe region for insertion of the second port by avoiding unwanted body wall and neurovascular trauma during insertion. A laparoscopic 10-mm Babcock or 10-mm DuVall forceps can be used for grasping the stomach from the second instrument port (Figure 14-5). These instruments can be safely used to manipulate the cranial abdominal organs and obtain an unobstructed view of the antrum of the stomach. If exposure of the stomach is still not ideal for the surgeon, the patient can be tilted in reverse Trendelenburg positioning to shift the abdominal viscera caudally. After it is clearly visualized, the antrum of the stomach is grasped with the forceps midway between the greater and lesser curvature of the stomach, approximately 5 to 7 cm oral to the pylorus. This site

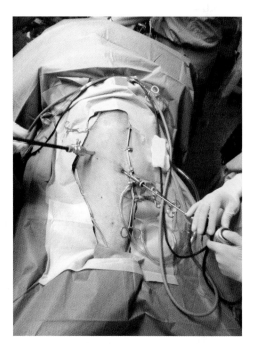

Figure 14-4 A 10-mm instrument port is placed for laparoscopic-assisted gastropexy adjacent to the lateral margin of the rectus abdominis on the patient's right side, approximately 3 to 5 cm caudal to the last rib. is placed for laparoscopic-assisted gastropexy. (Courtesy of Dr. Ameet Singh.)

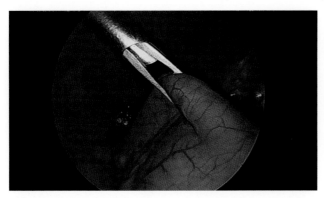

Figure 14-5 10-mm DuVall forceps can be used for grasping the stomach from the instrument port. (Courtesy of Dr. Ameet Singh.)

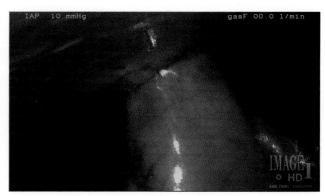

Figure 14-7 Laparoscopic view of completed gastropexy.

also becomes the location for the incisional gastropexy. After the surgeon has grasped the antrum securely, the pneumoperitoneum is evacuated. The forceps and antrum are exteriorized by removing the cannula and extending the port incision to 4 to 5 cm in an orientation parallel to the last rib (Figure 14-6). This dissection of the body wall can be accomplished with a number of techniques that use either sharp dissection or electrosurgical dissection. Alternatively, a muscle-splitting approach to the external and internal abdominal oblique muscles by incising parallel to the orientation of their fibers has also been described.[36] The transversus abdominis is the final layer of the inner abdominal wall to be sectioned before the stomach can be exteriorized. Stay sutures can be placed on this muscle layer to aid in retraction. During the antral exteriorization, care is taken to avoid twisting the stomach because this can lead to unwanted outcomes postoperatively. After the antral portion

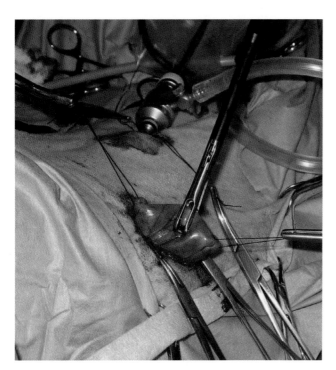

Figure 14-6 The forceps and antrum are exteriorized by removing the cannula and extending the port incision to 4 to 5 cm in an orientation parallel to the last rib. (Courtesy of Dr. Philipp Mayhew.)

of the stomach is visualized, a full-thickness or partial-thickness stay suture of 2-0 to 0 absorbable or nonabsorbable monofilament suture is placed in the exposed antral stomach wall. The laparoscopic grasping forceps can then be released. A second stay suture is placed 4 to 5 cm orally or aborally. The relative positions of these sutures define the extent of the proposed gastropexy.

An incision 2 to 5 cm long (depending on patient size) is made through the seromuscular layer of the antrum along the long axis of the stomach. Care is taken to avoid the larger blood vessels emerging from the greater and lesser curvatures. The submucosa is dissected from the seromuscular layer to ensure that the sutures are not placed through the mucosa into the lumen. Two simple, continuous lines of 2-0 or 0 monofilament, absorbable suture are placed to appose both margins of the seromuscular layer in the antrum to the transversus abdominis muscle. Before closure, the full-thickness stay sutures that were placed are removed. Transected abdominal oblique musculature is closed with interrupted or continuous absorbable suture material. The remainder of the incision is closed in routine fashion.

After completion, the pneumoperitoneum is briefly reestablished through the subumbilical port, and the gastropexy is visualized laparoscopically from the subumbilical port to ensure that optimal positioning and orientation has been achieved and that excessive hemorrhage or body wall defects are not present (Figure 14-7). After evacuating the remaining pneumoperitoneum, the subumbilical midline cannula is removed, and the port site incision is closed in routine fashion.

Intracorporeally Sutured Laparoscopic Gastropexy (and Modification with Novel Suture Devices)

The intracorporeally sutured laparoscopic gastropexy was originally described by Mayhew and Brown in 2009.[31] To perform the totally laparoscopic intracorporeally sutured technique, the patient is placed in dorsal recumbency, and the surgeon stands on the left side of the patient (Figure 14-8). To safely complete this technique, specialized equipment is required. The suturing can be completed using standard suture on a curved needle or on specialized ski-type needles. Novel suture devices have been developed to reduce the time required for standard knot ties (e.g., Endo Stitch; Covidien, Mansfield, MA), but in one study, the use of this device did not improve surgical time in dogs.[31] Additionally, the newer barbed suture types have also now been used for this indication in dogs (e.g., V-Loc suture, Covidien/Medtronic, Salem, CT; Quill, Angiotech Pharmaceuticals, Vancouver, Canada). Apart from the standard laparoscopic equipment used for the "assisted" technique, for

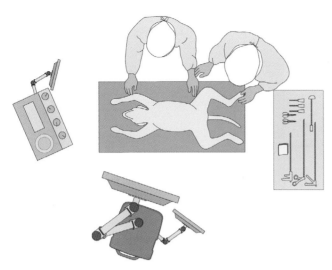

Figure 14-8 Operating room layout for an intracorporeally sutured gastropexy.

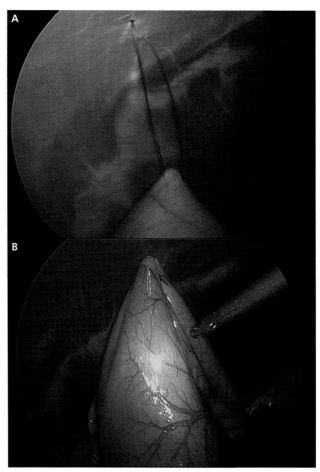

Figure 14-10 A stay suture placed percutaneously is passed full thickness through the antrum of the stomach (**A**). The suture is then pulled up to approximate the antrum to the body wall and secured in that position by clamping a pair of forceps on the suture exteriorly (**B**).

intracorporeally sutured gastropexy, two laparoscopic needle holders (e.g., Szabo-Berci 5-mm, 33-cm laparoscopic parrot-jaw or flamingo tongue needle holders, Karl Storz Endoscopy) are required to complete the suturing successfully unless a suture-assist device is used.

Initially, a telescope port is placed on the linea alba at a subumbilical location as previously described. Two other 6-mm instrument ports are then placed on the ventral midline, their location varying depending on the size and breed of the dog in relation to the available working space (Figure 14-9). The locations of the second and third ports can vary and depend on patient size. The second port can be placed 4 cm caudal to the xiphoid process, and the third can be placed midway between the cranial and umbilical port.

The intracorporeally sutured technique is started first by using a length of 2-0 nylon suture on a 38-mm reverse-cutting 3/8-circle needle that is passed percutaneously at the intended site of the gastropexy 2 to 3 cm caudal to the last rib and 5 to 8 cm lateral to midline. The needle is grasped with a laparoscopic needle holder within the peritoneal cavity and a deep, full-thickness bite through the antrum of the stomach is taken. The suture is passed back

through the abdominal wall adjacent to its previous point of entry (Figure 14-10). This stay suture is used as a temporary anchor to appose the stomach to the body wall during incising and suturing by placing Kelly forceps on the two ends of the stay suture on the exterior aspect of the body wall (Figure 14-11). The first incision is made in the transversus abdominis muscle using laparoscopic

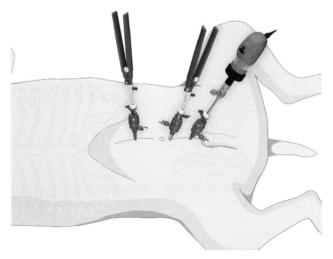

Figure 14-9 Instrument and port placement for the intracorporeally sutured laparoscopic gastropexy.

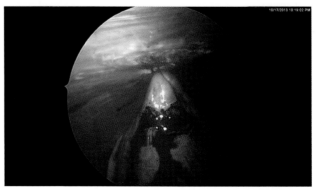

Figure 14-11 Partial-thickness incisions made on the seromuscular layer of the stomach and the transversus abdominis in preparation for intracorporeal suturing.

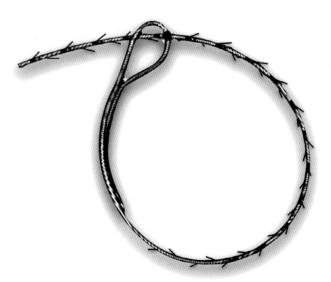

Figure 14-12 Knotless suture relies on the barbs cut into the suture to maintain tension during a continuous pattern.

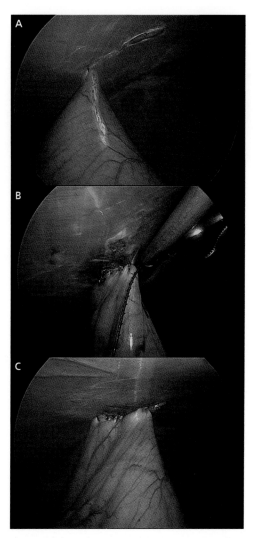

Figure 14-13 Monopolar electrosurgery is used to score a 3- to 4-cm line into both the transversus abdominis and adjacent seromuscular layer of the antrum (**A**). Continuous bites are then taken with the knotless-barbed suture, with slight tension being applied to each bite so the barbs can seed maintaining suture tension (**B**). View of the gastropexy after knotless suture application (**C**).

Metzenbaum scissors or a monopolar J- or L-hook probe. A partial-thickness incision is then made in the seromuscular layer of the stomach using laparoscopic Metzenbaum scissors. These incisions should be 3 to 5 cm long and be adjacent to each other in an orientation parallel to the ventral midline (Figure 14-12).[31]

An approximately 30-cm length of 2-0 or 0 polydioxanone on a curved or ski-type needle is passed into the peritoneal cavity by passing the needle through the body wall adjacent to the gastropexy site. First, suture the lateral wall of the incision in the transversus abdominis muscle and incised seromuscular layer of the antrum using a simple continuous pattern. While tying knots, evacuate the pneumoperitoneum to decrease tension and ensure secure knots and tight suture lines. After the lateral margins of the incision have been sutured, introduce a second piece of suture and suture the medial margins to complete the gastropexy. After suturing is complete, remove the stay suture. The three midline ports are closed in routine fashion after the pneumoperitoneum has been evacuated.[31]

 If a knotless suture (Figure 14-13, Video Clip 14-1) is used, a percutaneous stay suture is needed to appose the antrum to the proposed gastropexy site on the adjacent body wall as has been described. The barbed suture is then percutaneously placed adjacent to this stay suture and pulled into the abdominal cavity. Because this is a knotless suture, a short length of 6 to 9 inches is typically sufficient,[34] or a double-armed barbed suture can be used.[33] Two methods can be used to create a gastropexy with knotless suture laparoscopically, one that requires incisions into the stomach and transversus and another technique that does not make incisions. For the first technique, before starting knotless suturing, incisions are made internally on the transversus abdominus and antrum of the stomach in the same manner as described by Mayhew and Brown.[31] An alternative technique solely uses monopolar electrocautery to score a 3- to 4-cm line into both the transversus abdominis and adjacent seromuscular layer of the antrum (see Figure 14-13).[34]

The knotless continuous suture line is started by passing the point of the needle percutaneously into the abdomen. The entire strand of suture is pulled into the abdomen, and the first bites are taken at the most lateral aspect of the gastropexy and include both the transversus abdominis and seromuscular layer of the stomach. After these bites are made, the needle is then passed through a loop

that has been premanufactured on the end of the suture. After the needle is passed through the loop, the suture is pulled and cinched tightly against the tissue in a snare-like fashion. The subsequent continuous bites are then taken with slight tension being applied to each bite (see Figure 14-13). After each bite, the suture is pulled snugly and carefully, enabling the unidirectional barbs to seed into the tissue; this ultimately prevents any loosening of the suture line. After the continuous line is of appropriate length, an additional bite is taken in a reverse direction, and then a final bite is taken directing the needle externally. When the needle is seen penetrating the dermal layer, the assistant surgeon can grasp it externally and pull it snugly. The suture is cut flush with the skin, and the gastropexy is visualized internally with the scope (see Figure 14-13). Despite this latter technique not involving the traditional full-thickness incisions, follow-up by ultrasonography has been performed in a number of cases with experience to date suggesting that a permanent gastropexy can be created using this technique, although this still represents early data, and further evaluation is ongoing.[34]

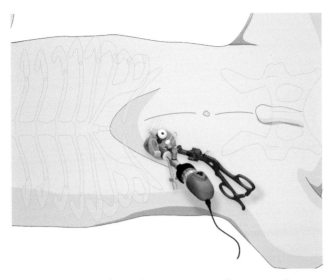

Figure 14-14 For a single-port laparoscopic-assisted gastropexy, placement of the single-port device is shown at the anticipated site of the gastropexy.

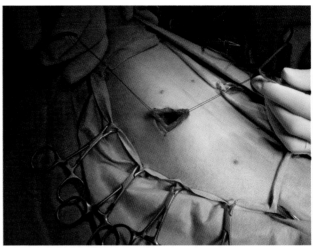

Figure 14-15 Stay sutures are placed in the cauterized or cut edges of the transversus abdominis muscle to aid in countertraction for port insertion.

These techniques are more technically challenging than laparoscopic-assisted gastropexy and require the use of some specialized equipment (i.e., the laparoscopic needle holders). Totally laparoscopic techniques are more time consuming, but they may be associated with less postoperative discomfort because they avoid the paramedian incision used in the laparoscopic-assisted technique and therefore reduce tissue trauma.[31]

Single-Port Access Gastropexy (Including Combined Procedures)

The single-port access laparoscopic gastropexy was originally described by Runge and Mayhew in 2013 (Figure 14-14).[38] This technique is particularly relevant to female dogs that need concurrent sterilization or male dogs that have retained testicles because these procedures can be performed concomitantly. A 2- to 3-cm skin incision is made starting just lateral to the rectus abdominis muscle and approximately 2 to 5 cm caudal to the right 13th rib. Dissection through the oblique and transverse abdominal musculature is continued using a combination of monopolar electrosurgery and sharp dissection. Stay sutures are placed in the cauterized or cut edges of the transversus abdominis muscle (Figure 14-15). This technique has principally been described using the SILS single-port device (e.g., SILS Port, Covidien), although the other single-port devices described in Chapter 6 could also be used for this purpose (Figure 14-16). When using the SILS device, it is inserted into the incision by clamping two curved Rochester Carmalt forceps at the base of the soft multitrocar port in a staggered fashion. The base of the port is then coated with a liberal quantity of sterile lubricant to facilitate insertion. The cauterized or cut edges of the transversus abdominis muscle are grasped with two large rat-toothed tissue forceps to provide counterpressure during port insertion. The tips of the Rochester Carmalt forceps are clamped on the single port and then directed into the incision. The curved Carmalt forceps are used to allow the bottom half of the SILS port to fit snugly within the incision. The clamps are then released to allow the bottom portion of the port to expand and seat in position. Three 5-mm cannulae supplied with the SILS port are inserted into the three corresponding holes in the port with the aid of a 5-mm blunt obturator. A small quantity of sterile lubricant is applied to the ends of the obturator

to facilitate insertion into the SILS port. The heights of the cannulae are then staggered, which can aid in avoiding instrument interference during the procedure. Insufflator tubing is attached to the SILS insufflation port, and the abdomen is insufflated to 8 to 10 mm Hg with CO_2 using a pressure-regulating mechanical insufflator. A 5-mm, 30-degree laparoscope (Hopkins II, Karl Storz Endoscopy) is inserted into a cannula and oriented caudally to view the abdomen, and a limited abdominal exploration is performed. The 5-mm straight or articulating grasper (SILS Clinch XL, Covidien, or Cambridge Endo, Farmington, MA) is inserted though one of the cannulae. With the articulating grasper, a 90-degree positional bend at the distal third of the instrument can be created with the tip deflecting toward an ovary or cryptorchid testicle if ovariectomy or cryptorchidectomy is indicated in the patient. After it has been grasped, the tissue is suspended with the bent portion of the articulating instrument still deflected. An ovariectomy or cryptorchidectomy can then be performed, and upon completion of the procedure, the port is removed from the body wall after the tissue has been excised as has been previously described.[38]

After ovaries or cryptorchid testicles have been removed by exteriorization of the SILS device with the tissue sample still

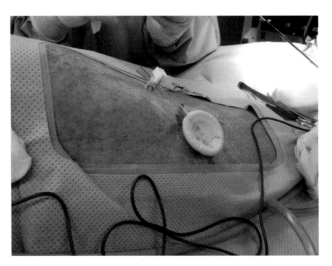

Figure 14-16 Single port device in place at the designated gastropexy site.

attached, the SILS port is reinserted through the same incision. Two 5-mm cannulae and one 12-mm cannula are inserted through the device, and the abdomen is reinsufflated. The table is tilted in a slight reverse Trendelenburg position to facilitate exposure of the greater curvature of the stomach. A 30-degree telescope is inserted into one of the 5-mm cannulae, and standard rigid 10-mm DuVall forceps are then inserted through the 12-mm cannula and directed toward the antrum of the stomach. A relatively avascular region near the pyloric antrum is grasped atraumatically midway between the greater and lesser curvatures for use as the site for incisional gastropexy. Holding firmly with the atraumatic 10-mm DuVall forceps, the stomach is carefully exteriorized by first removing the 30-degree telescope and then the two remaining 5-mm cannulae. As insufflation is lost, the SILS port is digitally dislodged from the incision with the 10-mm DuVall forceps maintaining traction on the stomach. The stomach is exteriorized through the abdominal incision. Stay sutures are securely placed to maintain orientation of the stomach axis. Incisional gastropexy is then completed as has previously been described for conventional laparoscopic-assisted incisional gastropexy. After completing the incisional gastropexy, the 2-cm multitrocar portal site is closed in the same fashion as has been described for the laparoscopic-assisted technique.

Complications and Prognosis

In the hands of skilled laparoscopic surgeons, intraoperative complications are rare. However, access-related lesions such as splenic laceration are well-known complications in any laparoscopic surgery. In the current published literature on laparoscopic and laparoscopic-assisted gastropexy, no major intraoperative or postoperative complications have been reported.[31-33,35-37,46] Minor reported complications include stomach perforation during dissection,[32] splenic puncture on cannula introduction,[31-33,38] minor hemorrhage,[33] incorrect port placement,[38] residual subcutaneous emphysema,[32] regurgitation or vomiting,[31,37] seroma formation,[37] incisional fistula,[44] and incisional infection.[31] Given the low risk of major complications, the prognosis is excellent in the short and long terms.

Postoperative Care

One night of postoperative hospitalization is recommended to allow pain management and monitoring for any gastrointestinal issues. Immediate postoperative management focuses on pain control. A suggested postoperative analgesic regimen includes injectable opioids for analgesia administered for 6 to 12 hours postoperatively followed by tramadol hydrochloride at 2 to 4 mg/kg for 3 to 5 days. Mild sedatives may also be indicated depending on patient anxiety and temperament. Water can be provided postoperatively when the patient is alert and standing with a small meal offered 8 to 12 hours later.

The patient should be discharged with an E-collar and instructions for approximately 14 days of activity restrictions to allow proper skin and gastropexy site healing. Additionally, typical recommendations to reduce the chance of future bloat incidences should continue to be implemented, including providing several small meals versus once-daily feeding, reducing the speed of eating, avoiding foods with a particle diameter smaller than 30 mm, not feeding from a raised bowl, limiting stresses, and avoiding breeding animals with first-degree relatives that had GDV.

If the integrity of the gastropexy is in question, focal abdominal ultrasonography can be performed 6 to 12 months after surgery to confirm the persistence of the gastropexy. The laparoscopic-assisted gastropexy will usually be within 3 to 4 cm of the skin incision.

 All videos cited in this chapter can be found on the book's companion website at **www.wiley.com/go/fransson/ laparoscopy**

References

1 Aronson, L.R., Brockman, D.J., Brown, D.C. (2000) Gastrointestinal emergencies. Vet Clin North Am Sm Anim Pract 30, 555-579.
2 Burrows, C.G., Ignaszewski, A. (1990) Canine gastric dilation-volvulus. J Small Anim Pract 31, 495-501.
3 Brockman, J.D., Washabau, R.J., Drobatz, K.J. (1995) Canine gastric dilation-volvulus syndrome in a veterinary critical care unit: 295 cases (1986-1992). J Am Vet Med Assoc 207, 460-464.
4 Glickman LT, Glickman NW, Perez CM et al. (1994) Analysis of risk factors for gastric dilation and dilation-volvulus in dogs. J Am Vet Med Assoc 204, 1965-1971.
5 Glickman, L.T., Lantz, G.C., Schellenberg, D.B., et al. (1998) A prospective study of survival and recurrence following the acute gastric dilation-volvulus syndrome in 136 dogs. J Am Anim Hosp Assoc 34, 253-259.
6 Beck, J.J., Staatz, A.J., Pelsue, D.H., et al. (2006) Risk factors associated with short-term outcome and development of perioperative complications in dogs undergoing surgery because of gastric-dilation-volvulus: 166 cases (1992-2003). J Am Vet Med Assoc 229, 1934-1939.
7 Mackenzie, G., Barnhart, M., Kennedy, S., et al. (2010) A retrospective study of factors influencing survival following surgery for gastric dilatation-volvulus syndrome in 306 dogs. J Am Anim Hosp Assoc 46, 97-102.
8 Brourman, J.D., Schertel, E.R., Allen, D.A., et al. (1996) Factors associated with perioperative mortality in dogs with surgically managed gastric dilatation-volvulus: 137 cases (1988-1993). J Am Vet Med Assoc 208, 1855-1858.
9 Glickman, L.T., Glickman, N.W., Schellenberg, D.B., et al. (1997) Multiple risk factors for the gastric dilatation-volvulus syndrome in dogs: a practitioner/owner case-control study. J Am Anim Hosp Assoc 33, 197-204.
10 Glickman, L.T., Glickman, N.W., Lantz, G.C., et al. (2000a) Incidence of breed-related risk factors for gastric-dilatation-volvulus in dogs. J Am Vet Med Assoc 216, 40-45.
11 Evans, K.M., Adams, V.J. (2010) Mortality and morbidity due to gastric dilatation-volvulus syndrome in pedigree dogs in the UK. J Small Anim Pract 51, 376-381.
12 Ward, M.P., Patronek, G.J., Glickman, L.T. (2003) Benefits of prophylactic gastropexy for dogs at risk of gastric dilatation-volvulus. Prev Med 60, 319-329.
13 Theyse, L.F., van de Brom, W.E., van Sluijs, F.J. (1998) Small size of food particles and age as risk factors for gastric dilatation volvulus in Great Danes. Vet Rec 143, 48-50.
14 Fallah, A.M., Lumb, W.V., Nelson, A.W., et al. (1982) Circumcostal gastropexy in the dog. A preliminary study. Vet Surg 11, 9-12.
15 Glickman, L.T., Glickman, N.W., Schellenberg, D.B., et al. (2000b) Non-dietary risk factors for gastric dilatation-volvulus in large and giant breed dogs. J Am Vet Med Assoc 217, 1492-1499.
16 Schaible, R.H., Ziech, J., Glickman, N.W., et al. (1997) Predisposition to gastric-dilation-volvulus in relation to genetics of thoracic confirmation in Irish Setters. J Am Anim Hosp Assoc 33, 379-383.
17 Glickman, L., Emerick, T., Glickman, N., et al. (1996) Radiological assessment of the relationship between thoracic conformation and the risk of gastric dilatation-volvulus in dogs. Vet Rad Ultrasound 37, 174-180.
18 Braun, L., Lester, S., Kuzma, A.B., et al. (1996) Gastric dilatation-volvulus in the dog with histological evidence of pre-existing inflammatory bowel disease: a retrospective study of 23 cases. J Am Anim Hosp Assoc 32, 287-290.
19 De Battisti, A., Toscano, M.J., Formaggini, L. (2012) Gastric foreign body as a risk factor for gastric dilatation and volvulus in dogs. J Am Vet Med Assoc 241;1190-1193.
20 Sartor, A.J., Bentley, A.M., Brown, D.C. (2013) Association between previous splenectomy and gastric dilatation-volvulus in dogs: 453 cases (2004-2009). J Am Vet Med Assoc 242;1381-1384.
21 Raghavan, M., Glickman, N.W., Glickman, L.T. (2006) The effect of ingredients in dry dog foods on the risk of gastric dilatation-volvulus in dogs. J Am Anim Hosp Assoc 42, 28-36.
22 Elwood, C.M. (1998) Risk factors for gastric dilatation in Irish setter dogs. J Small Anim Pract 39, 185-190.

23 Pipan, M., Brown, D.C., Battaglia, C.L., et al. (2012) An internet-based survey of risk factors for surgical gastric dilatation-volvulus in dogs. J Am Vet Med Assoc 240, 1456-1462.

24 Schulman, A.J., Lusk, R., Lippincott, C.L., et al. (1986) Muscular flap gastropexy: a new surgical technique to prevent recurrences of gastric dilation-volvulus syndrome. J Am Anim Hosp Assoc 22, 339-346.

25 Tanno, F., Weber, U., Wacker, C.H., et al. (1998) Ultrasonographic comparison of adhesions induced by two different methods of gastropexy in the dog. J Small Anim Pract 39, 432-436.

26 Frendin, J., Funkquist, B. (1990) Fundic gastropexy for prevention of recurrence of gastric volvulus. J Small Anim Pract 31, 78-82.

27 Pritchard, D. (1977) Prevention of acute gastric dilation by gastrojejunostomy. Canine Pract 4, 51-55.

28 Christie, T.R., Smith, C.W. (1976) Gastrocolopexy for prevention of recurrent gastric volvulus. J Am Anim Hosp Assoc 12, 173-176.

29 Steelman-Szymeczek, S.M., Stebbins, M.E., Hardie, E.M. (2003) Clinical evaluation of a right-sided prophylactic gastropexy via a grid approach. J Am Anim Hosp Assoc 39, 397-402.

30 Dujowich, M., Reimer, S.B. (2008) Evaluation of an endoscopically assisted gastropexy technique in dogs. Am J Vet Res 69, 537-541.

31 Dujowich, M., Keller, M.E., Reimer, S.B. (2010) Evaluation of short- and long-term complications after endoscopically assisted gastropexy in dogs. J Am Vet Med Assoc 236, 177-182.

32 Mayhew, P.D., Brown, D.C. (2009) Prospective evaluation of two intracorporeally sutured prophylactic laparoscopic gastropexy techniques compared with laparoscopic-assisted gastropexy in dogs. Vet Surg 38, 738-746.

33 Hardie, R.J., Flanders, J.A., Schmidt, P., et al. (1996) Biomechanical and histological evaluation of a laparoscopic stapled gastropexy technique in dogs. Vet Surg 25, 127-133.

34 Spah, C.E., Elkins, A.D., Wehrenberg, A., et al. (2013) Evaluation of two novel self-anchoring barbed sutures in a prophylactic laparoscopic gastropexy compared with intracorporeal tied knots. Vet Surg 42, 932-942.

35 Runge, J.J., Holt, D.E. (2013) Initial experience utilizing V-Loc suture for total intracorporeally sutured laparoscopic gastropexy in dogs. In Proceedings of the Veterinary Endoscopy Society Symposium, Key Largo FL.

36 Mathon, D.H., Dossin, O., Palierne, S., et al. (2009) A laparoscopic-sutured gastropexy technique in dogs: mechanical and functional evaluation. Vet Surg 38, 967-974.

37 Rawlings, C.A., Foutz, T.L., Mahaffey, M.B., et al. (2001) A rapid and strong laparoscopic-assisted gastropexy in dogs. Am J Vet Res 62, 871-875.

38 Rivier, P., Furneaux, R., Viguier, E. (2011) Combined laparoscopic ovariectomy and laparoscopic-assisted gastropexy in dogs susceptible to gastric dilation-volvulus. Can Vet J 52, 62-66.

39 Runge, J.J., Mayhew, P.D. (2013) Evaluation of single port access gastropexy and ovariectomy using articulating instruments and angled telescopes in dogs. Vet Surg 42, 807-813.

40 Waschak, M.J., Payne, J.T., Pope, E.R., et al. (1997) Evaluation of percutaneous gastrostomy as a technique for permanent gastropexy. Vet Surg 26, 235-241.

41 Benitez, M.E., Schmiedt, C.W., Radlinsky, M.G., et al. (2013) Efficacy of incisional gastropexy for prevention of GDV in dogs. J Am Anim Hosp Assoc 49, 185-189.

42 Leib, M.S., Konde, L.J., Wingfield, W.E., et al. (1985) Circumcostal gastropexy for preventing recurrence of gastric dilatation-volvulus in the dog: an evaluation of 30 cases. J Am Vet Med Assoc 187, 245-248.

43 Eggertsdottir, A.V., Stigen, O., Lonaas, L., et al. (2001) Comparison of the recurrence rate of gastric dilation with or without volvulus in dogs after circumcostal gastropexy versus gastrocolopexy. Vet Surg 30, 546-551.

44 Wacker, C.A., Weber, U.T., Tanno, F., et al. (1998) Ultrasonographic evaluation of adhesions induced by incisional gastropexy in 16 dogs. J Small Anim Pract 39, 379-384.

45 Rawlings, C.A., Mahaffey, M.B., Bement, S. (2002) Prospective evaluation of laparoscopic-assisted gastropexy in dogs susceptible to gastric dilatation. J Am Vet Med Assoc 221, 1576-1581.

46 Runge, J.J., Mayhew, P.D., Case, J.B., et al. (2014) Single-port cryptorchidectomy in dogs and cats: 25 cases (2009-2014). J Am Vet Med Assoc 245, 1258-1265.

47 Fox, S.M., Ellison, G.W., Miller, G.J., et al. (1985) Observations on the mechanical failure of three gastropexy techniques. J Am Anim Hosp Assoc 21, 729-734.

48 Coolman, B.R., Marretta, S.M., Pijanowski, G.J., et al. (1999) Evaluation of a skin stapler for belt-loop gastropexy in dogs. J Am Anim Hosp Assoc 35, 440-444.

49 Wilson, E.R., Henderson, R.A., Montgomery, R.D., et al. (1996) A comparison of laparoscopic and belt-loop gastropexy in dogs. Vet Surg 25, 221-227.

15 Laparoscopic Splenectomy

Stephanie L. Shaver and Philipp D. Mayhew

Key Points

- Laparoscopic splenectomy (LS) may provide improved patient outcomes compared with open splenectomy for a subset of patients with certain forms of splenic disease.
- Careful case selection is imperative to achieve success with LS.
- Patients with small- to moderate-sized splenic masses without hemoperitoneum and those with generalized splenomegaly may be candidates for LS.
- Use of a tilt table or manual shifting of the patient into right lateral recumbency may aid in final dissection of the mesenteric attachments to the head of the spleen.

In human medicine, laparoscopic splenectomy (LS) was first performed in the early 1990s, and since then has been increasingly used, becoming the gold standard for treatment in many cases.[1-4] LS is most commonly indicated for hematologic conditions, such as idiopathic thrombocytopenia purpura and lymphoproliferative, hemolytic, and myeloproliferative disorders[4,5]; however, LS has also been successfully performed in a number of traumatic cases.[6] The decision to perform LS in humans depends on a number of factors. Splenic size is a major determinant of whether LS is considered in patients with spleens measuring up to longitudinal lengths of 20 to 25 cm generally being considered candidates for LS.[3,5,7] Massive splenomegaly or megasplenism, as it is sometimes called, is generally a relative contraindication, and several studies have documented increasing splenic size as an independent predictor for complications .[5,8] It should be remembered that the normal canine spleen is a significantly larger organ relative to body size than it is in humans (the normal human spleen measures approximately 13 cm in length), meaning that guidelines for LS in humans should probably be considered with caution in companion animals. Other relative contraindications to LS in humans are ascites, uncorrected coagulopathy, and severe portal hypertension in which the presence of multiple venous collateral vessels can be challenging to deal with laparoscopically.[9,10]

Several important advantages in outcomes have been documented for LS compared with open splenectomy in humans.

Patients undergoing LS experience less postoperative pain; have shorter duration of hospitalization; and have fewer wound, pulmonary, and infectious complications than those undergoing the open procedure.[4,11] However, multiple studies have also documented that surgical time is longer for LS compared with open splenectomy.[4,11]

The classical description of the LS procedure in humans is a four-port procedure with the patient in right lateral decubitus position (right lateral recumbency) on a flexed table.[5] More recently, descriptions of other surgical platforms for LS have been reported, including hand-assisted techniques,[12] single-port techniques,[13,14] robotic splenectomy,[15] and even investigations of splenic access using natural orifice transluminal endosurgery (NOTES).[16]

Splenectomy in dogs is performed for diagnosis and treatment of benign and malignant splenic masses, torsion, infarction, diffuse neoplastic disease, trauma, and immune-mediated disease. One of the earliest reports of LS in the human literature used porcine and canine models to develop the procedure before its widespread implementation in human patients.[17] This report describes a four- to seven-port procedure with quite prolonged surgical times reported, although little morbidity was described. Since then, refinements to the technique have been described experimentally using either a three-port or single-incision laparoscopic approach.[18,19] A single clinical case report of successful multiple-port LS for treatment of splenic hemangiosarcoma has been

---

Small Animal Laparoscopy and Thoracoscopy, First Edition. Edited by Boel A. Fransson and Philipp D. Mayhew.
© 2015 by ACVS Foundation. Published 2015 by John Wiley & Sons, Inc.
Companion website: www.wiley.com/go/fransson/laparoscopy

reported in a dog,[21] and a case series of three cats that underwent LS was also recently documented.[22] More recently, a small case series describing the short-term outcome of dogs that underwent multiple-port LS procedures for a variety of underlying causes was described.[23]

Preoperative Considerations

Surgical Anatomy

The spleen is a relatively large organ in dogs and is located on the left side of the abdomen. The dorsal extremity, or head of the spleen, rests between the fundus of the stomach and the cranial portion of the left kidney; this is the least freely moveable portion of the spleen. It is suspended by part of the greater omentum, arising from the left crus of the diaphragm, which forms the phrenicosplenic ligament. This omental tissue also forms a wide gastrosplenic ligament, which attaches the hilus of the spleen to the greater curvature of the stomach. The ventral extremity of the spleen, or tail, has less restrictive omental attachments and is variable in position. Blood supply is from the splenic artery, which in most dogs originates from the celiac artery (but in a small number of dogs, the splenic artery can originate from the cranial mesenteric artery.[24] This blood supply branches into approximately 25 branches that fan out at the splenic hilum. Venous drainage from the spleen is through the splenic vein, which drains into the gastrosplenic vein. Care needs to be taken especially in cats to avoid iatrogenic damage to the pancreas which runs in close proximity to the splenic hilus within the mesentery. In dogs, the organs are more distant, but in both species, blood supply to the left limb of the pancreas, which emanates from branches of the splenic artery and veins, needs to be protected to avoid vascular insult to that area of pancreas.

Total splenectomy in canine patients is often performed through a standard ventral midline laparotomy with ligation of vessels along the splenic hilus; alternatively, ligation of the left gastroepiploic artery, short gastric arteries, and splenic artery and vein distal to the pancreatic blood supply may also be performed. Descriptions of LS have been specific to the former surgical technique (hilar splenectomy) because the hilar vessels are readily identifiable from a laparoscopic approach.

Diagnostic Workup and Imaging

Identification of a splenic mass or lesion should prompt thorough evaluation of systemic health, including complete blood count, serum biochemistry profile, and urinalysis. Particular attention to red blood cell parameters and platelet counts is useful to determine ongoing or recent hemorrhage, as well as evaluation of immune-mediated or hemophagocytic disorders. When concern exists regarding coagulation ability, diagnostics to evaluate coagulation or platelet function should be evaluated preoperatively.

Thoracic radiographs are a necessary component of a comprehensive workup to evaluate for the presence of pulmonary metastatic disease. Echocardiography may be considered to look for a mass associated with the right atrium or atrial appendage, particularly when splenic hemangiosarcoma is thought to be a likely differential because concurrent cardiac involvement is known to occur in a significant number of cases.[25,26] Computed tomography (CT) of the thorax is another diagnostic imaging modality that has higher sensitivity for detection of pulmonary metastatic disease[27] and may allow identification of some larger cardiac tumors.

Abdominal ultrasonography is considered essential before LS for appropriate patient selection and surgical planning. Documentation of splenic size and presence of masses, concurrent hemoperitoneum or other abdominal effusion, and presence of concurrent intraabdominal disease is critical for determining the appropriateness of LS, as well as overall patient prognosis and outcome. Abdominal CT is recommended over ultrasonography in human medicine.[9] CT may give a better sense of splenic size and shape; however, the degree of variability in splenic vasculature and ligamentous attachments seen in humans may make this information more essential in human medicine than in veterinary patients. Contrast-enhanced CT has been evaluated as a modality for differentiating splenic masses in dogs, and certain features, such as attenuation characteristics, were found to be helpful in differentiating benign from malignant lesions.[28] Magnetic resonance imaging has also been used for evaluation of splenic masses in dogs and was found to have very high sensitivity and specificity for differentiation of benign from malignant disease.[29]

Fine-needle aspirates (FNA) of the spleen, liver, lymph nodes, or other intraabdominal abnormalities may be of utility in determining the etiology of disease before surgical intervention. Although FNA is a relatively safe and well-tolerated procedure that may shed light on the underlying disease process, splenic cytology alone has a reported accuracy rate of only 61.3% in one study,[30] and in another, complete agreement between cytologic and histologic diagnoses was only found in 51.4% of cases.[31] Nonetheless, because of a positive predictive value of 86.7% for neoplastic disease, these findings may still be of use in guiding treatment decisions.

Patient Selection

In human medicine, some authors suggest that LS should be used in all elective splenectomy cases unless portal hypertension, ascites, or traumatic splenic injury is present.[9] Relative contraindications are controversial and include obesity and massive splenomegaly (>25 cm longitudinal length). Hand-assisted LS has been suggested as an alternative approach in cases of massive splenomegaly.[12]

At this time, recommendations for appropriate patient selection in veterinary medicine are empirical but include the absence of hemoperitoneum, the absence of massive splenomegaly, and splenic masses smaller than 6 cm in diameter. A case report describes the successful excision of a 3-cm splenic hemangiosarcoma in a canine patient via LS,[21] and a case series of dogs that underwent LS for splenic masses up to 6 cm in size has been published.[23] Very large splenic masses are likely to hinder both visualization and the ability to manipulate the spleen with a laparoscopic approach. Large lesions may also be more friable and may rupture more easily during manipulation, although these are unconfirmed hypotheses at this time. Dogs with concurrent hemoperitoneum are currently not considered appropriate candidates for LS because of impaired visualization in the presence of free abdominal fluid and the need to obtain rapid hemostasis. Despite LS having been described for traumatic splenic rupture in humans,[6] including a description of a technique for rapid control of the splenic hilum, no reports exist of acute hemorrhage control in LS in small animal patients. Dogs with large splenic masses are also prone to formation of extensive omental adhesions, which increases the difficulty of laparoscopic dissection. Because techniques for LS will progress in veterinary medicine, these concerns may be mitigated through improved instrumentation and surgeon proficiency with LS in the future.

Prognostic Factors

Currently, no studies are available in the veterinary literature that have evaluated risk factors for conversion or complications in companion animal species. In humans, increasing body mass index, the presence of hematologic malignancy, and increasing splenic longitudinal diameter were all risk factors for complications in LS, and the first of these two factors were independent risk factors for conversion in one large multicenter study.[8] Larger studies are necessary to evaluate these prognostic factors in small animal LS.

Patient Preparation

Surgical Preparation

Preoperative preparation for LS is routine with recommended fasting overnight to avoid gastric distension at surgery. The patient's bladder should ideally be expressed immediately before entering the operating room to ensure maximal working space within the peritoneal cavity. Perioperative antibiotics are administered intravenously during surgery (cefazolin 22 mg/kg every 90–120 minutes). The abdomen should be clipped for standard exploratory laparotomy from 3 to 5 cm cranial to the xiphoid process as far caudally as the pubis and laterally to the proximal third of the body wall on both sides. The possibility of conversion to an open approach should always be considered.

Operating Room Setup and Patient Positioning

Different approaches for LS in dogs and cats have been described, but these authors favor placement of the patient in dorsal recumbency and positioning the patient in such a way that rotation into an oblique right lateral position during the surgical procedure can be performed. The surgeon and surgeon's assistant both stand on the patient's right side, and the endoscopic tower is placed straight across from them on the patient's left side (Figure 15-1). The authors have found that, especially in the totally LS procedure, during dissection of the head of the spleen, it can be very helpful to either tilt the operating room table toward the patient's right-hand side or to roll the dog into lateral recumbency or near-lateral recumbency to improve access to the area of the splenic head and short gastric vessels.

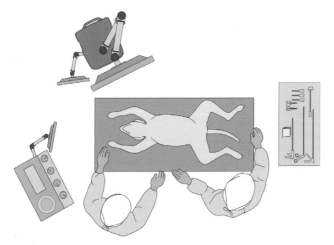

Figure 15-1 The operating room is set up for laparoscopic splenectomy with the surgeons on the patient's right side and the endoscopic tower located straight across from them on the left side.

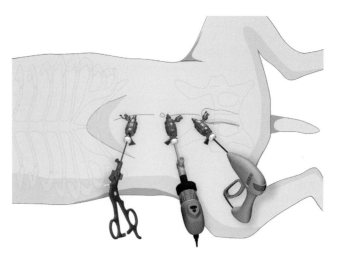

Figure 15-2 For multiport laparoscopic splenectomy, the procedure is initiated in dorsal recumbency with ports inserted on the ventral midline as shown. During dissection of the splenic head and gastrosplenic ligament, it can be helpful to allow the dog to rotate into right lateral recumbency.

Portal Position and Creation of Working Space

Multiple-port laparoscopic splenectomy (MLS) is the most commonly described surgical technique with fewer reports in human and veterinary medicine addressing single-incision laparoscopic surgery (SILS), laparoscopic-assisted, or hand-assisted splenectomy. MLS in humans is described using both anterior and posterior approaches, although variations on a right lateral approach currently appear to be the most commonly used position.[9,10,32] This technique uses three to five ports placed below the left costal margin. In veterinary descriptions, MLS has been performed using a variety of techniques. Dogs are generally positioned in either dorsal recumbency or 30 to 45 degrees right lateral oblique.[19,20,23] Nearly all descriptions are of a three-port technique, but the location of these ports varies among authors, and no definitive location has been identified as superior to any other. Reported port placements in dogs include cranial to the umbilicus, subumbilical, and right caudolateral abdomen[19]; cranial to the umbilicus, right paramedian at the level of the umbilicus, and cranial to the pubis[18]; umbilicus, cranial to the prepuce, and left caudolateral abdomen[21]; and three ventral midline ports.[20] Although all of these approaches were effective in the reports documenting their use, the authors prefer a three-port approach for MLS with all ports located on the ventral midline (Figure 15-2). A subumbilical telescope port is placed with this technique, and instrument ports are located cranial and caudal to the camera. The distance between the ports is variable, but in the authors' experience, placing the cranial port approximately halfway between the xiphoid and umbilicus and the caudal port approximately halfway between umbilicus and pubis is a general guideline, but it may require adjustment to account for splenic and patient size. Two cats have also successfully undergone MLS using this general approach.[22]

A single-incision laparoscopic splenectomy (SILS-LS) technique has also been performed by the authors group in a number of dogs using a single-port device centered on the umbilicus (Figure 15-3). A laparoscopic-assisted splenectomy (LAS) has recently been described in which the spleen is removed through a wound-protector device (Figure 15-4) (Alexis; Applied Medical, Rancho Santa Margarita, CA). This device is placed on the umbilicus and allows the spleen to be exteriorized through it.[33]

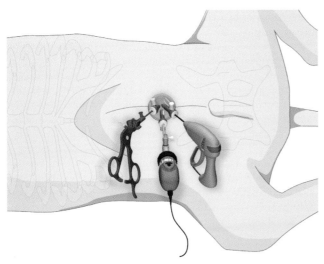

Figure 15-3 A single-incision laparoscopic device has been placed over the umbilicus for performing a single-incision laparoscopic splenectomy procedure.

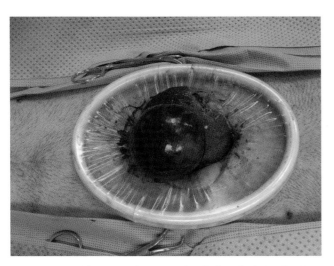

Figure 15-4 An Alexis wound retractor (Applied Medical, Rancho Santa Margarita, CA) has been placed for performing a laparoscopic-assisted splenectomy.

Surgical Techniques

Surgical Instrumentation

Certain essential instrumentation is required if LS is to be performed in a safe and efficient manner. Three to four trocar–cannula assemblies are required to complete the MLS procedure. Threaded cannulae are helpful to avoid accidental cannula withdrawal during instrument exchanges. For SILS-LS, one of the commercially available single-port laparoscopic devices such as the SILS port (Covidien, Mansfield, MA) device, the Triport (Olympus, Center Valley, PA), or the EndoCone (Karl Storz Endoscopy, Goleta, CA) will be required. For the LAS procedure described, an Alexis wound retractor (Applied Medica, Rancho Santa Margarita, CA) is used to create a protected "assist" incision on the ventral midline through which the spleen can be exteriorized.[22,33] Instrumentation available should include a blunt probe, Babcock grasping forceps, and one of the many laparoscopic retractors available such as a fan retractor or

a Cuschieri retractor. A vessel-sealing device is ideal for sealing and dividing all but the very largest of the splenic hilar vessels. Vessels up to 7 mm can be safely sealed using the common bipolar vessel-sealing devices such as the Ligasure (Covidien) and Enseal (Ethicon Endosurgery, Cincinnati, OH) Use of the Ligasure device has been described in a small cohort of dogs undergoing open splenectomy for resection of splenic masses with good success.[34] Although endoscopic staplers can be used for hilar resection, their use in veterinary clinical patients has not been reported for this indication. In human patients, vascular staplers are used more often for LS, but the use of vessel-sealing devices has been shown to be associated with less surgical time and a reduction in blood loss and transfusion rate.[2,35] Specimen retrieval bags should always be used to retrieve the spleen in the totally laparoscopic technique because confirmation of benign disease is rarely possible before histopathologic evaluation, and the risk of intraabdominal or port site metastasis can be reduced by use of these devices.

Multiport Laparoscopic Splenectomy

After establishing a camera port, the abdomen is insufflated with carbon dioxide to create a pneumoperitoneum of approximately 8 to 12 mm Hg for adequate working space. The instrument port size is variable, but the authors prefer having at least one 10- to 12-mm port to allow for introduction of a specimen retrieval bag at the conclusion of the procedure. The spleen must usually be manipulated to expose the splenic hilus with use of a blunt probe or fan retractor, but care must be taken to avoid puncturing the splenic capsule with overzealous manipulation (Figure 15-5). When using a blunt probe, the spleen should always be manipulated with the body of the instrument rather than the tip, which can penetrate the thin splenic capsule easily. After the hilar vessels are identified, transection of vessels may be performed, generally starting from the mobile tail of the spleen and working toward the head. Sealing and dividing of the hilar vessels can be achieved in a variety of ways, although the use of a bipolar or harmonic vessel-sealing device is strongly recommended (Figure 15-6, Video Clip 15-1). These devices have been used in open canine splenectomy[34] with success and are routinely used in human LS.[2,35] Other modalities that can be used include laparoscopic hemoclips and vascular stapling devices. Because of the large numbers of splenic vessels, hemoclips are likely to be laborious to use for this application and are likely to extend surgical time compared with the use of a vessel-sealing device, a finding that has been confirmed in a canine ovariohysterectomy model.[36] The use of vascular staplers for sealing the splenic hilum is used extensively in humans, although the use of multiple stapler cartridges is

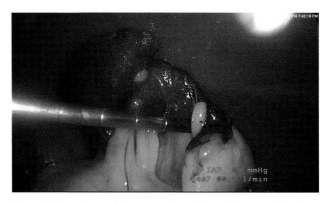

Figure 15-5 During totally laparoscopic multiport splenectomy, the spleen is retracted laterally to expose the splenic hilum.

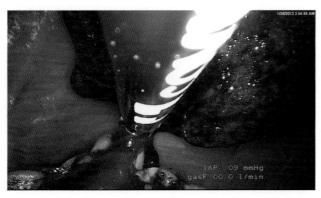

Figure 15-6 A vessel-sealing device can be seen sealing and dividing the final attachments at the splenic head. A small amount of hemorrhage can be seen because of minor inadvertent trauma to the splenic capsule during dissection.

likely to be necessary in medium to large breed dogs, which may increase the costs of the procedure considerably.

As sealing and dividing of the splenic hilum progresses, rotation of the patient into an oblique or complete right lateral recumbency facilitates exposure of the gastrosplenic ligament and short gastric vessels at the splenic head. After complete dissection of the spleen, additional laparoscopic procedures, such as laparoscopic liver biopsy, may be performed as indicated. Before exteriorizing the spleen, a specimen retrieval bag is introduced through the large cannula, and the spleen is manipulated into the bag using a blunt probe or laparoscopic Babcock forceps. Standard-sized specimen retrieval bags are likely to be of adequate size for most spleens in cats and smaller breed dogs. However, in medium to large dogs or in smaller dogs with significant splenomegaly, the use of an extra-large specimen retrieval bag may be necessary (e.g., Inzii retrieval system, Applied Medical). It should be noted that some of these larger specimen retrieval bags require a 12-mm cannula for placement. After the spleen has been mobilized into the bag, the midline incision is elongated into a mini-laparotomy (length varies on splenic size), and the specimen retrieval bag is withdrawn (Video Clip 15-2). The authors often position two of the three ventral midline ports 5 to 7 cm apart so that they can be joined during retrieval of the spleen in medium to large breed dogs. In smaller dogs and cats, the spleen can often be retrieved through a smaller 2- to 4-cm "assist" incision. In one report of LS in cats, a wound retraction device (Alexis wound retractor) was used to retrieve the spleen without placement of a specimen retrieval bag, which can be challenging in the small confines of the feline abdomen.[22] These wound retractors will act like specimen retrieval devices to protect the wound edges from contamination during extraction. After the specimen has been retrieved, the telescope is replaced into the abdomen one more time to evaluate for any ongoing hemorrhage before removal of the ports and routine abdominal closure. In humans, morcellation of the spleen is sometimes performed to reduce the size of the incision required to remove the spleen. Although LS in humans is most often performed for non-neoplastic disease, morcellation is still used for neoplasms, perhaps most commonly for removal of benign uterine tumors and benign or malignant renal tumors. In a controlled, blinded study evaluating histopathologic diagnoses of uterine tissue before and after morcellation, neoplasia was missed in one fifth of morcellated specimens.[37] In a similar study of nephrectomy cases, the same diagnosis, grade, and stage were identified for all morcellated samples compared with nonmorcellated

ones.[38] Other complications of morcellation have been described in human medicine, such as the rare development of parasitic myomas after minimally invasive hysterectomy resulting from dissemination of tissue throughout the peritoneum after morcellation.[39] Damage to retrieval devices secondary to morcellation has also been rarely implicated in spread or recurrence of disease.[40] Splenic morcellation has not been described in LS in companion animal species, and complications and the effect on histopathologic evaluation of the recovered tissue are unknown at this time.

Laparoscopic-Assisted Splenectomy

Hand-assisted laparoscopic splenectomy (HALS) has been described in humans. This approach uses a special hand-assist port that allows the surgeon to introduce his or her hand into the abdomen to aid in manipulation of the spleen without loss of pneumoperitoneum. In a retrospective study comparing HALS with MLS in human medicine, the HALS group had larger spleens; was more likely to have a malignant diagnosis; and on average, had lengthier operative times and a longer hospital stay.[12] When controlling for splenic weight and malignancy, however, there were no significant differences between the HALS and MLS groups. A similar technique to HALS has been reported in a cohort of dogs[33] and a single cat[22] and has been termed *laparoscopic-assisted splenectomy*. In this procedure, an initial laparoscopic exploration can be performed through either a single-port device centered on the umbilicus or through two ports located close to each other on the ventral midline close to the umbilicus. If indicated, liver biopsies can be taken before the creation of an "assist" insertion on the ventral midline.[33] An Alexis wound retractor is then placed (size depends on the size of the mass and the patient, but generally, the 2- to 4-cm, 2.5- to 6-cm, or 5- to 9-cm sizes are most appropriate) into the "assist" incision, and the spleen is manually elevated out of the incision (see Figure 15-4). Digital retraction is generally used, but gentle retraction with atraumatic laparoscopic forceps can also be used as long as any mass lesions are not grasped. As the spleen is exteriorized, the hilar vasculature and mesenteric attachments are sealed and divided using a vessel-sealing device or one of the other modalities described earlier (Figure 15-7). Closure of the incision after splenectomy is complete is performed routinely.

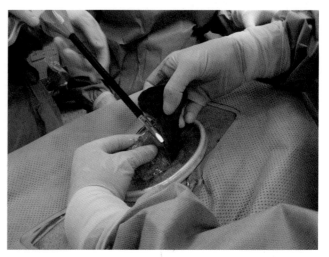

Figure 15-7 During laparoscopic-assisted splenectomy, the spleen is manually exteriorized through the "assist" incision, and the hilar vessels are sealed as they are exteriorized using a vessel-sealing device.

Single-Incision Laparoscopic Splenectomy

Splenectomy via SILS-LS has been gaining traction in human medicine as an approach with possible advantages over traditional MLS.[14] Advantages identified in the literature include decreased pain scores and shorter operative times; however, one study did identify increased blood loss associated with SILS-LS.[41] A systematic review of the technique concludes that SILS-LS appears safe and effective in the highly selected patient population in which it has been performed, but further study is needed before encouraging wide acceptance of this approach[14] SILS-LS has been experimentally described in 12 dogs, with a control group of 6 dogs undergoing MLS; this study found that operative time and incision length were both significantly shorter in the SILS-LS group, without significant differences in patient outcome; conversion was not required with either approach.[20] The authors have performed SILS-LS splenectomy in a number of clinical cases and have found it a very useful technique in smaller animals in which the spleen is smaller and can be removed through the incision that the SILS port was placed into at the end of the procedure. Using the SILS port, the procedure progresses in very similar fashion to the MLS technique, but instrument trajectory is more parallel to the telescope compared with the MLS technique. This can make splenic retraction and elevation more challenging, although the authors have been successful with this approach in most cases.

Complications and Prognosis

In humans, a total LS complication rate of 15.5%, compared with 26.6% for open splenectomy, was noted in a large meta-analysis of 2119 LS cases and 821 open splenectomy cases.[4] LS was associated with fewer pulmonary, wound, and infectious complications than open splenectomy; however, more hemorrhagic complications were documented in LS patients. Other complications described in the human literature have not been documented in veterinary patients, including delayed hemorrhage, subphrenic abscess, and ischemic bowel injury.[10]

Hemorrhage is the major intraoperative complication of concern with LS. Reported sources of hemorrhage in canine LS include injury to the spleen with initial trocar–cannula placement,[18] inadequate sealing of vessels during electrocoagulation,[19] tears to the splenic capsule during manipulation,[21] or disruption of small omental vessels.[23] In no reported case in veterinary medicine has this hemorrhage been hemodynamically significant or severe enough to warrant conversion, although only small numbers of clinical cases have been reported to date. Described bleeding has been self-limiting or readily treatable with application of a vessel-sealing device. In one study, blood loss was less significant in the LS group compared with open splenectomy.[18]

As with all laparoscopic procedures, the need for conversion is a possible complication. Conversion has only been described in one case in the veterinary literature,[23] during which conversion was elected because of lengthy surgical time in a patient with multiple omental adhesions and abundant falciform fat that limited visualization. Conversion is relatively uncommon in the human literature as well, with a meta-analysis reporting a conversion rate of 5.7% to 6.6% of patients.[4]

Infection or inflammation of the surgical wound in LS cases was six times lower compared with the surgical incision from open splenectomy in one report.[18] In the authors' case series, incisional bruising was the only postoperative complication and was described in two of eight cases.[23]

Postoperative Care

Recovery after LS has generally been rapid and with few complications; however, patient selection and small numbers make it difficult to draw definitive conclusions. Pain scores in one study were significantly lower in the LS group than the open group at 24 hours after surgery; however, observers were not blinded to the surgical procedure performed.[18] In the reported literature, dogs were initially maintained on μ-agonist opioids every 4 hours for approximately the first 12 hours postoperatively and then transitioned to oral tramadol (2–4 mg/kg every 8–12 hours) and/or carprofen (2 mg/kg every 12 hours), resulting in apparently adequate analgesia and patient comfort.[21,23] All dogs were discharged with oral analgesics to be administered at home if deemed necessary by the owner.

Perioperative antibiotics were discontinued after surgery, and additional medications or treatments (gastroprotectants, intravenous fluids) were administered at the discretion of the clinician. In the 11 clinical cases described, 9 patients were discharged the day after surgery and 2 patients after an additional day of hospitalization for reasons unrelated to LS. Outcome in clinical patients has been excellent, with no long-term complications related to LS documented to date.

 All videos cited in this chapter can be found on the book's companion website at **www.wiley.com/go/fransson/ laparoscopy**

References

1 Podevin, G., Victor, A., De Napoli, S., et al. (2011) Laparoscopic splenectomy: comparison between anterior and lateral approaches. J Laparoendosc Adv Surg Tech 21 (9), 865-868.

2 Gelmini, R., Romano, F., Quaranta, N., et al. (2006) Sutureless and stapleless laparoscopic splenectomy using radiofrequency: LigaSure device. Surg Endosc 20, 991-994.

3 Feldman, L.S., Demyttenaere, S.V., Polyhronopoulos, G.N., et al. (2008) Refining the selection criteria for laparoscopic versus open splenectomy for splenomegaly. J Laparoendosc Adv Surg Tech 18, 13-19.

4 Winslow, E.R., Brunt, L.M. (2002) Perioperative outcomes of laparoscopic versus open splenectomy: a meta-analysis with an emphasis on complications. Surgery 134, 647-655.

5 Feldman, L.S. (2011) Laparoscopic splenectomy: standardized approach. World J Surg 35, 1487-1495.

6 Carobbi, A., Romagnani, F., Antonelli, G., et al. (2010) Laparoscopic splenectomy for severe blunt trauma: initial experience of ten consecutive cases with a fast hemostatic technique. Surg Endosc 24, 1325-1330.

7 Ardestani, A., Tavakkoli, A. (2013) Laparoscopic versus open splenectomy: the impact of spleen size on outcomes. J Laparoendosc Adv Surg Tech 23, 760-764.

8 Casaccia, M., Torelli, P., Pasa, A., et al. (2010) Putative predictive parameters for the outcome of laparoscopic splenectomy. Ann Surg 251, 287-291.

9 Fisichella, P.M., Wong, Y.M., Pappas, S.G., et al. (2014) Laparoscopic splenectomy: perioperative management, surgical technique, and results. J Gastrointest Surg 18, 404-410.

10 Corcione, F., Pirozzi, F., Aragiusto, G., et al. (2012) Laparoscopic splenectomy: experience of a single center in a series of 300 cases. Surg Endosc 26, 2870-2876.

11 Kucuk, C., Sozuer, E., Ok, E., et al. (2005) Laparoscopic versus open splenectomy in the management of benign and malignant hematologic diseases: a ten year single center experience. J Laparoendosc Adv Surg Tech 15, 135-139.

12 Altaf, A.M.S., Ellsmere, J., Bonjer, H.J., et al. (2012) Morbidity of hand-assisted laparoscopic splenectomy compared to conventional laparoscopic splenectomy: a 6 year review. Can J Surg 55(4), 227-232.

13 Liang, Z.W., Cheng, Y., Jiang, Z.S., et al. (2014) Transumbilical single-incision endoscopic splenectomy: report of ten cases. World J Gastroenterol 20, 258-263.

14 Fan, Y., Wu, S.D., Kong, J., et al. (2014) Feasibility and safety of single-incision laparoscopic splenectomy: a systematic review. J Surg Res 186, 354-362.

15 Gelmini, R., Franzoni, C., Spaziani, A., et al. (2011) Laparoscopic splenectomy: conventional versus robotic approach-A comparative study. J Laparoendosc Adv Surg Tech 21, 393-398.

16 Tagaya, N., Kubota, K. (2009) NOTES; approach to the liver and spleen. J Hepatobiliary Pancreat Surg 16, 283-287.

17 Thibault, C., Mamazza, J., Létourneau, R., et al. (1992) Laparoscopic splenectomy: operative technique and preliminary report. Surg Laparosc Endosc 2 (3), 248-253.

18 Stedile, R., Beck, C.A., Schiochet, F., et al. (2009) Laparoscopic versus open splenectomy in dogs. Pesquisa Vet Brasil 29, 653-660.

19 Bakhtiari, J., Tavakoli, A., Khalaj, A, et al. (2011) Minimally invasive total splenectomy in dogs: a clinical report. Int J Vet Res 5, 9-12.

20 Khalaj, A., Bakhtiari, J., Niasari-Naslaji, A. (2012) Comparison between single and three portal laparoscopic splenectomy in dogs. BMC Vet Res 8, 161.

21 Collard, F., Nadeau, M.E., Carmel, E.N. (2010) Laparoscopic splenectomy for treatment of splenic hemangiosarcoma in a dog. Vet Surg 39, 870-872.

22 O'Donnell, E., Mayhew, P., Culp, W.T.N., et al. (2013) Laparoscopic splenectomy: operative technique and outcome in three cats. J Fel Med Surg 15, 48-52.

23 Shaver, S. L., Mayhew, P.D., Steffey, M.A., et al. (2014) Short-term outcome of multiple port laparoscopic splenectomy in 10 dogs. Vet Surg DOI:10.1111/j.1532-950X.2014.12312.x

24 Bezuidenhout, A.J. (2013) The lymphatic system. In: EvansHE (ed.) Miller's Anatomy of the Dog, 4th edn. Saunders, St. Louis, pp. 535-562.

25 Yamamoto, S., Hoshi, K., Hirakawa, A., et al.(2013) Epidemiological, clinical and pathological features of primary cardiac hemangiosarcoma in dogs: a review of 51 cases. J Vet Med Sci 75, 1433-1441.

26 Boston, S.E., Higginson, G., Monteith, G. (2011) Concurrent splenic and right atrial mass at presentation in dogs with HSA: a retrospective study. J Am Anim Hosp Assoc 47, 336-341.

27 Nemanic, S., London, C.A., Wisner, E.R. (2006) Comparison of thoracic radiographs and single breath-hold helical CT for detection of pulmonary nodules in dogs with metastatic neoplasia. J Vet Intern Med 20, 508-515.

28 Fife, W.D., Samii, V.F., Drost, W.T., et al. (2004) Comparison between malignant and nonmalignant splenic masses in dogs using contrast-enhanced computed tomography. Vet Radiol Ultrasound 45, 289-297.

29 Clifford, C.A., Pretorius, E.S., Weisse, C., et al. (2004) Magnetic resonance imaging of focal splenic and hepatic lesions in the dog. J Vet Intern Med 18, 330-338.

30 Ballegeer, E.A., Forrest, L.J., Dickinson, R.M., et al. (2007) Correlation of ultrasound appearance of lesions and cytologic and histologic diagnosis in splenic aspirates from dogs and cats: 32 cases (2002-2005). J Am Vet Med Assoc 230, 690-696.

31 Watson, A.T., Penninck, D., Knoll, J.S., et al. (2011) Safety and correlation of test results of combined ultrasound-guided and fine-needle aspiration and needle core biopsy of the canine spleen. Vet Radiol Ultrasound 52 (3), 317-322.

32 Corcione, F., Esposito, C., Cuccurullo, D., et al. (2002) Technical standardization of laparoscopic splenectomy: experience with 105 cases. Surg Endosc 16, 972-974.

33 Singh, A., Runge, J.J., Case, J.B., et al. (2014) Laparoscopic-assisted splenectomy in dogs: 7 cases (2011-2013). Proceedings of the 11th Annual Veterinary Endoscopy Society Meeting Florence, Italy.

34 Rivier, P., Monnet, E. (2011) Use of a vessel sealant device for splenectomy in dogs. Vet Surg 40, 102-105.

35 Romano, F., Gelmini, R., Caprotti, R., et al. (2007) Laparoscopic splenectomy: Ligasure versus EndoGIA: a comparative study. J Laparoendosc Adv Surg Tech 17, 763-767.

36 Mayhew, P.D., Brown, D.C. (2007) Comparison of three techniques for ovarian pedicle hemostasis during laparoscopic-assisted ovariohysterectomy. Vet Surg 36, 541-547.

37 Rivard, C., Salhadar, A., Kenton, K. (2012) New challenges in detecting, grading, and staging endometrial cancer after uterine morcellation. J Minim Invasive Gynecol 9(3), 313-316.

38 Landman, J., Lento, P., Hassen, W., et al. (2000) Feasibility of pathological evaluation of morcellated kidneys after radical nephrectomy. J Urol 164 (6), 2086-2089.

39 Larraín, D., Rabischong, B., Khoo, C.K., et al. (2010) "Iatrogenic" parasitic myomas: unusual late complication of laparoscopic morcellation procedures. J Minim Invasive Gynecol 17 (6), 719-724.

40 Lansdale, N., Marven, S., Welch, J., et al. (2007) Intra-abdominal splenosis following laparoscopic splenectomy causing recurrence in a child with chronic immune thrombocytopenic purpura. J Laparoendosc Adv Surg Tech A 17 (3), 387-390.

41 Choi, K.K., Kim, M.J., Park, H., et al. (2013) Single- incision laparoscopic splenectomy versus conventional multiport laparoscopic splenectomy: a retrospective comparison of outcomes. Surg Innov 20, 40.

16 Liver Biopsy and Cholecystocentesis

Ameet Singh

Key Points

- Laparoscopic liver biopsy (LLB) and cholecystocentesis are quick, safe, and minimally invasive methods for obtaining samples of diagnostic quality in dogs and cats.
- Contraindications are few for LLB, and this technique is associated with an extremely low complication rate even in patients with coagulopathy and ascites.
- Methods to minimize hemorrhage from liver biopsy sites can be performed laparoscopically if marked coagulopathy exists.
- Single-port platforms for laparoscopy can be used to perform liver biopsy or cholecystocentesis.

In veterinary medicine, liver biopsy is a commonly performed procedure because many diseases of the hepatobiliary system do not require surgical intervention. Biopsy can provide a definitive diagnosis, which can guide additional diagnostic or therapeutic measures. In addition, liver biopsy can provide important prognostic information for the clinician and pet owner. Indications for liver biopsy are numerous and may include elevated hepatic enzyme activities for more than 30 days, investigation of ultrasonographically identified lesions, abnormal liver size, and staging for neoplastic disease.[1-4] Several techniques for liver biopsy have been described in the veterinary literature such as percutaneous cutting needle biopsy, with or without ultrasound guidance,[5] laparoscopic biopsy,[1,2,6-9] or biopsies harvested at the time of celiotomy.[1,3] Each technique for liver biopsy carries its own potential for complications and limitations, with bleeding the most commonly described. Bleeding can be further exacerbated in patients with hepatobiliary disease[10]; therefore, the technique of liver biopsy must be selected carefully, taking into account the potential risks for the individual patient.

Laparoscopy is a minimally invasive technique for procedures of the abdomen and provides numerous advantages over open celiotomy, including improved illumination and detail of abdominal organs, reduced postoperative pain, and rapid return to function for patients.[11-13] Diagnostic laparoscopy is commonly performed in human and veterinary medicine and can be used to obtain high-quality tissue biopsies, assess the resectability of lesions, and stage neoplasia.[6,7,14,15]

Percutaneous cutting needle biopsy, with or without ultrasound guidance, is also a minimally invasive technique for liver biopsy.[5] However, this technique has been associated with reduced diagnostic efficacy compared with wedge biopsy of the liver obtained at the time of celiotomy or postmortem.[16] In one study, morphologic diagnosis obtained via cutting needle biopsy agreed with the definitive diagnosis obtained via wedge biopsy in only 48% of cases.[16] The discordance between biopsy techniques was attributed to the median surface area of the cutting needle liver biopsy, which was one quarter the size obtained via wedge biopsy, resulting in reduced numbers of portal triads and hepatic acini in the cutting needle biopsy specimen.[16] The minimum number of portal triads required in a biopsy specimen to obtain an accurate morphologic diagnosis in veterinary medicine has not been established; however, a previous report suggested that more than six to eight were adequate in human patients.[17] Feline patients undergoing cutting needle biopsy are at risk for vagotonic shock after rapid fire of the biopsy needle, and some authors have suggested avoiding this method in this species.[3]

The use of laparoscopy for liver biopsy maintains the minimally invasive advantage of the cutting needle technique but is able to obtain diagnostic biopsy samples similar to what can be obtained at the time of celiotomy.[2,6,8,9] Furthermore, the liver biopsy sites can be selected under direct laparoscopic visualization of liver lobes, and hemorrhage can be monitored and addressed if required by the surgeon. In a canine experimental study comparing various techniques for liver biopsy, laparoscopic liver biopsy (LLB) of the

Small Animal Laparoscopy and Thoracoscopy, First Edition. Edited by Boel A. Fransson and Philipp D. Mayhew.
© 2015 by ACVS Foundation. Published 2015 by John Wiley & Sons, Inc.
Companion website: www.wiley.com/go/fransson/laparoscopy

left lateral lobe produced biopsy specimens that were adequate for histologic investigation with 16.8 ± 1.43 and 18.1 ± 2.51 portal triads from peripheral and central locations, respectively.[2] An additional finding in this study was that regardless of technique for liver biopsy, hemorrhage was minimal (<2 mL), and normal coagulation occurred rapidly.[2] These results must be interpreted with caution because these were healthy experimental dogs without evidence of hepatobiliary disease. A retrospective study of dogs undergoing LLB found that this method was associated with minimal morbidity and mortality and produced adequate samples for histologic interpretation.[8] The authors suggested submission of multiple LLB specimens for histologic interpretation because disagreement in diagnosis was found in 14% of cases.[8] The results from another recent study evaluating dogs undergoing LLB as the sole diagnostic procedure performed corroborated safety results with the findings by Petre.[9]

Cholecystocentesis is a diagnostic procedure most commonly performed during investigation of hepatobiliary diseases of bacterial origin.[3,18,19] In cats, cholangitis or cholangiohepatitis is one of the most commonly diagnosed hepatobiliary diseases with ascending bacterial infection most commonly implicated as the inciting cause.[20,21] Treatment is based on appropriate bacterial culture and susceptibility testing, and percutaneous, ultrasound-guided cholecystocentesis has been shown to be a safe, minimally invasive, and effective procedure in dogs[22,23] and cats.[18] Laparoscopic cholecystocentesis (LC) provides an additional minimally invasive technique for bile sampling and can be performed concurrently at the time of LLB or other laparoscopic procedures. Advantages of LC include the use of laparoscopic guidance for needle placement into the gallbladder and having the ability to monitor for bile leak or hemorrhage into the peritoneal cavity. Diagnostic laparoscopy can also allow for investigation of the extrahepatic biliary tract and any other abnormalities in the abdomen. Studies comparing the safety and efficacy of percutaneous, ultrasound-guided cholecystocentesis with LC are lacking in the veterinary literature.

Extrahepatic biliary obstruction (EHBO) can result in devastating metabolic abnormalities, such as coagulopathy, reduced Kupffer cell function, increased circulating endotoxins, and intra- and postoperative hypotension in dogs and cats.[24-29] Surgery for EHBO is associated with prolonged operative times and high mortality rates,[24,25,27] and preoperative biliary drainage has been considered as a therapeutic option to improve postoperative outcomes.[29,30] A clinical study in three dogs reported the successful treatment of EHBO secondary to pancreatitis with percutaneous ultrasound-guided cholecystocentesis.[23] In humans, controversy exists as to the benefit of preoperative biliary drainage via cholecystocentesis (laparoscopic or ultrasound guided) because bile has many important functions in the gastrointestinal tract.[31-33] In veterinary medicine, most often a one-stage, definitive surgical procedure (biliary rerouting or cholecystostomy tube placement) is performed in cases with EHBO. However, the development of endoscopic retrograde cholangiography or laparoscopic evaluation of the extrahepatic biliary tract may result in a larger number of cases in which LC may represent the ideal treatment option for the treatment of EHBO.

Preoperative Considerations

Surgical Anatomy

The parenchyma of the liver is divided into six lobes (from left to right): left lateral, left medial, quadrate, right medial, right lateral, and caudate. The caudate lobe is further subdivided into the caudate and papillary processes. Deep fissuring separates each lobe and allows the lobes to stack upon each other during movement, preventing tearing of the parenchyma. The liver is fixed at its cranial aspect by the coronary and left and right triangular ligaments and to the ventral portion of the abdominal wall and sternal portion of the diaphragm by the falciform ligament. Minor support is provided by the hepatorenal ligament, which attaches the right kidney to the renal fossa of the caudate lobe. The caudal aspect of the liver lobes, opposite to the hilar aspect, is relatively movable and provides a suitable target for LLB when diffuse hepatopathies are present. The hepatogastric ligament contains the bile duct, portal vein, and hepatic artery but does not provide additional support to the liver. The gallbladder (Figure 16-1) is a pear-shaped structure that resides in a fossa between the quadrate and right medial liver lobes. The cystic duct connects the gallbladder to the common bile duct, where a variable number of hepatic ducts also insert. The common bile duct then traverses within the hepatoduodenal ligament and inserts into the major duodenal papilla in dogs and cats. It is important to note the unique anatomy of the feline extrahepatic biliary tract in which the major pancreatic duct joins the common bile duct before its opening to the duodenum in the majority of cats.[24,34] This intimate association makes cats more susceptible to EHBO with pancreatitis; in dogs, the minor pancreatic duct, which inserts into the duodenum at the minor duodenal papilla, distal to the insertion of the common bile duct, is the predominant duct.[35] The liver has a unique dual blood supply in which 80% percent of its blood volume and 50% of its oxygen supply is provided by the portal vein and 20% of its blood volume and the remaining half of oxygen is provided by the hepatic artery which is a branch of the celiac artery. The cystic artery provides blood supply to the gallbladder, which is a branch of the hepatic artery.[35]

Preoperative Diagnostic Evaluation

In many patients undergoing LLB or LC, a thorough diagnostic evaluation has already been performed and has led the clinician to search for a histopathologic diagnosis from a liver biopsy sample. This evaluation frequently includes serum biochemistry, complete blood count, urinalysis, and diagnostic imaging of the abdomen. Elevated hepatobiliary enzymes are commonly present in patients undergoing LLB. Abdominal radiography can provide information on liver size and whether loss of serosal detail is present that is consistent with free peritoneal fluid. In addition, radiography may identify choleliths that could be causing EHBO depending on

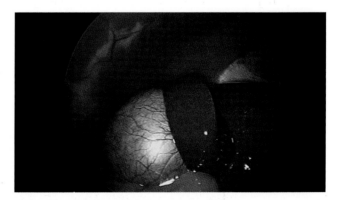

Figure 16-1 Laparoscopic view of the gallbladder, left of the adjacent quadrate liver lobe (patient positioned in dorsal recumbency).

their location within the biliary tract. Abdominal ultrasonography is critical in evaluating the liver parenchyma and size as well as gallbladder and common bile duct wall thickness, appearance of contents, size, and distension. In general, the decision to perform liver biopsy or cholecystocentesis is made after information gained from these diagnostic tests.

Because the potential for hemorrhage from liver biopsy or cholecystocentesis site(s) is higher in patients with hepatic dysfunction,[10] all patients should have coagulation testing (prothrombin time and partial thromboplastin time with or without buccal mucosal bleeding time) before LLB. Depending on the suspected underlying cause, three-view thoracic radiographs can be considered to rule out metastatic disease.

Patient Selection

Many patients requiring liver biopsy or cholecystocentesis are debilitated and metabolically compromised as a result of hepatobiliary dysfunction, resulting in coagulopathies and even development of ascites. Laparoscopy represents the ideal technique for liver biopsy in these patients because it is a minimally invasive and relatively quick procedure that reduces hemorrhage potential compared with open celiotomy. In addition, coagulation can be confirmed at biopsy sites, and this method provides samples from multiple lobes of suitable quality for histopathologic evaluation.[2,6,8,9] Contraindications for LLB and LC are few. Liver biopsy is contraindicated in patients with thrombocytopenia (<80,000 platelets/mL) or marked prolongation of coagulation times because the risk for hemorrhage after biopsy is increased.[5] However, in most patients undergoing LLB, clinical bleeding is rarely seen even in the face of abnormalities in coagulation testing.[8,9] It has previously been shown that hemorrhage from liver biopsy is not correlated with coagulation times.[3] If concerns are present, LLB can be performed with a technique thought to result in minimal hemorrhage (bipolar or ultrasonic vessel-sealing device, or pretied or extracorporeally tied loop ligature).[6,36]

Ascites can form in patients with severe hepatic dysfunction and portal hypertension and does not constitute an absolute contraindication for LLB. In the author's opinion, laparoscopy represents the ideal method for liver biopsy in patients with ascites because these patients are often debilitated and coagulopathic; a method of rapidly obtaining a liver biopsy of diagnostic quality is needed. Removal of ascitic fluid at the time of LLB is not recommended or required. Albumin diffuses into the peritoneal space in patients with ascites, and abrupt removal of this fluid will result in exacerbation of hypoalbuminemia and rapid reaccumulation of ascites.[3] Many of the contraindications for LLB are also present for LC. In addition, LC will be unsuccessful in improving bile flow in cases of gallbladder mucocele because the thick, sludge consistency of bile will prevent it from being aspirated through a small-gauge needle. Caution should be exercised when considering LC for EHBO. In cases of confirmed gallbladder mucocele, the surgeon should consider definitive therapy (laparoscopic or open cholecystectomy).

Patient Preparation

Preparation for Surgery

Dogs or cats undergoing LLB or LC should have a wide clip of the abdomen beginning approximately 5 cm cranial to the xiphoid process and extended caudally to beyond the prepuce or to the level of the vulva. The clip should be taken laterally to the dorsal half

to third of the abdominal wall to allow for paramedian port placement. The clipped area is then prepared for surgery using standard aseptic techniques.

Operating Room Setup and Patient Positioning

For LLB or LC, the patient is placed in dorsal recumbency. The surgeon and assistants should stand behind the patient with the endoscopic tower positioned toward the head of the patient (Figure 16-2). Positioning the patient with the head elevated 15 to 30 degrees in relation to the body (reverse Trendelenburg) can be considered to allow for abdominal organs to fall away from the liver caudally, improving visualization of the cranial abdomen. In most instances, this strategy is not required because the hepatobiliary system is readily visualized with patients placed in dorsal recumbency and is not commonly performed by the author.

Portal Position and Creation of Working Space

A two-port technique is most commonly used for LLB and LC, and additional ports may be placed if concurrent procedures are to be performed. The LLB or LC procedure can also be performed using a single-port technique using either an operating laparoscope or a commercially available single-port device (e.g. SILS port; Covidien, Mansfield, MA) in dogs weighing more than 10 kg. For the multiport technique with the patient placed in dorsal recumbency, a modified Hasson technique or Veress needle is used to place a 6-mm subumbilical camera port with either a smooth or threaded cannula. If using an operating laparoscope, a 10-mm cannula is usually placed subumbilically. If a single-port technique is used, depending on the device used, a 25-mm incision is created (for use with the SILS port) through the skin, subcutaneous tissues, and linea alba just caudal to the umbilicus to allow for placement of the single-port device (Figure 16-3). If using the SILS port, the device is inserted into the abdomen with the aid of two Carmalt forceps.[15] Pneumoperitoneum is created with carbon dioxide (CO_2) from a mechanical insufflator to an intraabdominal pressure of 10 to 15 mm Hg in dogs[37] and 8 mm Hg in cats.[38] A 5-mm × 29-cm, 0- or 30-degree laparoscope is inserted, and an initial evaluation of visible abdominal structures is performed. If using the multiport technique, a second 6-mm instrument port is placed midway between the camera port and the xiphoid process. The instrument port can be placed in a variety of locations depending on surgeon preference

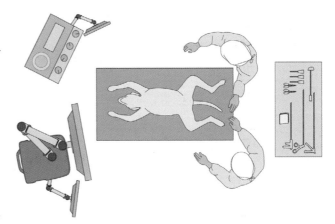

Figure 16-2 Operating room setup, including equipment, surgeon(s), and patient position for performing laparoscopic liver biopsy or laparoscopic cholecystocentesis.

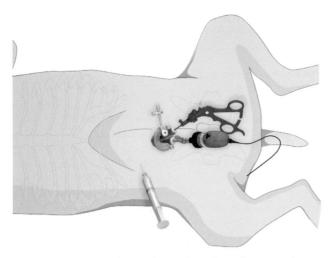

Figure 16-3 Placement of the single-port device for performing single-port liver biopsy or cholecystocentesis. The cholecystocentesis needle can be placed in the right cranial quadrant.

with other common locations being in the right or left paramedian region of the cranial abdomen (Figure 16-4).

Surgical Technique

Instrumentation for Laparoscopic Liver Biopsy and Laparoscopic Cholecystocentesis

A 5-mm, blunt palpation probe and a cup or punch biopsy forceps are all that is required to perform LLB. Other methods of harvesting an LLB include an ultrasonic vessel-sealing device (Harmonic scalpel; Ethicon Endosurgery, Cincinnati, OH)[6]; bipolar vessel-sealing device (Ligasure, Covidien); and a pretied (Endoloop, Ethicon Endosurgery) or extracorporeally tied loop ligature of monofilament, absorbable suture material.[36] The method selected for LLB is performed based on surgeon's preference, location of liver tissue to be biopsied, and concern for hemorrhage. Some surgeons prefer to use precut pieces of hemostatic gelatin sponge (Vetspon; Novartis Animal Health Inc., Greensboro, NC), which can be grasped

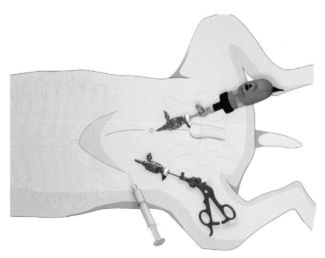

Figure 16-4 Location for placement of two 6-mm ports for performing multiport liver biopsy or cholecystocentesis. The cholecystocentesis needle can be placed in the right cranial quadrant.

by laparoscopic forceps and placed at the biopsy site to promote hemostasis. In addition to the laparoscopic instruments described for performing LLB, laparoscopic atraumatic grasping forceps; a 20- to 22-gauge, 3- to 6-inch spinal needle; and a 12-cc syringe are required for performing LC.

Procedure

After introduction of a blunt palpation probe into the abdomen under laparoscopic guidance, brief exploration of visible abdominal structures is performed. The hepatobiliary system is then evaluated in a systematic fashion to ensure both diaphragmatic (ventral) and visceral surfaces of all liver lobes, gallbladder, and common bile duct are visualized. The diaphragmatic (ventral) surfaces of the liver lobes are more readily apparent with the patient positioned in dorsal recumbency with lesions present on the visceral surfaces being more challenging to visualize. Subjective assessment of liver size and gross appearance can be made. The blunt probe is used to elevate and manipulate each liver lobe, which are inspected for pathology to identify locations for LLB (Figure 16-5). Care must be taken when using the blunt probe to manipulate liver lobes so as not to perforate the surface; the shaft of the probe is used for lobe elevation. The gallbladder is visualized, palpated, and elevated to reveal the common bile duct, which is subjectively evaluated for distention and pathology (Figure 16-6). When focal lesions are to be evaluated for surgical resectability or LLB, preoperative diagnostic imaging is essential to guide the surgeons as lesions may not be readily visible during laparoscopic examination. Tilting the patient into either left or right lateral recumbency may allow for improved visualization of laterally based liver lobes.

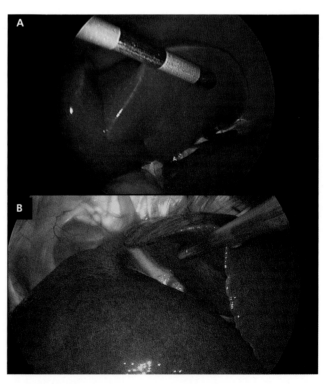

Figure 16-5 Laparoscopic view of left medial lobe elevation using a blunt probe to evaluate its visceral surface (**A**). The left lateral liver lobe and its hilus is also visible; the axial aspect of the left medial lobe is inspected (**B**). (Courtesy of Dr. Jeffrey J. Runge.)

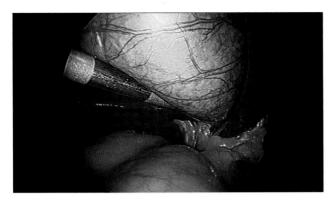

Figure 16-6 The gallbladder is elevated using a blunt probe in this laparoscopic image to allow for evaluation of the common bile duct.

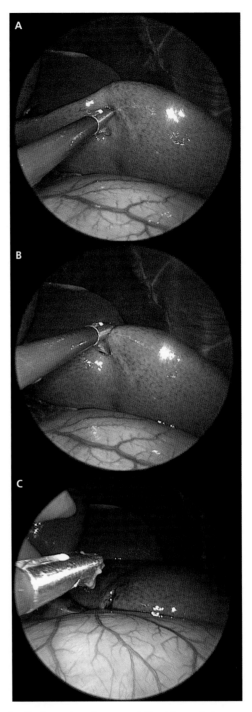

Figure 16-7 For harvesting a laparoscopic liver biopsy, the laparoscopic cup biopsy forceps are first placed under the edge of a liver lobe (**A**). The forceps are opened and allowed to slip forward to the margin of the lobe so that the liver falls into the open jaws of the biopsy forceps (**B**). The biopsy is then harvested by closing the jaws and twisting and pulling the forceps away from the liver (**C**). (Courtesy of Dr. Philipp D. Mayhew.)

When a diffuse hepatopathy is present and multiple LLBs are performed, sampling of the distal edge of multiple lobes is recommended.[8] Cup or punch biopsy forceps are passed into the abdomen under laparoscopic guidance and are inserted below the liver lobe to be biopsied in a closed configuration. The forceps are then opened and gently withdrawn, allowing the edge of the lobe to fall into the jaws of the forceps, which are then closed (Figure 16-7). The forceps are held closed for about 30 seconds to promote hemostasis and then twisted and gently pulled from the surrounding tissue. The blunt palpation probe is then immediately passed into the abdomen under laparoscopic guidance and pressed into the biopsy site to promote hemostasis (Figure 16-8) (Video Clips 16-1 and 16-2). Depending on the extent of fibrotic parenchymal changes, the surgeon may need additional force to retrieve the biopsy specimen in advanced disease.

For hepatic lesions or masses not located at the periphery of the liver lobe, the cup or punch biopsy forceps are opened and gently pushed into the desired area for biopsy and closed ensuring tissue harvest. The jaws are closed, held for approximately 30 seconds, and then twisted and gently pulled from the surrounding tissue. The blunt palpation probe is then passed into the abdomen and gently pressed into the biopsy site to promote hemostasis (Video Clip 16-3). Some surgeons place precut pieces of hemostatic gelatin sponge (Gelfoam), which can be grasped by laparoscopic forceps and placed at the biopsy site to promote hemostasis (Video Clip 16-4). The surgeon must exhibit extreme caution when performing LLB of large focal masses because the potential for brisk hemorrhage exists. As with any laparoscopic procedure, the surgeon must always be prepared for conversion to open celiotomy, if necessary.

If a single-port technique is performed for LLB, the blunt palpation probe, biopsy forceps, and laparoscope are inserted into the single-port device concurrently. An LLB is obtained using the technique described earlier, and the blunt palpation probe is immediately pressed into the biopsy site (Video Clip 16-5).

If the surgeon is concerned about hemorrhage at the biopsy site, a vessel-sealing device or ultrasonic-activated scalpel can be used to obtain the LLB from the distal tip of a lobe. Alternatively, a pretied or extracorporeally tied loop ligature can be used to minimize hemorrhage. A second 6-mm instrument portal is required for this method (if a multiport technique is performed) and can be placed using standard techniques under laparoscopic guidance. The pretied or extracorporeally tied loop ligature is passed into the abdomen through one of the instrument ports.

Laparoscopic Kelly forceps are then passed into the abdomen from the second instrument port and passed through the loop and opened to grasp liver tissue at the tip of the lobe to be biopsied. Sufficient tissue (~0.5 cm) should be grasped to provide a sufficient LLB. The knot from the pretied or extracorporeally tied loop is then advanced with a knot pusher and secured proximal to the

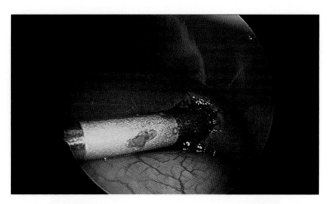

Figure 16-8 A blunt probe is placed at the site of laparoscopic liver biopsy to promote hemostasis.

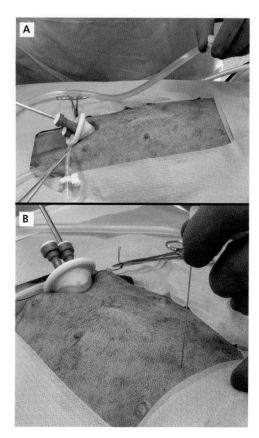

Figure 16-9 **A** and **B,** A SILS port has been placed for laparoscopic liver biopsy and cholecystocentesis in a dog. A spinal needle has been placed caudal to the xiphoid process for percutaneous entry into the peritoneal space.

laparoscopic Kelly forceps, which are removed after knot placement. Laparoscopic Metzenbaum scissors are used to incise the hepatic tissue distal to the knot with care to not inadvertently traumatize the knot. Laparoscopic Kelly forceps are reintroduced with laparoscopic guidance to carefully retrieve the biopsy sample.

As discussed previously, ascites is not an absolute contraindication for performing LLB. Minimizing fluid loss is essential in preventing exacerbation of hypoalbuminemia and subsequent ascites development. Depending on the amount of ascitic fluid present, sufficient working space may be present for performing LLB, or low-level CO_2 insufflation only may be needed. Biopsies are obtained using previously described techniques (Video clip 16-6). After completion of LLB, the surgeon must ensure proper closure of all portal sites to prevent ascitic fluid extravasation into the subcutaneous tissues.

Laparoscopic cholecystocentesis is most commonly performed using a two-port technique. A blunt palpation probe is passed into the abdomen under laparoscopic guidance and used to manipulate the gallbladder and associated quadrate lobe to approximately midcranial abdomen, if not already present in that location. A spinal needle is selected depending on size of the patient. The author commonly uses a 22-gauge spinal needle in small dogs and cats and a 20-gauge needle in large dogs. The length of needle selected should ensure that the gallbladder can be accessed. The needle is inserted caudal to the diaphragm (Figure 16-9) and advanced at such an angle to enter the gallbladder (Figure 16-10) or first enter the quadrate lobe and then the gallbladder. The blunt palpation probe can be maintained intracorporeally and is used to provide counterpressure on the gallbladder during needle puncture; alternatively, an atraumatic grasping forceps can be used to stabilize the gallbladder during LC (see Figure 16-10) (Video Clip 16-7). The inner stylet is removed, and a 12-cc syringe is fixed to the needle hub and bile aspirated. Puncture into the quadrate lobe of the liver before gallbladder puncture is recommended by some surgeons to prevent bile leak into the peritoneum. Direct gallbladder puncture can also be performed and has not been associated with clinically significant bile leak.[19] Its has also been suggested to remove as much bile as possible when performing cholecystocentesis to minimize the chances of bile leak by reducing intracholecystic pressure.[19]

After the surgeon has verified clot formation on all biopsy sites, and no leak from the gallbladder if LC has been performed, the instruments, laparoscope, and cannulae are withdrawn from the abdomen, ensuring maximal removal of intracorporeal CO_2. Local

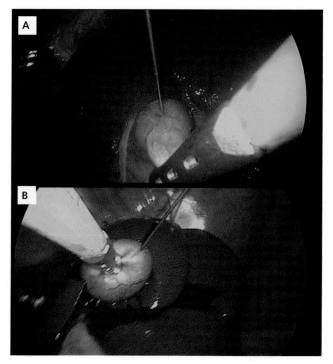

Figure 16-10 **A** and **B,** Laparoscopic image of spinal needle entry into gallbladder for cholecystocentesis. Atraumatic grasping forceps have been used to stabilize the gallbladder. (Courtesy of Dr. Jeffrey J. Runge.)

anesthesia is infiltrated into the fascia or muscle at the port sites, which are then closed in a routine fashion.

Complications

In a recent retrospective study in dogs undergoing LLB in addition to other procedures, complications, defined as conversion to open laparotomy or anemia requiring blood transfusion, were identified in 6 of 80 (7.5%) dogs.[8] Three dogs required conversion to laparotomy, and three required blood transfusion; however, all of these dogs were noted to be anemic before surgery.[8] Seventy-six of 80 (95%) of dogs survived until discharged with a median hospitalization time of 1 day (range, 1–5 days).[8] A platelet count of less than 150,000 platelets/mL was found to be significantly associated with complications in this study.[8] In another study evaluating dogs undergoing LLB as the sole diagnostic procedure, only 2 of 109 (1.9%) dogs had complications, which were converted to open laparotomy as a result of splenic laceration.[9] Despite a large number of dogs having coagulopathy, thrombocytopenia, and even ascites, because of hepatobiliary dysfunction, results of clinical studies indicate that LLB is a safe procedure with an extremely low complication rate.

Complications associated with LC have not been evaluated in the veterinary literature. The surgeon must ensure penetration of the needle into the peritoneal cavity caudal to the insertion of the diaphragm to prevent iatrogenic pneumothorax. Bile leak into the peritoneal space from the cholecystocentesis site can be minimized by first entering the quadrate lobe of the liver before gallbladder puncture or removing as much bile as possible, thereby reducing intracholecystic pressure. However, direct gallbladder puncture has not been shown to result in clinically significant bile leak into the peritoneal cavity.[3,19]

Postoperative Care

The majority of dogs and cats undergoing LLB and LC have a rapid return to preoperative status because these are generally quick procedures associated with short general anesthesia times. In addition to the port site local analgesic block, systemic analgesia commonly administered to these patients includes tramadol hydrochloride 2 to 4 mg/kg orally every 8 hours[39] and/or buprenorphine 0.01 mg/kg IV or intramuscularly every 6 hours in cats[40] or dogs.[41] Nonsteroidal antiinflammatory drugs are avoided by the author in patients undergoing LLB or LC because of hepatic dysfunction and subsequent altered drug metabolism possibly being present.

Patients undergoing LLB or LC that are considered stable preoperatively are commonly discharged the same day of the procedure at the author's institution. Some patients require additional supportive care as a result of ongoing hepatobiliary disease and are hospitalized until their condition stabilizes.

Instructions must be provided to owners to monitor for evidence of port site infection, which include inflammation, redness, swelling, pain upon palpation, and discharge. Recently, it was shown that incidence of surgical site infections may be reduced with the use of minimally invasive surgical techniques compared with their open counterparts.[42]

 All videos cited in this chapter can be found on the book's companion website at **www.wiley.com/go/fransson/ laparoscopy**

References

1 Rawlings, C.A., Howerth, E.W. (2004) Obtaining quality biopsies of the liver and kidney. J Am Vet Med Assoc 40, 353-358.

2 Vasanjee, S.C., Bubenik, L.J., Hosgood, G., et al. (2006) Evaluation of hemorrhage, sample size, and collateral damage for five hepatic biopsy methods in dogs. Vet Surg 35, 86-93.

3 Rothuizen, J., Twedt, D.C. (2009) Liver biopsy techniques. Vet Clin North Am Small Anim Pract 39, 469-480.

4 Mayhew, P.D., Weisse, C. (2012) Liver and biliary system. In: Tobias, K.M, Johnston, S.A. (eds.) Veterinary Surgery: Small Animal. Elsevier Saunders, St. Louis, pp. 1601-1623.

5 Bigge, L.A., Brown, D.J., Penninck, D.G. (2001) Correlation between coagulation profile findings and bleeding complications after ultrasound-guided biopsies: 433 cases (1993-1996). J Am Anim Hosp Assoc 37, 228-233.

6 Barnes, R.F., Greenfield, C.L., Schaeffer, D.J., et al. (2006) Comparison of biopsy samples obtained using standard endoscopic instruments and the harmonic scalpel during laparoscopic and laparoscopic assisted surgery in normal dogs. Vet Surg 35, 243-251.

7 Mayhew, P.D. (2009) Techniques for laparoscopic and laparoscopic-assisted biopsy of abdominal organs. Compend Contin Educ Pract Vet 31, 170-176.

8 Petre, S.L., McClaran, J.K., Bergman, P.J., et al. (2012) Safety and efficacy of laparoscopic hepatic biopsy in dogs: 80 cases (2004-2009). J Am Vet Med Assoc 240, 181-185.

9 McDevitt, H., Brown, D.C., Giuffrida, M., et al. (2014) Complications and conversion rates associated with laparoscopic liver biopsies in dogs: 106 cases (2005-2013) Proceedings of the ACVS Symposium, San Diego.

10 Kavanagh, C., Shaw, S., Webster, C.R.L. (2011) Coagulation in hepatobiliary disease. J Vet Emerg Crit Care 21, 589-604.

11 Devitt, C.M., Cox, R.E., Hailey, J.J. (2005) Duration, complications, stress, and pain of open ovariohysterectomy versus a simple method of laparoscopic-assisted ovariohysterectomy in dogs. J Am Vet Med Assoc 227, 921-927.

12 Hancock, R., Lanz, O.I., Waldron, D.R., et al. (2005) Comparison of postoperative pain after ovariohysterectomy by harmonic scalpel-assisted laparoscopy compared with median celiotomy and ligation in dogs. Vet Surg 34, 273-282.

13 Culp, W.T., Mayhew, P.D., Brown, D.C. (2009) The effect of laparoscopic versus open ovariectomy on postsurgical activity in small dogs. Vet Surg 38, 811-817.

14 Gower, S.B., Mayhew, P.D. (2011) A wound retraction device for laparoscopic-assisted intestinal surgery in dogs and cats. Vet Surg 40, 485-488.

15 Case, J.B., Ellison, G. (2013) Single incision laparoscopic-assisted intestinal surgery (SILAIS) in 7 dogs and 1 cat. Vet Surg 42, 629-634.

16 Cole, T.L., Center, S.A., Flood, S.N., et al. (2002) Diagnostic comparison of needle and wedge biopsy specimens of the liver in dogs and cats. J Am Vet Med Assoc 220, 1483-1489.

17 Bravo, A.A., Sheth, S.C., Chopra, S. (2001) Liver biopsy. N Engl J Med 344, 495-500.

18 Savary-Bataille, K.C.M., Bunch, S.E., Spaulding, K.A., et al. (2003) Percutaneous ultrasound guided cholecystocentesis in healthy cats. J Vet Intern Med 17, 298-303.

19 Robertson, E., Twedt, D. Webb, C. (2014) Diagnostic laparoscopy in the cat: rationale and equipment. J Feline Med Surg 16, 5-16.

20 Day, D.G. (1995) Feline cholangiohepatitis complex. Vet Clin North Am Small Anim Pract 25, 375-385.

21 Wagner, K.A., Hartmann, F.A., Trepanier, L.A. (2007) Bacterial culture results from liver, gall bladder, or bile in 248 dogs and cats evaluated for hepatobiliary disease: 1998-2003. J Vet Int Med 21, 417-424.

22 Voros, K., Sterczer, A., Manczur, F., et al. (2002) Percutaneous ultrasound-guided cholecystocentesis in dogs. Acta Vet Hung 50, 385-393.

23 Herman, B.A., Brawer, R.S., Murtaugh, R.J., et al. (2005) Therapeutic percutaneous ultrasound-guided cholecystocentesis in three dogs with extrahepatic biliary obstruction and pancreatitis. J Am Vet Med Assoc 227, 1782-1786.

24 Mayhew, P.D., Holt, D.E., McLear, R.C., et al. (2002) Pathogenesis and outcome of extrahepatic biliary obstruction in cats. J Small Anim Pract 43, 247-253.

25 Mehler, S.J., Mayhew, P.D., Drobatz, K.J., et al. (2004) Variables associated with outcome in dogs undergoing extrahepatic biliary surgery: 60 cases (1988-2002). Vet Surg 33, 644-649.

26 Minter, R.M., Fan, M.H., Sun, J., et al. (2005) Altered Kupffer cell function in biliary obstruction. J Surg 138, 236-245.

27 Amsellem, P.M., Seim, H.B. 3rd, MacPhail, C.M., et al. (2006) Long-term survival and risk factors associated with biliary surgery in dogs: 34 cases (1994-2004). J Am Vet Med Assoc 229, 1451-1457.

28 Buote, N.J., Mitchell, S.L., Penninck, D., et al. (2006) Cholecystoenterostomy for treatment of extrahepatic biliary tract obstruction in cats: 22 cases (1994-2003). J Am Vet Med Assoc 228, 1376-1382.

29 Lehner, C., McAnulty, J. (2010) Management of extrahepatic biliary obstruction: a role for temporary percutaneous biliary drainage. Compend Contin Educ Vet 32, E1.

30 Murphy, S.M., Rodriguez, J.D., McAnulty, J.F. (2007) Minimally invasive cholecystostomy in the dog: evaluation of placement techniques and use in extrahepatic biliary obstruction. Vet Surg 36, 675-683.

31 Qiu, Y.D., Bai, J.L., Xu, F.G., et al. (2011) Effect of preoperative biliary drainage on malignant obstructive jaundice: a meta-analysis. World J Gastroenterol 17, 391-396.

32 Fang, Y., Gurusamy, K.S., Wang, Q., et al. (2012) Pre-operative biliary drainage for obstructive jaundice. Cochrane Database Syst Rev 9, CDOO5444.

33 Sun, J., Liu, G., Yuan, Y., et al. (2013) Operable severe obstructive jaundice: how should we use pre-operative biliary drainage? S Afr J Surg 51, 127-130.

34 Bacon, N.J., White, R.A.S. (2003) Extrahepatic biliary tract surgery in the cat: a case series and review. J Small Anim Pract 44, 231-235.

35 Evans, H.E. (1993) The digestive apparatus and abdomen. In: Evans, H.E. (ed.) Miller's Anatomy of the Dog, 3rd edn. Saunders, Philadelphia, pp. 385-463.

36 Cuddy, L.C., Risselada, M., Ellison, G.W. (2013) Clinical evaluation of a pre-tied ligating loop for liver biopsy and liver lobectomy. J Small Anim Pract 54, 61-66.

37 Duke, T., Steinacher, S.L., Remedios, A.M. (1996) Cardiopulmonary effects of using carbon dioxide for laparoscopic surgery in dogs. Vet Surg 25, 77-82.

38 Mayhew, P.D., Pascoe, P.J., Kass, P.H., et al. (2013) Effects of pneumoperitoneum induced at various pressures on cardiorespiratory function and working space during laparoscopy in cats. Am J Vet Res 74, 1340-1346.

39 Kukanich, B. (2013) Outpatient oral analgesics in dogs and cats beyond nonsteroidal anti-inflammatory drugs: an evidence-based approach. Vet Clin North Am Small Anim Pract 43, 1109-1125.

40 Giordano, T., Steagall, P.V., Ferreira, T.H., et al. (2010) Postoperative analgesic effects of intravenous, intramuscular, subcutaneous or oral transmucosal buprenorphine administered to cats undergoing ovariohysterectomy. Vet Anaesth Analg 37, 357-366.

41 Linton, D.D., Wilson, M.G., Newbound, G.C., et al. (2012) The effectiveness of a long-acting transdermal fentanyl solution compared to buprenorphine for the control of postoperative pain in dogs in a randomized, multicentered clinical study. J Vet Pharmacol Ther 35, 53-64.

42 Mayhew, P.D., Freeman, L., Kwan, T., et al. (2012) Comparison of surgical site infection rates in clean and clean-contaminated wounds in dogs and cats after minimally invasive versus open surgery: 179 cases (2007-2008). J Am Vet Med Assoc 240, 193-198.

17 Laparoscopic Cholecystectomy

Philipp D. Mayhew and Ameet Singh

Key Points

- Laparoscopic cholecystectomy (LC) is an advanced laparoscopic procedure that requires experience and the correct instrumentation to be performed successfully.
- Careful case selection is paramount to success with this procedure.
- Uncomplicated gallbladder mucocele with no evidence of extrahepatic bile duct obstruction or discontinuity of the biliary tree is the most common indication for LC in dogs.
- LC can be performed using a multiport or single-port approach in dogs.

Laparoscopic cholecystectomy (LC) was first introduced into the armamentarium of human hepatobiliary surgeons by the German surgeon Erich Muhe in 1985. The procedure is widely credited with giving rise to the modern era of minimally invasive surgery in the human field and became widespread very quickly as general surgeons rapidly adopted the technique. In North America, the laparoscopic approach is currently used for approximately 90% of cholecystectomy procedures performed. The principal indications for the procedure in humans are for gallstone-related disease. Humans with symptomatic gallstones generally have straightforward indications for LC. Currently, there are very few indications in humans for open cholecystectomy (OC) with only suspected gallbladder neoplasia and some less common complex choledochal defects remaining as indications for an open approach.[1] Intraoperative complications in LC requiring conversion remain as an occasional cause of OC in humans with large meta-analyses of LC demonstrating conversion rates around 2% to 10%[2-5]

One of the major contributing factors for the rapid acceptance and paradigm shift toward LC for the treatment of gallbladder disease was that significant improvements in outcomes have been documented. A large meta-analysis of 38 trials concluded that LC is associated with shorter hospital stays and diminished convalescence compared with OC for symptomatic cholelithiasis.[6] There has, however, been controversy in the human literature with regard to whether complications rates associated with LC surpass those

seen in OC. During the development of the procedure in the late 1980s and early 1990s, concern for a greater incidence of biliary leaks, principally arising from common duct lacerations, was suspected. However, in more recent years, studies have found that biliary leaks occur in as few as 0.4% to 0.7% of cases, and no difference in complications rates were noted in one large meta-analysis of open and laparoscopic cases.[6,7] It should be remembered, however, that as with most technically challenging procedures, surgical experience and case volume have been shown to affect the outcomes of the procedure in humans with high-volume surgeons achieving superior results to those with lower volumes.[8]

In small animals, surgical disease of the extrahepatic biliary tract is far less common than in humans primarily because of the uncommon occurrence of gallstone-related disease and primary gallbladder neoplasia. Therefore, few case reports exist discussing LC for management of clinical feline or canine patients with gallbladder disease.[9] In many small animal patients with primary disease of the gallbladder, the presence of bile peritonitis or extrahepatic biliary tract obstruction (EHBO) likely rules out the ability to perform LC at this point in time. Therefore, of the range of pathologies seen in small animal patients, uncomplicated gallbladder mucoceles (GBMs), and patients with symptomatic cholelithiasis without choledochal stones may be good indications for LC.[9] In the overall population of dogs, the prognosis for successful surgical treatment of GBM is fair but associated with perioperative mortality rates of

---

Small Animal Laparoscopy and Thoracoscopy, First Edition. Edited by Boel A. Fransson and Philipp D. Mayhew.
© 2015 by ACVS Foundation. Published 2015 by John Wiley & Sons, Inc.
Companion website: www.wiley.com/go/fransson/laparoscopy

22% to 40%.[10–14] This high mortality rate is most likely attributable to the clinical consequences of EHBO and peritonitis in a proportion of cases and the fact that in many cases, these dogs are systemically highly compromised at time of hospital admission. Intra- and persistent postoperative hypotension has been reported in a large proportion of cases undergoing surgery for EHBO, further complicating perioperative outcomes.[15–17] However, in approximately 20% of cases, GBMs are detected as an incidental finding without the presence of obstructive disease or peritonitis present, and these cases may form a cohort of dogs that are amenable to management with LC.[11] It remains controversial whether dogs with GBMs that do not exhibit clinical signs related to the biliary system should undergo cholecystectomy, but this course of therapy does have the advantage of removing the diseased gallbladder at a time when the patient is stable and without the complications of EHBO and peritonitis that may be present at a future time. Recently, medical management of two dogs with GBM appeared to reverse the mucus buildup in the gallbladder of these dogs.[17] However, it is not known at this time which dogs should be candidates for cholecystectomy and which can be treated medically with careful monitoring. Future studies are required to evaluate these potential therapeutic options for this cohort of patients.

Cholelithiasis is uncommon in small animal patients and sometimes an incidental finding. There are currently no reports of management of cholelithiasis using LC, but it is thought that choleliths originate in the gallbladder, so if present and associated with significant morbidity, cholecystectomy may be indicated. However, approximately 50% of dogs with cholelithiasis in one study had choledocholiths with or without calculi in the gallbladder, so the application of LC in this cohort of patients needs to be considered in light of the possibility that choledocholiths could be missed and lead to ongoing or future EHBO.[18]

Preoperative Considerations

Surgical Anatomy

The gallbladder lies within the hepatic fossa that is bordered by the right medial and quadrate lobes of the liver. There is a variably well-adhered attachment of the gallbladder fundus and body to the hepatic parenchyma of these lobes. The neck of the gallbladder tapers to the beginning of the cystic duct. The cystic duct extends from the gallbladder neck to the point at which the first hepatic duct joins. It is just distal to the junction of the first hepatic duct that ligation of the cystic duct takes place during LC. The common bile duct continues toward its insertion into the duodenum at the major duodenal papilla in dogs and cats and receives tributary hepatic ducts that number two to eight in dogs.[19] The blood supply to the gallbladder is through the cystic artery that is a branch of the hepatic artery. The cystic artery lies in close association with the cystic duct, and the two structures are usually ligated together during LC.

Preoperative Diagnostic Evaluation

Candidates for LC should receive a thorough diagnostic evaluation before undergoing the procedure. Comorbidities need to be ruled out, and a thorough evaluation of the pathology of the hepatobiliary tract needs to be obtained. A complete blood count and biochemical evaluation along with a urinalysis should be obtained. Elevations in hepatobiliary enzymes and total bilirubin are commonly found in dogs with gallbladder disease and should be noted. There may be an

association between certain endocrinopathies and GBM formation in dogs with one study demonstrating that 21% of dogs with GBM were diagnosed with concurrent hyperadrenocorticism.[20] Changes associated with hyperadrenocorticism, such as elevations of alkaline phosphatase and cholesterol, present on preoperative blood work in the presence of consistent clinical signs should prompt an endocrinologic evaluation for the condition. Evaluation of coagulation status is also warranted in this patient population despite the incidence of significant coagulopathy being relatively low because significant hemorrhage is possible during dissection.[21]

Diagnostic imaging is an equally important part of the preoperative diagnostic evaluation. Thoracic radiographs are indicated to rule out clinically significant comorbidities in the thorax. Abdominal radiographs are usually nonspecific, although most choleliths in cats and dogs are radiopaque as they are most often composed of calcium bilirubinate (most common in dogs) or calcium carbonate (most common in cats).[18,19] Abdominal ultrasonography is a vital part of the preoperative diagnostic evaluation and can provide critical evaluation of gallbladder wall thickness, size, presence of choleliths, pericholecystic inflammation, and degree to which mucus is filling the lumen in cases with GBM.[22] Ultrasonographic characteristics of GBM have been described and often include enlargement of the gallbladder with a typical immobile stellate or finely striated ultrasonographic appearance ("kiwi" gallbladder).[10] Characteristics of the cystic and common bile ducts such as diameter (normal common bile duct diameter in cats and dogs is ~3–4 mm), discontinuity, and presence or absence of choledocholithiasis or masses involving the area can usually be diagnosed. Changes can be monitored over time with repeated ultrasound examinations providing vital information on whether changes are progressive or static. This is important information because extrahepatic biliary tract distension can remain after an episode of EHBO, so the presence of distension does not always indicate current obstruction.

Patient Selection

Because so few LCs have been reported to date in veterinary patients, case selection has not been thoroughly evaluated and is largely based on anecdote. In dogs with GBM, it is suggested that EHBO is a contraindication for LC at this point in time because of the risk of persistent postoperative EHBO. The thick, sludgy bile that is produced in the gallbladder readily moves down into the common bile duct and hepatic ducts, and in patients with evidence of obstruction, it is recommended that a technique that allows flushing of the bile from the common duct be performed. This is despite a recent study that failed to show a significant difference in outcome in dogs undergoing cholecystectomy for GBM that had common bile duct flushing compared with those that did not.[14] Common bile duct flushing has not been reported to date in conjunction with LC. In general, if the serum total bilirubin is significantly elevated or if there is ultrasonographic evidence of obstruction demonstrated by significant common bile duct or gallbladder enlargement, the authors suggest that an OC be pursued. In the future, if development of endoscopic retrograde cholangiography (ERC) or laparoscopic common bile duct exploration can be perfected in these species, the prospect of performing LC in animals without a patent common bile duct may become an option. ERC has been documented in healthy research animals but not yet in a significant population of clinical patients with EHBO.[23,24]

A further contraindication to LC in patients with gallbladder disease is evidence of bile peritonitis. If discontinuity of the extrahepatic biliary tract is present, thorough evaluation for leakage of bile from one or more sites should be performed, and this may be challenging to do laparoscopically. Additionally, because of the ability of bile salts to contribute to severe chemical peritonitis and the high mortality rate associated with bile peritonitis (especially when bacterial infection is present) in small animal patients, thorough lavage of the entire peritoneal cavity should be performed.[9,25] Despite some reports in humans of laparoscopic treatment of bile peritonitis,[26,27] it is unknown whether lavage can be performed as effectively laparoscopically as it can via a celiotomy approach. Future studies may find that less invasive peritoneal drainage techniques are adequate for management of dogs with bile peritonitis, but at present, data have not been reported in small animal patients.

In dogs and cats with symptomatic or asymptomatic cholelithiasis, LC may potentially be indicated. Again, obstructive disease and the presence of bile peritonitis should be ruled out in these patients before proceeding with LC. The presence of choleliths in the common bile duct is a contraindication for LC given the need to remove the stones by retrograde flushing or choledochotomy. Necrotizing cholecystitis may be an indication for LC, although many of these canine patients present with rupture of the biliary system and bile peritonitis at presentation, so LC should be used with caution in this cohort of patients.[28]

Patient Preparation

Surgical Preparation

In preparation for LC in dogs and cats, a wide clip of the entire abdomen from 5 cm cranial to the xiphoid process to the caudal prepuce or vulva caudally is recommended. Laterally, the patient should be clipped to the dorsal third of the abdominal wall to allow dorsally positioned ports to be placed. The entire area is aseptically scrubbed for surgery.

Operating Room Setup and Patient Positioning

The endoscopic tower is generally positioned at the head of the patient with the anesthesia machine and anesthesia staff located to one side (Figure 17-1). It can be helpful to position the dog or cat close to the end of the surgery table to allow the surgeons to stand behind the patient. This can aid in manipulation of the instruments, which are angled cranially toward the hepatic fossa throughout the procedure. The patient is positioned in dorsal recumbency. Reverse

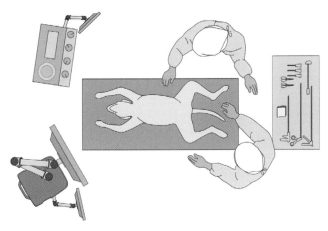

Figure 17-1 Operating room setup for laparoscopic cholecystectomy. The endoscopic tower is positioned at the head of the patient.

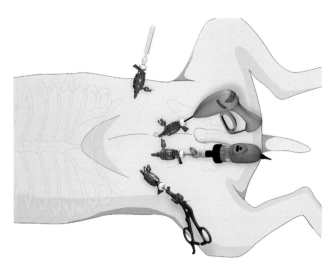

Figure 17-2 Port placement for the four-port approach described. Note the left-sided instrument port that is positioned cranially and dorsally for placement of the fan retractor that will retract the gallbladder cranially during cystic duct dissection.

Trendelenburg (head-up) positioning can be considered to allow the stomach and small intestines to fall caudally away from the liver. However, the authors do not consider this positioning to be mandatory and have generally performed the procedure in a fairly neutral position.

Portal Position and Creation of Working Space

A variety of approaches can be used for LC, including multiport approaches as well as single-port approaches. The multiport technique has been described using a four-port technique.[9] If the multiport technique is performed, the use of threaded cannulae is recommended because the technique involves many instrument exchanges, making cannula withdrawal a common problem if unthreaded cannulae are used. A subumbilical camera port is placed using either a modified Hasson technique or a Veress needle. Pneumoperitoneum is induced using carbon dioxide from a mechanical insufflator. Two further ports are placed in the right cranial quadrant in a triangulating pattern around the anticipated location of the gallbladder (Figure 17-2). A fourth port is then placed just behind the costal arch on the left side at mid-abdominal level. This fourth portal will be used to place a fan retractor to elevate the gallbladder ventrally to allow visualization of the common bile duct. Other types of retractors can also be used if a fan retractor is unavailable. Generally, three of the ports placed are sized to accept 5-mm instrumentation, and one is usually placed to accommodate 10-mm instrumentation to allow 10-mm clip appliers or specimen retrieval devices to be used. After all ports are in position, the telescope can either be retained in the subumbilical port or placed in one of the instrument ports in the right cranial quadrant. This choice is dictated by the quality of the visualization obtained from each port.

When a single-port cholecystectomy is considered, the single-port device is usually placed at the level of the umbilicus (Figure 17-3). Because retraction of the gallbladder can be challenging using only three ports, an additional separate port can be established in the cranial abdominal quadrant for use with a fan retractor as described for the multiport technique. Although this may contravene the strict single-port definition, this can greatly facilitate the procedure. As experience with single port LC increases, it may be possible to dispense with the use of additional ports.

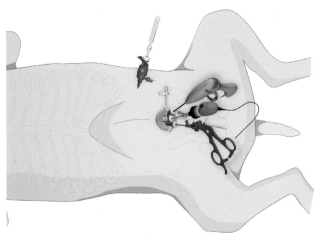

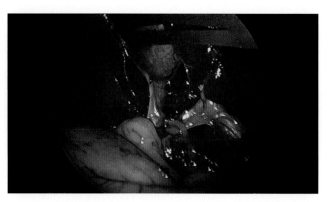

Figure 17-4 The fan retractor can be seen at the top of the image retracting the body of the gallbladder. This allows a clear view of the cystic duct area for ligation.

Figure 17-3 Port placement for single-port cholecystectomy. The single-port device is positioned at the level of the umbilicus.

Surgical Technique

Instrumentation for Laparoscopic Cholecystectomy

As for most laparoscopic interventions laparoscopic Metzenbaum scissors, suture-cutting scissors (hook scissors), Kelly forceps, Babcock forceps, cup or punch biopsy forceps, and a blunt probe are required. Laparoscopic right-angled forceps of both 5- and 10-mm dimensions are helpful for dissection around the cranial aspect of the cystic duct before ligation. Despite 5-mm right-angled forceps being adequate in most cases, it may not be possible to dissect the cranial aspect completely without the use of a 10-mm version in larger animals. A variety of types and sizes of laparoscopic retractor are available, including fan retractors, self-retaining retractors, and inflatable retractors. If intracorporeal suturing of the cystic duct is planned, then laparoscopic needle holders (e.g., Szabo-Berci) will be necessary. If extracorporeally assembled knots will be used, a laparoscopic knot pusher is used. Laparoscopic clip appliers can be used for sealing of the cystic duct in some cases. A bipolar or ultrasonic vessel-sealing device is very helpful for dissection of the gallbladder from the hepatic fossa. Monopolar electrosurgery may also be helpful for fine dissection of tissue planes that are difficult to maneuver the tip of a vessel-sealing device into. A suction and irrigation device is also necessary to aspirate away any accumulations of blood during dissection and to aspirate bile from the gallbladder before exteriorization of the gallbladder. Nondisposable laparoscopic suction devices that incorporate a trumpet valve (Karl Storz Veterinary Endoscopy, Goleta, CA) can be finely regulated and work well for this application. Disposable suction irrigators (e.g., Surgiwand, Covidien, Mansfield, MA) are also very useful for this purpose but can be expensive. Specimen retrieval bags are used in LC to aid in retrieval of the gallbladder after dissection is complete and can be obtained from a variety of medical device companies. When single-port LC is performed the use of a specimen retrieval bag may be unnecessary as the gallbladder can often be retrieved through the single port incision that has been created.

To aid in single-port LC or even for use with the multiport technique, the use of articulating instrumentation is becoming more commonplace. The advantage of these devices lies in their ability to create different trajectories into dissection planes that can be very helpful during advanced laparoscopic procedures.

Procedure

Initially, a limited exploration of the abdomen is performed with particular attention being paid to the liver, the gallbladder, and the extrahepatic biliary tree. In many cases, the anatomic relationships of the hepatobiliary organs can be normal, but omental adhesions to the gallbladder or gallbladder adhesions to the body wall or diaphragm are common findings in dogs and cats with gallbladder disease and are not always detected on preoperative diagnostic imaging. Diaphragmatic adhesions can sometimes be gently dissected with a blunt probe or endopeanut (Video Clip 17-1). Omental adhesions can be more challenging because they may obscure visualization of the common bile duct and cystic duct. If adhesions to the more apical portions of the gallbladder only are present, it may be possible to section these adhesions with the vessel-sealing device and complete the procedure without conversion to an open approach. Another incidental finding that can be present can be the presence of bile pigments in the abdominal cavity or around the gallbladder. Suspicion for biliary tract perforation in these cases should be raised, and consideration should be given to converting these cases to avoid missing a site of bile leakage and to provide thorough lavage of the abdomen.

The technique for LC previously described involves dissection of the gallbladder after dissection, ligation, and sealing of the cystic duct.[9] An alternative is to dissect the gallbladder out of the fossa before sealing the cystic duct. When cystic duct dissection is performed, the retractor is first used to elevate the gallbladder ventrally to expose the cystic duct (Figure 17-4). Right-angled or Kelly forceps are used to dissect a plane cranial to the cystic duct to free the duct for either suture passage or clip application (Figure 17-5, Video Clip 17-2). This dissection is usually associated with some hemorrhage, which is generally self-limiting. The optimal method of cystic duct ligation has not been established and may vary depending on the pathology present in the particular patient. Use of extracorporeally tied sutures has been described but is somewhat laborious and has been associated with extended surgical times.[9] For this technique, right-angled forceps are used to pass a length of 2-0 to 3-0 polydioxanone through the cannula and into position on the duct. A second pair of right-angled forceps is passed around the duct and used to grasp the polydioxanone and bring it around the duct. The suture is then withdrawn through the same cannula that was used to draw it into the abdomen. A laparoscopic slip knot is prepared extracorporeally and passed down the cannula and into position on the duct using a knot pusher. A variety of laparoscopic slip knots have been

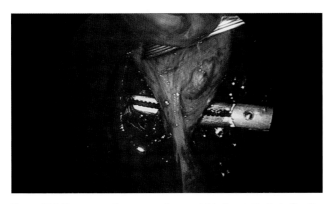

Figure 17-5 Forceps can be seen passing cranial to the cystic duct after dissection of the plane between the cystic duct and the hepatic parenchyma has been completed.

described in the literature, although the 4S modified Roeder knot has been found to be biomechanically superior to others tested.[29] Other options for cystic duct ligation include intracorporeally tied ligatures, application of a variety of types of laparoscopic clips, and the use of vessel-sealing devices for cystic duct closure. Intracorporeal suturing is an acquired skill that requires a learning curve before it can be performed proficiently. It also requires the use of a pair of laparoscopic needle holders to manipulate the suture intracorporeally. However, with practice, this can become an efficient and safe means of cystic duct ligation (Video Clip 17-3). The use of laparoscopic clips is controversial and has not been studied for canine LC in clinical cases. The application of hemoclips is simple and fast, but care needs to be taken that the clip spans the entire width of the cystic duct (Figure 17-6). To bolster clip application, a preformed loop ligature (e.g., Endoloop, Ethicon Endosurgery, Cincinnati, OH), extracorporeally prepared, or intracorporeally tied ligature can be applied on the cystic duct distal to the clips after sectioning and removal of the gallbladder. Particular care is required when some mild duct thickening or distension is present because in these cases, clips may have a higher incidence of failure, resulting in postoperative bile leaks. An additional option for cystic duct closure is the use of self-locking polymer clips (Hem-o-lok; Teleflex Medical, Research Triangle Park, NC). These have been used for LC in clinical canine patients with success (Dr. Ikuya Ehara, personal communication). If these clips are used, it is recommended that two clips are placed on the more proximal aspect of the cystic duct to avoid clip slippage and that one is placed on the gallbladder side to avoid bile spillage (Figure 17-7). Hem-o-lok clips are available in

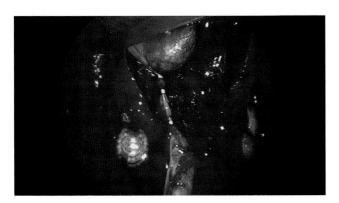

Figure 17-6 Hemostatic clips can be seen in position on the cystic duct before sectioning of the duct.

different sizes, and before application, an estimation of the width of the cystic duct should be made to select the appropriate size. Although not designed to seal nonvascular luminal structures, vessel-sealing devices have been evaluated for sealing of the cystic duct. A recent canine cadaver study compared the use of a vessel-sealant device with large endoclips for sealing grossly normal cystic ducts and found no difference in failure pressure between the two devices.[30] However, in porcine models of acute failure, the seal created with either the LigaSure (Covidien) or Harmonic (Ethicon) scalpel vessel-sealing devices failed at far inferior pressures compared with 10-mm clips, and in the chronic model that evaluated pigs over a 1-week period from the time of application, bile leakage was seen in 25% to 50% of the animals in the week after surgery.[31] Until further testing is performed in clinical patients, we urge caution in using vessel-sealing devices to seal the cystic duct in small animal patients, especially in the face of cystic duct thickening or distension.

Irrespective of which cystic duct ligation technique is used, we suggest that triple ligation of the duct is used with the duct

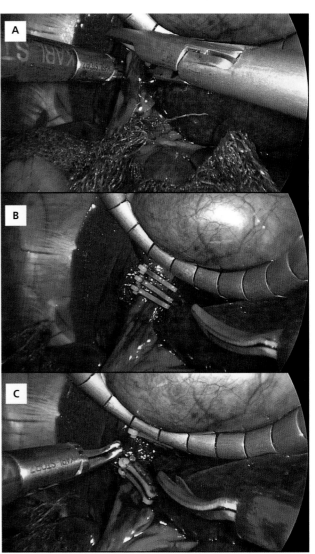

Figure 17-7 The Hem-o-lok applicator can be seen with the clip in position before application (**A**). In total, three clips have been placed on the cystic duct before transection (**B**). The cystic duct has been transected between the two most distal clips (**C**). (Courtesy of Dr Ikuya Ehara.)

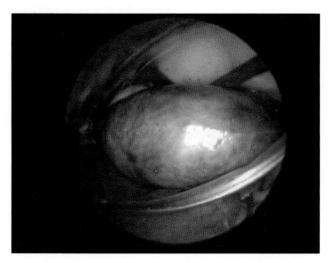

Figure 17-8 The gallbladder can be seen within the specimen retrieval device before exteriorization.

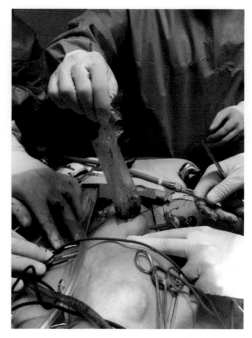

Figure 17-9 The specimen retrieval bag has been partially exteriorized with the gallbladder still within it. Before complete exteriorization, the gallbladder may be suctioned of bile to facilitate its removal without having to enlarge the port incision.

transected between the two most distal seal or ligation sites. After the cystic duct has been transected with laparoscopic scissors (Video Clip 17-4), the dissection of the gallbladder from the fossa can be initiated. To minimize hemorrhage, dissection is preferred with a vessel-sealing device or a combination of vessel-sealing and monopolar electrosurgery. During dissection of the gallbladder, grasping of the gallbladder wall is discouraged because in cases with significant gallbladder disease, extreme friability of the wall can contribute to perforation. If perforation of the gallbladder does occur, sealing of

the perforation can be attempted with laparoscopic clips (Video Clip 17-5). If significant bile leakage occurs, consideration should be given to converting the procedure to an open approach.

After dissection of the gallbladder from the hepatic fossa is complete, exteriorization of the organ is aided by drainage of the bile from within its lumen. This has been described by first inserting a specimen retrieval bag into one of the ports (most of these devices require passage through a 10-mm port). The gallbladder is placed into the specimen retrieval device, which is then closed within the abdomen (Figure 17-8). The cannula is withdrawn from the body wall, and the specimen retrieval bag containing the gallbladder is partially exteriorized through the port incision (Figure 17-9). At this point, a small incision can be made into the gallbladder with the bag partially opened to aspirate the remaining bile from the gallbladder. This allows the gallbladder to collapse down to a point where the remainder of the organ inside the bag can be removed through the 10-mm port incision or a slight enlargement of the

incision if this is deemed necessary (Video Clip 17-6). In this way, spillage or contamination of the surgical site is usually avoided.

After gallbladder removal, the 10-mm port site is closed in routine fashion before reestablishment of the pneumoperitoneum. The area of the hepatic fossa is reevaluated for any evidence of ongoing hemorrhage or biliary leakage. At this point, the surgical site can be liberally lavaged and the fluid reaspirated using a suction and irrigation device. If indicated, a laparoscopic liver biopsy is easily harvested at this point to assess the liver for diffuse hepatopathies that can be present in patients with surgical diseases of the gallbladder. Subsequently, the remaining cannulae are removed after purging of the pneumoperitoneum for the final time, and routine closure of the remaining port incisions can be performed.

Complications and Prognosis

A thorough evaluation of complication rates in small animal LC is not possible at this time given the paucity of literature on the subject. No significant complications were documented in a report of six dogs that was previously published, although two dogs were mentioned in this study in which conversion to an open approach was performed before initiating LC because brown bile staining was seen on tissues within the abdominal cavity, and bile peritonitis was suspected.[9] Iatrogenic perforation of the bile duct or gallbladder is possible during either ligation of the common bile duct or dissection of the gallbladder from the hepatic fossa. If leakage can be controlled and the procedure safely completed, conversion is unnecessary. However, if there is any doubt regarding the integrity of the biliary tract, conversion should be considered to diminish the risk of postoperative bile leakage. Leakage of bile from the cystic duct stump is also possible with LC, and care needs to be taken to ensure secure closure of this structure. Persistence of EHBO should also be considered as a possible postoperative complication in dogs with GBMs or cholelithiasis. Without choledochal lavage in dogs that undergo LC, there should always be awareness that ongoing EHBO from residual mucus or choleliths could be a possibility. Hemorrhage from the hepatic fossa is a possible complication after LC. Care should be taken before termination of the LC procedure to inspect the hepatic fossa to rule out ongoing hemorrhage. Postoperative elevation in liver enzymes after LC was seen in one study in dogs, although a similar change may well occur after OC and may be associated with the inherent hepatic parenchymal dissection that occurs after both open and LC.[9]

Postoperative Care

Patients that have undergone LC are likely to be less painful than those having undergone OC, although this has not been documented in a controlled study in small animals. Despite this, postoperative analgesic management remains critically important. Generally, small animals undergoing LC are administered intravenous doses of opioid drugs (buprenorphine 0.01 mg/kg every 6 hours or oxymorphone 0.05 mg/kg every 4 hours) for 24 to 48 hours postoperatively. Tramadol hydrochloride can also be administered by mouth for 3 to 5 days at 2 to 4 mg/kg every 6 hours in dogs and 4 mg/kg every 12 hours in cats. Cats can also be treated with transmucosal buprenorphine administered at 0.02 mg/kg sublingually every 6 hours for 2 to 4 days. Because hepatopathies and hyperadrenocorticism are common comorbidities in dogs with GBMs, use of nonsteroidal antiinflammatory drugs is best avoided in this patient population.

Careful examination of the port-site incisions is important in the postoperative period. Despite port-site infection being a rare complication in veterinary patients undergoing minimally invasive procedures, port-site infection can occur, and early detection will facilitate treatment.[9] When infection occurs, empirical antibiotic therapy can be initiated with clavulanic acid–potentiated amoxicillin (13.75 mg/kg every 12 hours by mouth for 7 days) until results of bacterial culture and sensitivity are available. Ongoing treatment of ongoing hepatopathies or biliary tract disease may also call for the use of other medications and will be dictated by the patient's specific underlying disease processes.

Ongoing monitoring for evidence of extrahepatic leakage or obstruction is important. It is recommended that a biochemical screen be performed within 48 hours of surgery and again 2 week after surgery to rule out these problems.

 All videos cited in this chapter can be found on the book's companion website at **www.wiley.com/go/fransson/ laparoscopy**

References

1 Visser, B.C., Parks, R.W., Garden, O.J. (2008) Open cholecystectomy in the laparoendoscopic era. Am J Surg 195, 108-114.

2 MacFadyen, B.V. Jr, Vecchio, R., Ricardo, A.E., et al. (1998) Bile duct injury after laparoscopic cholecystectomy. Surg Endosc 12, 315-321.

3 Rosen, M., Brody, F., Ponsky, J. (2002) Predictive factors for conversion of laparoscopic cholecystectomy. Am J Surg 184, 254-258.

4 Livingston, E.H., Rege, R.V. (2004) A nationwide study of conversion from laparoscopic to open cholecystectomy. Am J Surg 188, 205-211.

5 Shamiyeh, A., Danis, J., Wayand, W., et al. (2007) A 14-year analysis of laparoscopic cholecystectomy. Conversion—when and why? Surg Laparosc Endosc Percutan Tech 17, 271-276.

6 Keus, F., de Jong, J.A., Gooszen, H.G., et al. (2006) Laparoscopic versus open cholecystectomy for patients with symptomatic cholecystolithiasis. Cochrane Database Syst Rev 4, CD006231.

7 Adamsen, S., Hansen, O.H., Funch-Jensen, P., et al. (1997) Bile duct injury during laparoscopic cholecystectomy: a prospective nationwide series. J Am Coll Surg 184, 571-578.

8 Csikesz, N.G., Singla, A., Murphy, M.M., et al. (2010) Surgeon volume metrics in laparoscopic cholecystectomy. Dig Dis Sci 55, 2398.

9 Mayhew, P.D., Mehler, S.J., Radhakrishnan, A. (2008) Laparoscopic cholecystectomy of uncomplicated gall bladder mucocele in six dogs. Vet Surg 37, 625-630.

10 Besso, J.G., Wrigley, R.H., Gliatto, J.M., et al. (2000) Ultrasonographic appearance and clinical findings in 14 dogs with gallbladder mucocele. Vet Radiol Ultrasound 41, 261-271.

11 Pike, F.S., Berg, J., King, N.W., et al. (2004) Gall bladder mucocele in dogs: 30 cases (2000-2002) J Am Vet Med Assoc 224, 1615-1622.

12 Worley, D.R., Hottinger, H.A., Lawrence, H.J. (2004) Surgical management of gallbladder mucoceles in dogs: 22 cases (1999-2003). J Am Vet Med Assoc 225, 1418-1422.

13 Aguirre, A.L., Center, S.A., Randolph, J.F., et al. (2007) Gallbladder disease in Shetland Sheepdogs: 38 cases (1995-2005) J Am Vet Med Assoc 231, 79-88.

14 Malek, S., Sinclair, E., Hosgood, G., et al. (2013) Clinical findings and prognostic factors for dogs undergoing cholecystectomy for gall bladder mucocele. Vet Surg 42, 418-426.

15 Mehler, S.J., Mayhew, P.D., Drobatz, K.J., et al. (2004) Variables associated with outcome in dogs undergoing extrahepatic biliary surgery: 60 cases (1988-2002). Vet Surg 33, 644-664.

16 Buote, N.J., Mitchell, S.L., Penninck, D., et al. (2006) Cholecystoenterostomy for treatment of extrahepatic biliary tract obstruction in cats: 22 cases (1994-2003). J Am Vet Med Assoc 228:1376-1382.

17 Walter, R., Dunn, M.E., d'Anjou, M.A., et al. (2008) Nonsurgical resolution of gallbladder mucocele in two dogs. J Am Vet Med Assoc 232, 1688-1693.

18 Kirpensteijn, J., Fingland, R.B., Ulrich, T., et al. (1993) Cholelithiasis in dogs (29 cases (1980-1990). J Am Vet Med Assoc 202, 1137-1142.

19 Evans, H.E. (1993) The digestive apparatus and abdomen. In: Evans, H.E. (ed.) Miller's Anatomy of the Dog, 3rd edn. Saunders, Philadelphia, pp. 385-463.

20 Mesich, M.L., Mayhew, P.D., Paek, M., et al. (2009) Gall bladder mucocele and their association with endocrinopathies in dogs: a retrospective case-control study. J Small Anim Pract 50, 63-65.

21 Eich, C.S., Ludwig, L.L. (2002) The surgical treatment of cholelithiasis in cats: a study of nine cases, J Am Anim Hosp Assoc 38, 290-296.

22 Crews, L.J., Feeney, D.A., Jessen, C.R., et al. (2009) Clinical, ultrasonographic, and laboratory findings associated with gallbladder disease and rupture in dogs: 45 cases (1997-2007). J Am Vet Med Assoc 234, 359-366.

23 Spillmann, T., Happonen, I., Kahkonen, T., et al. (2005) Endoscopic retrograde cholangio-pancreatography in healthy beagles. Vet Radiol Ultrasound 46, 97-104.

24 Berent, A., Weisse, C., Schattner, M., et al. (2015) Initial experience with endoscopic retrograde cholangiography and endoscopic retrograde biliary stenting for treatment of extrahepatic bile duct obstruction in dogs. J Am Vet Med Assoc 246, 436-446.

25 Ludwig, L.L., McLoughlin, M.A., Graves, T.K., et al. (1997) Surgical treatment of bile peritonitis in 24 dogs and 2 cats: a retrospective study (1987-1994). J Am Vet Med Assoc 26, 90-98.

26 Griffen, M., Ochoa, J., Boulanger, B.R. (2000) A minimally invasive approach to bile peritonitis after blunt liver injury. Am Surg 66, 309-331.

27 Franklin, G.A., Richardson, J.D., Brown, A.L., et al. (2007) Prevention of bile peritonitis by laparoscopic evacuation and lavage after non-operative treatment of liver injuries. Am Surg 73, 611-616.

28 Church, E.M., Matthiesen, D.T. (1988) Surgical treatment of 23 dogs with necrotizing cholecystitis, J Am Anim Hosp Assoc 24, 305-310.

29 Shettko, D.L., Frisbie, D.D., Hendrickson, D.A. (2004) A comparison of knot security of commonly used hand-tied laparoscopic slipknots. Vet Surg 33, 521-524.

30 Marvel, S., Monnet, E. (2014) Use of a vessel-sealant device for cystic duct ligation in the dog. Vet Surg 43, 983-987.

31 Hope, W.W., Padma, S., Newcomb, W.L. (2010) An evaluation of electrosurgical vessel-sealing devices in biliary tract surgery in a porcine model. HPB (Oxford) 12, 703-708.

18 Laparoscopic Adrenalectomy

Philipp D. Mayhew and Jolle Kirpensteijn

> **Key Points**
>
> - Laparoscopic adrenalectomy (LA) can be performed in cats and dogs for both left- and right-sided tumors.
> - Noninvasive modestly sized adrenal tumors are usually very amenable to resection using a laparoscopic approach.
> - Although associated with a low level of morbidity and conversion to open surgery in experienced hands, LA is a challenging procedure and should only be attempted by surgeons with considerable experience in open adrenalectomy and laparoscopic surgery.

Among advanced laparoscopic procedures in human medicine, laparoscopic adrenalectomy (LA) has become a standard of care procedure for resection of most primary adrenal tumors. There is now gathering evidence that LA may represent a very reasonable option for resection of noninvasive adrenal tumors in small animal patients.

The first description of LA in humans emerged in 1992 at which time it was suggested that LA may help to decrease postsurgical pain and morbidity compared with open adrenalectomy (OA).[1] Since that time, widespread adoption of LA has occurred, and progressively, the indications for the laparoscopic approach have widened. Initial recommendations for treatment of smaller lesions have now been revised to include larger masses as experience with the technique has increased. Although the laparoscopic management of benign adrenal neoplasia is generally accepted, laparoscopic management of adrenocortical carcinoma (ACC) remains highly controversial in humans. Care needs to be taken in extrapolating information from humans to veterinary species; however, ACC is a highly malignant neoplasm in humans, with nodal and distant metastases present in 26.5% and 21.6%, respectively, at the time of diagnosis.[2] In dogs, ACC is a less malignant tumor with distant metastasis reported to occur in only 5% to 14% of cases[3-5] and histopathologic differentiation between these lesions not always clearly defined. In humans, some studies suggest equal results between LA and OA after resection of ACC, but others have found that recurrence and disease-free interval are inferior to results obtained with OA.[6-8] Initial concerns regarding the use of LA for human pheochromocytoma resection

included the hypothesis that increased hemodynamic instability might be associated with laparoscopic manipulation of the tumor.[9] These concerns, however, appear to have been disproven and even superseded in favor of the many other advantages that LA has afforded the patient.[10,11]

Although a four-port approach had been initially described as the standard procedure for LA in humans, an evolution is taking place with regard to minimally invasive surgical approaches. Both retroperitoneal and transperitoneal surgical approaches have been described. A retroperitoneal approach involves the distension of a balloon device within the retroperitoneal space to create a working space adjacent to the adrenal mass. This is followed by the establishment of a pneumoretroperitoneum. Three to four ports are placed to complete the dissection. Recent reports document significant advantages to the retroperitoneal approach over the transperitoneal approach in terms of blood loss and hospital stay,[12] but other reports have not been able to confirm these advantages.[13] It appears that the choice between retroperitoneal approaches and transperitoneal approaches is largely surgeon preference in human medicine, and even in very large meta-analyses of outcomes, it has proved difficult to discern whether one technique has an advantage over the other.[12,13] There are currently no published descriptions of the laparoscopic retroperitoneal approach to the adrenal gland in small animals. However, in the authors' experience, the retroperitoneal approach can be performed in dogs, and further evaluation of this approach in small animals is warranted in the future.

Small Animal Laparoscopy and Thoracoscopy, First Edition. Edited by Boel A. Fransson and Philipp D. Mayhew.
© 2015 by ACVS Foundation. Published 2015 by John Wiley & Sons, Inc.
Companion website: www.wiley.com/go/fransson/laparoscopy

The advance of single-port or reduced port surgery in human surgery has continued unabated over the past 5 years, and single-port LA has now also been described in humans in multiple reports.[14] In one meta-analysis of the outcomes of nine studies comparing single-port adrenalectomy with traditional LA, the single-port group had lower postoperative visual analog scale pain scores but increased surgical time.[14] Other important variables such as blood loss, conversion rate, and complication rates were no different between groups. Single-port surgery in small animals has been gaining popularity recently for a variety of procedures, although descriptions of its use for adrenalectomy have yet to be published.

With just over 20 years of experience of LA in the human literature, there is now a large body of data allowing comparison of LA with OA. The literature regarding benign disease is quite categorical in its endorsement of the laparoscopic approach over OA. Significant advantages of LA have been documented in multiple human studies and include decreases in postoperative pneumonia, sepsis, renal insufficiency, wound infection, cardiac arrest, hospital stay, intensive care unit admission rate, and cost.[15,16]

Adrenal incidentaloma presents an interesting diagnostic and therapeutic conundrum in humans and increasingly in veterinary patients. In human medicine, a National Institutes of Health (NIH) consensus statement on adrenal incidentaloma suggests that all incidentally discovered adrenal masses should have an endocrinologic evaluation for functionality. It further states that all functional tumors and those larger than 4 to 6 cm in diameter should most likely undergo surgical resection.[17] The incidence and nature of adrenal incidentaloma in small animal patients are largely unknown at this time, so similar statements cannot be made in relation to optimal management of these lesions.

Adrenalectomy in dogs, cats, and ferrets is indicated principally for the removal of primary adrenal neoplasms, most commonly adrenocortical adenomas, adenocarcinomas, and pheochromocytomas. Occasionally, other pathologies seen in dogs include embryonal cyst remnants, metastatic lesions, and adrenal abscesses. In cats, functional adrenocortical tumors are most commonly aldosterone or progesterone secreting with pheochromocytomas described very rarely. Adrenalectomy is often performed in pet ferrets, in which a high incidence of adrenal neoplasia occurs, although a laparoscopic approach for adrenalectomy has not been reported in this species to date. Recently, the first reports of LA in dogs and cats have been published with promising results. The first report documented the results of seven dogs that were all cushingoid and diagnosed with ACCs.[18] This study demonstrated that both left- and right-sided adrenal masses were resectable with all procedures completed uneventfully and without conversion to an open approach. The principal intraoperative complication seen was capsular rupture, which occurred in some early cases, prompting the authors to prophylactically suction the necrotic centers from these dogs after creation of a capsular window in the mass. Despite two dogs dying in the postoperative period, this study demonstrated the feasibility of the LA procedure in canine patients with naturally occurring adrenal neoplasia.[18] A second study documenting nine dogs with adrenal neoplasia also demonstrated very good success of the technique without the need for conversion to an open approach and with few intraoperative complications.[19] A single feline case report has been published of a patient with an aldosterone-secreting tumor, which was successfully resected laparoscopically and lived over 4 years postoperatively.[20] Recently, a comparative study of 48 dogs with noninvasive adrenocortical lesions, of which 23 underwent

LA and 25 underwent OA, was reported.[21] This study documented a significantly shorter surgical time and hospitalization time for dogs undergoing LA compared with OA. Despite perioperative pancreatitis and the mortality rate being higher in the OA group compared with the LA group, these differences were not statistically significant. Only one dog in this study required conversion from LA to OA, and all dogs in the LA group survived at least 1 month postoperatively. Bilateral adrenalectomy is sometimes required for management of bilateral adrenal masses, and although this intervention has been performed by the authors laparoscopically in a staged fashion, we have not performed this as a single-stage laparoscopic procedure. Despite being feasible, bilateral adrenalectomy renders dogs acutely deficient of both corticosteroids and mineralocorticoids, and careful pretreatment of these dogs is vital as detailed later.

Preoperative Considerations

Surgical Anatomy

Knowledge of the surgical anatomy of the region is critical for success in adrenalectomy whether or not a laparoscopic approach is being chosen. The adrenal glands are paired organs located cranial to their respective kidneys and adjacent to the vena cava. The right adrenal gland has a capsule, which is continuous with the external tunic of the vena cava, making resection of the right gland somewhat more challenging than the left gland, whose capsule does not normally contact the vena cava directly unless significantly enlarged. Blood supply to the adrenal gland comes from many branching arteries surrounding the gland including the phrenic, abdominal, and renal arteries, among others.[22] The phrenicoabdominal artery branches off the aorta and shortly thereafter divides into the phrenic and cranial abdominal arteries. Although the phrenic artery branches cranially toward the diaphragm, the cranial abdominal artery turns caudally under the cranial pole of the kidney before perforating the epaxial musculature. It is in this location on the lateral aspect the adrenal gland that the cranial abdominal artery is often encountered during LA. The phrenicoabdominal vein (PV) bisects the two poles of the gland on its ventral aspect before entering the vena cava. The PV is clearly visible during LA and can act as a useful landmark to orient the surgeon. The left renal vein follows a course from the renal hilus, running cranially and medially toward its insertion onto the vena cava. In many dogs with left-sided adrenal masses, the renal vein will be closely associated with the most caudal aspect of the mass as well as its medial border, which in some cases might be compressing the renal vein against the vena cava. On the right side, the renal vein follows a shorter, more perpendicular course from the renal hilus to its insertion into the vena cava and also is frequently in close association with adrenal masses involving the caudal pole of the gland.

Preoperative Diagnostic Evaluation

Endocrine testing and diagnostic imaging are critical components of the preoperative evaluation of an adrenal mass and form the basis of decision-making regarding surgical resection, surgical approach, and perioperative treatment. Endocrine function testing is variable in different institutions but is aimed at evaluating the tumor for potential glucocorticoid, catecholamine, aldosterone and sex hormone secreting capability.

A thorough history and clinical examination are obtained with particular attention paid to the typical clinical findings of hyperadrenocorticism (HAC). A history and clinical examination that is suggestive of HAC should prompt further endocrine testing. A complete blood count, biochemistry panel, urinalysis, urine corticoid:creatinine ratio (UCCR), and noninvasive blood pressure measurement are reasonable next steps, although results of these tests will not be specific for HAC or a catecholamine-releasing tumor. The UCCR is often used as a screening test because it is relatively inexpensive and simple for owners to perform. Recent recommendations suggest that two tests performed on consecutive days at least 2 days after a visit to a veterinarian using a morning free-catch urine sample yields a very high sensitivity (99%) but a lower sensitivity (77%).[23] In the absence of clinical signs and in the presence of a UCCR below the reference range, no further endocrine testing is performed, and a non–cortisol-secreting tumor is assumed to be present. If clinical signs are present and the UCCR is elevated, a low-dose dexamethasone test (LDDST) is recommended to confirm adrenal-dependent HAC. If suppression to less than 50% of baseline occurs after an LDDST in a dog with HAC, the pituitary form of the disease is present.[23] Conversely, if no suppression occurs after an LDDST, it does not completely confirm a cortisol-secreting adrenal tumor because approximately 25% of pituitary-dependent cases do not suppress after a LDDST.[23] Therefore, in cases in which no suppression occurs after an LDDST, measurement of endogenous adrenocorticotropic hormone (ACTH) concentration, a high-dose dexamethasone suppression test, or abdominal ultrasonography (AUS) is recommended. AUS in dogs with adrenal-dependent HAC often demonstrates an adrenal mass with loss of normal gland architecture along with an atrophied contralateral gland.

Preoperative diagnosis for pheochromocytoma remains challenging because of the nonspecific nature of the clinical signs (trembling, weakness, collapse) and the historical lack of a blood test with high sensitivity and specificity for the condition. Hypertension is an inconsistent finding in dogs with pheochromocytoma with only 43% of dogs affected in one study.[24] Recently, one report has documented excellent sensitivity and specificity for plasma-free normetanephrine in differentiating dogs with pheochromocytoma from dogs with adrenocortical tumors, healthy dogs, and dogs with non-adrenal illness.[25] A further study evaluated urinary normetanephrine-to-creatinine ratios and demonstrated a high sensitivity and specificity for pheochromocytoma compared with dogs with HAC and healthy dogs.[26] Serum inhibin has also recently been evaluated as a potential differentiator of adrenal neoplasia in dogs given that it is produced by adrenocortical tumors but not by pheochromocytomas in humans. It was found to be a highly sensitive marker for differentiating pheochromocytomas from either adrenal- or pituitary-dependent HAC in dogs, although it was not capable of differentiating between the different forms of HAC.[27]

Cats are principally affected by aldosterone-secreting adrenal tumors, a syndrome that is typically characterized by hyperaldosteronemia, hypokalemia, and hypertension. The clinical signs associated with the condition commonly include hypokalemic polymyopathy (cervical ventroflexion and weakness can be present) and systemic hypertension. Surgical resection of these tumors is the preferred treatment, and one case of LA for resection of an aldosterone-secreting tumor has been reported in the literature.[20]

Progesterone-secreting adrenal tumors have also rarely been diagnosed in both dogs and cats.[28] Progesterone is a potent inhibitor of insulin as well as a precursor of cortisol, and therefore these animals can present either with symptoms related to unregulated diabetes mellitus or signs associated with steroid excess such as alopecia and thin, fragile skin. Cyclic estrus-like behavior has also been noted in one spayed cat with a sex-hormone secreting ACC.[29]

Preoperative medical management of adrenal neoplasia is now considered a critical part of optimal perioperative management and is administered in the same fashion whether or not a laparoscopic approach is chosen. In the case of cortisol-secreting adrenocortical tumors, administration of trilostane may be initiated at 0.5 to 1 mg/kg orally (PO) twice a day and increased as necessary to achieve adequate control based on clinical signs and results of an ACTH stimulation test. The recommendation is to treat for 2 to 3 weeks before surgery. Supplementation with corticosteroids before initiation of surgery to avoid a hypoadrenocortical episode in the recovery period is important. A suitable choice is dexamethasone (0.1–0.2 mg/kg intravenously [IV]), which will not interfere with the results of an ACTH stimulation test, which is usually performed 6 to 12 hours after surgery to check adrenal reserve function. In animals in which pheochromocytoma is suspected or cannot be ruled out, pretreatment with an α-adrenergic blocker, such as phenoxybenzamine (escalating dose up to 1–1.5 mg/kg PO), is strongly encouraged for 2 to 3 weeks after surgery until the animal is normotensive. This drug has been shown to improve outcomes in dogs undergoing adrenalectomy.[30] In cats with functional adrenocortical tumors, it has been suggested that treatment with trilostane be initiated until the skin abnormalities accompanying the condition in this species resolve.[31] Cats with aldosterone-secreting tumors should have their metabolic and electrolyte disturbances corrected before surgery.

Diagnostic Imaging

Imaging plays a critical part in the workup of patients with adrenal tumors. Imaging is crucial to rule out vascular invasion, which is currently a contraindication for a laparoscopic approach. Additionally, assessment of the size and location of the mass is important in good case selection for LA. Ultrasonography has been shown to have a sensitivity and specificity of 80% and 90%, respectively, for detection of vascular invasion and tumor thrombus.[4] The sensitivity and specificity of contrast-enhanced computed tomography (CE-CT) for detection of tumor thrombus were reported to be 92% and 100% respectively in another study.[32] Ultrasonography usually detects moderate to large tumor thrombi in the vena cava or renal vasculature and is often used as a screening test to provide noninvasive prognostic information for owners as the presence of both tumor thrombus within the cava as well as the extent of thrombus are prognostic in adrenal neoplasia.[33] If LA appears to be an option based on the results of ultrasonography, we usually recommend a CE-CT to further rule out minor vascular invasion and to evaluate the anatomical margins of the tumor. Approximately 20% to 48% of adrenal neoplasms exhibit vascular invasion into the vena cava, PVs, or renal vasculature, with pheochromocytomas more likely to invade than adrenocortical tumors.[4,24,33] Pheochromocytomas have been shown to be invasive in 48% to 55% of cases, with adrenocortical tumors invasive in 2% to 21% of cases.[4,24] Invasion into the PV alone is not, in the authors' opinion, an exclusion criterion for LA because the PV is sealed at the point of entry into the vena cava and thus will incorporate excision of the thrombus with the tumor. CE-CT can help to delineate very small thrombi that are entering the vena cava that may not be detectable at surgery when a laparoscopic approach is used (Figure 18-1). Other factors to note on the CE-CT are the relationships of the renal vasculature to the mass (Figure 18-2). Caudal pole masses can be closely associated with the renal vein, making them more challenging to resect. Knowledge of

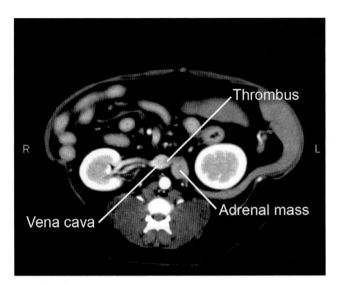

Figure 18-1 In this contrast-enhanced computed tomography image, a small thrombus can be seen entering the vena cava from the left phrenicoabdominal vein. This is an indication for an open approach to be used because a vascular dissection may be required to remove the adrenal mass and thrombus en bloc.

these relationships can aid in case selection in the early part of the learning curve as well as facilitate intraoperative decision making.

Patient Selection

As one of the more advanced laparoscopic procedures, it is recommend that LA be performed by surgeons with previous experience with OA. Additionally, working experience with other laparoscopic procedures is crucial because the dissection involved in LA is more complex and often more critical than in many other simpler laparo-

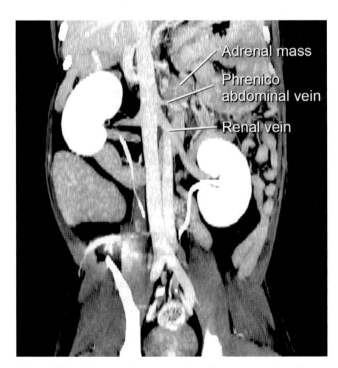

Figure 18-2 In this coronal reconstruction of a contrast-enhanced computed tomography image, a left-sided adrenal mass can clearly be seen in the cranial pole of the gland. The relationships to the phrenicoabdominal vein, vena cava, and the renal vasculature can also be appreciated.

scopic interventions. Poor hand–eye coordination or depth perception could have serious consequences during LA.

The LA technique has been performed in dogs from 2.7 to 40 kg and in cats from 4.3 to 7.3 kg.[18-21] As patient size increases, the available working space generally increases, facilitating the procedure. However, other challenges, such as the retraction of larger and heavier regional organs, can affect the technical ease of the procedure as patient size increases, although optimal positioning of the patient can mitigate some of these problems. Body condition score may dictate the amount of fat deposition around the adrenal glands, although this appears to be a greater problem in cats that commonly have larger perirenal fat pads compared with dogs.

Characteristics of the adrenal mass should be carefully considered during the early learning curve. It is critical to rule out vascular invasion because this may not be readily recognizable during surgery and could lead to migration of the thrombus if it goes unnoticed. Lesion size is often discussed in the human LA literature as a case selection criterion, and a progressive enlargement of lesions that are attempted laparoscopically has occurred in recent years. In veterinary patients, lesions up to 5 to 7 cm maximal diameter have been resected, although these large lesions are more challenging.[18,19,21] The authors recommend that smaller lesions (1–4 cm) be attempted early in the learning curve until greater experience with the technique is gained. In the future, it may be that larger lesions are shown to be readily resectable laparoscopically. Right-sided lesions may be more challenging to resect than left-sided lesion because of the close attachment of the right gland to the vena cava, but both right- and left-sided lesions have been resected in multiple studies.[18-21] Many adrenal neoplasms are located predominantly in the cranial pole or the caudal pole, and it is the authors' subjective impression that the cranial pole lesions are simpler to resect, mainly because of their less intimate relationship to the renal artery and vein. Lesions that are closely associated with the renal vein can create a more challenging dissection that may not be necessary when the lesion originates in the cranial pole.

Spontaneous adrenal rupture with consequent hemorrhage is seen occasionally in dogs. Acute hemorrhage is challenging in that diffuse retroperitoneal hemorrhage is often present and can make recognition of regional anatomy challenging.[34,35] In some cases in which some time has passed since the bleeding episode occurred, an organized thrombus may be present. In these cases, the dissection planes are usually more detectable, although en-bloc dissection of the mass with the thrombus can require very extensive dissection in the retroperitoneal space in and around the kidney. Cases with spontaneous adrenal rupture and hemorrhage would likely represent a challenging laparoscopic dissection in dogs and have not been described in the literature to date.

Patient Preparation

Surgical Preparation

After induction of general anesthesia, instrumentation for appropriate anesthetic monitoring is performed. When LA is performed in lateral recumbency, a wide area is clipped extending from the midthorax cranially to the hindlimb caudally on the affected side. Proximally, the clip is extended to the level of the transverse spinous processes, and it extends to the mid-abdominal area on the contralateral side, allowing for a conversion to a ventral midline celiotomy if deemed necessary. When performed in sternal recumbency, the patient is clipped from the midthorax to the pelvic area and laterally from the spinous process to the abdominal midline. For a bilateral adrenalectomy, a 360-degree clip is applied.

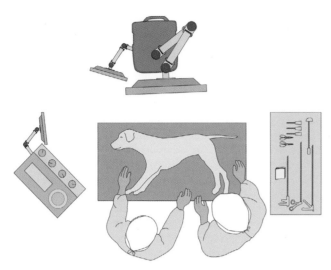

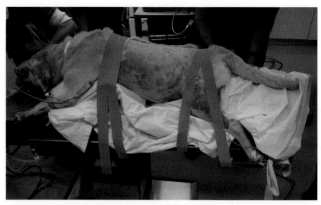

Figure 18-4 For sternal positioning, padding is placed in between the front and back legs to elevate the thorax and pelvis and allow the abdomen to "hang" to allow gravitational movement of organs away from the surgical site.

Figure 18-3 Both surgeons stand on the side of the patient's ventral abdomen (when the procedure is performed in lateral recumbency) with the endoscopic tower directly across from them on the contralateral side. The same general operating room layout is used when the patient is positioned in sternal recumbency with both surgeons standing on the side ipsilateral to the lesion.

Operating Room Setup and Patient Positioning

The surgeon and surgical assistant (laparoscope holder) should stand on the side of the table that faces the animal's ventral abdomen, with the endoscopic tower placed directly opposite the surgeon on the other side of the patient (Figure 18-3). In sternal position, both the surgeon and the assistant are located on the side of the adrenal gland. A bilateral approach is possible if two laparoscopic units are available.

There are a number of ways in which a dog or cat can be positioned for LA, and advantages and disadvantages to both approaches exist. Initial descriptions of LA in the literature describe the use of lateral recumbency with a foam wedge placed under the back to elevate the erector spinae muscle group to tilt the dog toward the side on which the surgeon is standing.[18] This "semi-sternal" positioning can also be created using a mechanical tilt table that is tilted over toward the surgeon standing on the side of the table facing the dog's ventrum. These positions aid the procedure in allowing the surrounding organs to fall ventrally away from the adrenal gland. In lateral or semi-sternal positioning, impingement of regional organs is a bigger problem on the left than the right in the primary author's experience, where sometimes the spleen and the stomach (especially if gas filled) can partially cover the mass. Simple retraction of these organs will often facilitate improved visualization. On the right side, impingement onto the mass from an enlarged liver lobe can be a problem. In many cases, the procedure can proceed despite a small amount of interference from the liver lobes. The intestines can sometimes cover the adrenal gland initially during the procedure, but simple movement of the intestinal loops in a ventral direction with a blunt probe usually resolves this problem.

In a fully sternal position, the dog is placed on its sternum with a cushion between its hind legs lifting the pelvis off the table (Figure 18-4). The two hind legs are placed besides the cushion in a splayed leg position. The purpose of this recumbency is to lift the abdomen as far from the table as possible, preferably in a hanging position. This often requires taping the dog in the unscrubbed areas to handles of the table to increase stability (see Figure 18-4). The sternal position makes the organs "suspend" in the abdomen and eliminates the need for pushing organs away during the procedure. The visibility of the adrenal gland can be improved with this posi-

tioning technique. If the kidney is closely associated with the adrenal gland, cutting the retroperitoneal attachment cranially or over the full length of the kidney will also increase visibility. In this way, the surgeon creates an open retroperitoneal approach.

Portal Position and Creation of Working Space

For LA in lateral or semi-sternal positioning, a three- or four-port technique can be used. When using a 30-degree laparoscope, it is recommended that the camera portal be placed 2 to 5 cm lateral to the umbilicus on the affected side. This allows a compromise between being able to get a good angle of view of the mass during dissection and not having the camera portal in such a proximal body wall position so that the laparoscope has to be held at an almost vertical angle during the procedure which can lead to rapid fatigue of the surgical assistant. When a 0-degree laparoscope is used, a somewhat more dorsal position might be necessary to ensure a good field of vision of the mass during dissection because there is no ability to deflect the angle of view down onto the mass. Initial laparoscope port placement at this paramedian location can be performed using either the Veress needle or a modified Hasson technique. Instrument ports are placed in a triangulating pattern around the location of the adrenal gland (Figure 18-5). The use of

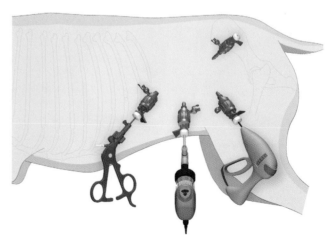

Figure 18-5 For laparoscopic adrenalectomy in lateral recumbency, three ports are usually placed in a triangulating fashion around the site of the adrenal gland. Note the telescope portal is located 3 to 5 cm lateral to the umbilicus. A fourth port can be added if extra retraction is necessary.

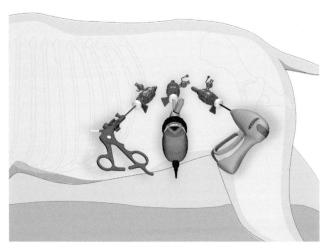

Figure 18-6 Port placement for laparoscopic adrenalectomy in sternal recumbency. The telescope portal is best placed just above the level of the instrument ports.

threaded ports is encouraged because they provide increased resistance to pull-out during the many instrument exchanges that are necessary during the procedure. Instruments should not be placed too close together to avoid interference during dissection. For a left-sided lesion, place a trocar–cannula assembly suitable for passage of 5-mm instrumentation 5 to 10 cm cranial to and 5 to 8 cm lateral to the subumbilical port on the left side in a location just caudal to the costal arch. It is important that the port remain caudal to the last rib to avoid inadvertent penetration of the thoracic cavity. Place a second instrument port 5 to 10 cm caudal and 5 to 8 cm lateral to the subumbilical port in the lower left quadrant. One of these three ports is usually established using a cannula suitable for passage of 10-mm instrumentation, which allows passage of a 10-mm clip applier (if needed) and specimen retrieval bag. If a right-sided adrenalectomy is being performed, the ports are placed at similar locations but on the opposite side.

For LA in sternal recumbency, ports are placed in a semicircular line starting halfway up the ribcage and ending at the middle of the ilial wing. The circle is pointing upward (Figure 18-6). The first trocar inserted is the camera port on the highest point of the circle, 1 to 2 cm under the epaxial abdominal muscles and preferably cranial to the left kidney (if palpable). The authors prefer to use an open approach using a threaded trocar under endoscopic visualization. As soon as the abdomen is entered, carbon dioxide is insufflated, and one or two cannulae are inserted cranial and caudal to the telescope port using the same line (i.e., slightly ventral to the camera). For a sternal approach, either a 30- or 0-degree telescope can be used. The 30-degree telescope needs to be placed a bit more dorsal than the 0-degree telescope. For a retroperitoneal approach, the 30-degree telescope is preferred.

The right adrenal approach is similar but placed a bit more cranial. Visualization can be improved by cutting the nephrohepatic ligament. A retroperitoneal approach is preferred for a right-sided large adrenal gland.

For single-port adrenalectomy, a single-port device is placed 2 to 5 cm lateral to the umbilicus, and a 2 to 3 cm incision is made into which the device is placed. The margins of the incision are elevated with retractors and the device is passed into the peritoneal cavity. Using a 30-degree telescope and two instrument ports the mass is dissected out in similar fashion as is described for the multiport

approach, although triangulation is significantly diminished, making this approach somewhat more challenging in the early phase of learning. Straight or articulating instruments can be used if available.

Surgical Technique

Instrumentation for Laparoscopic Adrenalectomy

Beyond the basic equipment housed on an endoscopy tower, a number of instruments are very useful to enable successful completion of the LA procedure. The use of a 30-degree laparoscope is helpful to allow an optimal viewing angle to be obtained, although LA can be performed using a 0-degree laparoscope. Cannulae of various sizes are helpful. Although most minimally invasive surgeons consider 5-mm instrumentation to provide a good balance among instrument size, cannula size, and image quality, 10- or 3-mm instrumentation can also be used. Placement of at least one cannula that can accommodate 10-mm instruments is helpful after dissection is complete if withdrawal in a commercial specimen retrieval bag is planned because these devices are mostly 10 mm in diameter. Relatively few laparoscopic instruments are essential for LA, but a blunt probe, laparoscopic Babcock forceps, and Kelly and right-angle dissection forceps can be very helpful in aiding dissection. Endopeanuts can be used to place pressure against the mass in an atraumatic way, sometimes obviating the need to grasp the tumor capsule directly. Hemostasis can be achieved in a number of ways, but use of a vessel sealer is strongly advised to facilitate the procedure and shorten surgical time. Bipolar vessel-sealing systems (LigaSure, Covidien, Mansfield, MA or Enseal, Ethicon Endosurgery, Cincinnati, OH) as well as ultrasonic vessel sealers (Harmonic, Ethicon Endosurgery) all now have handpieces with fine tips, which are very helpful for delicate tissue dissection and sealing in narrow tissue planes. Monopolar j- or l-hook electrosurgery can also be helpful in dissection of tissue planes around adrenal tumors, and the authors have found this especially helpful during dissection of the plane between the mass and the vena cava and renal veins, where it can often be difficult to place the larger tips of the vessel-sealing devices (Figure 18-7). However, it should be remembered that monopolar electrosurgery generates higher temperatures and greater lateral thermal spread than vessel-sealing devices and so should be used with significant caution around large vascular structures.[36] Activation for very short periods is strongly encouraged.

Suction devices with or without the capability to irrigate simultaneously are very helpful for LA to aspirate small accumulations of

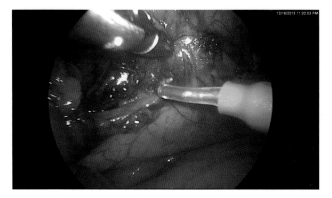

Figure 18-7 A laparoscopic j-hook monopolar electrosurgical probe is being used to gently dissect the plane between the vena cava and the adrenal capsule. The authors have found this especially useful in right adrenal tumors that are intimately attached to the vena cava.

hemorrhage that can obscure tissue planes. Also, when iatrogenic rupture of the capsule has occurred, suction of the contents of the tumor that spill out is essential to prevent further contamination. Both disposable (e.g., Surgiwand, Covidien) and nondisposable suction devices exist. In common with all laparoscopic suction devices, fine control over the amount of suction delivered is critical to avoid aspiration of the pneumoperitoneum with consequent repeated loss of working space. Nondisposable suction devices with incorporated trumpet valves (Trumpet valve 30804, Karl Storz Endoscopy, Goleta, CA) work very well for this purpose.

Finally, it is strongly recommended that adrenal masses be exteriorized in a specimen retrieval bag after dissection is completed. These often very friable masses fragment easily during exteriorization if a bag is not used with the possible consequence of leaving tumor fragments in the abdomen or body wall during exteriorization. For smaller masses, the inverted cut thumb of a large surgical glove works well as a specimen retrieval bag, although the risk of bursting a glove finger is a serious complication that should be considered. For larger masses, it may be necessary to use a commercially available specimen retrieval bag that is available from a variety of medical device companies. Commercial specimen retrieval bags are much easier to manipulate samples into because the attached handle allows easy "scooping" of the sample into it as opposed to the cut thumbs of surgical gloves, which require that instruments are used to manipulate the specimen into the bag while simultaneously holding the bag open so that the sample can be manipulated inside. This process is facilitated if the thumb is firstly inverted before insertion into the abdomen because this will cause the cut end to spring open rather than collapse.

Surgical Technique

For multiport transperitoneal LA, three ports are positioned initially as described. A brief exploratory laparoscopy can be performed at this stage to look for evidence of metastatic deposits in the abdomen, although thorough exploration of the abdomen is usually precluded by the lateral or sternal positioning of the patient. Exploration of the abdomen is facilitated if the surgical table allows changing the position of the animal intraoperatively. In most canine patients, the adrenal mass is usually immediately visible upon placing the camera into the abdominal cavity (Figure 18-8). If the mass is not immediately apparent, retraction of organs away from the kidney and adrenal gland is performed using a blunt probe. If the adrenal gland is still not visible, it is most likely surrounded by a fat pad located retroperitoneally. Care should be taken to always move regional organs away in an atraumatic

fashion using the body of the blunt probe rather than the tip, which in the case of the spleen especially can cause iatrogenic injury with consequent hemorrhage. On the left side, ventral retraction of the spleen is sometimes necessary, and rarely a gas-filled stomach can obscure the surgical field. Sometimes the ipsilateral kidney can fall onto the adrenal gland; in these cases, a somewhat more laterally recumbent position can be used to avoid this problem. If necessary, a stomach tube can be passed to decompress the stomach. On the right side, organ interference with the surgical site is less common in these authors' experience. Hepatomegaly (especially in dogs with hypercortisolism) can cause the right-sided liver lobes to overlay the adrenal gland on the right, which can be problematic, although we have not encountered cases in which the liver lobes could not be worked around. Significant neovascularization in most adrenal tumors ensures that almost all planes of dissection are highly vascular. Even modest hemorrhage in the early stages of the procedure can cause great difficulty in discerning the appropriate tissue planes for dissection.

On the left side, the surgery is generally initiated by incision of the peritoneum over the caudal margin of the mass between the mass and the kidney. This incision can be made bluntly using Babcock forceps, right-angle forceps, or the tip of a fine-tipped vessel sealer. A blunt probe, Babcock forceps, or endopeanut is then used to aid in manipulation of the gland as the dissection progresses. With any adrenal gland resection, it is preferable not to grasp the mass during the dissection because the capsule is usually very delicate and prone to rupture. Fatty attachments are usually very friable, and even moderate retraction will usually lead to some hemorrhage. Although this hemorrhage is not usually hemodynamically significant, it obscures visualization and can be a source of frustration. Intermittent suctioning of small amounts of hemorrhage as well as fat around the gland helps improve visualization. If capsular rupture occurs, the tumor often has a toothpaste consistency that tends to run out after the capsule is perforated. Gentle suction can be used to decrease contamination after adrenal gland tumor rupture. As the plane between the mass and kidney is dissected, the renal vein usually becomes visible and can be traced cranially to its insertion into the vena cava (Figure 18-9). The dissection plane continues cranially between the renal vein and the mass where the PV is

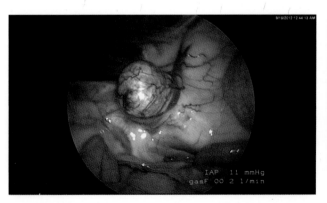

Figure 18-8 This left-sided adrenocortical mass was found upon entry into the abdomen. It can clearly be seen as primarily a cranial pole mass with a smaller caudal pole remnant attached caudal to the phrenicoabdominal vein. The relationship to the renal vein and caudal vena cava can also be seen.

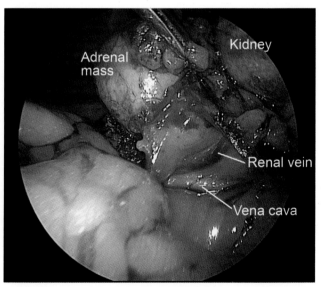

Figure 18-9 The course of the renal vein on the left side can clearly be seen running cranially and medially to join the vena cava. The caudal aspect of this mass will have to be carefully dissected off the renal vein.

soon encountered. The phrenicoabdominal (PA) vein and artery are large and must be identified and ligated. Vessel-sealing devices should reliably seal the PA vessels of small- to medium-sized dogs if the vessels are less than 5 to 7 mm in diameter (Video Clip 18-1). In larger dogs, hemoclips can be placed on these vessels but are now rarely used by the authors. After the PA vessels have been sealed and sectioned, the mass can usually be elevated up from the vena cava, and dissection dorsal to the gland can proceed. The PA vessels, after being sealed, can be used as a handle to manipulate the mass if great care is taken not to use excessive traction. Some larger masses can exhibit contact with or invasion into the epaxial muscles in this region, and these attachments require sectioning. It must be remembered that the PA vessels will be again encountered on the lateral aspect of the adrenal mass; the authors have on rare occasions encountered hemorrhage from the cranial abdominal artery as it passes on the lateral aspect of the mass under the cranial pole of the kidney. Care needs to be taken to seal these vessels because significant hemorrhage can result in they are traumatized during the final dissection of the mass on the lateral aspect.

Right-sided lesions present some unique challenges as the capsule of the right adrenal gland is continuous with the tunica externa of the vena cava. This results in an often very close relationship and more fibrous attachment between the mass and the vena cava. These authors prefer to initiate dissection on right-sided lesions by dissecting bluntly between the mass and the vena cava with either the fine tip of the vessel sealer or a right-angle dissector (Video Clip 18-2). In most cases, a plane can be established, but great care needs to be taken in ensuring that the wall of the vena cava is properly evaluated and not traumatized. The tip of a monopolar j-hook wand can also be used to separate out very fibrous bands of tissue, but care needs to be taken to ensure that thermal damage to the caval wall is not caused (see Figure 18-7). After the plane between the vena cava has been dissected, the plane between the mass and the renal vein needs to be dissected (see Video Clip 18-2). In some cases, there is little contact between the mass and the renal vein, but in others (especially caudal pole tumors), the vein can be intimately attached to the tumor or the tumor can be dorsal to the vein, requiring it to be gently teased away from the mass (Figure 18-10). In right-sided lesions, care also needs to be taken to ensure that diaphragmatic penetration does not occur during dissection of the dorsal aspects of the gland. There is considerable proximity of these structures in this location, and penetration can be suspected by visualization of the diaphragm bellowing caudally.

After the mass has been completely separated from its last tissue attachments, the mass is grasped and held while a specimen retrieval device is passed into the abdomen. After the mass has been manipulated into the bag, it is usually necessary to enlarge one of the portal incisions slightly to withdraw the bag with the mass inside unless the mass is very small (Figure 18-11). During mass removal, if the device is pulled out of a small incision with significant force, rupture of the capsule occurs, commonly precluding a histopathologic assessment of whether the tumor capsule is intact. The surgical site should ideally be thoroughly lavaged with sterile saline and closely inspected for ongoing hemorrhage before decompression of the pneumoperitoneum and routine closure of all port sites.

For retroperitoneal LA, after insufflation of the abdomen, the kidney is visualized, and the retroperitoneal space entered through the peritoneal fascia dorsal and cranial to the kidney. A trocar is inserted, and the abdomen is desufflated. After insertion of the camera, the retroperitoneal space is slowly insufflated, and the adrenal gland is approach from a dorsocaudal direction. Alternatively, this space can

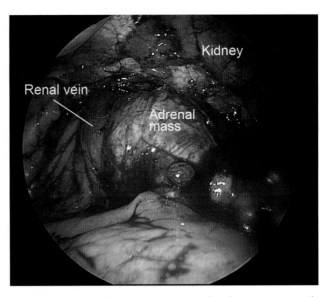

Figure 18-10 This right-sided caudal pole adrenal mass is intimately attached to the renal vein, which has been compressed by the mass. The renal vein was carefully dissected off the mass. These cases represent the most challenging cohort of cases for laparoscopic adrenalectomy.

be approached by a relative dorsal blind placement of the first trocar without insufflation or under ultrasonographic guidance.

Feline Laparoscopic Adrenalectomy

Only small numbers of feline laparoscopic adrenalectomies have been performed by the authors' group, but early experience suggests that some important differences exist, making the procedure potentially more challenging in cats.[20] The use of small lightweight cannulae and instruments is recommended in this species. A 3-mm laparoscope is ideal, if available, along with 3-mm instrumentation and lightweight cannulae, although at least one 5-mm cannula is necessary for placement of the vessel-sealing device. However, in some cats, especially those with right-sided lesions, the dissection plane between the mass and vena cava may be too limited to fit the

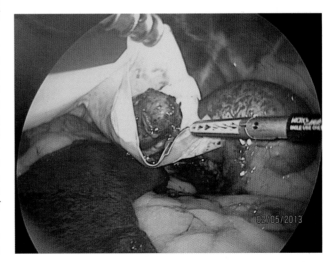

Figure 18-11 The inverted thumb of a large-sized surgical glove has been used here as an inexpensive specimen retrieval device. The adrenal tumor has been manipulated inside the glove before its exteriorization through one of the portals.

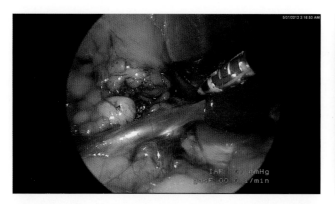

Figure 18-12 This aldosterone-secreting tumor in a cat can be seen lying dorsal to the vena cava. Dissection in this case was approached from both the medial and lateral aspect and was facilitated by the use of 3-mm instrumentation.

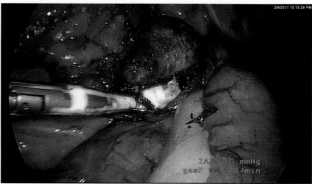

Figure 18-13 In this right-sided lesion, the capsule of the mass has been iatrogenically penetrated by the vessel-sealing device, and white "toothpaste-like" material can clearly be seen oozing from the tumor. This material was aspirated using a suction device before continuing with the procedure.

tip of a 5-mm vessel sealer into. Most cats with primary adrenal neoplasia have aldosterone-secreting adenomas or adenocarcinomas. However, some have either cortisol- or progesterone-secreting masses, which can cause extreme body wall fragility. The procedure in these cats can be challenging because tearing of the body wall tissues around the cannula can lead to chronic loss of pneumoperitoneum. The feline adrenal gland is sometimes hidden in the large perirenal fat pad that exists in this species. Most of the lesions we have operated have been quite small, and in some cases, some dissection into the fat cranial to the kidney was necessary to identify the mass on the left side. The feline gland on the right side is sometimes located more dorsal to the vena cava rather than lateral to it, and this may be evident if a preoperative CT scan is performed (Video Clip 18-3). This makes dissection even more challenging, and partial dissection from both lateral and medial aspects of the gland has been necessary in some cases (Figure 18-12). Advanced imaging is strongly encouraged in cats to assess the location and margins of the tumor and to aid the surgeon in deciding whether a laparoscopic approach is appropriate.

Complications and Prognosis

Several important complications can occur after LA, some of which are specific to the laparoscopic approach and some of which can be seen irrespective of the surgical approach. Intraoperative complications in dogs undergoing adrenalectomy are mostly related to hemorrhage and capsule rupture. If penetration of one of the principal vessels (vena cava, renal vein and artery) occurs, resulting in profuse hemorrhage, conversion to an open approach should be performed immediately to arrest hemorrhage and attempt repair of the bleeding vessel. If bleeding occurs from smaller vessels or the adrenal capsule, which is much more common, it may be possible to suction enough blood to visualize the bleeding vessel and then clamp or clip it. Bleeding from the PA vessels can sometimes occur lateral to the adrenal gland, and in this area, bleeding can usually be controlled without conversion to an open approach. Most commonly, "nuisance" hemorrhage occurs that, although not usually hemodynamically significant, can often prevent optimal visualization of the surgical field, which can result in prolonged surgical time.

Capsular penetration is a potential intraoperative complication with any form or adrenalectomy. It is unknown whether it is more likely to occur after LA compared with OA. Capsular penetration can easily be visualized at surgery during LA because of the superior magnification provided by the laparoscope (Figure 18-13). However, the significance of capsular penetration is unknown at this time. Despite being reported as a complication in all of the canine clinical reports of LA to date, no study has reported recurrence of the tumor or recurrence of clinical signs in cases with functional tumors.[18,19,21] In the future, longer term oncologic follow-up periods may help to define whether capsular rupture represents a clinically important complication.

Intraoperative complications specific to pheochromocytomas resection mostly relate to their catecholamine-releasing ability and its effect on systemic vascular resistance, blood pressure, and cardiac rhythm. Initial reports in humans suggested that hemodynamic instability with laparoscopic pheochromocytoma resection might be greater than when open resection was performed, but this hypothesis has not gained widespread support in the literature.[9] Although the authors strongly encourage preoperative treatment with phenoxybenzamine in small animal patients with suspected pheochromocytoma, their experience with laparoscopic resection in these patients has not been obviously different than OA in these cases, although no controlled studies exist to corroborate that experience in small animal patients. Despite the greater tendency for pheochromocytomas to be invasive into the local vasculature, careful preoperative diagnostic imaging of these patients should make complications related to this phenomenon no more common when a LA is used.

Other intraoperative complications can include iatrogenic damage to regional organs such as the kidneys, liver, spleen, or pancreas. Inadvertent penetration of the diaphragm with consequent pneumothorax can occur, especially on the right side, where adrenal masses are usually located closer to the diaphragmatic insertion.

Several complications are common to both the laparoscopic and open procedure, although it remains to be seen whether it can be shown that a laparoscopic approach may minimize some of these morbidities as has been shown in humans.[15,16] Thromboembolism is a potentially fatal complication and has been seen after both open[4] and laparoscopic[18] adrenalectomy in dogs and necessitates careful monitoring. Preoperative treatment of patients with cortisol-secreting tumors may help to decrease the incidence of postoperative thromboembolism in dogs undergoing adrenalectomy. Pancreatitis has been reported as a potentially fatal postoperative complication after adrenalectomy. Extensive manipulation and retraction of the pancreas is often necessary with OA but is largely avoided with LA. One study comparing LA with OA demonstrated a higher incidence of postoperative pancreatitis in a cohort of dogs with adrenocortical masses undergoing the open procedure (2 of 25 affected) compared with those undergoing LA (0 of 23), although this difference was not statistically significant, and further studies will be required to confirm this hypothesis.[21]

The long-term oncologic outcome of LA compared with OA has not yet been evaluated in veterinary patients. In humans, it is clear that for benign disease, whether or not it is hormonally active (including pheochromocytoma), the long-term recurrence rates are no different between OA and LA.[11,37] Long-term outcomes for ACC in humans are very controversial with some studies suggesting inferior long-term recurrence rates after LA but others suggesting that outcomes are equal.[6,7] Recurrence of adrenal neoplasia in dogs is anecdotally very rare, although it is possible that it goes underdiagnosed because of a lack of follow-up in many cases. However, there are no reported cases of recurrent adrenal neoplasia after LA to date.

Postoperative Care

Postoperative analgesia after LA can be in the form of intermittent IV or constant-rate infusion administration of an opioid drug (hydromorphone hydrochloride, 0.1 mg/kg IV every 4 hours; oxymorphone hydrochloride, 0.1 mg/kg IV every 4 hours; or buprenorphine hydrochloride, 0.01 mg/ kg IV every 6 hours). Tramadol hydrochloride can be prescribed upon discharge from the hospital (2–4 mg/kg PO every 8 hours for 3–5 days) in most dogs. Nonsteroidal antiinflammatory drugs can be administered in dogs with no suspicion of HAC (Deracoxib, 1 mg/kg PO, every 24 hours for 3–7 days, or carprofen 2.2 mg/kg PO, every 24 hours for 3–7 days), although the authors use these drugs very judiciously in this patient population. In one study, the median time spent in the hospital postoperatively was 48 hours (range, 22–70 hours), and this was significantly shorter compared with when the procedure is performed through a traditional celiotomy.[21]

Patients with functional adrenocortical tumors must be monitored in the postoperative period for hypoadrenocorticism. Ongoing therapy with corticosteroids should be continued for 2 to 3 weeks postoperatively until the results of ACTH stimulation tests confirm normal corticosteroid production from the contralateral adrenal gland.

 All videos cited in this chapter can be found on the book's companion website at **www.wiley.com/go/fransson/ laparoscopy**

References

1 Gagner, M., Lacroix, A., Bolte, C. (1992) Laparoscopic adrenalectomy in Cushing's syndrome and pheochromocytoma. N Engl J Med 327, 1033.
2 Bilimoria, K.Y., Shen, W.T., Elaraj, D., et al. (2008) Adrenocortical carcinoma in the United States. Cancer 113, 130-136.
3 Anderson, C.R., Birchard, S.J., Powers, B.E., et al. (2001) Surgical treatment of adrenocortical tumors: 21 cases (1990-1996). J Am Anim Hosp Assoc 37, 93.
4 Kyles, A.E., Feldman, E.C., De Cock, H.E.V., et al. (2003) Surgical management of adrenal gland tumors with and without associated tumor thrombi in dogs: 40 cases. J Am Vet Med Assoc 223, 654-662.
5 Schwartz, P., Kovak, J.R., Koprowski, A., et al. (2008) Evaluation of prognostic factors in the surgical treatment of adrenal gland tumors in dogs: 41 cases (1999-2005). J Am Vet Med Assoc 232, 77-84.
6 Brix, D., Allolio, B., Fenske, W., et al. (2010) Laparoscopic versus open adrenalectomy for adrenocortical carcinoma: surgical and oncological outcome in 152 patients. Eur Urol 58, 609-615.
7 Miller, B.S., Ammori, J.B., Gauger, P.G., et al. (2010) Laparoscopic resection is inappropriate in patients with known or suspected adrenocortical carcinoma. World J Surg 34, 1380-1385.
8 Miller, B.S., Gauger, P.G., Hammer, G.D., et al. (2012) Resection of adrenocortical carcinoma is less complete and local recurrence occurs sooner and more often after laparoscopic adrenalectomy than after open adrenalectomy. Surgery 152, 1150-1157.
9 Tiberio, G.A., Baiocchi, G.L., Arru, L., et al. (2008) Prospective randomized comparison of laparoscopic versus open adrenalectomy for sporadic pheochromocytoma, Surg Endosc 22, 1435.
10 Fernandez-Cruz, L., Taura, P., Saenz, A., et al. (1996) Laparoscopic approach to pheochromocytoma: hemodynamic changes and catecholamine secretion. World J Surg 20, 672-768.
11 Humphrey, R., Gray, D., Paulter, S., et al. (2008) Laparoscopic compared with open adrenalectomy for resection of pheochromocytoma: a review of 47 cases. Can J Surg 51, 276-280.
12 Wei, C., Fei, L., Dingnan, C., et al. (2013) Retroperitoneal versus transperitoneal laparoscopic adrenalectomy in adrenal tumor: a meta-analysis. Surg Laparosc Endosc Percutan Tech 23, 121-127.
13 Nigri, G., Rosman, A.S., Petrucciani, N., et al. (2013) Meta-analysis of trials comparing laparoscopic transperitoneal and retroperitoneal adrenalectomy. Surgery 153, 111-119.
14 Wang, L., Wu, Z., Li, M., et al. (2013) Laparoendoscopic single-site adrenalectomy versus conventional laparoscopic surgery: a systematic review and meta-analysis of observational studies. J Endourol 27, 743-750.
15 Lee, J., El-Tamer, M., Schifftner, T., et al. (2008) Open and laparoscopic adrenalectomy: analysis of the national surgical improvement program. J Am Coll Surg 206, 953-961.
16 Shaligram, A., Unnirevi, J., Meyer A., et al. (2012) Perioperative outcomes after adrenalectomy for malignant neoplasm in laparoscopic era: a multicenter retrospective study. Surg Laparosc Endosc Percutan Tech 22, 523-525.
17 National Institutes of Health. (2002) NIH state-of-the-science statement on management of the clinically inapparent adrenal mass ("incidentaloma") NIH Consens State Sci Statements 19, 1-25.
18 Pelaez, M.J., Bouvy, B.M., Dupre, G.P. (2008) Laparoscopic adrenalectomy for treatment of unilateral adrenocortical carcinomas: techniques, complications and results in seven dogs. Vet Surg 37, 444-453.
19 Naan, E.C., Kirpensteijn, J., Dupre, G.P., et al. (2013) Innovative approach to laparoscopic adrenalectomy for treatment of unilateral adrenal gland tumors in dogs. Vet Surg 42, 710-715.
20 Smith, R.R., Mayhew, P.D., Berent, A.C. (2012) Laparoscopic adrenalectomy for management of an aldosterone-secreting tumor in a cat. J Am Vet Med Assoc 241, 368-372.
21 Mayhew, P.D., Culp, W.T.N., Hunt, G.B., et al. (2014) Comparison of perioperative morbidity and mortality rates in dogs with non-invasive adrenocortical masses undergoing laparoscopic versus open adrenalecomy. J Am Vet Med Assoc 245,1028-35.
22 Hullinger, R.L. (1993) The endocrine system. In: Evans, H.E. (ed.) Miller's Anatomy of the Dog, 3rd edn. Saunders, St. Louis, pp. 559-585.
23 Behrend, E.N., Kooistra, H.S., Nelson R, et al. (2013) Diagnosis of spontaneous canine hyperadrenocorticism: 2012 ACVIM consensus statement (small animal). J Vet Intern Med 27, 1292-1304.
24 Barthez, P.Y., Marks, S.L., Woo, J., et al. (1997) Pheochromocytoma in dogs: 61 cases (1984-1995). J Vet Intern Med 11, 272-278.
25 Gostelow, R., Bridger, N., Syme, H.M. (2013) Plasma-free metanephrine and free normetanephrine measurement for the diagnosis of pheochromocytoma in dogs. J Vet Intern Med 27, 83-90.
26 Quante, S., Boretti, F.S., Kook, P.H., et al. (2010) Urinary catecholamine and metanephrine to creatinine ratios in dogs with hyperadrenocorticism or pheochromocytoma and in healthy dogs. J Vet Intern Med 24, 1093-1097.
27 Bromel, C., Nelson, N.W., Feldman, E.C., et al. (2013) Serum inhibin concentration in dogs with adrenal gland disease and in healthy dogs. J Vet Intern Med 27, 76-82.
28 Syme, H.M., Scott-Moncrieff, J.C., Treadwell, N.G., et al. (2001) Hyperadrenocorticism associated with excessive sex hormone production by an adrenocortical tumor in two dogs. J Am Vet Med Assoc 219, 1725-1728.
29 Meler, E.N., Scott-Moncrieff, J.C., Peter, A.T., et al. (2011) Cyclic estrous-like behavior in a spayed cat associated with excessive sex-hormone production by an adrenocortical carcinoma. J Fel Med Surg 13, 473-478.
30 Herrera, M.A., Mehl, M.L., Kass, P.H., et al. (2008) Predictive factors and the effect of phenoxybenzamine on outcome in dogs undergoing adrenalectomy for pheochromocytoma. J Vet Intern Med 22, 1333-1339.
31 Chiaramonte, D., Greco, D.S. (2007) Feline adrenal disorders. Clin Tech Small Anim Pract 22, 26.
32 Schultz, R.M., Wisner, E.R., Johnson, E.G., et al. (2009) Contrast-enhanced computed tomography as a preoperative indicator of vascular invasion from adrenal masses in dogs. Vet Radiol Ultrasound 50, 625-629.
33 Barrera, J.S., Bernard, A.F., Ehrhart, E.J., et al. (2013) Evaluation of risk factors for outcome associated with adrenal gland tumors with or without invasion of the caudal vena cava and treated via adrenalectomy in dogs: 86 cases (1993-2009). J Am Vet Med Assoc 242, 1715-1721.

34 Whittemore, J.C., Preston, C.A., Kyles, A.E., et al. (2001) Nontraumatic rupture of an adrenal gland tumor causing intra-abdominal or retroperitoneal hemorrhage in four dogs. J Am Vet Med Assoc 93, 329-333.

35 Lang, J.M., Schertel, E., Kennedy, S., et al. (2011) Elective and emergency surgical management of adrenal gland tumors: 60 cases (1999-2006). J Am Anim Hosp Assoc 47, 428-435.

36 Sutton, P.A., Awad, S., Perkins, A.C., et al. (2010) Comparison of lateral thermal spread using monopolar and bipolar diathermy, the Harmonic scalpel and the Ligasure. Br J Surg 97, 428-433.

37 Brunt, L.M., Moley, J.F., Doherty, G.M., et al. (2001) Outcomes analysis in patients undergoing laparoscopic adrenalectomy for hormonally active adrenal tumors. Surgery 130, 629-635.

19 Laparoscopic Surgery of the Pancreas

Floryne O. Buishand, Sebastiaan A. van Nimwegen, and Jolle Kirpensteijn

---

Key Points

- The pancreas can be reached laparoscopically via either a classic ventral midline or a left-, or right-sided flank approach.
- Placing patients in sternal recumbency may improve access to the pancreas in a lateral approach.
- The pancreas should be handled as gently as possible to prevent postoperative pancreatitis.
- The pancreatic blood supply should always be identified during surgery, and extreme caution should be taken to prevent damage to the pancreaticoduodenal arteries and the ductal system.

Currently, except for laparoscopic or laparoscopic-assisted pancreatic biopsies, the use of laparoscopic surgery of the pancreas in companion animal patients has not been reported. In the human medical field, the complexity and morbidity associated with pancreatic surgery have resulted in a relatively slow uptake of laparoscopic surgery. There are no consensus guidelines on the role of laparoscopic pancreatic surgery.[1] Although there are no randomized controlled trials in human medicine, several recent large series and comparative studies on the short- and long-term outcomes of laparoscopic pancreatic surgery have demonstrated clear advantages over the open approach.[2,3] Extrapolating this to veterinary medicine provides significant impetus for extending the role of laparoscopy in pancreatic surgery.

Preoperative Considerations

Relevant Pathophysiology

The pancreas consists of 98% exocrine and 2% endocrine tissue. The acinar cells of the exocrine pancreas secrete amylase, proteases, and lipases. These enzymes are responsible for the digestion of carbohydrate, protein, and fat. Besides enzymes, pancreatic juice contains bicarbonate for neutralization of gastric acid, factors that facilitate absorption of cobalamin, zinc and colipase C, and antibacterial factors.

The most common disease of the exocrine pancreas is pancreatitis. The pathogenesis, underlying causes, and risk factors for pancreatitis are not well known, and most cases are considered idiopathic in origin.[4] Regardless of the underlying cause, after initiation of pancreatitis, autodigestion of the gland starts to occur. The most common clinical signs of pancreatitis in dogs are anorexia, vomiting, weakness, abdominal pain, and diarrhea.[5] In cats, anorexia and lethargy are most common; vomiting only occurs in a minority of cases, and diarrhea is usually not observed.[6]

Pancreatic abscesses are mucopurulent necrotic exudates within the pancreatic parenchyma that can also extend into adjacent tissues.[7] Because pancreatic abscesses are usually a sequela to pancreatitis, their clinical signs parallel those of pancreatitis.

Pancreatic pseudocysts are collections of pancreatic secretions, debris, and blood in a nonepithelialized fibrous tissue sac.[8] Pseudocysts most likely form after premature activation of digestive enzymes, resulting in autodigestion of pancreatic parenchyma, leading to inflammation and necrosis. Pancreatic pseudocysts may be asymptomatic, or animals may be presented with clinical signs of pancreatitis. If parts of the pancreas are devoid of a pancreatic duct, for example, as a result of leaving a distal part of the pancreas intact during partial resection, this can also cause pancreatic cyst or abscess formation.

Pancreatic (adeno)carcinomas are highly malignant tumors that originate from acinar or ductal epithelial cells. These tumors most

---

Small Animal Laparoscopy and Thoracoscopy, First Edition. Edited by Boel A. Fransson and Philipp D. Mayhew.
© 2015 by ACVS Foundation. Published 2015 by John Wiley & Sons, Inc.
Companion website: www.wiley.com/go/fransson/laparoscopy

commonly occur in older animals that present with weight loss, anorexia, abdominal pain, ascites, vomiting, and icterus. Benign pancreatic adenomas are extremely rare and are often incidental findings.[9]

Scattered through the exocrine pancreas are the islets of Langerhans that form the endocrine part of the pancreas. Islets are composed of five distinct cell types : α cells that secrete glucagon, β cells that create insulin, δ cells that secrete somatostatin, and ε cells that secrete ghrelin, and PP cells that secrete pancreatic polypeptide. The main function of the endocrine pancreas is to regulate glucose metabolism through insulin and glucagon secretion.

The most common disease of the endocrine pancreas is insulinoma, an insulin-secreting β cell tumor.[10,11] These tumors hypersecrete insulin, leading to hyperinsulinemia. The resulting hypoglycemia causes clinical signs such as seizures, generalized weakness, posterior paresis, lethargy, ataxia, and muscle tremors. Insulinomas and other endocrine tumors of the pancreas are extremely rare in cats.

Other tumors of the endocrine pancreas are very rare and include gastrinomas and glucagonomas.[12,13] Gastrinomas are malignant islet tumors of dogs and cats. The secretion of excessive amounts of gastrin results in gastric acid hypersecretion and is associated with gastric and intestinal ulceration and associated clinical signs. Glucagonomas are glucagon-secreting carcinomas of α cells in dogs. Serum glucagon increases and causes a decrease in plasma amino acids, albumin and albumin-bound zinc, and essential fatty acids. These changes probably contribute to the cutaneous manifestation of glucagonoma syndrome: erosions, ulceration and hyperkeratosis of footpads, and crusting and alopecia around mucocutaneous junctions.

Surgical Anatomy

The pancreas of dogs and cats is divided in a right and a left lobe that unite at the pancreatic body (Figure 19-1). The right or duodenal lobe is located within the mesdoduodenum. In contrast to the canine pancreas, the distal third of the feline (and ferret) right lobe curves cranially, giving it a hooklike appearance, which ends close to the caudal vena cava. The distal or caudal part of the right lobe lies relatively unattached to the duodenum. More cranially, toward the pancreatic duct and the corpus, the pancreas is tightly associated to the duodenum and the common bile duct, which runs adjacent to the duodenum. The corpus of the pancreas is closely related to the pylorus and proximal duodenum cranially. The portal vein crosses the corpus or proximal left lobe dorsally, close to where the cranial pancreaticoduodenal artery and gastroduodenal vein enter the pancreatic body, crossed on their right side by the common bile duct.[14,15] The left lobe, which is positioned high in the dorsal leaf of the omentum, begins just caudal to the pylorus and extends along the greater curvature of the stomach to the dorsal extremity of the spleen. The dorsal surface is associated with, from right to left, the portal vein, caudal vena cava, left gastric vein, and splenic vein. The arterial blood supply to the pancreas is tripartite. The largest artery is the cranial pancreaticoduodenal artery, a terminal branch of the gastroduodenal artery. The cranial pancreaticoduodenal artery enters the body of the pancreas, courses through the right pancreatic lobe, and supplies the duodenum after exiting the pancreas. The pancreatic artery, which branches from the splenic artery in 80% of dogs, supplies the left lobe of the pancreas. In 20% of dogs, the pancreatic artery originates from the cranial mesenteric artery. The third and smallest source of arterial inflow is the caudal pancreaticoduodenal artery that arises from the cranial mesenteric artery and supplies and courses through the distal portion of the right pancreatic lobe. The cranial and caudal pancreaticoduodenal arteries anastomose within the right lobe of the pancreas. The pancreaticoduodenal vein drains the right lobe of the pancreas into the gastroduodenal vein. The body and left lobe are drained via the splenic vein.[16]

Pancreatic duct anatomy differs between dogs and cats. Dogs typically have two pancreatic ducts (see Figure 19-1). The large accessory pancreatic duct carries secretions from the right pancreatic lobe to the minor duodenal papilla. The smaller pancreatic duct transports secretions from the left lobe and enters the major duodenal papilla next to the common bile duct, approximately 5 cm from

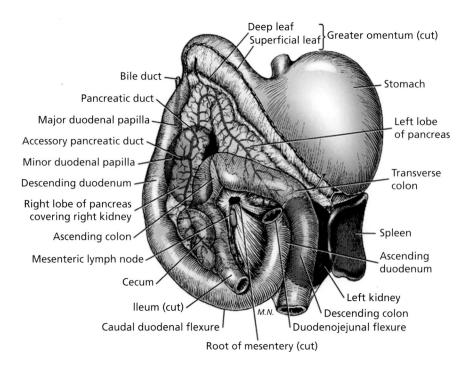

Deep leaf
Superficial leaf } Greater omentum (cut)
Bile duct
Pancreatic duct
Major duodenal papilla
Accessory pancreatic duct
Minor duodenal papilla
Descending duodenum
Right lobe of pancreas covering right kidney
Ascending colon
Mesenteric lymph node
Cecum
Ileum (cut)
Caudal duodenal flexure
Root of mesentery (cut)
M.N.
Stomach
Left lobe of pancreas
Transverse colon
Spleen
Ascending duodenum
Left kidney
Descending colon
Duodenojejunal flexure

Figure 19-1 Anatomy of the pancreas and surrounding structures. (From Evans, H.E. (1993) The digestive apparatus and abdomen: the pancreas. In: Evans, H.E., Evans, S.A. (eds.) Miller's Anatomy of the Dog, 3rd edn. Saunders, Philadelphia, pp. 458-460. Reproduced with permission from Elsevier.)

the pylorus. Some dogs only have an accessory pancreatic duct, and another reported variation is the presence of three duodenal openings. In 80% of cats, a single pancreatic duct is present that joins the common bile duct before entering the major duodenal papilla. In the remaining 20% of cats, an accessory pancreatic duct is present, which, as in dogs, opens into the minor duodenal papilla.

Multiple lymph nodes drain the pancreas. Knowledge of location of these lymph nodes is important in cases of malignant disease. Lymph nodes known to drain the pancreas are the pancreaticoduodenal, splenic, mesenteric, and hepatic. Other lymph nodes that most likely also drain the pancreas are the colic and gastric lymph nodes.

The pancreas is directly innervated by vagal nerve fibers. The celiac and superior mesenteric plexus innervate the blood vessels of the pancreas.

Diagnostic Workup and Imaging

For laparoscopic pancreatic surgery, no different workup is necessary compared with open surgery.[1]

In most cases, the diagnosis of pancreatitis is based on the clinical signs, together with increased serum pancreatic lipase levels. On ultrasound examination, the echogenicity of the pancreas can be decreased or increased caused by pancreatic fibrosis. The echogenicity of the surrounding mesentery is often hyperechoic in acute pancreatitis as a result of inflammation.[17] Pancreatic biopsy can be performed to confirm the diagnosis with histology. Ultrasonography may reveal a mass lesion within the pancreas, which is fluid filled in case of a pancreatic pseudocyst, or an abscess. Pancreatic adenocarcinomas present as mass lesions as well and histopathology of pancreatic biopsy specimens is required to distinguish between neoplasia and pancreatitis. Imaging alone may not differentiate pseudocysts from abscesses. To make a definitive diagnosis, fluid acquired by percutaneous fine-needle aspiration (FNA) should be examined. However, FNA of cavitary pancreatic masses is not without risk, and this risk must be weighed against the advantage of a preoperative diagnosis.

The presumptive diagnosis of canine insulinoma is commonly based on signalment and history combined with the fulfillment of Whipple's triad: (1) presence of clinical signs associated with hypoglycemia, (2) fasting blood glucose concentration less than 2.2 mmol/L (<40 mg/dL), and (3) relief of clinical signs after glucose administration or feeding. Although the presence of Whipple's triad diagnoses hypoglycemia, it is not definitive for insulinoma. The next step is to exclude differential diagnoses by determining the plasma insulin concentration. In insulinoma cases, circulating insulin concentrations are typically within the reference range or higher despite hypoglycemia. The simultaneous occurrence of blood glucose less than 3.4 mmol/L (<62.5 mg/dL) and plasma insulin greater than 70 pmol/L is diagnostic for insulinoma.[18] Use of diagnostic imaging techniques, including transabdominal ultrasonography, computed tomography (CT), single-photon emission computed tomography (SPECT), and somatostatin receptor scintigraphy (SRS), have been reported in the identification and preoperative staging of insulinoma. Ultrasonography was found to have a low sensitivity in detecting canine insulinoma[19] with only 5 of 14 primary insulinomas correctly identified and no lymph node metastases detected. Similar results were obtained using SPECT. CT has proved to be the most sensitive method, correctly identifying 10 of 14 primary tumors and 2 of 5 lymph node metastases. Conventional pre- and postcontrast CT was not found to be a very specific method because it also identified many false-positive lesions. More

recently, dual-phase CT angiography (CTA) techniques have been developed, and the accurate use of dynamic CTA for the presurgical localization of insulinoma in four dogs has been reported.[20,21] With CTA, after an intravenous (IV) injection of contrast medium, final CT images are acquired during the arterial and venous phases. CT images of canine insulinoma are hyperattenuating at the arterial phase in 55% of cases[21] compared with the normal pancreas. Finally, a recent case study by Choi *et al.* has investigated the potential of positron emission tomography CT (PET-CT) to detect an insulinoma in a dog.[22] They used the radiopharmaceutical ^{18}F-FDG, which is a glucose-derivative. PET-CT failed to detect both the primary tumor and the extent of the metastatic lesions in this case. The limited utility of FDG PET-CT in detection of canine insulinomas may be attributable to the low level of glucose turnover. Because it was used only in one case, further studies on FDG PET-CT in canine insulinomas are warranted, including time activity and dose-response studies of ^{18}F-FDG to establish the optimal scan condition for detecting canine insulinomas.

As with insulinomas, ultrasonography frequently fails to detect gastrinomas or glucagonomas. The diagnosis of gastrinoma is usually based on clinical signs in combination with hypergastrinemia in fasted patients. Furthermore, endoscopic examination of the stomach and duodenum often reveals ulceration, and SRS has been successfully used to diagnose metastatic gastrinoma in one dog.[23] The use of CT scanning has been reported for the diagnosis of lymph node, splenic, and hepatic canine glucagonoma metastases.[24] Biopsies of cutaneous lesions in dogs with glucagonomas demonstrate histologic changes characteristic of metabolic epidermal necrosis. In 90% of canine cases with metabolic epidermal necrosis, however, the skin condition is associated with severe liver dysfunction rather than the presence of a glucagonoma. Furthermore, plasma glucagon levels can also be increased in hepatocutaneous syndrome without the presence of a glucagonoma. Therefore, liver disease and other dermatological differential diagnoses need to be ruled out before the diagnosis of glucagonoma can be made.

Patient Selection

Pancreatic biopsies for the identification of pancreatitis are preferably taken laparoscopically. Laparoscopic partial pancreatectomy is indicated in cases with isolated pancreatic masses, pseudocysts, or abscesses located in the distal two thirds of either the right or left pancreatic lobe. If complete excision of a pancreatic abscess is not possible, it should be surgically drained and omentalized using either an open or laparoscopic technique. If focal lesions are located close to the pancreatic body, local enucleation can be attempted. In case of lesions located in the pancreatic body, laparotomy is still preferred over laparoscopic surgery in most cases, but novel positioning techniques of the patient may allow successful laparoscopic approaches. Open surgery is the preferred technique in cases in which pancreatic tumors have extensive metastases to abdominal lymph nodes or the liver, requiring extensive exploration and palpation of organs. However, selected abdominal lymph nodes are accessible using a laparoscopic technique.

Prognostic Factors

No data are available in small animal medicine that compare minimally invasive versus open pancreatic surgery; therefore, it is presumed that prognostic factors will not differ between the two approaches when they are performed correctly.

An overall survival rate of 63% of dogs with acute pancreatitis treated surgically has been reported.[23] The severity of symptoms at initial diagnosis was not correlated with clinical outcome. The prognosis for dogs with pancreatic abscesses is guarded with postoperative survival rates of 14% to 55%. The prognosis for dogs that had surgery (including repeated percutaneous aspiration) of pancreatic pseudocysts is better and resulted in a survival rate of 75%.

At the authors' institution, dogs with insulinomas have a mean postoperative survival time of 25 months (3–41 months). Dogs with a negative insulinoma Ki67 index or with their insulinoma confined to the pancreas and with primary tumors smaller than 2 cm survive significantly longer postoperatively than dogs with a positive Ki67 index or with insulinomas that have spread to lymph nodes and distant sites or larger tumors.[11] Furthermore, dogs that are hyperglycemic or normoglycemic immediately postoperatively survive significantly longer than dogs with hypoglycemia postoperatively. The prognosis for other pancreatic neoplasms is poor. In cases where surgery is feasible in pancreatic adenocarcinoma cases, most dogs only survive 3 months postoperatively. Regarding canine glucagonoma and gastrinoma, only a limited number of cases have been reported with varying outcomes after surgery.[24,25]

Patient Preparation

Surgical Preparation
Dry food should be withheld 12 hours before surgery. Canned food can be fed until 6 hours before surgery. In case of insulinomas and if dogs are clinically hypoglycemic, liquid, easily digestible food preparations should be given until 1 to 2 hours before surgery. If clinical signs of hypoglycemia occur in the immediate preoperative period, the dog should be administered a glucose solution intravenously (1–5 mL of 50% dextrose administered over 10 minutes based on clinical effect) to stabilize blood glucose concentration before surgery. In cases of pancreatitis, it is important to pay attention to factors that could increase the complication rate, including hypoproteinemia, disseminated intravascular coagulation, and diabetes mellitus. Any abnormalities in fluid and electrolyte balance, coagulation, oncotic pressure, or plasma glucose levels should be corrected preoperatively.

For a ventral midline laparoscopic approach, the abdomen should be clipped from the xiphoid process to the pubis. Laterally, the patient should be clipped to approximately the mid-abdomen level as for open pancreatic surgery. It is important to perform wide clipping and aseptic preparation because it might be necessary intraoperatively to convert to an open procedure or change the position of the dog. The authors prefer a 360-degree clip to allow an approach from all sides for complicated laparoscopic pancreatic surgery. For a flank approach only, the left or right caudal hemithorax and the lateral abdomen should be clipped and prepared for aseptic surgery.

There are no indications in laparoscopic pancreatic surgery for the use of prophylactic antibiotics. Only in febrile patients with septic complications of pancreatitis, prophylactic antibiotics should be used. However, septic complications are rare in cases of pancreatitis, and these cases should preferably be approached using open instead of minimally invasive surgery.

Patient Positioning
The operating room layout for laparoscopic pancreatic surgery is shown in Figure 19-2. According to the literature, animals should be positioned in dorsal or left lateral recumbency.[25-28] However, in the authors' experience, sternal recumbency provides good access to the right lobe and the distal part of the left lobe of the pancreas

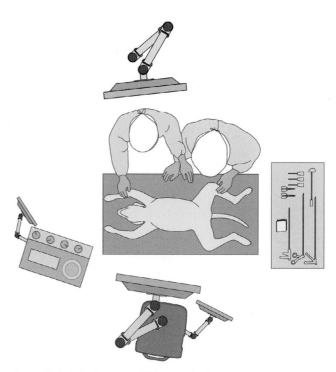

Figure 19-2 Operating room (OR) layout for laparoscopic pancreatic surgery. If available, a second monitor in the OR facilitates changing sides during surgery without loss of alignment between surgical field and monitor.

when a right- or left-sided flank approach is used, comparable to the lateral laparoscopic approach to the adrenal glands.[29] For the left lateral approach, the sternum and pelvic area are tightly supported using two moldable vacuum or gel-foam cushions, one under the sternum and one between the pelvic limbs supporting the pubic bone while the abdomen hangs more or less free in between (Figure 19-3). Ideally, the animal is positioned on a motorized tilt table so that tilting to the left and to the right, as well as head-up and head-down (Trendelenburg) positions can be used. A good overview of the abdominal cavity is ensured because gravity can be used to move the abdominal organs away from the surgery site (Figure 19-4). The right leg and corpus of the pancreas

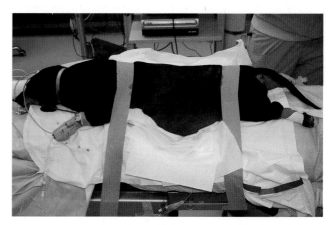

Figure 19-3 Patient positioning for laparoscopic flank approach. The thorax and pelvis are supported using moldable vacuum cushions so that the abdomen is free and the abdominal organs can move ventrally. The table can be tilted head up or down and sideways to improve access.

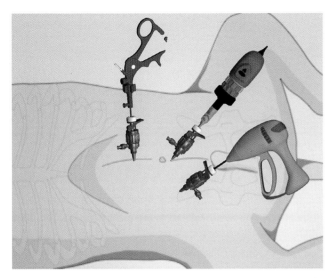

Figure 19-4 Portal placement for ventral approach to the pancreas. The initial portal is subumbilical. Subsequent portals are placed according to intraabdominal findings.

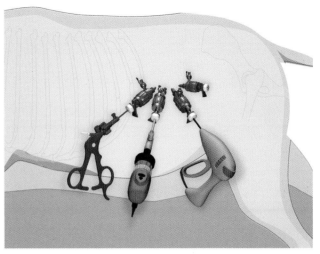

Figure 19-5 Port placement for laparoscopic flank approach. The initial portal is just caudal to the last rib. Subsequent portals are placed according to intraabdominal findings.

can be approached by a sternal-oblique right lateral approach, (30–45 degrees sternal–left lateral oblique recumbency). The corpus and proximal left lobe of the pancreas are the most difficult areas to approach. A ventral approach with the patient in dorsal recumbency has commonly been recommended. In this position, it is crucial to be able to tilt the animal to the right or to the left. Additionally, a reverse Trendelenburg (head-up) position may improve visibility of the cranial part of the abdomen by gravity-dependent caudal displacement of the intestines. However, access to the corpus and left lobe can still be difficult because of their position deep to the other abdominal organs. A right lateral approach with the patient in sternal–left lateral oblique position may provide better access to the corpus and proximal left lobe (see later).

Portal Type and Position

Ventral Approach

A classic ventral laparoscopic approach of the pancreas in dogs and cats has been reported using three portals (see Figure 19-4).[25,26,28,30] The first portal should be placed in the midline to reduce muscle trauma, just caudal to the umbilicus (subumbilical) to avoid the falciform ligament. Two additional portals are usually placed in paramedian locations, lateral to the third mammary glands. Some surgeons prefer to use three midline portals. Note that for procedures other than exploration or biopsy, a fourth portal may be necessary for constant retraction of organs while performing surgery using atraumatic graspers or a fan retractor. The authors prefer to start with a midline subumbilical camera portal and choose additional portal locations based on intraabdominal findings (see Figure 19-4).

Lateral Approach (Left or Right Sided)

The initial camera portal is made 1 to 3 cm caudal to the last rib and 3 to 5 cm ventral to the transverse spinous processes or epaxial musculature (Figure 19-5), a position just cranio-latero-ventral to the kidney. This position is slightly more ventral compared with the approach to the adrenal gland.[29] Subsequent portals are placed according to the intraabdominal situation and surgical procedure, enabling a proper triangulated laparoscopic approach.

Creation of Working Space

Pneumoperitoneum and Abdominal Access

For both a ventral or lateral approach, pneumoperitoneum is established through either a modified Hasson technique or using a Veress needle. The authors prefer an open modified Hasson technique using blunt threaded cannulae (Ternamian Endotip; Karl Storz Endoscopy, Goleta, CA) for visual guidance of abdominal entry and stay sutures in the external abdominal fascia. An intraabdominal carbon dioxide pressure of 8 to 10 mm Hg is usually sufficient to create a suitable surgical working space in dogs. In very small dogs and cats, pressure can often be reduced to 4 to 6 mm Hg.[31] A 5-mm, 0- or 30-degree telescope is commonly used except in very small dogs and cats, in which smaller instruments are preferred.[25,31]

Ventral Approach in Dorsal Recumbency

At rest in dorsal recumbency, none or only a small portion of the right pancreatic lobe is visible (Figure 19-6 depicts normal anatomy in dorsal recumbency). To access the right lobe of the pancreas, the patient is best tilted over to the left side as far as possible (30 degrees or more). The duodenum is located by gently moving the intestines to the left. Both sides of the right lobe of the pancreas can be inspected by pulling the duodenum ventromedially or grasping and lifting it upward (Figure 19-7). The dorsal side of the corpus and left lobe can be approached by grasping and elevating the greater omentum and stomach cranially (see Figure 19-7). The corpus and proximal part of the left lobe can be visualized more easily than the rest of the left lobe because moving the omentum and stomach cranially becomes more difficult further to the left side. It may help to tilt the dog far to the left side and head up (reverse Trendelenburg position) so that the omentum and spleen move to the left and can be more easily retracted cranially while the intestines move left and caudal. The dorsal surface of the distal left lobe may also be accessed by tilting the patient to the right and moving the omentum and spleen craniomedially. To visualize the ventral surface of the corpus and left pancreatic lobe, the ventral leaf of the omentum is perforated in an avascular part, and the stomach is pulled cranially in a reverse Trendelenburg position. This can be quite difficult and does not always lead to sufficient visualization of the pancreas.

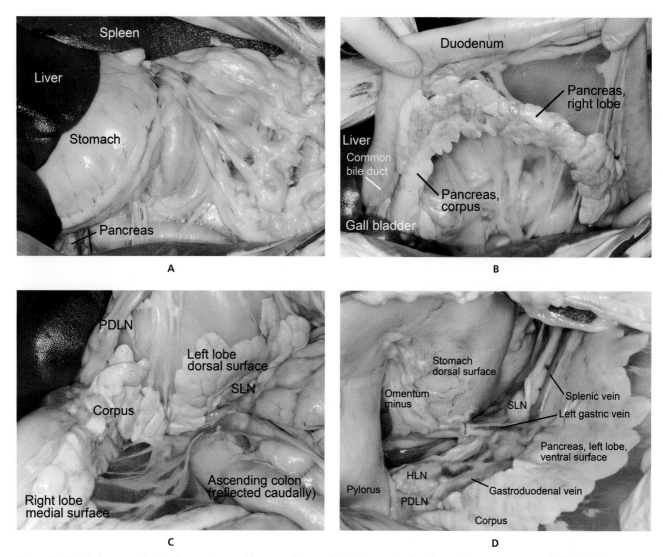

Figure 19-6 Surgical anatomy in dorsal recumbency with a ventral approach. **A,** Anatomy in dorsal recumbency in situ. **B,** Right limb of the pancreas. Lateral view when lifting up the duodenum. **C,** View on the dorsal surface of the pancreas. The stomach and greater omentum are lifted upward and cranially, and the transverse colon is retracted caudally, showing the left lobe, right lobe, and corpus pancreatis. PDLN, pancreaticoduodenal lymph node; SLN, splenic lymph node. **D,** View of the ventral surface of the left lobe and left part of the corpus of the pancreas through a window in the ventral leaf of the greater omentum. HLN, hepatic lymph node.

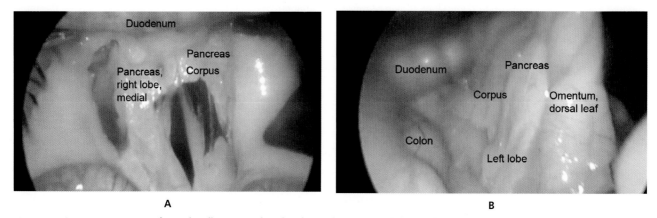

Figure 19-7 Laparoscopic images of ventral midline approach in dorsal recumbency. **A,** Medial view of the right lobe and corpus of the pancreas by gently holding the descending duodenum upward through a ventral midline laparoscopic approach in a Chihuahua in dorsal recumbency and tilted to the left side, using 6 mm Hg of intraabdominal carbon dioxide pressure. **B,** Laparoscopic view of the dorsal surface of the corpus and left lobe of the pancreas by holding the omentum upward and retracting the colon caudally through a ventral midline approach with the dog in a reverse Trendelenburg position and tilted to the left side.

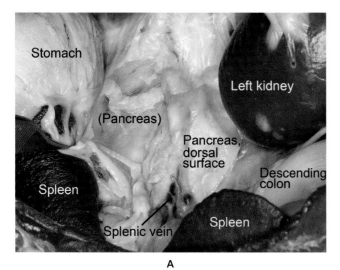

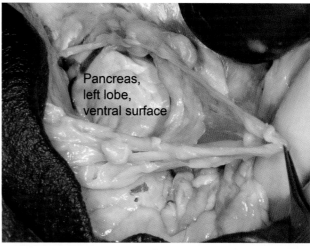

A   **B**

Figure 19-8 Normal surgical anatomy of left sided flank approach in sternal recumbency. **A,** Normal anatomy of left lateral flank approach in a dog in sternal recumbency. The most distal tip of the left pancreatic lobe is visible from the dorsal side of the dorsal leaf of the omentum. The ventral side is vaguely visible through the semitransparent omentum just cranially. An extended view of the dorsal surface of the pancreas is limited because of the splenic part of the omentum running caudally toward the mesocolon. **B,** The ventral surface of the left pancreatic lobe can be approached by bluntly opening the omental bursa in an avascular part.

Left Lateral Approach

With the patient in sternal recumbency, a left-sided laparoscopic flank approach gives access to the space dorsocaudal to the antrum of the stomach, dorsal to the head of the spleen, ventrolateral to the left kidney and adrenal gland. (Figure 19-8 depicts normal left lateral surgical anatomy of the canine pancreas in sternal recumbency.) In the left lateral approach, the left pancreatic lobe is located cranioventrally to the left kidney (see Figure 19-8). Only a limited part of the dorsal surface may be visible right away. A larger part of the lobe is approachable by retracting the omentum cranially, which usually exposes the pancreas, shining through the transparent omentum. Blunt perforation of the omentum in an avascular part gives access to the lobe (see Figure 19-8). Figure 19-9 shows the left flank laparoscopic approach to a large mass in the proximal left lobe of the pancreas. The distal part of the lobe was atrophied. Although accessible, the mass was too adhered to the large veins in the area to be safely resected laparoscopically. Fat deposition in the ligaments further complicates visibility. This section of the pancreas together with the corpus is the most difficult to access laparoscopically.

Right Lateral Approach

For the right lateral laparoscopic flank approach, the animal is placed in sternal recumbency and tilted 30 to 45 degrees to the left side. The normal right lateral flank anatomy is shown in Figure 19-10. For the laparoscopic approach, the initial portal is made 1 to 3 cm caudal to the last rib, 3 to 5 cm ventral to the transverse processes of the lumbar vertebrae. This gives access to the space lateroventral to the right kidney, dorsal to the pylorus, caudolateral to the liver, and lateral to the mesoduodenum. The complete right pancreatic lobe can be visualized and accessed. At rest, the lateral surface lies in full view (see Figure 19-10A). The proximal part of the right lobe, the corpus, and the proximal part of the left lobe can be accessed by carefully retracting the liver craniodorsally (see Figure 19-10B). The proximal left lobe can be followed until the portal vein. The medial surface of the right lobe, the dorsal surface of the corpus, and the proximal part of the left lobe can be approached by lifting the duodenum upward (see Figure 19-10C). Most of the draining lymph nodes of the pancreas are also accessible in the

right-sided approach (see Figure 19-10). The example of a laparoscopic approach in Figure 19-11 shows an insulinoma in the dorsal edge of the corpus with adjoining metastatic lymph node in a dog. A ventral midline laparoscopic approach in the same dog in dorsal recumbency is also shown (see Figure 19-11F) giving proper access to the tumor-containing corpus but not to the metastatic lymph node.

Surgical Technique

Specific Instrumentation
Required
- Curved endoscopic dissecting forceps
- Endoscopic grasping forceps, including Babcock
- Vessel-sealing device (e.g., Ligasure/ForceTriad, Covidien/Medtronic, Salem, CT or Harmonic Scalpel, Ethicon Endosurgery, Cincinnati, OH)

Alternatives
- 5-mm cup biopsy forceps
- Pretied loop ligature
- Hemostatic clips
- Endoscopic Metzenbaum scissors
- Other bipolar vessel-sealing devices

Facilitating Instruments
- Specimen retrieval bag for neoplastic lesions
- Fan retractors
- Endoscopic suction and irrigation instrument

Surgical Technique
Pancreatic Biopsy
In case of diffuse pancreatitis, the tip of the right limb of the pancreas is preferably sampled because it is most easily accessible. The right lobe is easily approached by either a ventral approach with the patient in dorsal recumbency or a right-sided flank approach with the patient in sterno-oblique recumbency. Biopsies are preferably

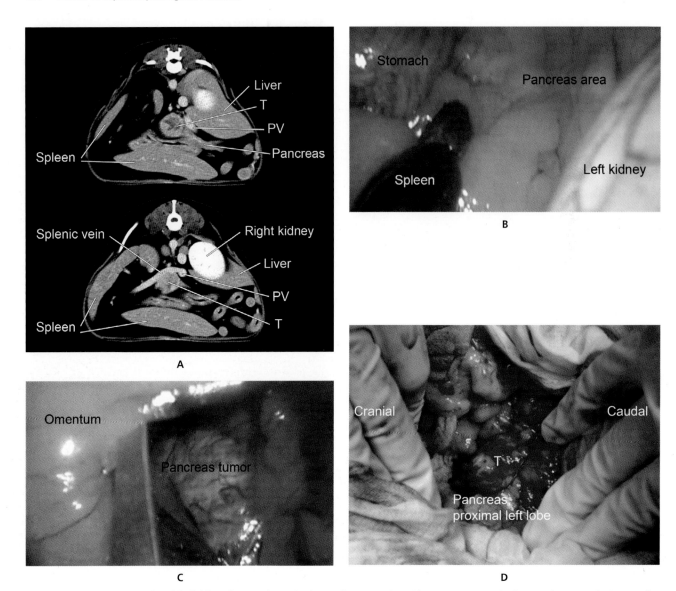

Figure 19-9 Laparoscopic images of the left lateral approach in sternal recumbency in a dog with pancreatic mass. **A,** Computed tomography images after intravenous contrast injection of a mass (T) in the proximal left lobe of the pancreas. The mass seems closely related to the portal (PV), splenic, and left gastric veins. The distal part of the left lobe is absent. **B,** Laparoscopic view through a left flank portal craniolateral to the left kidney showing the kidney, stomach, and spleen. **C,** Laparoscopic left-sided flank approach to the mass of the proximal left lobe of the pancreas, as seen in A. **D,** The same mass as in C through a standard ventral open laparotomy approach. Because of size, location in the proximal left lobe, and especially tight adherence to the splenic vein, laparoscopic removal was considered impossible.

taken from the edge of the pancreas to avoid the ductal system and larger vessels. The most common technique is the use of a cup or punch biopsy forceps. After placing the forceps at a distal edge of the pancreas (in case of generalized pancreatic pathology) or on a focal lesion, the forceps are closed, and a pause of 10 to 30 seconds is introduced to achieve hemostasis of crushed blood vessels. The forceps are then gently tugged away from the organ. Pancreatic biopsy for diagnosis of pancreatic disease is safe in dogs and cats, and biopsies taken with cup forceps did not negatively affect pancreatic health in both dogs and cats in prospective studies in healthy animals.[28,32-34] Another technique for pancreatic biopsy is the use of a pretied loop ligature. A pretied loop ligature can be placed proximal to the biopsy site or a small lesion to be excised. When tightened, the loop crushes through the pancreatic parenchyma, ligat-

ing vessels and ducts. Thereafter, the pancreatic tissue distal to the ligature can be transected using endoscopic Metzenbaum scissors. The loop ligature can also be used for excision of the distal tip of the pancreatic lobe after careful dissection from surrounding tissue.

Excision of Pancreatic Lesions

Larger lesions or lesions not located at the tip of a pancreatic lobe can be treated by a nodulectomy or partial pancreatectomy approach. For nodulectomy or partial pancreatectomy, the use of a vessel sealer and divider device is highly recommended for both dissecting the pancreatic tissue free from surrounding tissues as for dissection and excision of pancreatic parenchyma.[35] The use of a LigaSure vessel sealer and divider for pancreatic surgery was safe and effective, decreased surgery duration, and improved surgical performance in

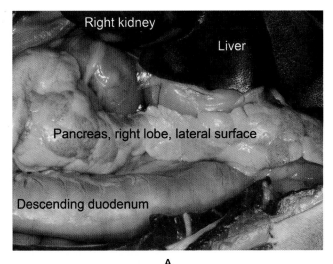

A

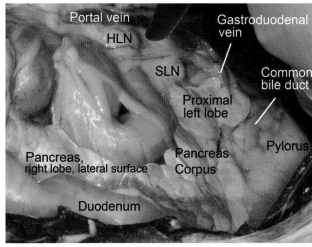

B

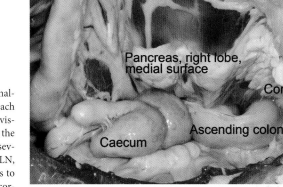

C

Figure 19-10 Normal anatomy of the right flank approach in sternal-oblique recumbency. **A,** Normal in situ anatomy of the right flank approach in sternal-oblique recumbency. The complete right pancreatic lobe is visible from the lateral side. **B,** Craniodorsal retraction of the liver exposes the corpus and proximal left lobe of the pancreas, portal vein, splenic vein, several lymph nodes, and common bile duct. HLN: hepatic lymph node; SLN, splenic lymph node. **C,** Dorsal retraction of the duodenum gives access to the medial surface of the right pancreatic lobe and dorsal surface of the corpus and proximal left lobe.

lesions with difficult access compared with conventional pancreatic surgery techniques.[35] In case of a focal lesion located in the middle of either pancreatic lobe, a partial pancreatectomy is usually preferred over nodulectomy to avoid postoperative pancreatitis or cyst formation. If a nodulectomy would be performed, the distal part of the pancreas may still have an adequate blood supply but often has no ductal structure that leads to the duodenum, which may increase the risk of local pancreatitis or sterile pancreatic abscess formation. The distal part of the lobe that will be removed is fixated using endoscopic grasping forceps while LigaSure forceps are used to carefully dissect the pancreatic tissue, including the lesion, free from surrounding tissues. Special attention should be paid to the vital structures surrounding the pancreatic tissue, such as the pancreatic ducts, pancreaticoduodenal arteries, gastroduodenal vein, and common bile duct associated with the right pancreatic lobe and the portal and splenic vein, and pancreatic, hepatic, and splenic artery associated with the left pancreatic lobe. Dissection is continued until the distal part of the pancreatic lobe, including the lesion, is dissected free. The partial pancreatectomy is completed by sealing and dividing the pancreatic parenchyma proximal to the

lesion. The extent of the surgical margin depends on the type of lesion and distance to vital structures.

If the lesion is located close to the pancreatic body, a marginal excision should be carried out by dissecting close to the lesion. This is only feasible if the lesion is quite small and comprises only one third of the circumference of the pancreatic lobe.

If minor bleeding persists at a biopsy or surgery site, placing pieces of absorbable gelatin sponge on the area is usually sufficient. When using a vessel-sealing device for surgery, most bleeding can also be adequately coagulated. Other options are the use of endoscopic vascular clips or a pretied loop ligature. The use of an endoscopic linear stapler for partial pancreatectomy has also been described in dogs.[36]

Challenges to the Technique

The pancreatic tissue should be handled as gently as possible to prevent postoperative pancreatitis. Grasping forceps may never be placed on pancreatic tissue that will remain in the patient. Extreme caution should also be taken to prevent damage to the ductal system and the pancreaticoduodenal arteries in case a mass has to be

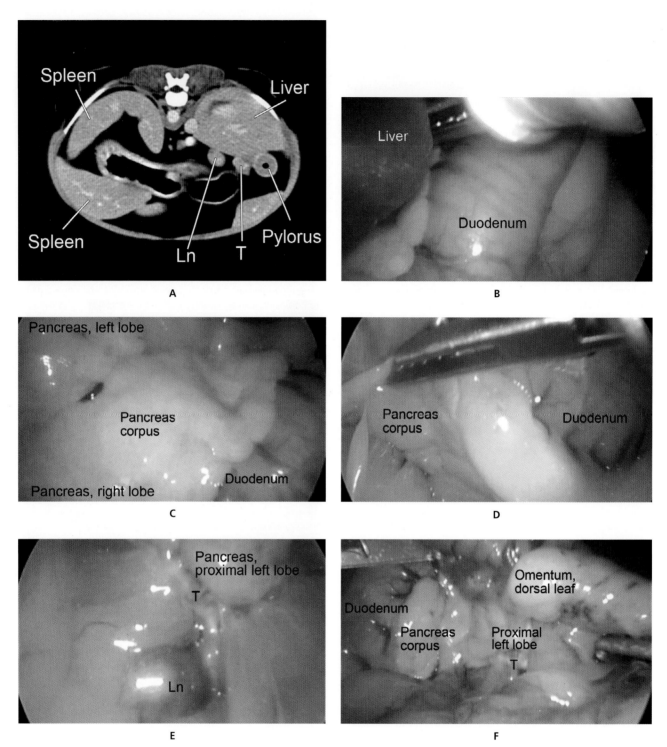

Figure 19-11 Laparoscopic images of the right lateral approach in sternal recumbency and ventral midline approach in dorsal recumbency in a dog with insulinoma. **A,** Computed tomography image of insulinoma (T) in the dorsal edge of the pancreatic corpus and an adjoining metastatic lymph node (Ln). **B,** Right lateral flank laparoscopic approach in sternal-oblique recumbency. The liver has to be manipulated craniodorsally so the corpus of the pancreas can be visualized. **C,** Corpus and proximal left lobe of the pancreas, dorsal surface. **D,** Dorsal retraction of the duodenum gives access to the ventral surface of the corpus and proximal left lobe. **E,** A small insulinoma (T) is located at the edge of the corpus/proximal left lobe. A metastatic lymph node (Ln) lies just distal to it. **F,** The same insulinoma (T) at the edge of the corpus/proximal left lobe of the pancreas as seen from a ventral midline laparoscopic approach with the patient in dorsal recumbency. The omentum is retracted cranially. The metastatic lymph node is not easily visualized in this approach.

resected from the portions of the pancreas that are the closest to the pancreatic body. The pancreatic blood supply and important surrounding structures should always be identified during surgery and preferably before surgery using advanced imaging modalities, so that the specific surgical procedure is carried out knowing the precise anatomic relations and considering the areas of increased risk of complications. In case of insulinoma surgery, excessive manipulation of the tumor during surgery should be minimized because this can trigger increased insulin secretion, leading to more profound hypoglycemia. Furthermore, in cases of insulinoma, profound fat deposition in the ligaments surrounding the pancreas can greatly reduce visibility of important tissue structures. Apart from accessing the tumor itself, it may be difficult to evaluate local lymph nodes and liver parenchyma for metastasis. Extensive preoperative staging using advanced imaging techniques is therefore mandatory in case of a laparoscopic approach for insulinoma.

Access to the corpus and the left pancreatic lobe can be difficult, and it may be necessary to change approaches during surgery to enhance access to specific lesions. Laparoscopic pancreatic surgery requires advanced endoscopic surgery skills, and as for all advanced endoscopic surgery procedures, one should always consider the possibility of conversion to an open laparotomy approach.

Complications and Prognosis

Complications that have been described for open pancreatic surgery in small animals include pancreatitis, formation of a pancreatic fistula, and persistent bleeding from the pancreatic parenchyma. There are no reports on complications after laparoscopic pancreatic surgery in small animals. However, in the human literature, it has been described that patients who underwent laparoscopic distal pancreatectomy or laparoscopic pancreatic enucleation had significantly decreased blood loss and comparable postoperative morbidity compared with patients who underwent open pancreatic surgery.[1]

Postoperative Care

Pain Control

Local infiltration of portal sites or intraperitoneal application of bupivacaine may reduce postoperative pain,[37-41] but there is no general consensus on its clinical efficacy in both human and veterinary medicine at this time.

At the authors' institution, 5 to 20 μg/kg/hr IV constant-rate infusion (CRI) of fentanyl is often used together with isoflurane during maintenance of anesthesia in patients undergoing pancreatic surgery. In the postoperative period, fentanyl can be continued at an IV dosage of 5 to 10 μg/kg/hr. One day after surgery, fentanyl is usually discontinued and replaced by 0.3 mg/kg IV methadone every 4 hours or 10 to 20 μg/kg IV buprenorphine every 6 hours until discharge. In severely painful patients, 3 to 5 μg/kg/min IV CRI of ketamine can be added. On discharge, if no signs of pancreatitis are present in otherwise healthy patients, 2 mg/kg of oral (PO) carprofen twice a day is usually prescribed.[35] Alternatively, 3 to 5 mg/kg PO tramadol every 6 to 8 hours can be used after discharge if nonsteroidal antiinflammatory drugs are contraindicated.

Prophylactic Measures

Historically, it has been suggested that oral food should be withheld for 24 to 48 hours after surgery to reduce pancreatic secretions.

However, there is no good evidence to suggest that this is necessary. In the authors' experience, offering a bland, well-balanced diet right after surgery is well tolerated by most patients. If a patient refuses to eat, balanced electrolyte solutions should be administered intravenously until oral intake of food and water resumes. Furthermore, when patients show clinical signs of pancreatitis that persist for more than 24 hours after surgery, further diagnostics, including serum lipase activity, should be performed. Also, in patients with vomiting and inappetence, additional therapy with ranitidine, maropitant, and metoclopramide is indicated for several days.[16]

After insulinoma resection, blood glucose levels should be closely monitored. If glucose levels are very low (<2 mmol/L) and the patient refuses to eat and demonstrates clinical signs of hypoglycemia, the dog should be stabilized using a balanced electrolyte solution with 5% dextrose intravenously. Moreover, therapy with diazoxide (5–30 mg/kg twice daily) should be initiated. IV glucose can be discontinued if the animal has a stable and normal glucose level or in case the animal becomes hyperglycemic. In some dogs, hyperglycemia may occur because of atrophy of the normal β cells by feedback inhibition. Hyperglycemia might be transient and resolve with time. If hyperglycemia is persistent, administration of insulin is required. In most cases, normal pancreatic endocrine function should eventually resume; however, some dogs require lifelong insulin therapy.[16]

Hospitalization Time

There are no data available on hospitalization times of small animal patients that underwent laparoscopic pancreatic surgery. A mean hospitalization time of 2 days has been reported for dogs that underwent open partial pancreatectomy using LigaSure for insulinoma resection.[35] In human medicine, significantly reduced hospital stays have been reported after laparoscopic distal pancreatectomies and laparoscopic pancreatic enucleations compared with open partial pancreatectomies and enucleations.[1,2,42] Therefore, it is expected that similar results will hold true for veterinary laparoscopic pancreatic surgery.

References

1 Subar, D., Gobardhan, P.D., Gayet, B. (2014) Laparoscopic pancreatic surgery. An overview of the literature and experiences of a single center. Best Pract Res Clin Gastroenterol 28, 123-132.

2 Briggs, C.D., Mann, C.D., Irving, G.R., et al. (2009) Systematic review of minimally invasive pancreatic resection. J Gastrointest Surg 13, 1129-1137.

3 Venkat, R., Edil, B.H., Schulick, R.D., et al. (2012) Laparoscopic distal pancreatectomy is associated with significantly less overall morbidity compared to the open technique: a systematic review and meta-analysis. Ann Surg 255, 1048-1059.

4 Steiner, J. (2010) Canine pancreatitis. In: Ettinger, S., Feldman, E. (eds.) Textbook of Veterinary Internal Medicine, vol 2, 4th edn. Saunders/Elsevier, St. Louis, pp. 1695-1703.

5 Hess, R., Saunders, H., Van Winkle, T. (1995) Clinical, clincopathologic, radiographic, and ultrasonographic abnormalities in dogs with fatal acute pancreatitis: 70 cases (1986-1995). J Am Vet Med Assoc 213, 665-670.

6 Ferreri, J.A., Hardam, E., Kimmel, S.E., et al. (2003) Clinical differentiation of acute necrotizing from chronic nonsuppurative pancreatitis in cats: 63 cases (1996-2001). J Am Vet Med Assoc 223, 469-474.

7 Anderson, J.R., Cornell, K.K., Parnell, N.K., et al. (2008) Pancreatic abscess in 36 dogs: a retrospective analysis of prognostic indicators. J Am Anim Hosp Assoc 44, 171-179.

8 Coleman, M., Robson, M. (2005) Pancreatic masses following pancreatitis: pancreatic pseudocysts, necrosis, and abscesses. Compend Contin Educ Pract Vet 27, 147-154.

9 Withrow, S. (2007) Exocrine pancreatic cancer. In: Withrow, S., Vail, D. (eds.) Small animal Clinical Oncology, vol 1 4th edn. Saunders/Elsevier, St. Louis, pp. 479-480.

10 Caywood, D., Klausner, J., Leary, T.O. (1988) Pancreatic insulin-secreting neoplasms: clinical, diagnostic, and prognostic features in 73 dogs. J Am Anim Hosp Assoc 24, 577-584.

11 Buishand, F.O., Kik, M., Kirpensteijn, J. (2010) Evaluation for clinic-pathological criteria and the Ki67 index as prognostic indicators in canine insulinoma. Vet J 185, 62-67.

12 Vergine, M., Pozzo, S., Pogliani, E., et al. (2005) Common bile duct obstruction due to a duodenal gastrinoma in a dog. Vet J 170, 141-143.

13 Mizuno, T., Hiraoka, H., Yoshioka, C., et al. (2009) Superficial necrolytic dermatitis associated with extrapancreatic glucagonoma in a dog. Vet Dermatol 20, 72-79.

14 Evans, H.E. (1993) The digestive apparatus and abdomen: the pancreas. In: Evans, H.E., Evans, S.A. (eds.) Miller's Anatomy of the Dog, 3rd edn. Saunders, Philadelphia, pp. 458-460.

15 Cáceres, A.V., Zwingenberger, A.L., Hardam, E., et al. (2006) Helical computed tomographic angiography of the normal canine pancreas. Vet Radiol Ultrasound 47, 270-278.

16 Buishand, F.O., Kirpensteijn, J. (2014) The pancreas. In: Williams, J., Niles, J. (eds.) BSAVA Manual of Canine and Feline Abdominal Surgery, 2nd edn. Wiley-Blackwell, Hoboken, NJ.

17 Hecht, S., Henry, G. (2007) Sonographic evaluation of the normal and abnormal pancreas. Clin Tech Small Anim Pract 22, 115-221.

18 Buishand, F.O., Kirpensteijn, J. (2013) Canine and feline insulinoma. In: Monnet, E. (ed.) Small Animal Soft Tissue Surgery, 1st edn. Wiley-Blackwell, Ames, IA, pp. 32-42.

19 Robben, J.H., Pollak, Y.W., Kirpensteijn, J., et al. (2005) Comparison of ultrasonography, computed tomography, and single-photon emission computed tomography for detection and localization of canine insulinoma. J Vet Intern Med 19, 15-22.

20 Iseri, T., Yamada, K., Chijiwa, J., et al. (2007) Dynamic computed tomography of the pancreas in normal dogs and in a dog with pancreatic insulinoma. Vet Radiol Ultrasound 48, 328-331.

21 Mai, W., Caceres, A.V. (2008) Dual-phase computed tomographic angiography in three dogs with pancreatic insulinoma. Vet Radiol Ultrasound 49, 141-148.

22 Choi, J., Keh, S., Kim, S., et al. (2012) Diagnostic imaging of malignant insulinoma in a dog. Korean J Vet Res 52, 205-208.

23 Altschul, M., Simpson, K.W., Dykes, N.L., et al. (1997) Evaluation of somatostatin analogues for the detection and treatment of gastrinoma in a dog. J Small Anim Pract 38, 286-291.

24 Oberkirchner, U., Linder, K.E., Zadrozny, L., et al. (2010) Successful treatment of canine necrolytic migratory erythema (superficial necrolytic dermatitis) due to metastatic glucagonoma with octreotide. Vet Dermatol 21, 510-516.

25 Van Nimwegen, S.A., Kirpensteijn, J. (2014) Endoscopic surgery in cats: laparoscopy. In: Langley-Hobbs, S.J., Demetriou, J.L., Ladlow, J.F. (eds.) Feline Soft Tissue and General Surgery. Elsevier/Saunders, Philadelphia, pp. 253-268.

26 Barnes, R.F., Greenfield, C.L., Schaeffer, D.J., et al. (2006) Comparison of biopsy samples obtained using standard endoscopic instruments and the harmonic scalpel during laparoscopic and laparoscopic-assisted surgery in normal dogs. Vet Surg 35, 243-251.

27 Mayhew, P. (2009) Techniques for laparoscopic and laparoscopic-assisted biopsy of abdominal organs. Compend Contin Educ Pract Vet 31, 170-176.

28 Cosford, K.L., Shmon, C.L., Myers, S.L., et al. (2010) Prospective evaluation of laparoscopic pancreatic biopsies in 11 healthy cats. J Vet Intern Med 24, 104-113.

29 Naan, E.C., Kirpensteijn, J., Dupré G.P., et al. (2013) Innovative approach to laparoscopic adrenalectomy for treatment of unilateral adrenal gland tumors in dogs. Vet Surg 42, 710-715.

30 Naitoh, T., Garcia-Ruiz, A., Vladisavljevic, S., et al. (2002) Gastrointestinal transit and stress response after laparoscopic versus conventional distal pancreatectomy in the canine model. Surg Endosc 16, 1627-1630.

31 van Nimwegen, S.A., Kirpensteijn, J. (2007) Laparoscopic ovariectomy in cats: comparison of laser and bipolar electrocoagulation. J Fel Med Surg 9, 397-403.

32 Harmoinen, J., Saari, S., Rinkinen, M., et al. (2002) Evaluation of pancreatic forceps biopsy by laparoscopy in healthy beagles. Vet Ther 3, 31-36.

33 Webb, C.B., Trott, C. (2008) Laparoscopic diagnosis of pancreatic disease in dogs and cats. J Vet Intern Med 22, 1263-1266.

34 Webb, C.B. (2008) Feline laparoscopy for gastrointestinal disease. Top Companion Anim Med 23, 193-199.

35 Wouters, E.G.H., Buishand, F.O., Kik, M., et al. (2011) Use of a bipolar vessel-sealing device in resection of canine insulinoma. J Small Anim Pract 52, 139-145.

36 Biel, M., Klumpp, S., Peppler, C., et al. (2011) Partial pancreatectomy using a linear stapler device for the treatment of pancreatic neoplasias in three dogs. Tierarztliche Praxis Ausgabe K: Kleintiere Heimtiere 39, 441-447.

37 Kim, Y.K., Lee, S.S., Suh, E.H., et al. (2012) Sprayed intraperitoneal bupivacaine reduces early postoperative pain behavior and biochemical stress response after laparoscopic ovariohysterectomy in dogs. Vet J 191, 188-192.

38 Coughlin, S.M., Karanicolas, P.J., Emmerton-Coughlin, H.M., et al. (2010) Better late than never? Impact of local analgesia timing on postoperative pain in laparoscopic surgery: a systematic review and metaanalysis. Surg Endosc 24, 3167-3176.

39 Kahokehr, A., Sammour, T., Srinivasa, S. et al. (2011) Systematic review and meta-analysis of intraperitoneal local anaesthetic for pain reduction after laparoscopic gastric procedures. Br J Surg 98: 29-36.

40 Marks, J.L., Ata, B., Tulandi, T. (2012) Systematic review and metaanalysis of intraperitoneal instillation of local anesthetics for reduction of pain after gynecologic laparoscopy. J Minim Invasive Gynecol 19, 545-553.

41 Møiniche, S., Jørgensen, H., Wetterslev, J., et al. (2000) Local anesthetic infiltration for postoperative pain relief after laparoscopy: a qualitative and quantitative systematic review of intraperitoneal, port-site infiltration and mesosalpinx block. Anesth Analg 90, 899-912.

42 Crippa, S., Bassi, C., Salvia, R., et al. (2007) Enucleation of pancreatic neoplasms. Br J Surg 94, 1254-1259.

20 Laparoscopic Renal Biopsy

Keith Richter and Sheri Ross

Key Points

- Primary indications for kidney biopsy are severe, unresponsive, or progressive proteinuria and unexplained acute or rapidly progressive kidney injury.
- It is important to obtain samples from only the renal cortex to maximize the information obtained from the biopsy and avoid bleeding complications.
- Laparoscopy is a safe and effective method of procuring renal tissue for biopsy.
- Renal biopsies should be evaluated with light, immunofluorescence, and electron microscopy by an experienced nephropathologist.
- Patients should be monitored for 24 hours after the procedure to identify major complications such as hemorrhage.

Renal biopsy analysis is emerging as an important diagnostic step for evaluating dogs and cats with a variety of renal diseases, particularly those associated with proteinuria, unexplained renomegaly, suspected systemic diseases with renal involvement (e.g., Lyme disease or systemic lupus erythematosus), and infiltrative renal diseases. Proper biopsy evaluation may give insight into etiology, treatment options, and prognosis.

Recent advances in imaging technology, the use of multiple imaging modalities, and newer biopsy methods have resulted in improvement in veterinary clinician's' ability to safely procure renal tissue for evaluation. There are several means of obtaining renal samples, including fine-needle aspiration (FNA), percutaneous methods (blind, ultrasound guided, and computed tomography [CT] guided), laparoscopy, and laparotomy. All techniques have both advantages and disadvantages, which should be carefully considered before choosing the appropriate sampling method for an individual patient. Laparoscopic renal biopsy has emerged as a noninvasive and safe method and has been described in humans[1-5] and dogs.[6-10] This chapter discusses the details of laparoscopic renal biopsy.

Indications for Renal Biopsy

In veterinary medicine, renal biopsy is indicated in patients in which a histologic diagnosis is likely to influence the therapeutic management of the patient or provide significant prognostic information. Therefore, primary indications for kidney biopsy are substantial,

unresponsive, or progressive proteinuria and unexplained acute or rapidly progressive kidney injury.[11,12] It is important to realize that these indications are not absolute and that in some cases, clinical and laboratory data may suggest a predictable histologic pattern and therefore kidney biopsy may not be required. Common indications and contraindications for renal biopsy are listed in Box 20-1.

In patients with chronic kidney disease (CKD), particularly those in stage 4, it is unlikely that renal biopsy will alter the diagnosis, prognosis, or therapy of the patient.[13] Although comparative data are not available in veterinary medicine, in human medicine, patients with end-stage renal disease are more likely to have clinically significant complications associated with renal biopsy.[14]

In patients with severe acute kidney injury (AKI) or those with AKI not responding as expected to medical management, kidney biopsy may be helpful in determining the underlying etiology and thus in directing specific therapy. More commonly, kidney biopsies are obtained in cases of AKI for prognostic purposes. The overall appearance of the tissue; the integrity of the basement membrane; and the degree of regeneration, if present, may all help the clinician determine if the patient is able to recover from the injury. This information is very important to owners who are faced with continuing intensive and expensive therapies, such as hemodialysis, when supporting patients with AKI.

In veterinary medicine, renal biopsies are most commonly obtained percutaneously under ultrasound guidance. Possible reasons why a clinician might choose a laparoscopic approach

Small Animal Laparoscopy and Thoracoscopy, First Edition. Edited by Boel A. Fransson and Philipp D. Mayhew.
© 2015 by ACVS Foundation. Published 2015 by John Wiley & Sons, Inc.
Companion website: www.wiley.com/go/fransson/laparoscopy

Box 20-1 Indications and Contraindication for Renal Biopsy

Indications for Renal Biopsy

Persistent, progressive, or nonresponsive proteinuria
Acute severe or progressive kidney injury
Suspected infiltrative renal disease
Renal mass
Suspected systemic diseases with renal involvement

Contraindications for Renal Biopsy

Chronic kidney disease, stage IV
Severe anemia
Refractory coagulopathy
Uncontrolled hypertension
Hydronephrosis
Uncontrolled pyelonephritis
Cystic renal disease
Poor patient immobilization
Inexperienced operator

over other percutaneous methods include failed ultrasound-guided biopsy (including procurement of samples that contain mainly medullary tissue), lack of ultrasound skills, unavailability of ultrasound, and severe obesity or patients with other anatomic anomalies that would make a percutaneous approach difficult or dangerous. Other potential reasons to consider laparoscopy over ultrasound-guided biopsy include coagulopathy (in which case absolute precision can be achieved with laparoscopy and hemostasis can be achieved under direct vision in a controlled fashion) and when other organs need to be sampled at the same time (in particular the liver, in which case needle biopsies are often inadequate for accurate interpretation). In one study in dogs, laparoscopy was shown to be superior to ultrasound-guided biopsy in terms of the number of glomeruli obtained and resulted in fewer complications.[7] Despite those findings, there is strong institutional bias in the relative success of ultrasound-guided biopsy, usually related to the skills of the ultrasonographer. This is demonstrated by the results of another study in which renal biopsies obtained at other institutions had no difference in quality when comparing ultrasound-guided and laparoscopy-guided biopsies.[10] In another study, 96% of samples obtained from 25 dogs undergoing laparoscopic renal biopsy were classified as excellent, with only minor complications.[8]

Preoperative Considerations

Before biopsy, the patient must be assessed thoroughly to identify factors that could increase the risk of complications of renal biopsy. One of the most important complications is postbiopsy hemorrhage, which can be life threatening in some cases. However, the best preprocedure predictor of renal hemorrhage is unclear. In one study of dogs and cats undergoing ultrasound-guided percutaneous renal and hepatic biopsy, patients with thrombocytopenia were at increased risk for major complications compared with patients with normal platelet numbers.[15] In this study, 8.9% (15 of 168) of patients undergoing renal biopsy had major complications. This suggests that delaying the biopsy until the platelet numbers improve might be warranted, but often this is not clinically feasible. The clinician must therefore weigh the benefits of the information gained from the biopsy with the risk of major bleeding complications. Because coagulation status should be assessed, the minimum data

base should include prothrombin time, activated partial thromboplastin time, and a platelet count. Other methods of coagulation assessment may be better predictors of hemorrhage, including assessing proteins induced by vitamin K antagonism (PIVKA) and thrombelastography. Although these methods may have advantages in other clinical situations (e.g., patients with hepatic disease, hypercoagulable patients, and other critically ill patients), they have not been described in patients before renal biopsy. If it is deemed necessary to obtain a biopsy in a patient with thrombocytopenia or a coagulopathy, the clinician should use the smallest needle and fewest numbers of samples necessary to obtain a diagnostic sample. Higher numbers of biopsies increases the risk of a drop in hematocrit, especially after the second sample.[15] The clinician should also be prepared to monitor patients with coagulopathies or thrombocytopenia closely and have compatible blood products available if needed.

Another risk factor for hemorrhage is systemic hypertension, a common finding in patients with renal disease.[16] Studies quantifying the risk of systemic arterial hypertension in patients undergoing renal biopsy are lacking in dogs and cats. However, it seems prudent to attempt to normalize arterial pressure before renal biopsy.

Patients undergoing renal biopsy must be placed under general anesthesia, and therefore every effort should be made to normalize any metabolic or cardiovascular abnormalities that may be present. The patient's hydration status must be carefully assessed because patients with renal disease are commonly over- or underhydrated. In patients that are underhydrated, intravenous fluid support should be administered before general anesthesia, especially if they are hypotensive. In patients that are overhydrated, fluid therapy should be more judicious or discontinued, and if the patient is oliguric or anuric, stabilization with hemodialysis should be considered.

Before undergoing laparoscopy, the patient should have an ultrasound examination to evaluate the internal architecture of the kidney. Relative contraindications to laparoscopy-guided needle biopsy include renal cysts, ureteral obstruction, and hydronephrosis. These can be readily detected via ultrasonography. In addition, ultrasonography can detect focal renal lesions (e.g., masses, infiltrative areas) to allow selection of the proper kidney and region to be biopsied.

Patient Preparation

After routine preparation, the patient is placed under general anesthesia. It is important that the bladder be voided before the procedure to avoid inadvertent bladder puncture during trocar placement. Most of the ventral abdomen should be clipped and surgically prepared, allowing the clinician the option to biopsy either kidney. For the unlikely possibility that the gross findings determine the opposite kidney should be biopsied (e.g., adhesions or other anatomic factors that create poor visualization), advance preparation of the patient makes it possible to turn the animal over to access the opposite kidney. Most animals needing a renal biopsy have diffuse and bilateral disease, so it does not matter which kidney is biopsied. In most animals, the left kidney lies in a more caudal location and is therefore easier to sample, in which case the procedure is performed in right lateral recumbency or right dorsolateral recumbency, with the patient placed at a 45-degree angle. If there is focal disease in the right kidney (as determined by ultrasonography or CT), then the animal is placed in opposite recumbency. The operating room setup is depicted in Figure 20-1.

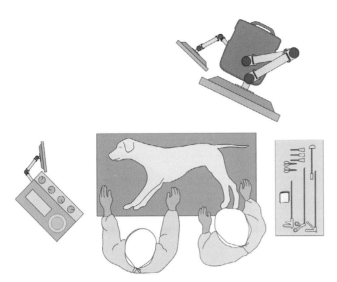

Figure 20-1 Operating room setup for laparoscopic renal biopsy procedure.

Instrument Placement

Laparoscopic access is established 2 cm lateral and 2 cm caudal to the umbilicus (Figure 20-2) with pneumoperitoneum pressure of 12 to 15 mm Hg. This location provides an appropriate working distance. Because of the caudal access, emptying the bladder before the procedure is imperative. Access is usually suitable for examination of both the liver and kidney, if required. When the liver is examined, the animal is tilted at a 45-degree oblique angle, and when the kidney is examined, the animal can be left in that position or repositioned in lateral recumbency during the procedure. Usually the right side of the liver is evaluated (including the biliary tree and

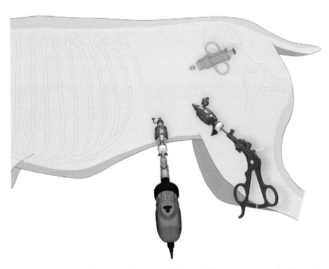

Figure 20-2 Port placement for renal biopsy. The scope cannula is positioned 2 cm caudal and 2 cm lateral to the umbilicus. If the liver and kidney are to be evaluated and changes are bilateral, a right-sided approach is advantageous because the liver is harder to visualize from the left side. However, if only kidney biopsies are to be procured, the left kidney is more caudal and easier to biopsy. A second cannula is optional but may be placed a few centimeters lateral to the scope portal for retraction using a blunt probe. The biopsy needle portal is placed transcutaneously at the cranial or caudal pole of the kidney.

right limb of the pancreas), necessitating examination of the right kidney if a single entry site for the scope is desired. However, if the left kidney needs to be evaluated, the clinician should not hesitate to remove the equipment after hepatic evaluation, turn the animal over, and reinsert the equipment in the required location.

In some cases, a second cannula is helpful for introduction of a blunt probe. This insertion site is located a few centimeters lateral to the cannula used to introduce the scope. The blunt probe can be helpful for retraction of overlying omentum or bowel if obscuring visualization of the kidney. It can also be useful to apply direct pressure to the biopsy site if there is excessive hemorrhage. In rare instances, laparoscopic retractors may be necessary to isolate the kidney from surrounding omentum, bowel, or other viscera. These can be deployed through the accessory cannula.

Selection of the Biopsy Needle

For renal biopsy, a completely automated biopsy needle (Box 20-2) is preferred over manual or semiautomated. Completely automated needles use a spring-loaded mechanism to thrust the inner obturator (with a side-notch biopsy tray) into the kidney followed by the outer cutting sheath in a fraction of a second. These needles can be operated with one hand while the other hand operates the scope or camera to allow precise placement of the biopsy instrument. There is minimal displacement of the kidney, a shorter intraparenchymal phase, and a more reliable yield of tissue. Using the rapid cutting action, the renal tissue tends to be less fragmented. Semiautomated needles (see Box 20-2) require manual thrusting of the internal obturator into the kidney followed by an automatic thrusting of the outer sheath by a spring-loaded mechanism. These needles have the advantage of control over the final tip position because the tip of the needle can be precisely localized before the outer cutting sheath is deployed. However, this is mainly an advantage with ultrasound-guided needle biopsy because the tip can no longer be visualized laparoscopically when it is within the kidney, thus making fully automated needles preferable. Manually operated needles require two hands to deploy when the needle has entered the kidney, necessitating an assistant to hold the scope. More important, though, manual cutting needles provide inferior samples compared with fully automated needles. More recently, a novel end-cut needle has been developed (BioPince; Angiotech, Vancouver, British Columbia, Canada). Rather than the side-notch style of the needles described earlier, this needle has an end-cut design in which the

Box 20-2 Examples of completely automated, semi-automated, manual, and novel end-cut biopsy needles

Completely Automated

Monopty needle (C.R. Bard, Tempe, AZ)
Max-Core needle (C.R. Bard)
Magnum needle (C.R. Bard)
Achieve needle (CareFusion, San Diego, CA)

Semi-Automated

Temno needle (CareFusion)
Vet-Core needle (Smiths Medical PM, Norwell, MA)

Manual

Tru-Cut needle (CareFusion)

End Cut

BioPince needle (Angiotech, Vancouver, British Columbia, Canada)

entire lumen and almost the whole length of advancement of the needle are used to capture the specimen. A coaxial pincer, which slides through a slit at the tip of the device, cuts and encloses the full core specimen. In humans undergoing renal biopsy, this 16-gauge needle type provided superior samples and fewer major complications than a 14-gauge fully automated side-notch style needle.[17] However, in 100 dogs, high-quality biopsies were obtained with both 18-gauge end-cut needles and 18-gauge semiautomated side-notch style needles.[18] In general, most completely automated biopsy needles yield diagnostic quality biopsy specimens, and the choice of instrument should remain one of personal preference.

The size of the biopsy needle is another important consideration. A single puncture with a 14- or 16-gauge needle is generally adequate for conventional histopathology alone. Optimally, however, individual samples are obtained for light, immunofluorescence, and electron microscopy, thus necessitating at least two core samples. In dogs, 14- and 16-gauge needles have yielded higher glomeruli numbers, adequate in more than 96% of cases, but 18 gauge needles showed less glomeruli and more crush artifact.[7,8] In human patients, larger needles (14 and 16 gauge) have been shown superior,[19,20] but controversy exists.[21] In general, the authors prefer 16-gauge needles. This appears to provide the best balance of diagnostic yield without excessive bleeding.

Biopsy Technique

The kidneys should be examined for position, contour, and relationship to other structures. The kidneys are often covered with omentum, so that a blunt probe (or biopsy needle) inserted through a second puncture is used to "sweep" the omentum in a caudal direction to uncover the kidney. In obese patients, perirenal fat often obscures visualization of much of the kidney. Generally, the gross examination is noncontributory, and the main value of the examination is to direct a biopsy of the kidney.

The insertion site of the needle is selected after visualizing the kidney and is located at the closest spot on the body wall overlying the kidney. This can be ascertained by using a gloved finger and depressing the body wall repeatedly, noting where the finger causes an indentation as viewed from the laparoscopic camera. The finger is then moved in the proper direction until the depression is seen to be directly overlying the caudal pole or cranial pole of the kidney (avoiding the center of the kidney). The path of the needle should be planned to obtain as much cortical tissue as possible, usually perpendicular to the long axis of the kidney, avoiding as much of the medulla as possible and missing the renal pelvis (Figure 20-3). The needle is inserted through a small stab incision in the skin, typically made with a #11 blade. The needle is directly visualized and positioned either adjacent to the renal capsule or perhaps just immediately under the capsule (Figure 20-4). If it is inserted too far into the kidney, cortical tissue may be missed, or it may go completely through the kidney. If the patient is overinsufflated, the body wall may be too far from the kidney, making optimal needle placement difficult. If that is the case, the pneumoperitoneum is gradually decreased until there are less tension and a shorter distance between the body wall and kidney. This usually then allows appropriate needle placement. When the needle is properly positioned, it is activated to cut the biopsy. The author generally takes three to four samples for light microscopy, immunofluorescence microscopy, and electron microscopy (see later section on biopsy handling). Occasionally, more samples are obtained if there is minimal bleeding and there is a need for additional tissue. If there is

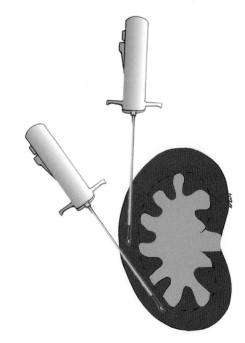

Figure 20-3 Graphic representation of acceptable needle path angles. The needle is positioned with the sample site within the renal cortex. Penetration of the renal pelvis is avoided because it renders nondiagnostic samples and greatly increases the risk for complications such as bleeding and urine leakage.

excessive bleeding, usually pressure with a blunt probe for a few minutes will control hemorrhage (Figure 20-5). Hemostatic agents (Gelfoam; Pfizer, New York, NY) can also be deployed using laparoscopic forceps and placed over the bleeding site (Figure 20-6). When the clinician is satisfied that hemorrhage is minimal, the procedure is completed by removing all instruments and pneumoperitoneum in the standard manner (see Chapter 9). Usually a single suture is placed in the body wall and skin at the laparoscopic port sites. Generally, no suture is needed at the needle insertion site.

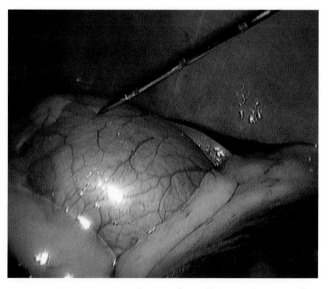

Figure 20-4 Laparoscopic visualization of a needle biopsy. (Courtesy of Dr. Philipp Mayhew, University of California, Davis.)

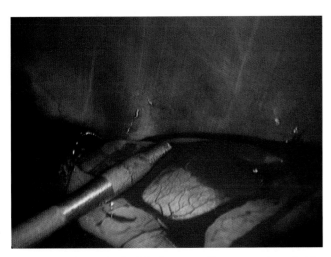

Figure 20-5 After removal of the biopsy needle, pressure is applied by a blunt probe to decrease the hemorrhage from the site. (Courtesy of Dr. Philipp Mayhew, University of California, Davis.)

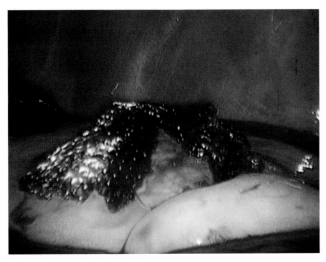

Figure 20-6 A hemostatic cellulose product has been applied to the biopsy site to aid in hemorrhage control. (Courtesy of Dr. Philipp Mayhew, University of California, Davis.)

Sample Handling and Submission

After a kidney biopsy has been obtained, it is crucial to ensure that it is of adequate diagnostic quality. Although the optimum number of glomeruli in a renal biopsy is not universally accepted, generally at least five glomeruli are required for adequate interpretation of light microscopy and a similar number for immunofluorescence and electron microscopy. When submitting samples for evaluation, the clinician should ensure that the biopsies are evaluated by experienced veterinary nephropathologists. Although light microscopy plays an important role in diagnosing renal disease, definitive diagnosis and complete characterization of the ultrastructure abnormalities of the glomerulus can only be obtained using a combination of light, immunohistochemistry, and electron microscopy. Standard light microscopy evaluation using only hematoxylin and eosin (H&E) staining is rarely sufficient to properly characterize most renal pathology.

Historically, the utility of renal biopsies in veterinary medicine has been limited by the availability of advanced evaluation techniques. Currently, there is an active International Veterinary Renal Pathology Group operating under the auspices of the World Small Animal Veterinary Association. The long-term goals of this initiative are to better characterize, understand, and evaluate glomerular diseases in dogs. Renal biopsy samples can be submitted to specific centers for thorough evaluation (International Veterinary Renal Pathology Service, Department of Veterinary Biosciences, The Ohio State University, Columbus, OH 43210; Contact: Dr Rachel Cianciolo, rachel.cianciolo@cvm.osu.edu; In Europe: Utrecht Veterinary Nephropathology Service, Utrecht University, Utrecht, The Netherlands; Contact: Dr Astrid M. van Dongen, a.m.vandongen@uu.nl). Before a renal biopsy, the clinician is encouraged to contact one of these centers to obtain a renal biopsy kit. These kits contain the required fixatives and instructions for proper sample submission.[22]

Extreme care must be used when handling renal biopsy samples to avoid crush artifact. Ideally, samples should be flushed from the biopsy instrument onto a glass slide using a gentle stream of chilled 0.9% saline. Any division of a biopsy core should be done with a sharp scalpel blade to minimize sample damage. In most cases of renal biopsy, a minimum of two good cortical samples should be obtained. The first sample should be submitted in 10% buffered formalin solution for light microscopy. The second sample could be divided into two sections (or a third sample obtained), ensuring that each contains glomeruli. The first section, for immunofluorescence microscopy, should be submitted in Michel's solution (ammonium sulfate-N-ethylmaleimide) which preserves immunoglobulins. The second section should be submitted in 3% glutaraldehyde in sodium phosphate buffer for electron microscopy.[22]

Light microscopy on renal samples is typically done on thin (3-μm) sections stained with H&E, as well as several other standard stains, including periodic acid-Schiff, Congo red, Jones methenamine silver, and Masson's trichrome.[12] Nephropathology is one of the few subspecialties that requires routine use of electron microscopy to obtain a definitive diagnosis, in particular with glomerular diseases. Likewise, the routine use of immunofluorescence to identify pathogenic immunoglobulin and complement molecules within the tissues is common in nephropathology. Renal biopsies are evaluated for immune deposits with immunofluorescence (IgM, IgG, IgA, C3, lambda light chains, and C1q).[22]

Complications Associated with Renal Biopsy

Potential complications of renal biopsy are listed in Box 20-3.

Box 20-3 Complications of Renal Biopsy

Nondiagnostic sample
Hemorrhage
Microscopic hematuria
Macroscopic hematuria
Perirenal hematoma
Hydronephrosis
Infarction or thrombosis
Laceration of renal artery, vein, or other vessel or organ
Laceration of the ureter
Scar formation and fibrosis
Renal pelvic or ureteral obstruction caused by a blood clot
Decreased renal function

Changes in renal architecture have been documented after renal biopsy. Infarction and fibrosis along needle tracts have been observed. Despite these anatomic changes, properly performed renal biopsies appear to have minimal effects on renal function in both dogs and cats.[23,24]

Postoperative Care

After a renal biopsy, the patient should be maintained on intravenous fluids for several hours to minimize the risk of blood clot formation in the renal pelvis and subsequent obstruction of the ureter. In our practice, patients are closely monitored for a minimum of 6 hours after kidney biopsy, and most are hospitalized overnight. In humans, 89% to 98% of reported complications occurred within the first 24 hours after the procedure.[14]

After the procedure has been completed and the patient has recovered from general anesthesia, serial packed cell volume (PCV) measurements are obtained, typically every 3 hours for 6 hours and then every 6 hours for the next 24 hours. Additionally, blood pressure, heart rate, respiratory rate, and pain level are monitored frequently. Before discharge, a recheck of the biopsy site with ultrasonography to assess for hematoma formation is typically performed. The owners are instructed to limit the patient's activity for the next 72 hours.

References

1 Anas, C.M., Hattori, R., Morita, Y., et al. (2008) Efficiency of laparoscopic-assisted renal biopsy. Clin Nephrol 70 (3), 203-209.

2 Jesus, C.M., Yamamoto, H., Kawano, P.R., et al. (2007) Retroperitoneoscopic renal biopsy in children. Int Braz J Urol 33 (4), 536-541; discussion 541-543.

3 Jackman, S.V., Bishoff, J.T. (2000) Laparoscopic retroperitoneal renal biopsy. J Endourol 14 (10), 833-838; discussion 838-839.

4 Shetye, K.R., Kavoussi, L.R., Ramakumar, S., et al. (2003) Laparoscopic renal biopsy: a 9-year experience. BJU Int 91 (9), 817-820.

5 Gimenez, L.F., Micali, S., Chen, R.N., et al. (1998) Laparoscopic renal biopsy. Kidney Int 54 (2), 525-529.

6 Grauer, G.F., Twedt, D.C., Mero, K.N. (1983) Evaluation of laparoscopy for obtaining renal biopsy specimens from dogs and cats. J Am Vet Med Assoc 183 (6), 677-679.

7 Rawlings, C.A., Diamond, H., Howerth, E.W., et al. (2003) Diagnostic quality of percutaneous kidney biopsy specimens obtained with laparoscopy versus ultrasound guidance in dogs. J Am Vet Med Assoc 223 (3), 317-321.

8 Nowicki, M., Rychlik, A., Nieradka, R., et al. (2010) Usefulness of laparoscopy guided renal biopsy in dogs. Pol J Vet Sci 13 (2), 363-371.

9 Vaden, S.L. (2005) Renal biopsy of dogs and cats. Clin Tech Small Anim Pract 20 (1), 11-22.

10 Vaden, S.L., Levine, J.F., Lees, G.E., et al. (2005) Renal biopsy: a retrospective study of methods and complications in 283 dogs and 65 cats. J Vet Intern Med 19 (6), 794-801.

11 Littman, M.P., Daminet, S., Grauer, G.F., et al. (2013) Consensus recommendations for the diagnostic investigation of dogs with suspected glomerular disease. J Vet Intern Med 27 (suppl 1), S19-S26.

12 Segev, G., Cowgill, L.D., Heiene, R., et al. (2013) Consensus recommendations for immunosuppressive treatment of dogs with glomerular disease based on established pathology. J Vet Intern Med 27 (suppl 1), S44-S54.

13 Vaden, S.L. (2004) Renal biopsy: methods and interpretation. Vet Clin North Am Small Anim Pract 34(4), 887-908.

14 Whittier, W.L., Korbet, S.M. (2004) Renal biopsy: update. Curr Opin Nephrol Hypertens 13(6), 661-665.

15 Bigge, L.A., Brown, D.J., Penninck, D.G. (2001) Correlation between coagulation profile findings and bleeding complications after ultrasound-guided biopsies: 434 cases (1993-1996). J Am Anim Hosp Assoc 37 (3), 228-233.

16 Syme, H. (2011) Hypertension in small animal kidney disease. Vet Clin North Am Small Anim Pract 41 (1), 63-89.

17 Constantin, A., Brisson, M.L., Kwan, J., Proulx, F. (2010) Percutaneous US-guided renal biopsy: a retrospective study comparing the 16-gauge end-cut and 14-gauge side-notch needles. J Vasc Interv Radiol 21 (3), 357-361.

18 Zatelli, A., D'Ippolito, P., Zini, E. (2005) Comparison of glomerular number and specimen length obtained from 100 dogs via percutaneous echo-assisted renal biopsy using two different needles. Vet Radiol Ultrasound 46 (5), 434-436.

19 Nicholson, M.L., Wheatley, T.J., Doughman, T.M., et al. (2000) A prospective randomized trial of three different sizes of core-cutting needle for renal transplant biopsy. Kidney Int 58(1), 390-395.

20 Mai, J., Yong, J., Dixson, H., et al. (2013) Is bigger better? A retrospective analysis of native renal biopsies with 16 gauge versus 18 gauge automatic needles. Nephrology (Carlton) 18 (7), 525-530.

21 Song, J.H., Cronan, J.J. (1998) Percutaneous biopsy in diffuse renal disease: comparison of 18- and 14-gauge automated biopsy devices. J Vasc Interv Radiol 9 (4), 651-655.

22 Cianciolo, R.E., Brown, C.A., Mohr, F.C., et al. (2013) Pathologic evaluation of canine renal biopsies: methods for identifying features that differentiate immune-mediated glomerulonephritides from other categories of glomerular diseases. J Vet Intern Med 27 (suppl 1), S10-S18.

23 Drost, W.T., Henry, G.A., Meinkoth, J.H., et al. (2000) The effects of a unilateral ultrasound-guided renal biopsy on renal function in healthy sedated cats. Vet Radiol Ultrasound 41 (1), 57-62.

24 Osborne, C.A., Low, D.G., Jessen, C.R. (1972) Renal parenchymal response to needle biopsy. Invest Urol 9, 463-469.

21 Laparoscopic Ureteronephrectomy

Philipp D. Mayhew

Key Points

- Before any ureteronephrectomy is performed, assessment of per kidney glomerular filtration rate should ideally be performed to evaluate the functional reserve of the remaining kidney.
- Transperitoneal laparoscopic ureteronephrectomy is a complex minimally invasive technique that should only be attempted by surgeons experienced in laparoscopic as well as open ureteronephrectomy.
- Before dissection of the renal hilus, early isolation and elevation of the proximal ureter can aid in dissection of the renal hilar vessels.
- Use of a vessel-sealing device greatly facilitates laparoscopic ureteronephrectomy and in most small- to medium-sized dogs can be used to seal and divide the renal artery and vein.

The laparoscopic approach to ureteronephrectomy was first described in humans in 1991 by Clayman.[1] Since that time, laparoscopic developments in urology have moved very rapidly in human medicine. Laparoscopic ureteronephrectomy is performed in human surgery as a treatment for a variety of conditions. Simple nephrectomy is used in the management of chronic pyelonephritis, obstructive calculus disease, traumatic injury, renovascular hypertension, and congenital dysplasia.[2,3] Radical nephrectomy, which generally includes removal of the kidney as well as the associated adrenal gland, lymph nodes, and surrounding tissues, is the treatment of choice for most renal cell carcinoma cases.[4-6]

Both retroperitoneal (RLU) and transperitoneal laparoscopic ureteronephrectomy (TLU) have been described in human patients, and comparative studies have not consistently shown superior outcomes for one technique over the other. Some evidence suggests that RLU may be associated with shorter surgical time.[7,8] Other authors have suggested that TLU may offer advantages when large lesions are operated.[9]

Analysis of perioperative outcomes for RLU and TLU in human patients have generally favored the laparoscopic approach over the open approach even for malignant disease. Reductions in blood loss, length of hospital stay, pain medication requirement, and time to return to normal activity have all been described.[10-12] Oncologic outcomes have been analyzed for a variety of stages of renal cancer and generally have shown equal outcomes in disease-free interval

and median survival between groups. This is true for renal cell carcinoma.[4-6,11] Transitional cell carcinoma of the upper urinary tract is rare in humans as well as small animal patients and has been associated with a high rate of urothelial recurrence when a complete ipsilateral urothelial resection is not performed. A laparoscopic approach for complete ureteronephrectomy with bladder cuff resection is considered a reasonable approach in human patients with transitional cell carcinoma.[13] Despite the many advantages seen in patient morbidity rates with RLU and TLU, surgical time is often longer with the laparoscopic approach versus the open approach.[11,12]

More recently, the development of a variety of newer surgical platforms for minimally invasive ureteronephrectomy has been published in the human literature. These include the laparoendoscopic single-site (LESS) approach using a variety of single-port devices and usually performed through the umbilicus.[14] Hand-assisted approaches have been promoted as a way to minimize surgical time compared with fully laparoscopic approaches and have been shown to have similar outcomes in terms of complications and postoperative pain.[15] Other proposed platforms include natural orifice transluminal endoscopic approaches[16] and robotic approaches.[17]

In small animal patients, ureteronephrectomy has generally been performed through a ventral midline celiotomy. With the advent of numerous nephron-sparing techniques to manage a variety of

---

Small Animal Laparoscopy and Thoracoscopy, First Edition. Edited by Boel A. Fransson and Philipp D. Mayhew.
© 2015 by ACVS Foundation. Published 2015 by John Wiley & Sons, Inc.
Companion website: www.wiley.com/go/fransson/laparoscopy

urologic disorders, ureteronephrectomy has thankfully become less commonplace. However, it remains an important treatment option in select canine and feline cases with primary renal neoplasia, hydronephrosis, end-stage chronic renal failure with chronic infection, renal dysplasia, nephrolithiasis, trauma, and idiopathic renal hematuria.[18,19]

Significant advantages to a laparoscopic approach in small animal patients have been reported in several comparative studies of laparoscopic versus open surgical techniques using ovariohysterectomy, ovariectomy, and gastropexy models. These include a reduction in postoperative pain and a more rapid return to normal activity in these patients.[20-22] One veterinary study has also shown some evidence that a minimally invasive approach may be associated with a lower infection rate compared to open surgery.[23]

In the veterinary literature, a limited amount of work has been published specifically on TLU in research models[24-28] and even less so in clinical patients.[28,29] Canine models of TLU have shown that surgical stress is diminished in the laparoscopic group compared with the open group.[25] In clinical studies, good success was obtained with the technique in clinical patients, although conversion due to of technical challenges was required in some cases.[28]

Preoperative Considerations

Surgical Anatomy

The canine and feline kidneys are paired organs that lie in the retroperitoneal space just ventral to the first four lumbar vertebrae. They lie lateral to the aorta and vena cava. The right kidney is located more cranial than the left and is often in contact with the caudate lobe of the liver. The adrenal gland is located just cranial to the kidneys, although a clear plane of dissection is almost always present between these organs. The renal hilus is the origin of the ureter, renal artery, and vein. The renal artery and vein are branches off the aorta and caudal vena cava but show significant natural variation among individuals with branching or multiple renal arteries and veins common in both species.[30,31] The cranial abdominal artery passes over the adrenal gland and then dives dorsal to the cranial pole of the kidney. This vessel can be encountered during TLU. Recently, a survey of anatomic variations in ureteral anatomy in cats has been performed showing that circumcaval ureters are common in cats, occurring in approximately one third of those evaluated.[32] The ureters lie dorsal to the internal spermatic vessels and the vas deferens over which they pass approximately 2 cm cranial to the bladder. In females, the ureters pass dorsal to the ureteroovarian artery and vein in a similar location. During resection of the more distal aspects of the ureter, dissection around these structures is necessary. The ureters join the lateral ligaments of the bladder before entering the bladder at the ureterovesicular junction on the dorsolateral surface of the bladder just caudal to the neck.

Preoperative Diagnostic Evaluation

Patients that might be candidates for TLU can have a plethora of underlying renal diseases. In many cases, they may be older patients with important comorbidities that need to be assessed. One of the most important parameters to evaluate is overall renal functional reserve because many renal pathologies are bilateral and affect the contralateral (unresected) kidney to varying extents. A complete blood count, biochemical screen, and urinalysis with urine culture and bacterial culture and sensitivity should be performed in all cases. Serum creatinine is a relatively insensitive test for detection of kidney damage, and significant elevations are only detected when 60% to 75% of nephrons have been lost. In patients in which TLU is being considered, a more sensitive test for early renal disease and especially the relative loss of filtration ability from each kidney is vital. This can be obtained using a variety of tests, including glomerular filtration rate (GFR) testing, determination of fractional excretion of electrolytes, or assays of urinary biomarkers. Global GFR calculation provides a summated measure of filtration from both kidneys and has been validated in dogs and cats using a variety of methods.[33] However, in patients in which TLU is being contemplated, a per-kidney GFR is more useful to predict the prognosis for renal function in the postoperative period. Per-kidney GFR can be calculated using scintigraphic means.[34,35] or contrast-enhanced computed tomography (CT).[36] If urinary tract infection is detected from a urinalysis performed preoperatively, treatment based on the results of culture and susceptibility testing should be initiated. If the patient's clinical status allows, preoperative treatment with an appropriate antibiotic is recommended for 1 to 2 weeks before surgery.

Diagnostic imaging of the urinary tract is also critical in these cases to evaluate the extent and severity of disease, to assess for comorbidities and metastatic disease in the case of malignancy, and to provide vital information for surgical planning. Plain radiography provides relatively insensitive information for assessment of renal pathology but may give a rough idea of kidney size and may highlight radiopaque lithiasis at different locations within the urinary tract. Abdominal ultrasonography is extremely useful for assessment of renal and ureteric pathology. The presence and extent of mass lesions, degree of hydronephrosis and hydroureter, and evidence of dysplasias should be detectable. It also allows ultrasound-guided aspiration of any lesions that are evident and recovery of samples for bacterial culture and susceptibility testing by cystocentesis or pyelocentesis. Contrast-enhanced computed tomography (CE-CT) is often recommended in small animals that are being considered for TLU because it provides the surgeon with an assessment of lesion dimensions, location, and the relationship of any mass lesions to surrounding organs. CE-CT also allows evaluation of any associated lymphadenopathy that may be clinically important for disease staging and surgical planning.

Patient Selection

Relatively little data are available for TLU in clinical patients, so making strict case selection guidelines at this point in the development of the technique is challenging.[28] The author suggests that case selection be made very carefully, especially in the early part of a surgeon's learning curve, because TLU represents one of the more challenging laparoscopic interventions. The author's group as well as others have found that laparoscopic removal of grossly normal kidneys in research animals or animals with diseased kidneys but without gross morphologic change to their kidneys is relatively simple and not associated with prolonged surgical times.[27,28] In clinical patients with distortion of the kidney by larger renal masses, hydronephrosis, or hydroureter, surgeons should select cases cautiously to avoid a high conversion rate and significant morbidity. At this time, appropriate case selection for TLU includes modestly sized primary renal neoplasms, chronic renal failure with infection, renal dysplasia, and idiopathic renal hematuria. Note that other options may be available for some of these conditions that may not necessitate TLU in these patients. Contraindications for TLU at this point in time include large renal masses (>5–7 cm), severe hydronephrosis or hydroureter, or pyelonephritis with abscessation or if there is any infection that extends beyond the renal capsule. In clinical cases, preoperative imaging with ultrasonography and preferably CT (or magnetic resonance imaging) is very helpful in ruling out conditions that might make a laparoscopic approach undesirable. As more experience is gained with the technique, the case selection criteria for TLU may change.

Patient Preparation

Surgical Preparation

The hair is liberally clipped from the lateral abdomen of the patient on the affected side. The clip extends from the transverse spinous processes of the spine to the mid-abdominal area on the contralateral side. Cranially, the clipped area extends to the midthorax, and caudally it extends to the perineal area. The whole area is aseptically prepared for surgery, including an aseptic wash of the prepuce in male dogs.

Operating Room Setup and Patient Positioning

The patient is initially placed in partial lateral recumbency so that aseptic preparation of the ventral midline can be included in the draped area, thus allowing conversion to a ventral midline celiotomy if deemed necessary. After draping, the dog can be allowed to fall into a completely laterally recumbent position to aid in access to the kidney and ureter. The surgeon and surgeon's assistant stand on the side of the patient facing the dog's abdomen, and the endoscopic tower is placed on the contralateral side of the patient (Figure 21-1). This enables the surgeons to visualize the kidney in a straight line from their position to the kidney in question and on to the video monitor on the endoscopy tower. For dissection of the renal hilus, the endoscopic tower is usually maintained directly across from the location where the surgeon is standing. As dissection of the ureter is performed, it may be easier to have an assistant move the endoscopic tower to a location closer to the caudal end of the patient because the telescope and instruments will be positioned in a more caudally directed trajectory.

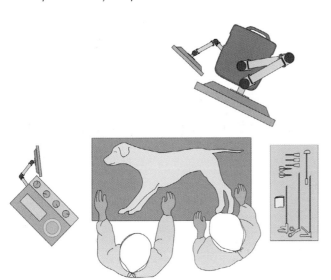

Figure 21-1 Operating room layout for laparoscopic ureteronephrectomy. During dissection of the renal hilus, the endoscopic tower is placed straight across from the surgeons on the other side of the table. During dissection of the distal ureter, it may be helpful to move the viewing monitor closer to the caudal end of the patient.

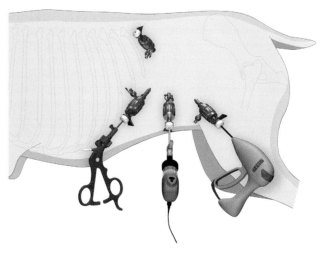

Figure 21-2 Port positioning for laparoscopic transperitoneal ureteronephrectomy. Three ports are usually sufficient, but a third instrument port can be placed over the anticipated location of the kidney when additional retraction of tissues may be necessary.

Portal Position and Creation of Working Space

The TLU procedure is usually performed using a three- or four-port technique. Three ports are usually adequate, but if additional retraction is required for any reason, a fourth port is placed. Abdominal access can be obtained using a Hasson or Veress needle technique, and a telescope portal is established either in a location just caudal to the umbilicus or 2 to 3 cm lateral to the umbilicus on the affected side. If a 30-degree telescope is available, the subumbilical position works well for the telescope portal. If a 0-degree telescope only is available, this location may not give an adequate view of the kidney; in that case, a more laterally positioned telescope portal is recommended. Care should be taken not to place the camera portal too dorsal, however, because when this is done, the surgeon's assistant will have to hold the telescope in a very elevated position, which can rapidly lead to fatigue.

After pneumoperitoneum has been established, two further instrument ports are placed, one at the mid-abdominal level just caudal to the last rib and one at the same level just cranial to the pelvic limb (Figure 21-2) The telescope portal size needs to be appropriate to the size of the telescope available. The instrument ports can be variable in size. However, if a 10-mm clip applier or 10-mm specimen retrieval bag is to be used, at least one of the instrument ports needs to be large enough to accommodate these sizes of instruments. The use of threaded ports can be helpful in TLU because a large number of instrument exchanges are usually necessary, and these ports help greatly in reducing the incidence of cannulae pulling out of the port incisions during exchanges.

Surgical Technique

Instrumentation for LA

The instrumentation necessary for TLU is similar to many of the other advanced laparoscopic techniques described. Three to four trocar–cannula assemblies are required, ranging usually from 5 to 10 mm in size depending on the instrumentation available. This author favors the use of a 30-degree telescope for TLU because it is very helpful to be able to view around anatomic structures, which can be more challenging with a 0-degree telescope. Instrumentation that is essential includes a blunt probe, Kelly or right-angled dissection forceps, and atraumatic grasping forceps. Electrosurgical capability is vital for TLU. A vessel-sealing device greatly simplifies the dissection in TLU because it allows blunt dissection of tissue planes followed by sealing and dividing without having to change instruments. This can reduce bleeding and shorten surgical time significantly. In smaller patients, the renal artery and veins can be sealed entirely with the vessel sealer, but as the size of these vessels increases, it may be necessary to use a different hemostatic modality because most bipolar vessel sealers are only indicated to seal vessels up to 7 mm in size. A variety of laparoscopic hemoclips are available from different companies. Using medium to large clips is essential for the larger renal hilar vessels. Polymer clips (Hem-o-lok; Teleflex Medical, Research Triangle Park, NC) are also available and have been used in both humans and canines for TLU with success.[27,37] Monopolar electrosurgery using a j- or l-hook probe can also be helpful in TLU for coagulation and cutting of smaller tissue planes that might be challenging to place the tip of the vessel-sealing device into. Extra- or intracorporeal suturing of the renal hilar vessels can also be used. A knot pusher is required for placement of extracorporeally assembled knots, and laparoscopic needle drivers are required for intracorporeal application of ligatures to the renal vasculature. These latter techniques tend to be more time consuming than the use of vessel sealers or clips applied to the renal vessels. A final option for hilar sealing is en-bloc sealing with endoscopic staplers. This technique has been shown to be safe and efficient in human patients and does not lead to arteriovenous fistula formation.[38,39] However, it is vital to ensure that the correct stapler dimensions are being used, with a 2.5-mm vascular cartridge being recommended (usually 45–60 mm long).

The kidney should always be removed in a specimen retrieval bag to minimize the risk of port site metastasis or infection; these bags are commercially available from a number of companies. Most specimen retrieval bags are placed through a cannula that accommodates 10-mm instrumentation.

Surgical Technique

Upon entering the peritoneal cavity, the surgeon should survey the kidney and the surrounding structures and optimize patient positioning to allow access to all the important anatomic landmarks. On the left side, the kidney is sometimes covered by the spleen or colon and, less commonly, a gas-filled stomach. In lateral recumbency, these structures will usually fall away from the kidney with gentle traction from a blunt probe. On the right side, the small intestine usually needs to be retracted medially to provide access to the kidney. Occasionally, on the right side, a liver lobe will obscure the cranial pole of the right kidney and will require some retraction, although this is less common. In cases in which retracted organs fall back into their original positions covering the kidney, the table should be tilted toward the surgeon, or a foam wedge can be placed under the patient's epaxial musculature to provide added gravitational force, allowing the organs to fall ventrally away from the kidney. The ureter is identified as well as the adrenal gland cranially. To initiate dissection of the kidney, a vessel-sealing or other electrosurgical device is used to dissect the kidney from its retroperitoneal attachments (Figure 21-3). Next, the ureter is dissected out close to its insertion into the renal pelvis. The advantage of early ureteral dissection is that it can then be used as a handle to provide mild traction on the kidney, which aids in identification of the renal hilus. Using Kelly or right-angled dissection forceps or the tip of the vessel-sealer, the renal vessels are

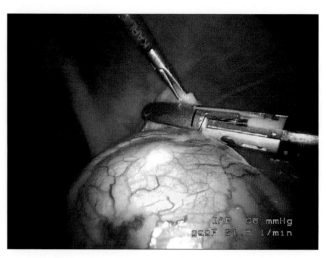

Figure 21-3 The vessel-sealing device can be seen dissecting and sealing the peritoneum and associated blood supply around the renal capsule.

skeletonized (Figure 21-4, Video Clip 21-1). If within the size limitations of the vessel-sealing device being used, the renal artery and vein can be sealed and divided using the vessel-sealing device alone (Figure 21-5). Alternatively, the artery and vein are triple clipped using laparoscopic hemoclips or polymer clips before being sectioned with a laparoscopic scissor (Figure 21-6, Video Clip 21-2). Remaining attachments of the kidney to the surrounding retroperitoneum are then sectioned using the vessel sealer. After the kidney is completely dissected out, tension is placed on the proximal ureter. This facilitates dissection of the remaining section of the ureter down to its insertion into the bladder (Figure 21-7). The surgeon may have to dissect on either side of the internal spermatic vessels and vas deferens in a male or the uretero-ovarian vessels in a female. After dissection up to the ureterovesicular junction is complete, the ureter can be triple clipped with hemoclips or double ligated with suture (Figure 21-8, Video Clip 21-1). At least two clips or ligatures should remain on the ureteral stump near the ureterovesicular junction. The resected specimen is placed into a specimen retrieval bag and removed through an enlargement

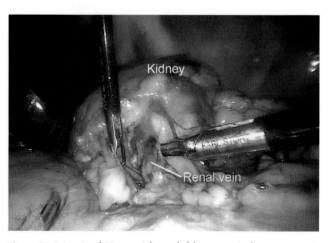

Figure 21-4 A pair of 10-mm right-angled laparoscopic forceps are positioned around the renal vein during the process of skeletonization of the renal vein and artery.

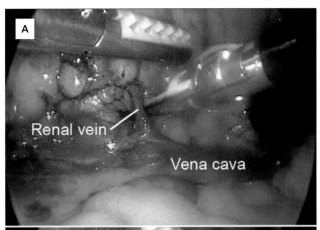

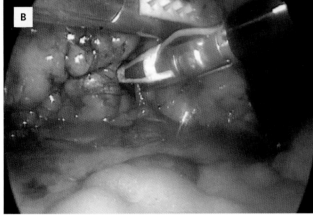

Figure 21-5 Feline laparoscopic ureteronephrectomy. A vessel-sealing device can be seen aiding in dissection of the renal vein (**A**), which is subsequently sealed and divided (**B**).

of one of the instrument ports (Figure 21-9). Before closure, the entire surgical site should be reexamined for any ongoing hemorrhage and lavaged with sterile saline that is then reaspirated using a suction device. Pneumoperitoneum is then purged from the peritoneal cavity, and the port sites are closed by placement of sutures in the muscular fascia of the body wall muscle followed by placement of intradermal sutures.

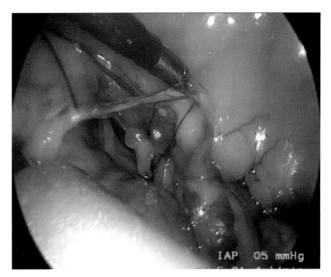

Figure 21-7 In this feline laparoscopic ureteronephrectomy, the ureter has been tensioned before laparoscopic hemoclips are applied close to the ureterovesicular junction.

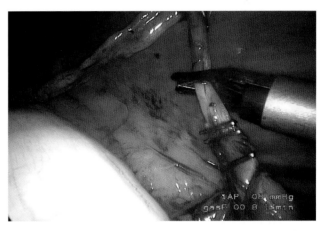

Figure 21-8 Laparoscopic hemoclips are being applied to the terminal portion of the ureter in this dog before sectioning close to the ureterovesicular junction.

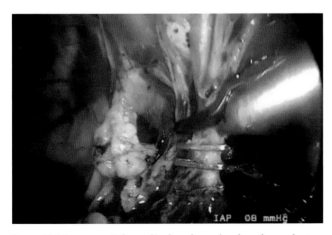

Figure 21-6 Laparoscopic hemoclips have been placed on the renal artery before its division.

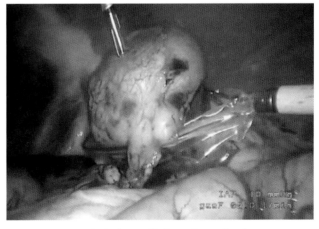

Figure 21-9 A completely dissected kidney is being placed into a specimen retrieval bag before removal from the abdomen.

Complications and Prognosis

Clinical reports of TLU in small animals are limited, resulting in a dearth of information regarding the intra- and postoperative complications associated with this technique. In one study in which TLU was performed in 16 healthy research dogs, no conversions to open surgery were required, and the complications noted were primarily access-related splenic lacerations ($n = 3$) and subcutaneous emphysema ($n = 2$).[27] The only other complication noted was specimen retrieval bag tearing, which occurred in only one case.[27] In the only article on clinical canine cases, two of nine dogs required conversion to an open approach.[28] In one dog, significant bleeding emanating from the phrenicoabdominal vein was not able to be adequately controlled, so conversion was opted for. In the second dog with a severe hydroureter, the kidney was adequately dissected, but the authors could not easily dissect the severely enlarged ureter close to the ureterovesicular junction without concern for leaving a substantial blind-ending pouch of ureter attached to the bladder. In a third dog in this study, bleeding from the renal hilar vessels during dissection and clipping resulted in hemorrhage but was adequately controlled, and conversion was not necessary. Iatrogenic damage to surrounding anatomy needs to be avoided during the procedure. Special care needs to be taken to avoid trauma to the large vessels in the area. Accidental rupture of the renal artery or vein should prompt immediate conversion to an open approach if the bleeding cannot be stopped immediately. However, many more minor forms of hemorrhage may be controllable without the need for conversion. The adrenal gland must be protected as long as it is not involved in the disease process. Iatrogenic damage to the contralateral ureter, a structure that can lie surprisingly close to the ureter being removed, is possible. This author likes to locate the contralateral ureter so that its position can be monitored throughout the procedure (Video Clip 21-3).

Postoperative complications common to all laparoscopic procedures include the possibility of port site infection, which has a very low incidence in small animals.[23] Seroma formation and subcutaneous emphysema can both occur but are usually self-limiting. Port site metastasis has been described in small numbers of human patients with renal carcinoma. Port site metastasis can be related to technical factors such as tumor fragmentation, morcellation, or lack of placement within a retrieval device but may also occur when these known risk factors are not involved.[40] Port site metastasis has not been reported in small animal patients after TLU, likely because of the small numbers of cases described.

The long-term outcome after TLU is mainly influenced by the underlying disease process, the presence of comorbidities, and the ability of the patient to compensate for the loss of renal function after TLU. Deterioration in renal function may be seen after either open or laparoscopic approaches, and progression of renal disease as a cause of death has been seen after both approaches also.[18,28] For this reason, whenever possible, alternative nephron-sparing techniques should be considered in small animal patients before any decision to perform ureteronephrectomy is taken.

Postoperative Care

Postoperative analgesia after TLU can be in the form of intermittent intravenous (IV) or constant-rate infusion administration of an opioid drug (hydromorphone hydrochloride, 0.1 mg/kg IV every 4 hours; oxymorphone hydrochloride, 0.1 mg/kg IV every 4 hours; or buprenorphine hydrochloride, 0.01 mg/kg IV every 6 hours).

Tramadol hydrochloride can be prescribed upon discharge from the hospital (2–4 mg/kg orally every 8 hours for 3–5 days) in most dogs. Nonsteroidal antiinflammatory drugs should generally be avoided in this patient population. Hospitalization time might vary depending on the underlying cause but is usually 2 or 3 days. Long-term monitoring of renal function is imperative in animals undergoing TLU.

All videos cited in this chapter can be found on the book's companion website at **www.wiley.com/go/fransson/laparoscopy**

References

1 Clayman, R.V., Kavoussi, L.R., Soper, N.J., et al. (1991) Laparoscopic nephrectomy: initial case report. J Urol 146, 278-282.
2 Traxer, O., Pearle, M.S. (2000) Laparoscopic nephrectomy for benign disease. Semin Laparosc Surg 7, 176-184.
3 Liao, J.C., Breda, A., Schulam, P.G. (2007) Laparoscopic renal surgery for benign disease. Curr Urol Rep 8, 12-18.
4 Bhayani, S.B., Clayman, R.V., Sundaram, C.P., et al. (2003) Surgical treatment of renal neoplasia: evolving toward a laparoscopic standard of care. Urology 62, 821-826.
5 Al-Qudah, H.S., Rodriguez, A.R., Sexton, W.J. (2007) Laparoscopic management of kidney cancer: updated review. Cancer Control 14, 218-230.
6 Deane, L.A., Clayman, R.V. (2007) Laparoscopic nephrectomy for renal cell cancer: radical and total. BJU International 99, 1251-1257.
7 Desai, M.M., Strzempkowski, B., Matin, S.F., et al. (2005) Prospective randomized comparison of transperitoneal versus retroperitoneal laparoscopic radical nephrectomy. J Urol 173, 38-41.
8 Kim, C., McKay, K., Docimo, S.G. (2009) Laparoscopic nephrectomy in children: systematic review of transperitoneal and retroperitoneal approaches. Urology 73, 280-284.
9 Taue, R., Izaki, H., Koizumi, T., et al. (2009) Transperitoneal versus retroperitoneal laparoscopic radical nephrectomy: a comparative study. Int J Urol 16, 263-267.
10 Rassweiler, J., Frede, T., Henkel, T.O., et al. (1998) Nephrectomy: a comparative study between the transperitoneal and retroperitoneal laparoscopic versus the open approach. Eur Urol 33, 489-496.
11 Dunn, M.D., Portis, A.J., Shalhav, A.L., et al. (2000) Laparoscopic versus open radical nephrectomy: a 9-year experience. J Urol 164, 1153-1159.
12 Beasley, K.A., Omar, M.A., Shaikh, A., et al. (2004) Laparoscopic versus open partial nephrectomy. Urology 64, 458-461.
13 Raman, J.D., Scherr, D.S. (2007) Management of patients with upper urinary tract transitional cell carcinoma. Urology 4, 432-443.
14 Kaouk, J.H., Autorino, R., Kim, F.J., et al. (2011) Laparoendoscopic single-site surgery in urology: worldwide multi-institutional analysis of 1076 cases. Eur Urol 60, 998-1005.
15 Silberstein, J., Parsons, J.K. (1998) Hand-assisted and total laparoscopic nephrectomy: a comparison. J Soc Laparoendosc Surg 13, 36-43.
16 Aminsharifi, A., Taddayun, A., Shakeri, S., et al. (2009) Hybrid natural orifice transluminal endoscopic surgery for nephrectomy with standard laparoendoscopic instruments: experience in a canine model. J Endourol 23, 1985-1989.
17 Ambani, S.N., Weizer, A.Z., Wolf, S., et al. (2014) Matched comparison of robotic vs laparoscopic nephroureterectomy: an initial experience. Urology 83, 345-349.
18 Gookin, J.L., Stone, E.A., Spaulding, K.A., et al. (1996) Unilateral nephrectomy in dogs with renal disease; 30 cases (1985-1994). J Am Vet Med Assoc 208, 2020-2026.
19 Fossum, T.W. (2007) Surgery of the kidney and ureter. In: Fossum, T.W. (ed.) Small Animal Surgery, 3rd edn. Mosby Elsevier, St. Louis, pp 635-662.
20 Devitt, C.M., Cox, R.E., Hailey, J.J. (2005) Duration, complications, stress, and pain of open ovariohysterectomy versus a simple method of laparoscopic-assisted ovariohysterectomy in dogs. J Am Vet Med Assoc 227, 921-927.
21 Culp, W.T.N., Mayhew, P.D., Brown, D.C. (2009) The effect of laparoscopic versus open ovariectomy on postsurgical activity in small dogs. Vet Surg 38, 811-817.
22 Mayhew, P.D., Brown, D.C. (2009) Prospective evaluation of two intracorporeally sutured prophylactic laparoscopic gastropexy techniques compared to laparoscopic-assisted gastropexy in dogs. Vet Surg 38, 738-746.
23 Mayhew, P.D., Freeman, L., Kwan, T., et al. (2012) Comparison of surgical site infection rates in clean and clean-contaminated wounds in dogs and cats after

minimally invasive versus open surgery: 179 cases (2007-2008). J Am Vet Med Assoc 240, 193-198.

24 Ravizzini, P.I., Shulsinger, D., Guarnizo, E., et al. (1999) Hand-assisted laparoscopic donor nephrectomy versus standard laparoscopic donor nephrectomy: a comparison study in the canine model. Tech Urol 5, 174-178.

25 Marcovich, R., Williams, A.L., Seifman, B.D., et al. (2001) A canine model to assess the biochemical stress response to laparoscopic and open surgery. J Endourol 15, 1005-1008.

26 Yoder, B., Wolf, J.S. (2005) Canine model of surgical stress response comparing standard laparoscopic, microlaparoscopic and hand-assisted laparoscopic nephrectomy. Urology 65, 600-603.

27 Kim, Y.K., Park, S.J., Lee, S.Y., et al. (2013) Laparoscopic nephrectomy in dogs: an initial experience of 16 experimental procedures. Vet J 98, 513-517.

28 Mayhew, P.D., Mehler, S.J., Mayhew, K.N., et al. (2013) Experimental and clinical evaluation of transperitoneal laparoscopic ureteronephrectomy in dogs. Vet Surg 42, 565-571.

29 Secchi, P., Valle, S.d.F., Brun, M.V., et al. (2010) Videolaparoscopic nephrectomy in the treatment of canine dioctophymosis. Acta Sci Vet 38, 85-892.

30 Christensen, G.C. (1952) Circulation of blood through the canine kidney. Am J Vet Res 13, 236-245.

31 Caceres, A.V., Zwingenberger, A.L., Aronson, L.R., et al. (2008) Characterization of normal feline renal vascular anatomy with dual-phase CT angiography. Vet Radiol Ultrasound 49, 350-356.

32 Belanger, R., Shmon, C.L., Gilbert, P.J., et al. (2014) Prevalence of circumcaval ureters and double caudal vena cava in cats. Am J Vet Res 75, 91-95.

33 Pressler, B.M. (2013) Clinical approach to advanced renal function testing in dogs and cats. Vet Clin Small Anim 43, 1193-1208.

34 Uribe, D., Krawiec, D.R., Twardock, A.R., et al. (1992) Quantitative renal scintigraphic determination of the glomerular filtration rate in cats with normal and abnormal kidney function, using 99mTc-diethylenetriaminepentaacetic acid. Am J Vet Res 53, 1101-1107.

35 Barthez, P.Y., Hornof, W.J., Cowgill, L.D., et al. (1998) Comparison between the scintigraphic uptake and plasma clearance of 99MTc-diethylenetriaminepentacetic acid (DTPA) for the evaluation of the glomerular filtration rate in dogs. Vet Radiol Ultrasound 39, 470-474.

36 O'Dell-Anderson, K.J., Twardock, R., Grimm, J.B., et al. (2006) Determination of glomerular filtration rate in dogs using contrast-enhanced computed tomography. Vet Radiol Ultrasound 47, 127-135.

37 Simforoosh, N., Sarhangnejad, R., Basiri, A., et al. (2012) Vascular clips are safe and a great cost effective technique for arterial and venous control in laparoscopic nephrectomy: single center experience with 1834 laparoscopic nephrectomies. J Endourol 26, 1009-1012.

38 Schatloff, O., Lindner, U., Lindner, A. (2010) Current status of en bloc stapling of the renal hilum during laparoscopic nephrectomy. J Laparoendosc Adv Surg Tech 20, 631-633.

39 Chung, J.H., Lee, S.W., Lee, K.S., et al. (2013) Safety of en bloc ligation of the renal hilum during laparoscopic radical nephrectomy for renal cell carcinoma: a randomized controlled trial. J Laparoendosc Adv Surg Tech 23, 489-494.

40 Song, J., Kim, E., Mobley, J., et al. (2014) Port site metastasis after surgery for renal cell carcinoma: harbinger of future metastasis. J Urol 192 (2), 364-368.

22 Laparoscopic-Assisted Nephrolith Removal

Eric Monnet

Key Points

- A 3-mm pyelolithotomy incision can be used for endoscopy of the renal pelvis and nephrolith removal.
- A 2.7-mm cystoscope was used for nephrolith removal.
- A 3-French infant feeding tube may be inserted next to the cystoscope for fluid egress.

Removal of kidney stones represents a surgical challenge. Stones can be removed by a nephrotomy or a pyelolithotomy. Nephrotomy has the potential to reduce kidney function by the damage to the renal parenchyma associated with surgical manipulation and transient ischemia.[1-4] Pyelolithotomy is a preferred technique because it does not interfere with the renal parenchyma and reduces the risk of compromised kidney function. However, it is only possible if the renal stones have migrated into the renal pelvis close to the proximal ureter.[5]

A laparoscopic-assisted approach may represent an alternative to remove stones that are not located in the renal pelvis but may migrate into the ureters and induce a urinary obstruction with hydroureter and hydronephrosis. The author has performed this procedure only in cats with chronic renal disease and uroliths in the ureter and the recesses of the renal pelvis. Kidney stones in cats can be isolated, but more often they are associated with stones in the ureter, inducing partial or complete urinary obstruction.

Preoperative Considerations

The most common clinical signs reported in cats with uroliths in the upper urinary tract are nonspecific, such as reduced appetite, lethargy, and weight loss.[6,7] Clinical signs may also be referable to uremia, such as vomiting, polyuria, and polydipsia, or directly to ureteral obstruction, such as stranguria, pollakiuria, hematuria, and abdominal pain.[6,7]

Clinical Evaluation

A complete blood count, chemistry profile, urinalysis, and urine culture should be performed. The blood urea nitrogen (BUN) and creatinine concentrations depend on the hydration status of the patient, kidney function, presence and extent of ureteral obstruction, and the function of the contralateral kidney. In one study of 163 cats with ureteral calculi, 83% of cats had a BUN or creatinine concentration above the reference range, and 33% were markedly azotemic (creatinine concentration >10 mg/dL; reference range, 1.1–2.2 mg/dL).[6,7] Seventy-six percent of cats with unilateral calculi were azotemic compared with 96% of cats with bilateral calculi. In addition, hyperphosphatemia was observed in 54%, hyperkalemia in 35%, and anemia in 48% of cats with ureteral calculi.[6,7] Urine should be evaluated for the presence of crystalluria, hematuria, and urinary tract infection.

Imaging

Most uroliths of the upper urinary tract are diagnosed using abdominal radiography and ultrasonography. When urolithiasis is diagnosed, the entire urinary tract should be evaluated for calculi.[6]

Plain Radiographs

Plain abdominal radiographs allow evaluation of renal size and shape; small radiopaque calculi and moderate to severe hydroureter may not be seen on plain abdominal radiographs.

Ultrasonography

Ureteral calculi can be imaged with abdominal ultrasonography. In one study in cats, the sensitivity of survey radiography alone for the diagnosis of ureteral calculi was 81%, sensitivity of ultrasonography alone was 77%, and sensitivity of a combination of survey radiography and ultrasonography was 90%.[6,7] In cats, ultrasonography has

---

Small Animal Laparoscopy and Thoracoscopy, First Edition. Edited by Boel A. Fransson and Philipp D. Mayhew.
© 2015 by ACVS Foundation. Published 2015 by John Wiley & Sons, Inc.
Companion website: www.wiley.com/go/fransson/laparoscopy

been associated with 100% sensitivity and 33% specificity for the diagnosis of obstruction of the ureter.[8] Abdominal ultrasonography is particularly useful for the evaluation of ureteral and renal pelvic dilation secondary to obstruction. Dilatation of the ureter, renal pelvis, or both was observed ultrasonographically in 92% of cats with ureteral calculi.[7]

Renal Scintigraphy

Technetium Tc 99m diethylenetriamine pentaacetic acid (DTPA) scintigraphy can be used to measure the glomerular filtration rate (GFR) of individual kidneys.[9-11] Total GFR in a normal dog should be between 2.53 and 5.41 mL/min/kg. Measurement of GFR is operator dependent.[10] The GFR in the obstructed kidney will be reduced, and scintigraphy cannot predict the GFR after relief of the obstruction. Measurement of the GFR of the contralateral kidney may assist in the decision to perform a nephrectomy on the obstructed kidney.

Patient Selection

Laparoscopic-assisted nephrolith removal has been attempted only in cats with small stones located in one or more recess of the renal pelvis (Figure 22-1). These stones represent a risk of recurrence of obstruction of the ureter because they may have migrated into the ureter.

Surgical Technique

Approach

After a midline laparotomy and a complete abdominal exploration, the affected kidney is exposed. The proximal ureter is dissected from the renal vasculature. The kidney is dissected from the retroperitoneal space and retracted medially.

Two stay sutures are placed in the proximal ureter close the renal parenchyma. A 3-mm-long incision is performed with a #11 blade in the proximal ureter. A 2.7-mm cystoscope is then introduced in the ureter and directed toward the renal pelvis. Warm sterile saline is connected to the cystoscope and instilled during the nephroscopy to keep the field clear of blood. It is not recommended to pressurize the sterile saline because doing so could induce a severe transient hydronephrosis. It is important that the ureterotomy is large enough

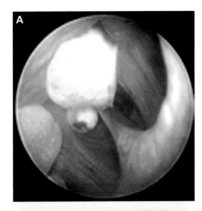
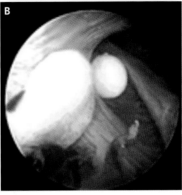

Figure 22-2 Intraoperative views (**A** and **B**) of stones wedged in different recesses of the renal pelvis.

to allow for the saline to flow around the cystoscope, egressing from the renal pelvis. If needed, a 3-French infant feeding tube can be inserted next to the cystoscope.

The recesses of the renal pelvis are all inspected with the cystoscope (Figure 22-2). A 3-French grasping forceps is then introduced through the working channel of the cystoscope to grasp and retrieve the stones one by one out of the renal pelvis.

After removal of all the stones, the renal pelvis is flushed with warm saline. The ureterotomy is then closed with either a simple continuous or simple interrupted suture. This authors prefers simple interrupted suture with 6-0 monofilament absorbable suture.

After completion of the surgery, the patient is diuresed overnight and monitored with continuous ECG and arterial pressure. Urine production is also monitored.

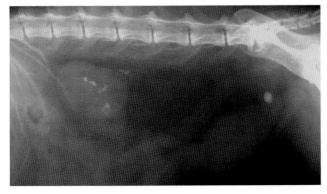

Figure 22-1 Lateral abdominal radiograph of a cat with several urinary stones in the ureters and kidney. The small stones in the kidney may migrate into the ureter after removal of the ureteral stone.

References

1 Gahring, D.R., Crowe, D.T., Powers, T.E., et al. (1977) Comparative renal function studies of nephrotomy closure with and without sutures in dogs. J Am Vet Med Assoc 171, 537-541.

2 Stone, E.A., Robertson, J.L., Metcalf, M.R. (2002) The effect of nephrotomy on renal function and morphology in dogs. Vet Surg 31 (4), 391-397.

3 Bolliger, C., Walshaw, R., Kruger, J.M., et al. (2005) Evaluation of the effects of nephrotomy on renal function in clinically normal cats. Am J Vet Res 66 (8), 1400-1407.

4 King, M.D., Waldron, D.R., Barber, D.L., et al. (2006) Effect of nephrotomy on renal function and morphology in normal cats. Vet Surg 35 (8), 749-758.

5 Greenwood, K.M., Rawlings, C. (1981) Removal of canine renal calculi by pyelolithotomy. Vet Surg 22, 12-21.

6 Kyles, A.E., Hardie, E.M., Wooden, B.G., et al. (2005) Clinical, clinicopathologic, radiographic, and ultrasonographic abnormalities in cats with ureteral calculi: 163 cases (1984-2002). J Am Vet Med Assoc 226 (6), 932-936.

7 Kyles, A.E., Hardie, E.M., Wooden, B.G., et al. (2005) Management and outcome of cats with ureteral calculi: 153 cases (1984-2002). J Am Vet Med Assoc 226 (6), 937-944.

8 Adin, C.A., Herrgesell, E.J., Nyland, T.G., et al. (2003) Antegrade pyelography for suspected ureteral obstruction in cats: 11 cases (1995-2001). J Am Vet Med Assoc 222 (11), 1576-1581.

9 Krawiec, D.R., Twardock, A.R., Badertscher, R.R., et al. (1988) Use of Tc-diethylen-etriaminepentaacetic acid for assessment of renal function in dogs with suspected renal disease. J Am Vet Med Assoc 192 (8), 1077-1079.

10 Kampa, N., Bostrom, I., Lord, P., et al. (2003) Day-to-day variability in glomeru-lar filtration rate in normal dogs by scintigraphic technique. J Vet Med A Physiol Pathol Clin Med 50 (1), 37-41.

11 Hecht, S., Lawson, S.M., Lane, I.F., et al. (2010) (99m)Tc-DTPA diuretic renal scin-tigraphy in dogs with nephroureterolithiasis. Can Vet J 51 (12), 1360-1366.

23

Laparoscopic-Assisted Cystoscopy for Urolith Removal and Mass Resection

Chloe Wormser, Jeffrey J. Runge, and Clarence A. Rawlings

Key Points

- Preoperative patient evaluation should aim to determine renal function and presence of urinary tract infection, as well as the characterization of the uroliths, including location, number, and size.
- All surgeons should be capable of converting to open surgery (cystotomy or urethrotomy) and be prepared to do so if any complications develop during urolith removal or mass resection.
- Ensure that all necessary equipment is available and in proper working order before starting the procedure.
- Laparoscopic-assisted cystoscopy can be readily used for polyp resection.

Preoperative Considerations

Introduction to Urolith Management

Despite advances in the prevention and management of urinary calculi in dogs and cats, urolithiasis remains a commonly encountered problem in companion animal medicine (Figures 23-1 and 23-2). Furthermore, changes in calculus management over the past decade have resulted in an increased percentage of uroliths that are difficult to manage medically.[1] Given that persistent urolithiasis can lead to cystitis, urinary tract infection (UTI), hematuria, or urethral obstruction, timely diagnosis and intervention are important to minimize morbidity and the perpetuation of lower urinary tract disease.

Surgical Management of Urolithiasis: Comparative Aspects

Bladder and urethral calculi account for 5% of human urinary stones in the Western world and usually occur in patients with underlying urologic disorders.[2,3] The most prevalent cause is bladder outlet obstruction due to benign prostatic hyperplasia, but UTI, neurogenic bladder disorders, urethral strictures, foreign bodies, and calculi migration from the upper urinary tract have also been described.[3]

Conversely, bladder stones are considered endemic among children in developing countries, representing up to 30% of diagnosed urinary calculi in this subpopulation.[4-7] Whereas the main component of stones seen in developed countries is struvite, the majority of stones in developing countries are composed of ammonium urate.[8] Although the pathogenesis and biochemical explanation for endemic stone formation remain unclear, there seems to be a correlation between urolithiasis and malnutrition, low animal protein intake, and vitamin A deficiency.[8-10]

In both children and adults, open surgery for removal of lower urinary tract stones has been almost entirely replaced by minimally invasive techniques. The transition to a minimally invasive approach has been prompted by the high number of complications reported with traditional open surgery for stone removal, including recurrent calculus formation, the need for serial surgeries, suture-induced stone formation, strictures, adhesions, bleeding, uroabdomen, pain, and other life-threatening conditions.[11-13] Indeed, open surgical removal of stones is currently described in only 0.3% to 4% of human patients with urolithiasis.[11]

Many stones can be removed using entirely noninvasive methods such as intra- or extracorporeal lithotripsy.[11,14,15] In stones not amenable to these techniques, transurethral disintegration and retrieval of bladder and urethral calculi is the current standard of care in adult urologic patients.[14-16] The narrow diameter of the urethra in pediatric patients precludes routine use of this technique, and instead percutaneous cystolithotomy is preferable.[14,17-19] This procedure is also used in adult patients with large solid stones and in

Small Animal Laparoscopy and Thoracoscopy, First Edition. Edited by Boel A. Fransson and Philipp D. Mayhew.
© 2015 by ACVS Foundation. Published 2015 by John Wiley & Sons, Inc.

Companion website: www.wiley.com/go/fransson/laparoscopy

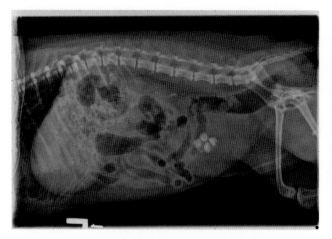

Figure 23-1 Abdominal radiograph of multiple uroliths in a dog.

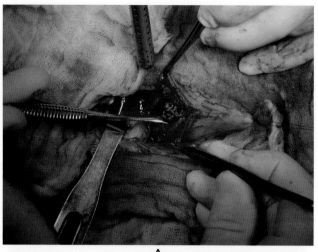

A

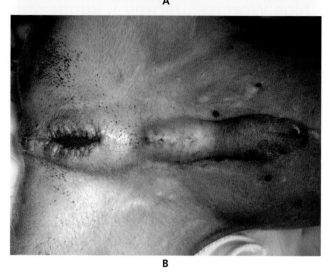

B

Figure 23-3 **A,** Open cystotomy on a male dog with a large cystic calculi. **B,** Urethrostomy in a male dog that had urethroliths.

circumstances that do not allow a transurethral approach, such as in patients with anatomic abnormalities.[19]

Veterinary Surgical Management of Urolithiasis

In small animals, surgical removal of uroliths by cystotomy or urethrotomy has been the traditional method of choice, and these procedures are still common (Figure 23-3). However, several studies have elucidated insufficiencies in the open cystotomy technique. In a 1992 study, calculi remained in the bladder after cystotomy in 10% of dogs and 20% of cats.[20] In a larger, more recent study, removal of uroliths was incomplete in 20% of dogs after cystotomy.[21] Furthermore, a 2008 study reported that 9.4% of recurrent stones in dogs were suture induced, indicating that cystotomy could, in fact, increase the risk of stone formation.[22] Recently, complications associated with traditional surgical cystotomy, regardless of closure method, were reported in 37% to 50% of cases, with a mean duration of hospitalization of 4 days.[23]

The above listed shortcomings of the open cystotomy procedure make less invasive alternatives with fewer complications, fewer long-term stone recurrences, more efficient stone removal, and shorter hospitalization times desirable. In small animals, minimally invasive treatment options for lower urinary tract stones include voiding urohydropulsion, intracorporeal lithotripsy, extracorporeal shock-wave lithotripsy, transurethral cystoscopic stone retrieval, laparoscopic-assisted cystotomy, and percutaneous cystolithotomy.

Pathophysiology of Uroliths in Dogs and Cats

Uroliths are organized concretions of primarily organic or inorganic crystalloid (the ionic component of crystals) and a much

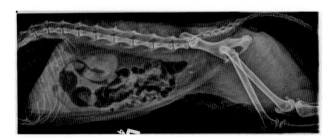

Figure 23-2 Abdominal radiograph of multiple uroliths in a cat.

smaller amount of organic matrix[24]. Urolith formation is dependent on a multitude of interrelated factors within the urine, including supersaturation with crystals, organic molecule contributions such as protein inhibitors or promoters of crystallization, urine pH, and presence of urine stasis. Not only does the interplay of these factors lead to urolith formation, but it also dictates urolith composition.[24,25] It is important to note that the presence of crystals within the urinary tract does not necessarily mean that the patient is at risk for urolithiasis.[24] Crystalluria in itself is not a disease, and no particular treatment is necessary unless concurrent urolithiasis is present or the patient has a history of past urolith formation.[24]

Epidemiology

Cats

Approximately 89% to 96% of all cats' uroliths submitted to urolith centers are composed of magnesium ammonium phosphate (struvite) or calcium oxalate.[26,27] Currently, struvite and oxalate stones occur with similar frequency in the feline lower urinary tract, although 75% to 87% of upper urinary tract stones (nephroliths and ureteroliths) are calcium oxalate.[26,27] An increase in oxalate urolithiasis from 1985 to 1994 is thought to be the result of widespread dietary acidification.[26] Changes in dietary management, with less emphasis on urinary acidification, may have affected urolith composition in recent years.[26] Less common uroliths recovered from cats include urate (3%–10%); calcium phosphate (0.1%–6%); and dried, solidified blood calculi (1%).[26,27] The signalment may help predict the composition of bladder calculi in feline patients. Specifically, male cats are more likely to have oxalate than struvite uroliths (1.6:1).[26,27] In contrast, female cats are slightly more likely to have struvite than oxalate uroliths (1.2:1).[26,27] Younger cats (younger than 4 years of age) have a higher frequency of struvite uroliths, middle-aged cats (4–7 years) have an equal proportion of struvite and oxalate uroliths, and cats older than 7 years of age are more likely to have oxalate uroliths. However, these differences are not dramatic.[26] Breed predilections have also been recognized, with oxalate uroliths twice as common as struvite uroliths in Persians and Himalayans.[26,27] Urate uroliths are more commonly recognized in Siamese cats than in other breeds.[26,27]

Dogs

Between 80% and 91% of all uroliths submitted from dogs are struvite or calcium oxalate.[28-30] Similar to cats, the frequency of oxalate uroliths has increased compared with struvite uroliths over recent years.[28] However, the frequency of struvite uroliths is still slightly higher than that of calcium oxalate uroliths (44%–45% vs. 35%–42%).[29,30] Whereas female dogs are 12 to 15 times more likely to have struvite uroliths compared with oxalate uroliths, male dogs are three times more likely to have oxalate uroliths.[28,29] Younger dogs are more likely to have struvite as opposed to oxalate uroliths.[28] Certain breeds are predisposed to developing uroliths, although the interactions among breed, sex, and age complicate prediction of composition. In contrast to cats, in which most upper urinary tract stones contain calcium, upper urinary tract uroliths in dogs are evenly distributed among struvite, calcium oxalate, and other urolith types.[1,31,32]

Surgical Anatomy

The lower urinary tract in male and female dogs can be generally divided into two regions, the bladder and the urethra. The urinary bladder can vary greatly in both size and location within the abdomen depending on the amount of urine it contains. The blood supply to the bladder comes from the cranial and caudal vesical arteries. The urinary bladder has sympathetic innervation from the hypogastric nerves and parasympathetic innervation from the pelvic nerves. The pudendal nerve provides somatic innervation to the external bladder sphincter and the striated musculature of the urethra.

Diagnostic Workup and Imaging

Patient evaluation should be aimed at determining renal function, the presence of UTI, and systemic organ function. With regard to uroliths, the number, size, and location of calculi should be determined.

History and Clinical Signs

Clinical signs associated with bladder calculi are similar to those seen with other diseases of the lower urinary tract and include hematuria, pollakiuria, stranguria, and dysuria. Uroliths and masses can cause a partial or complete urethral obstruction, which may result in bladder distension, abdominal pain, paradoxical incontinence, stranguria, and signs of postrenal azotemia (anorexia, vomiting, depression). Occasionally, bladder rupture and uroabdomen ensue.

Physical Examination Findings

With cystic calculi, the bladder wall may be thickened, and uroliths may be palpable. With urethral obstruction, the bladder is distended on abdominal palpation. Rectal examination may reveal palpable urethral calculi as well as a distended urethra when obstruction is present.

Laboratory Testing

A complete blood count and biochemical profile should be performed in any patient with history or clinical signs compatible with urolithiasis. Abnormalities may suggest a certain urolith type, such as the presence of hypercalcemia in patients with calcium oxalate or calcium phosphate urolithiasis. In cases of lower urinary tract obstruction, azotemia may be present. Azotemia should be addressed before calculus removal in all but the most urgent clinical cases. Confirmed renal dysfunction may require modification of the plan for calculus removal. Uroliths of both the upper and lower urinary tracts may cause or be associated with infection. Leukocytosis may be seen with pyelonephritis in some cases but is not typically associated with simple cystitis.[33]

A urinalysis should also be evaluated in patients with urinary disorders. Crystal solubility is affected by urine pH. Specifically, struvite uroliths are more likely to form in alkaline urine; calcium phosphate in alkaline to neutral urine; calcium oxalate and silica in neutral to acidic urine; and urate, xanthine, cystine, and brushite in acidic urine.[34] In patients without urinary tract disease, calcium oxalate and struvite crystals may form in urine samples that have been refrigerated or analyzed more than 4 to 6 hours after collection. However, in patients with uroliths, crystalluria in a fresh urine sample (<60 minutes) may provide some insight into urolith composition.

Uroliths are often associated with UTI. Therefore, urine sediment evaluation is of importance and may reveal pyuria or bacteriuria. Urine culture is indicated in all cases of urolithiasis. Infection has been documented in approximately 75% of dogs with cystic calculi when the results of urine, bladder mucosal biopsy, and urolith culture are combined.[35] Ideally, all stone retrieval procedures should be performed after a negative urine culture result has been documented or the patient has been receiving an appropriate antibiotic for at least 24 hours before intervention, although this is not always possible or completely necessary. It is the authors' opinion that surgery timing in relation to antibiotic treatment is determined on a patient-by-patient basis.

Further testing may be indicated for specific urolith types depending on clinical findings (e.g., tests for hyperadrenocorticism in patients with calcium oxalate urolithiasis), which is beyond the scope of this text.

Diagnostic Imaging

Survey Radiography

Calcium oxalate and struvite uroliths are generally radiopaque; as such, they are usually visible on survey radiographs.[36,37] However, 1.7% to 5.2% of these uroliths are not radiographically apparent. These undetected stones are typically small (<1 mm).[37] Urate, cysteine, and calcium phosphate calculi are variably radiopaque, and approximately 25% of survey radiographs are interpreted as negative for these uroliths.[36] The incidence of false-negative results with survey radiography is 13% for all urolith types combined.[37] Radiographic views must include the entire urethra such that urethral calculi are not overlooked. A false-positive radiographic diagnosis can occur because of end-on vessels, nipples, and other structures mistaken for uroliths. Thus, orthogonal radiographic projections should always be taken and compared.

Contrast Radiography

Negative-contrast (air) cystography is more sensitive than survey radiography for detection of calculi within the lower urinary tract, with a false-negative rate of 6.5%.[37] Double-contrast radiography further improves diagnostic accuracy, with a false-negative rate of 4.5%.[37] These techniques have been described in detail elsewhere.[38] Briefly, it is recommended that a pool of 200 mg/mL of contrast agent (1 part contrast to 1 part sterile saline) 5 mm deep (~1–5 mL) provides the best accuracy for determining whether calculi are present or absent.[37,39] Although double-contrast radiography is the most sensitive method for counting calculi, an accurate count is reported in only 53% of cases.[37]

Abdominal Ultrasonography

Abdominal ultrasonography is useful for the detection of both radiopaque and nonradiopaque calculi within the urinary bladder. Ultrasonography also helps obtain more information about renal structure and function. Urethral calculi, however, are difficult to visualize with ultrasonography unless they are lodged near the neck of the bladder. The false-negative rate of ultrasonography for detecting uroliths is 3.5%, making it more accurate than survey radiography and comparable to double-contrast radiography.[37]

Computed Tomography

Computed tomography (CT) is commonly used for detection of urinary tract stones in human urologic patients. A recent study showed that noncontrast CT could be used to predict stone composition in dogs on the basis of radiodensity, measured in Hounsfield units.[40]

Cystoscopy

Cystoscopy is increasingly used and constitutes a reliable method for urolith detection; it also allows for evaluation of the inner architecture of the bladder and urethra for inflammatory and neoplastic lesions. Cystoscopy is typically combined with minimally invasive therapies, including stone retrieval and biopsy.[41]

Patient and Technique Selection

Case selection is of critical importance when choosing between open surgery when uroliths are very large (Figure 23-4) or with minimally invasive urolith retrieval techniques when the urolith size does not require the need for conversion to an open cystotomy (Figure 23-5). Surgical failure and complications can often be avoided when careful attention is paid to both patient factors (signalment and concurrent disease) and stone characteristics (location, size).

Nearly all calculi in female dogs and cats can be removed by transurethral cystoscopy, laparoscopic-assisted cystotomy, or percutaneous cystolithotomy.[41] Most male dogs can be treated with laparoscopic-assisted cystotomy or percutaneous cystolithotomy. Transurethral cystoscopy is preferred for female cats and dogs because it is less invasive than laparoscopic-assisted techniques. However, the calculi must be small enough to be exteriorized by the transurethral route. Size criteria are continually being modified,

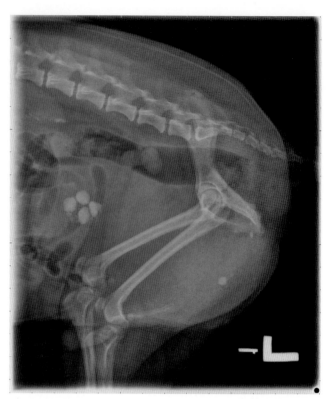

Figure 23-4 Radiograph of male dog with numerous large cystic and urethral calculi.

but in general, in female cats and dogs, calculi can be removed that are twice the diameter of the largest cystoscope appropriate for the patient. In male dogs, transurethral removal is limited to smaller calculi because the stones must pass the os penis region of the urethra. Calculi in male cats can be removed by laparoscopic-assisted cystoscopy and percutaneous cystolithotomy, but the urethra is likely too small for current transurethral cystoscopy techniques.

Transurethral cystoscopic calculus removal in female dogs has been enhanced in some specialty hospitals by cystoscopic lithotripsy.[42-46] This technique is indicated for calculi that are too large

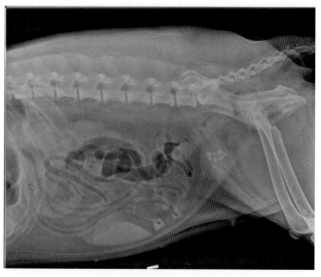

Figure 23-5 Radiograph of a female dog with multiple small cystic calculi.

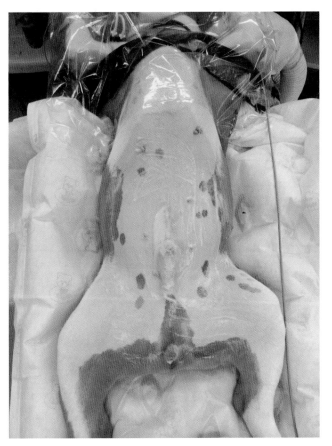
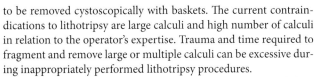

Figure 23-6 Male dog in dorsal recumbency clipped for laparoscopic-assisted cystoscopy.

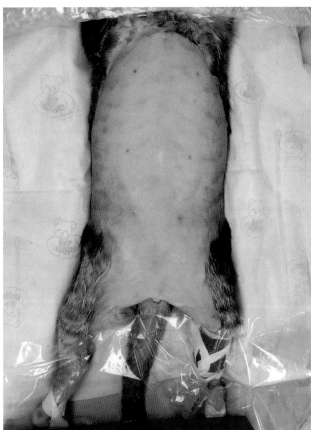

Figure 23-7 Male cat in dorsal recumbency clipped for laparoscopic-assisted cystoscopy.

to be removed cystoscopically with baskets. The current contraindications to lithotripsy are large calculi and high number of calculi in relation to the operator's expertise. Trauma and time required to fragment and remove large or multiple calculi can be excessive during inappropriately performed lithotripsy procedures.

Laparoscopic-assisted cystotomy and percutaneous cystolithotomy have proven to be effective methods to remove calculi from female and male dogs and cats.[47-49] The primary contraindication is the presence of large stones (i.e., several centimeters in diameter), requiring removal through a long abdominal incision. In contrast, a very large number of smaller calculi can be time consuming, but it is the authors' opinion that minimally invasive techniques are useful in such cases. These techniques, combined with the use of lavage and suction, can facilitate easy and thorough removal of a large number of stones, grit, and stone fragments.[41]

In the authors' opinion, traditional laparotomy and cystotomy are typically reserved for patients with very large calculi or those requiring additional complex abdominal procedures.[41] Most cases benefit from minimally invasive stone removal given the decreased morbidity and superior visualization associated with these techniques compared with open laparotomy and cystotomy.

Patient Preparation

Surgical Preparation
Patients should be fasted for at least 8 to 12 hours before surgery. This recommendation may vary depending on the age of the patient

or presence of concurrent illness. Perioperative antibiotics (cefazolin 22 mg/kg intravenously [IV]) are typically given at induction, with doses administered every 120 minutes for the duration of the surgical procedure. For the procedures outlined in this section, the patient is positioned in dorsal recumbency (Figures 23-6 and 23-7). The ventral abdomen is clipped and aseptically prepped. All patients should have a wide clip that can also accommodate an open cystotomy or urethrotomy procedure. This clip should extend caudally and include the entire prepuce or vulva, which are also draped in the surgical field to allow for cystoscopy, urethral catheterization, or both.

Surgical Technique(s)

Equipment
The basic scopes used to diagnose and remove calculi and perform mass resection and biopsy can be separated into two groups: (1) specifically manufactured cystoscopes and urethroscopes with integrated instruments channels and (2) standard nonoperating telescopes used in conjunction with minimally invasive instruments. Commonly used cystoscopes include the 2.7-mm rigid cystoscope and the 2.5-/2.8-mm flexible fiberoptic urethroscope. Cats and dogs weighing less than 5 kg may benefit from using a 1.9-mm cystoscope. Larger 3.5- or 4.0-mm cystoscopes are used for transurethral cystoscopy in female dogs. The flexible urethroscope is usually reserved for use in male dogs because it can accommodate the curve of the urethra.

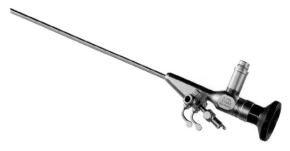

Figure 23-8 Multipurpose rigid endoscope (Karl Storz Endoscopy, Goleta, CA).

Equipment List
Commonly Used Cystoscopes Used for Laparoscopic-Assisted or Transurethral Cystoscopy in Canine and Feline Patients

1   Multipurpose rigid endoscope (Figure 23-8)
    HOPKINS II Forward-Oblique Telescope 30 degree (Karl Storz Endoscopy, Goleta, CA)
    Length, 18 cm
    Diameter, 2.7 mm
    Sheath, 14.5 French; working length, 15 cm; and working channel, 5 French
2   Pediatric operating cystoscope (Figure 23-9)
    Semi-rigid Operating Telescope 30 degree (Karl Storz Endoscopy)
    Diameter, 9.5 Fr
    Working length, 14 cm
    Working channel, 3 French
3   Flexible ureteroscopes (Figure 23-10)
    Flex –XC (Karl Storz Endoscopy)
    Diameter, 8.5 French
    Working length, 70 cm
    Working channel = 3.6 Fr

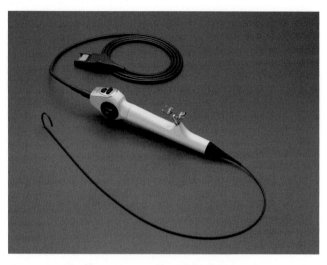

Figure 23-10 Flexible ureteroscope Flex XC (Karl Storz Endoscopy, Goleta, CA).

4   Flexible ureteroscopes (Figure 23-11)
    FLEX-X2 (Karl Storz Endoscopy)
    Diameter, 7.5 French
    Working length, 67 cm
    Working channel, 3.6 French

Commonly Used Ports and Trocar-Cannula Assemblies for Laparoscopic-Assisted Cystotomy Procedures

1   5-mm port with Luer lock attached to suction (Figure 23-12)
2   5-mm Ternamian cannula; EndoTIP (Karl Storz Endoscopy) (Figure 23-13)

Other

1   Stone basket (>70 cm length)
2   Stone basket (resterilizable) (Karl Storz Endoscopy) (Figure 23-14)
3   Grasper
4   Holmium:YAG laser tip for laser lithotripsy
5   Pressure bag for lavage
6   Red rubber catheters or Foley catheter
7   Hydrophilic guide (Weasel) wire (0.018, 0.035, and 0.045 mm)
8   360-degree wound retractor (Figure 23-15)

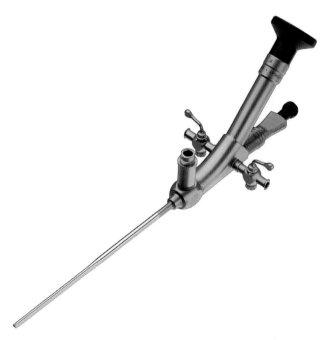

Figure 23-9 Pediatric operating cystoscope (Karl Storz Endoscopy, Goleta, CA).

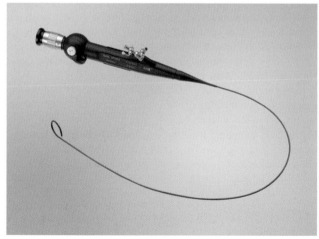

Figure 23-11 Flexible ureteroscope Flex X2 (Karl Storz Endoscopy, Goleta, CA).

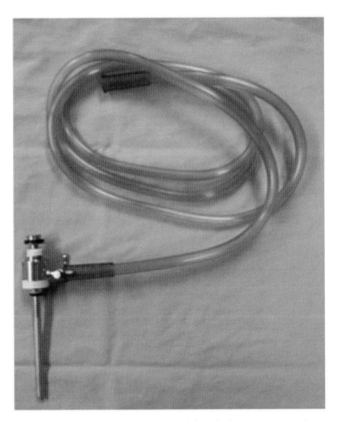

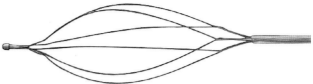

Figure 23-14 Stone basket (resterilizable) (Karl Storz Endoscopy, Goleta, CA).

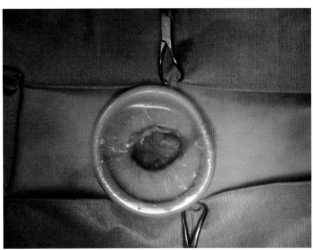

Figure 23-15 360-degree wound retractor device (Karl Storz Endoscopy, Goleta, CA).

Figure 23-12 Five-mm port with Luer lock (attached to suction tubing).

Surgical Techniques
Portal Position and Creation of Working Space
The location of port positions varies with the procedures; two- or single-port techniques may be used (Figures 23-16 and 23-17). The port positioning will be specifically described for each technique separately. Saline is commonly used to distend the bladder and to create working space for the procedure. The bladder can be easily distended, and the saline also allows for flushing of debris and blood to enhance visualization. The operating room setup is depicted in Figure 23-18.

Transurethral Cystoscopy
Transurethral cystoscopy as described by Rawlings *et al.*[41] allows for calculus removal using a stone basket and is therefore less

invasive than open cystotomy or other minimally invasive techniques. However, the calculi must be small enough for removal via the urethra. In general, basket removal can be attempted for calculi smaller than 3 mm in diameter in female cats and male dogs. In female dogs, calculi removed using this method should not exceed twice the diameter of the largest cystoscope the urethra can accommodate. Commonly used cystoscope sizes are 1.9 mm for female cats and dogs weighing less than 5 kg, 2.7 mm for medium-sized female dogs, and 3.5 or 4.0 mm for larger female dogs. The two smaller 1.9- and 2.7-mm cystoscope sizes can be

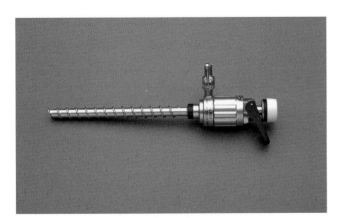

Figure 23-13 Five-mm Ternamian cannula.
(EndoTIP; Karl Storz Endoscopy, Goleta, CA).

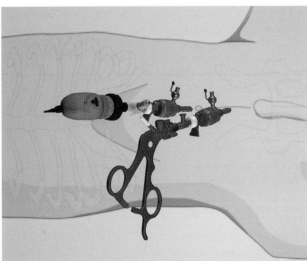

Figure 23-16 Location of port position for the two-port laparoscopic-assisted cystotomy technique.

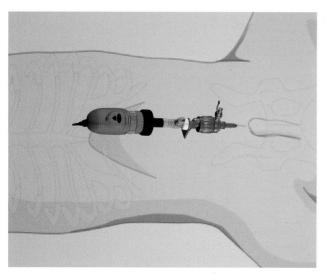

Figure 23-17 Location of port position for the percutaneous cystolithotomy or one-port techniques.

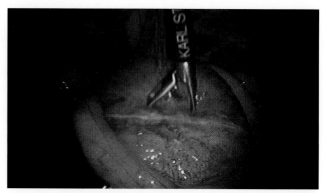

Figure 23-19 The bladder apex is grasped using laparoscopic Babcock forceps.

used to retrieve calculi in nearly all female dogs. A 1.9-mm cystoscope and a basket retrieval instrument have been used to remove calculi during cystoscopic examination of the urethra and bladder in male cats after perineal urethrostomy.[41] Basket retrieval devices (see Figure 23-14) with three or four wires are preferred. They should easily fit through the operating channel for the cystoscope. After diagnostic cystoscopy is used to examine the lower urinary tract and lavage the bladder, the basket is passed through the operating channel. Individual techniques vary, but it is the authors' preference to have the bladder only mildly distended and to keep the lavage flow rate low. This practice concentrates the calculi and reduces the swirling effect that can be produced by higher flow rates. Having the patient in dorsal recumbency and tilted with the head up (reversed Trendelenburg position) can also move the calculi toward the outflow tract. External abdominal manipulation of the bladder can be helpful. The basket is opened in the area of the calculi and gradually closed during cystoscopic examination to secure the basket around the stone. Only gentle pressure should be applied to the stone to minimize the likelihood of calculus fragmentation caused by basket compression. This procedure is repeated until all the calculi are removed. Vigorous flushing may be used to remove the smallest calculi.

Laparoscopic-Assisted Cystotomy

Laparoscopic-assisted cystotomy has been described in detail by Rawlings[41] and Rawlings *et al.*[47] (see Figure 23-16, Video Clip 23-1) The procedure is performed via a mini-laparotomy, the location of which is guided by visualization of the bladder through a laparoscopic cannula placed immediately caudal to the umbilicus. In this technique, the bladder is catheterized or aspirated to drain urine. After laparoscopic entry and pneumoperitoneum creation (described in detail elsewhere in this text), the bladder is visualized. Another cannula is placed at the level of the bladder apex, and the bladder is grasped using laparoscopic Babcock forceps (Figure 23-19, Video Clip 23-2). The port incision is enlarged to create a mini-laparotomy, and the bladder is partially exteriorized (Figure 23-20). A small cystotomy is performed, and the bladder wall is sutured to the skin of the abdominal incision using four isolated tension-relieving sutures (cruciate, or mattress patterns). A rigid cystoscope (2.7-mm except for cats and dogs weighing <5 kg, in which a 1.9-mm scope is preferred) is then inserted into the bladder for calculus retrieval. The cystoscope is used in combination with

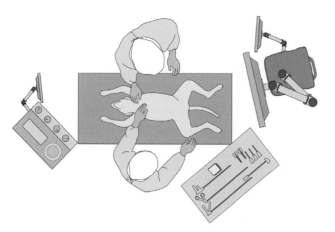

Figure 23-18 Operating room set-up for laparoscopic-assisted cystotomy or percutaneous cystolithotomy.

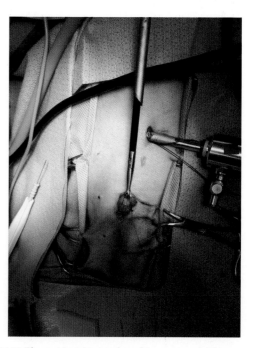

Figure 23-20 The port incision is enlarged to create a mini-laparotomy, and the bladder is partially exteriorized.

a basket retrieval instrument, which is passed through the cystoscope's operating channel.

After calculi are removed from the bladder, the urethra is examined with a rigid cystoscope (female dogs) or a flexible fiberoptic urethroscope (male dogs). Urethral calculi in male dogs can be removed by either retrograde flushing or a basket retrieval device. The cystotomy incision is closed routinely. Retracting a portion of the omentum to be sutured over the bladder incision has been recommended. Abdominal incisions are closed routinely.

Modified Laparoscopic-Assisted Cystotomy

Modifications of the above laparoscopic-assisted cystotomy technique have been described by Pinel et al.[49] (Video Clip 23-3). Modifications include creation of a temporary complete cystopexy with the abdominal wall instead of placement of stay sutures to secure the bladder (Figure 23-21). The cystopexy is thought to limit bladder manipulation and contamination of the peritoneal cavity with urine during surgery (Video Clip 23-4) Additionally, a 5-mm laparoscope can be used instead of a 2.7-/1.9-mm cystoscope to gain access to the bladder. When used with a cannula, this allows for the creation of a flow of saline to flush uroliths out of the bladder without the need for forceps (see Figure 23-12). Larger uroliths can be grasped with forceps introduced next to the cannula (Figure 23-22), which is technically less challenging than grasping uroliths with a retrieval device through the working channel of a cystoscope. The 5-mm laparoscope also provides a larger viewing window and greater image resolution compared with the 2.7-/1.9-mm cystoscope. Last, creation of retrograde saline flow using a urethral catheter as opposed to antegrade saline flow created with a cystoscope is described to help flush uroliths out of the bladder lumen.

Percutaneous Cystolithotomy

Percutaneous cystolithotomy (see Figure 23-17) has been described by one of the authors (JJR).[48] A small ventral midline incision (~1–1.5 cm) is made in the abdominal cavity just over the apex of the urinary bladder. A wound retraction device is used to expose the

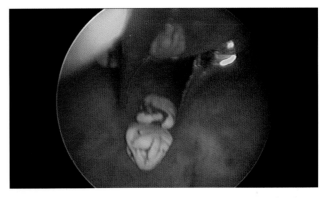

Figure 23-22 Larger uroliths can be grasped with forceps introduced next to the cannula.

urinary bladder (Figure 23-23). The bladder is palpated digitally and grasped with Babcock forceps. Three stay sutures are placed near the apex the bladder in a triangular arrangement. The sutures are used to hold the bladder in place and simultaneously place countertraction on the bladder while a laparoscopic threaded cannula is inserted into the bladder. The location of this threaded cannula placement is located caudal to the apex on the ventral aspect of the bladder centered within the triangulated stay sutures (Video Clip 23-5). The threaded cannula is inserted immediately after a small 2- to 3-mm incision is made using a #11 blade into the urinary bladder to enable insertion of the cannula (Figure 23-24). A rigid cystoscope or flexible ureteroscope is inserted through this port and into the bladder lumen or urethra, allowing for identification and removal of stones using a stone retrieval basket through the working channel of the cystoscope (Figure 23-25, Video Clip 23-6). For very small stones, suction can be placed into the threaded port, and the stones can be flushed and suctioned out of the port in retrograde fashion with saline being flushed through a urethral catheter. For stones that exceed the diameter of the port, a number of options exist to enable removal. For stones that exceed the diameter of the standard 5-mm instrument port, a number of options exist to enable removal. A 10-mm threaded cannula can be used to allow for larger stones, lithotripsy can be used to fragment the stones, or the stones can be manipulated through the small incision with the stone basket. After

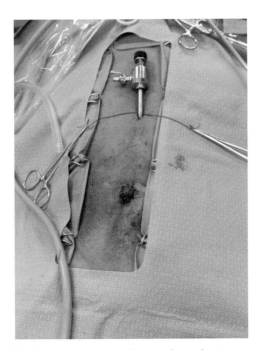

Figure 23-21 Complete cystopexy at the second cannula site.

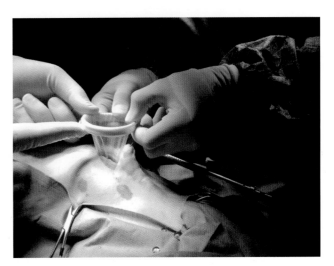

Figure 23-23 A wound retraction device properly positioned in the abdomen.

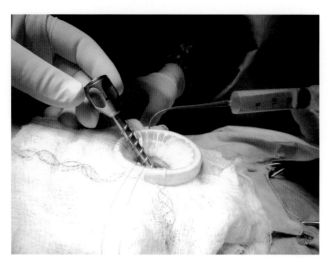

Figure 23-24 Threaded cannula inserted into the ventral apex region of the urinary bladder.

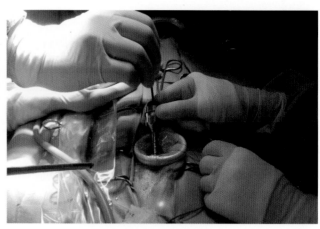

Figure 23-26 Flexible ureteroscope entering the threaded trocar on the ventral aspect of the bladder. The light of urethroscope can be seen transilluminating the urethra at the level of the os penis.

calculi removal from the bladder, the urethra is examined using a rigid cystoscope in female dogs or a flexible ureteroscope in male dogs (Figure 23-26). A basket retrieval device can be used to locate (Figure 23-27) and remove (Figure 23-28) any remaining urethral calculi through the working channel of the scope. The bladder wall is closed routinely using an interrupted appositional suture pattern and absorbable suture material.

Complications and Prognosis

It is these authors' opinion that the use of these minimally invasive techniques for urolith removal is safe and effective. Overall, these techniques have significantly improved the effectiveness of small animal urolith removal with very low complication rates. Excellent outcomes have been reported with use of laparoscopic-assisted cystotomy, modified laparoscopic-assisted cystotomy, and percutaneous cystolithotomy.[47-49] Complete stone removal rates are reported to be

approximately 96%,[48] and procedure times are dramatically shorter than those seen with other minimally invasive techniques such as laser lithotripsy, regardless of patient signalment or stone number.[48,50]

Regardless of the removal technique used, any urolith that is retrieved should be submitted for analysis. Quantitative analysis that provides relative percentage composition of each mineral type is preferred over qualitative analysis and helps guide postoperative management recommendations.

Postoperative Care

The hospitalization time for these minimally invasive urolith removal techniques is short, and surgery can often be offered on an outpatient basis. At least one lateral abdominal radiograph should

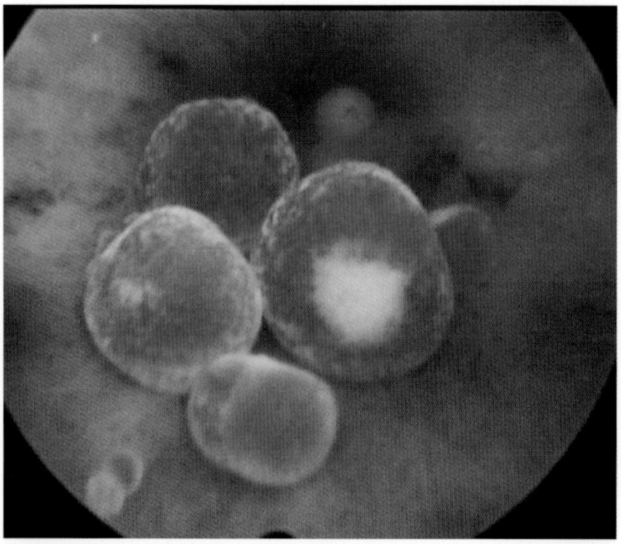

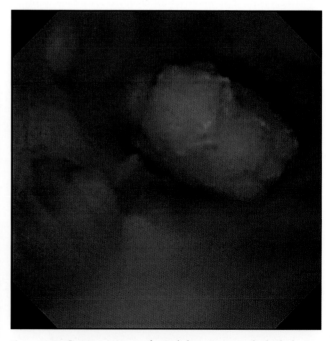

Figure 23-27 Cystoscopic image of a single large 7-mm urethral calculus in a dog that was seen on abdominal radiographs. Calculus was noted to be the level of the os penis. Multiple attempts at dislodging the calculi were unsuccessful.

Figure 23-25 Calculi visible in the trigonal region of the urinary bladder in a cat.

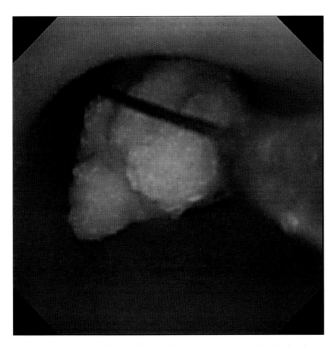

Figure 23-28 Same patient in Figure 23-27. The urethral calculus has been dislodged from the urethra and is being pulled in a retrograde manner back into the bladder and then out of the patient with a basket retrieval device.

be taken after calculus removal while the patient is anesthetized to confirm that all radiopaque calculi have been removed. Fluid therapy is recommended for the first 12 to 24 hours after surgery to help maintain renal function and to encourage voiding of residual blood and calculi fragments. Despite the minimally invasive approach, pain management is still a critical component of patient care. Common protocols include administration of an opioid during the initial recovery period and a nonsteroidal antiinflammatory drug or opioid for the first few days after surgery. Bupivacaine can be infused into the urethra for additional transient analgesia if desired. Dietary management to reduce the likelihood of calculus recurrence is typically delayed until the patient is fully recovered and the final calculi analysis is obtained. Nutritional therapy immediately postoperatively is targeted on supporting early healing.

Urinary calculi recurrence is common. Therefore, patients that are chronic calculi formers must be closely monitored by the owner and veterinarian for evidence of urinary tract dysfunction or blockage. In patients with a history of UTI, routine urinalysis and bacteriologic cultures should be performed. When feasible, dietary management should also be considered. In patients with calculi recurrence despite appropriate medical management, it is prudent to consider radiographic or ultrasonographic evaluation every 4 to 6 months for serial monitoring and early detection.

Bladder Tumor Biopsy and Polyp Resection

Tumors of the urinary bladder, both benign and malignant, are responsible for significant morbidity and mortality in veterinary patients. Accurate diagnosis of urinary bladder lesions is essential to guide prognosis and recommended treatment. Biopsy of suspicious bladder lesions is necessary for definitive diagnosis, especially because neoplastic lesions cannot be differentiated from non-neoplastic lesions based on appearance alone.

Preoperative Evaluation

A thorough workup in patients with suspect benign or malignant urinary bladder lesions is essential. This should include assessment of local tumor extent, evaluation for concurrent systemic illness, and staging for regional or distant metastatic disease. Serum biochemical analysis, complete blood count, urinalysis, and urine culture should be included in the diagnostic workup. Local tumor assessment can be performed using ultrasonography, contrast radiography, or cystoscopy. Ultrasonography can also be used for evaluation of locoregional metastasis, and cystoscopy provides visualization of the urethra in addition to the urinary bladder for extension of local disease. Thoracic radiographs for staging purposes should be taken in any patient with suspect malignant disease.

Cystoscopy for Bladder Mass Biopsy and Polyp Resection

Cystoscopy provides a minimally invasive means for evaluating patients with suspected bladder tumors because it allows for early detection and direct visualization of bladder mucosal lesions.[51] Cystoscopic biopsy can provide a definitive diagnosis, in particular with regards to differentiating neoplastic from non-neoplastic (polypoid) masses.[52] Cystoscopy and cystoscopic biopsy may also be used to monitor treatment success and disease progression in the context of urinary bladder neoplasia. Although these techniques are currently considered standard of care in human urologic patients,[52] their utilization in veterinary patients is currently in its infancy. Inflammatory polyps of the urinary bladder are the most commonly diagnosed non-neoplastic bladder lesions in dogs and occur as the result of inflammatory changes that can develop with recurrent UTIs or urinary tract stones. Polyp resection is often recommended to help attenuate inflammation and manage infections. In contrast to many neoplastic bladder lesions necessitating wide surgical excision or treatment options other than surgical intervention, marginal resection of polypoid lesions is appropriate.

Transurethral Cystoscopy for Bladder Mass Biopsy

Transurethral cystoscopy provides a minimally approach for evaluation of the urinary bladder and urethral mucosa and biopsy of suspicious lesions. The technique used is similar to that described by Rawlings et al.[41] (see previous section on transurethral cystoscopy for urolith retrieval). Biopsy forceps or graspers can be used to collect biopsy samples. After biopsy, the cystoscope should be used to evaluate for excessive hemorrhage.

Laparoscopic-Assisted Cystoscopy for Polyp Resection

A laparoscopic-assisted approach for resection of inflammatory polyps in the urinary bladder has been described by Rawlings et al.[51] After laparoscopic entry, the bladder is exteriorized using a technique similar to that described for laparoscopic-assisted cystoscopy for urinary calculi removal[47] (see previous section). A small cystotomy incision is made at the bladder apex for placement of a 2.7-mm, 30-degree cystoscope into the bladder lumen. Urine is evacuated through the cystoscope, and the urinary bladder is then lavaged with saline to provide a clear optical medium. The mucosal surface is examined, and the polypoid lesion is identified. The bladder is exteriorized through the abdominal incision, and an incision is made near the base of the polyp to resect the bladder wall containing the mass. Resection is performed under direct cystoscopic visualization using a #15 scalpel blade. After closure, the bladder is returned to the abdomen, the abdomen is reinsufflated, and the bladder closure site is omentalized.

All videos cited in this chapter can be found on the book's companion website at **www.wiley.com/go/fransson/laparoscopy**

References

1 Ling, G.V., Ruby, A.L., Johnson, D.L., et al. (1998) Renal calculi in dogs and cats: prevalence, mineral type, breed, age, and gender interrelationships (1981-1993). J Vet Intern Med 12 (1), 11-21.

2 Tzortzis, V., Aravantinos, E., Karatzas, A., et al. (2006) Percutaneous suprapubic cystolithotripsy under local anesthesia. Urology 68 (1), 38-41.

3 Schwartz, B.F., Stoller, M.L. (2000) The vesical calculus. Urol Clin North Am 27 (2), 333.

4 Borgmann, V., Nagel, R. (1982) Urolithiasis in childhood. A study of 181 cases. Urol Int 37 (3), 198-204.

5 Sarkissian, A., Babloyan, A., Arikyants, N., et al. (2001) Pediatric urolithiasis in Armenia: a study of 198 patients observed from 1991 to 1999. Pediatr Nephrol 16 (9), 728-732.

6 Holman, E., Khan, A.M., Flasko, T., et al. (2004) Endoscopic management of pediatric urolithiasis in a developing country. Urology 63 (1), 159-162; discussion 162.

7 Hulbert, J.C., Reddy, P.K., Gonzalez, R., et al. (1985) Percutaneous nephrostolithotomy: an alternative approach to the management of pediatric calculus disease. Pediatrics 76 (4), 610-612.

8 Ahmadnia, H., Kamalati, A., Younesi, M., et al. (2013) Percutaneous treatment of bladder stones in children: 10 years experience, is blind access safe? Pediatr Surg Int 29 (7), 725-728.

9 Vanwaeyenbergh, J., Vergauwe, D., Verbeeck, R.M. (1995) Infrared spectrometric analysis of endemic bladder stones in Niger. Eur Urol 27 (2), 154-159.

10 Kancha, R.K., Anasuya, A. (1992) Contribution of vitamin A deficiency to calculogenic risk factors of urine: studies in children. Biochem Med Metab Biol 47 (1), 1-9.

11 Wickham, J.E.A. (1993) Treatment of urinary tract stones. Br Med J 307 (6916), 1414-1417.

12 Urena, R., Mendez-Torres, F., Thomas, R. (2007) Complications of urinary stone surgery. Curr Clin Urol 511-553.

13 Carlin, B., Paik, M., Bodner, D., et al. (2001) Complications of urologic surgery prevention and management. In: Taneja, S., Smith, R., Erlich, R. (eds.) Complications of Urologic Surgery, 3rd edn. WB Saunders, Philadelphia, pp. 333-341.

14 Husain, I., Elfaqih, S.R., Shamsuddinf, A.B., Atassi, R. (1994) Primary extracorporeal shockwave lithotripsy in management of large bladder calculi. J Endourol 8 (3), 183-186.

15 Salah, M.A., Holman, E., Khan, A.M., Toth, C. (2005) Percutaneous cystolithotomy for pediatric endemic bladder stone: experience with 155 cases from 2 developing countries. J Pediatr Surg 40 (10), 1628-1631.

16 Losty, P., Surana, R., Odonnell, B. (1993) Limitations of extracorporeal shockwave lithotripsy for urinary-tract calculi in young-children. J Pediatr Surg 28 (8), 1037-1039.

17 Agrawal, M.S., Aron, M., Goyal, J., et al. (1999) Percutaneous suprapubic cystolithotripsy for vesical calculi in children. J Endourol 13 (3), 173-175.

18 Ikari, O., Netto, N.R., Dancona, C.A.L., Palma, P.C.R. (1993) Percutaneous treatment of bladder stones. J Urology 149 (6), 1499-500.

19 Wollin, T.A., Singal, R.K., Whelan, T., et al. (1999) Percutaneous suprapubic cystolithotripsy for treatment of large bladder calculi. J Endourol 13 (10), 739-744.

20 Lulich, J.P., Osborne, C.A., Thumchai, R., et al. (1998) Management of canine calcium oxalate urolith recurrence. Comp Contin Educ Pract 20 (2), 178.

21 Grant, D.C., Harper, T.A.M., Werre, S.R. (2010) Frequency of incomplete urolith removal, complications, and diagnostic imaging following cystotomy for removal of uroliths from the lower urinary tract in dogs: 128 cases (1994-2006). J Am Vet Med Assoc 236 (7), 763-766.

22 Appel, S.L., Lefebvre, S.L., Houston, D.M., et al. (2008) Evaluation of risk factors associated with suture-nidus cystoliths in dogs and cats: 176 cases (1999-2006). J Am Vet Med Assoc 233 (12), 1889-1895.

23 Thieman-Mankin, K.M., Ellison, G.W., Jeyapaul, C.J., Glotfelty-Ortiz, C.S. (2012) Comparison of short-term complication rates between dogs and cats undergoing appositional single-layer or inverting double-layer cystotomy closure: 144 cases (1993-2010). J Am Vet Med Assoc 240 (1), 65-68.

24 Westropp, J., Ruby, A., Campbell, S., et al. (2010) Canine and feline urolithiasis: pathophysiology, epidemiology and management. In: Bojrab, M., Monnet, E. (eds). Mechanisms of Disease in Small Animal Surgery, 3rd edn. Teton New Media, Jackson, WY, pp. 387-392.

25 Kyles, A., Monnet, E. (2013) Urolithiasis of the lower urinary tract. In: Monnet, E. (ed.) Small Animal Soft Tissue Surgery. Wiley-Blackwell, Denver, pp. 528-535.

26 Cannon, A.B., Westropp, J.L., Ruby, A.L., Kass, P.H. (2007) Evaluation of trends in urolith composition in cats: 5,230 cases (1985-2004). J Am Vet Med Assoc 231 (4), 570-576.

27 Houston, D.M., Moore, A.E., Favrin, M.G., Hoff, B. (2003) Feline urethral plugs and bladder uroliths: a review of 5484 submissions 1998-2003. Can Vet J 44 (12), 974-977.

28 Ling, G.V., Thurmond, M.C., Choi, Y.K., et al. (2003) Changes in proportion of canine urinary calculi composed of calcium oxalate or struvite in specimens analyzed from 1981 through 2001. J Vet Intern Med 17 (6), 817-823.

29 Houston, D.M., Rinkardt, N.E., Hilton, J. (2004) Evaluation of the efficacy of a commercial diet in the dissolution of feline struvite bladder uroliths. Vet Ther 5 (3), 187-201.

30 Osborne, C.A., Lulich, J.P., Polzin, D.J., et al. (1999) Analysis of 77,000 canine uroliths: perspectives from the Minnesota Urolith Center. Vet Clin North Am Small Anim Pract 29 (1), 17.

31 Ross, S.J., Osborne, C.A., Lulich, J.P., et al. (1999) Canine and feline nephrolithiasis: epidemiology, detection, and management. Vet Clin North Am Small Anim Pract 29 (1), 231.

32 Snyder, D.M., Steffey, M.A., Mehler, S.J., et al. (2005) Diagnosis and surgical management of ureteral calculi in dogs: 16 cases (1990-2003). N Z Vet J 53 (1), 19-25.

33 Bartges, J.W. (2004) Diagnosis of urinary tract infections. Vet Clin North Am Small Anim Pract 34 (4), 923.

34 Adams, L., Syme, H. (2005) Canine lower urinary tract disease. In: Ettinger, S.J., Feldman, E.C. (eds.) Textbook of Veterinary Internal Medicine. St. Louis, Elsevier Saunders 1850-1874.

35 Gatoria, I.S., Saini, N.S., Rai, T.S., Dwivedi, P.N. (2006) Comparison of three techniques for the diagnosis of urinary tract infections in dogs with urolithiasis. J Small Anim Pract 47 (12), 727-732.

36 Park, R., Wrigley, R. (2007) The urinary bladder. In: Thrall, D.E. (ed.) Textbook of Veterinary Diagnostic Radiology, 5th edn. Saunders Elsevier, St. Louis, pp. 708-724.

37 Weichselbaum, R.C., Feeney, D.A., Jessen, C.R., et al. (1999) Urocystolith detection: comparison of survey, contrast radiographic and ultrasonographic techniques in an in vitro bladder phantom. Vet Radiol Ultrasound 40 (4), 386-400.

38 Essman, S.C. (2005) Contrast cystography. Clin Tech Small Anim Pract 20 (1), 46-51.

39 Feeney, D.A., Weichselbaum, R.C., Jessen, C.R., Osborne, C.A. (1999) Imaging canine urocystoliths: detection and prediction of mineral content. Vet Clin North Am Small Anim Pract 29 (1), 59.

40 Pressler, B.M., Mohammadian, L.A., Li, E., et al. (2004) In vitro prediction of canine urolith mineral composition using computed tomographic mean beam attenuation measurements. Vet Radiol Ultrasound 45 (3), 189-197.

41 Rawlings, C.A. (2009) Endoscopic removal of urinary calculi. Compendium 31 (10), 476.

42 Lane, I.F. (2004) Lithotripsy: an update on urologic applications in small animals. Vet Clin North Am Small Anim Pract 34 (4), 1011.

43 Davidson, E.B., Ritchey, J.W., Higbee, R.D., et al. (2004) Laser lithotripsy for treatment of canine uroliths. Vet Surg 33 (1), 56-61.

44 Grant, D.C., Werre, S.R., Gevedon, M.L. (2008) Holmium : YAG laser lithotripsy for urolithiasis in dogs. J Vet Intern Med 22 (3), 534-539.

45 Adams, L.G., Berent, A.C., Moore, G.E., Bagley, D.H. (2008) Use of laser lithotripsy for fragmentation of uroliths in dogs: 73 cases (2005-2006). J Am Vet Med Assoc 232 (11), 1680-1687.

46 Defarges, A., Dunn, M. (2008) Use of electrohydraulic lithotripsy in 28 dogs with bladder and urethral calculi. J Vet Intern Med 22 (6), 1267-1273.

47 Rawlings, C.A., Mahaffey, M.B., Barsanti, J.A., Canalis, C. (2003) Use of laparoscopic-assisted cystoscopy for removal of urinary calculi in dogs. J Am Vet Med Assoc 222 (6), 759.

48 Runge, J.J., Berent, A.C., Mayhew, P.D., Weisse, C. (2011) Transvesicular percutaneous cystolithotomy for the retrieval of cystic and urethral calculi in dogs and cats: 27 cases (2006-2008). J Am Vet Med Assoc 239 (3), 344-349.

49 Pinel, C.B., Monnet, E., Reems, M.R. (2013) Laparoscopic-assisted cystotomy for urolith removal in dogs and cats: 23 cases. Can Vet J 54 (1), 36-41.

50 Defarges, A., Dunn, M., Berent, A. (2013) New alternatives for minimally invasive management of uroliths: lower urinary tract uroliths. Compend Contin Educ Vet 35 (1), E1.

51 Rawlings, C.A. (2007) Resection of inflammatory polyps in dogs using laparoscopic-assisted cystoscopy. J Am Anim Hosp Assoc 43 (6), 342-346.

52 Srikousthubha, Sukesh, C.V.R., Hingle, S. (2013) Profile of lesions in cystoscopic bladder biopsies: a histopathological study. J Clin Diagn Res 7 (8), 1609-1612.

24 Laparoscopic Ovariectomy and Ovariohysterectomy

Nicole J. Buote

> ### Key Points
>
> - A vessel-sealing device is extremely useful for performing these procedures safely and efficiently.
> - Newer flexible single-port devices allow for these procedures to be performed though one incision.
> - Laparoscopic ovariectomy is fast, simple to perform, and just as effective as laparoscopic ovariohysterectomy with regards to sterilization.
> - Laparoscopic ovariohysterectomy can be performed safely in cases with mild uterine horn pathology from mucometra or pyometra.
> - After ovarian exteriorization, it is always wise to check that the entire ovary has been removed.

Laparoscopic ovariectomy (LapOVE) and ovariohysterectomy (LapOVH) have become two of the most popular, if not the most commonly performed, minimally invasive soft tissue procedures in veterinary medicine in the United States.[1,2] Although laparoscopic reproductive procedures are performed commonly in women, usually these procedures leave the ovarian tissue behind and are mainly performed for reproductive control.[3,4] Not only do surgical specialists perform these types of sterilization procedures, but many general practitioners also enjoy offering the option to their clients. Currently, these procedures can be performed in cats and any size of dog, but originally they were held aside for medium to large breed dogs because of the difficulty with a small working space and rigid instruments in smaller patients.[5-8]

Laparoscopic procedures are not new to veterinary medicine, with the first sterilization technique being performed in 1985 for laparoscopic occlusion of the uterine horns by electrocoagulation in dogs and cats.[10] That study documented that it was possible to provide clinically healthy infertile patients years after the procedure if the separation point was at the uterotubal junction. This procedure may have sterilized the patients but did not stop unwanted sexual behavior or protect against pyometra or mammary carcinoma because the ovaries were left in situ. Work began in earnest in Europe to determine the efficacy and safety of OVE compared with OVH, and the former soon became the standard of care with regards to open surgery.[11] In the mid 1990s, LapOVE started to gain popularity in Europe. In the United States, open OVH is still the procedure of choice taught in veterinary schools but among laparoscopists LapOVE has now become the procedure of choice largely because it is simpler to perform.[12] Although there were case reports and small case series on artificial insemination in cats, vasectomy for dogs, and OVH for pyometra in two dogs, the majority of interest in these procedures in small animal medicine was not fully realized until the early 21st century.[13-15] The first case series in nine dogs that reported successful LapOVE was in 2003.[16] This manuscript highlighted some of the challenges to traditional open OVH, including decreased visualization with the risk of incomplete resection of ovarian tissue or ligation of ureters and trauma to tissues as the ovarian pedicle is strummed or torn down.[16] In women, laparoscopic hysterectomy is the treatment of choice in most cases and has even been shown to have the same efficacy as open surgery in treatment of cervical cancer with fewer postoperative complications.[4]

The data on decreased pain perception in patients undergoing LapOVH or LapOVE are clear.[17-20] One of the first papers studying this relationship cited complications with the LapOVH procedure and longer operative times than open OVH, but postoperative pain scores were significantly less with the minimally invasive technique.[17] This work has been continued by many other authors,[18-20] who have continued to determine that laparoscopic procedures consistently cause less discomfort in our patient population. A landmark paper by Devitt et al.[19] illustrated that LapOVH had clear biochemical and

Small Animal Laparoscopy and Thoracoscopy, First Edition. Edited by Boel A. Fransson and Philipp D. Mayhew.
© 2015 by ACVS Foundation. Published 2015 by John Wiley & Sons, Inc.
Companion website: www.wiley.com/go/fransson/laparoscopy

subjective pain score advantages over open OVH with no notable surgical complications. Other important work showed an increase in postoperative activity levels even in small breed dogs undergoing LapOVE versus open OVE as measured by accelerometry.[20]

Preoperative Considerations

Relevant Anatomy and Pathophysiology

The relevant anatomy for these procedures includes the ovaries, ovarian pedicles, suspensory ligaments, uterine horns, uterine body, and associated connective tissues (Figures 24-1 and 24-2). Although the anatomy is very familiar to most veterinarians, the magnification and view produced by high-quality telescopes provide amazing detail. Canine ovaries are usually completely concealed in the ovarian bursa, which commonly contains fat obscuring the view of the actual ovary. Feline ovaries are only covered by a bursa laterally and usually contain no fat, allowing for much better visualization. The ovary is attached to the dorsolateral abdominal wall by the mesovarium, which contains the ovarian blood vessels. The mesovarium is continuous with the suspensory ligament and caudally with the mesometrium. The uterus consists of the cervix, body, and uterine horns. The uterine horns range from 10 to 14 cm in length in dogs and 9 to 10 cm long in cats and lie completely within the peritoneal cavity. The mesometrium attaches the uterus to the dorsolateral body wall and contains the uterine arteries and veins.

Patient Selection

As stated previously, dogs and cats of all ages, sizes, and breeds can be good candidates for laparoscopic sterilization techniques. The size of the patient need not be a contraindication, but every laparoscopist should remember the increased difficulty in performing intraabdominal laparoscopic procedures with a small working space. This difficulty may translate into longer operative times in patients that are already prone to hypothermia because of their small size, so every precaution should be taken to keep patients warm, and surgeons should be prepared to convert if the procedure is not going smoothly. In older or obese patients, these procedures are extremely beneficial because the magnification allows for better confidence during pedicle ligation, and in the case of LapOVE, less

bleeding from fatty mesometrial tissue. Older or multiparous dogs or cats may have a greater blood supply to the ovaries and uterus, and along with increased tissue friability, these reasons make LapOVE or LapOVH a preferred option over open procedures in these patient populations.

There are very few relative contraindications to a LapOVH or LapOVE other than severe cardiopulmonary compromise or known diaphragmatic hernia, which would make carbon dioxide (CO_2) insufflation dangerous. However, even these situations have solutions in laparoscopy today, with techniques such as lift laparoscopy, which uses a specially designed metal ring threaded into the abdomen to lift the body wall away from the underlying organs to create working space, an option in these cases.[21] Other relative contraindications could be an active heat cycle, early pregnancy, or pyometra with moderate to large uterine distension. A pyometra or pregnancy can be considered a contraindication to a LapOVE but not to a LapOVH.[15,22] It has been shown that laparoscopic treatment of pyometra can be performed very safely if the uterine horns are only mildly distended.[15,22] In the author's experience, performing LapOVH in patients with large, heavy pyometras does not carry an obvious advantage over open OVH. This tissue is extremely friable, and the highly distended uterine horns are usually very close to the abdominal wall, increasing the risk of iatrogenic puncture with trocar–Veress needle placement. Appropriate case selection is key to a successful and safe procedure.

Diagnostic Workup

Any patient presenting for a LapOVE or LapOVH should have a complete physical examination and routine blood work depending on the age and relevant history of the patient. With young patients, special attention is paid to any visible congenital defects such as umbilical hernias because these may be an indication of other congenital defects that could complicate the procedure (diaphragmatic hernia, peritoneopericardial diaphragmatic hernia [PPDH]). Because of the insufflation used during these procedures, care must be taken to fully evaluate the respiratory system in any patient undergoing laparoscopy. Any predisposition to bleeding (e.g., Doberman Pinschers with von Willebrand's disease) should also be taken under consideration and appropriate testing and preoperative treatment performed if necessary.

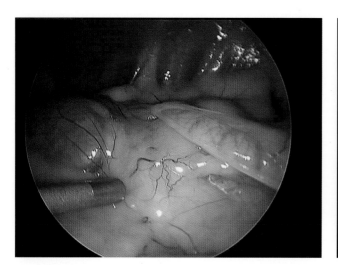

Figure 24-1 Intraoperative view from a 0-degree, 5-mm telescope view of the left ovary.

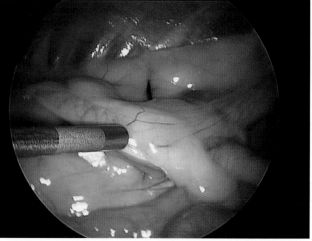

Figure 24-2 Intraoperative view from a 0-degree, 5-mm telescope of the left uterine horn.

Patient Preparation

Surgical preparation for any surgical patient begins the night before the procedure with appropriate fasting (at least 8–12 hours before the procedure). Water is allowed overnight but withdrawn the morning of surgery, and if there are oral medications that are crucial to the patient's health, they are given with the tiniest amount of food possible. After the patient presents to the hospital and a physical examination and appropriate blood work have been performed, a premedication is given and an intravenous (IV) catheter placed. Depending on the timing of surgery, walking laparoscopy patients to encourage urination before the procedure is very helpful because a large bladder can limit working space during caudal abdominal procedures.[8]

In cases in which transabdominal ovarian suspension is not used, the extent of the ventral abdomen that is clipped is similar for LapOVE and LapOVH and similar to that performed for an open OVH, extending to just lateral to the nipple line on each side, just cranial to the pubis and just caudal to the rib cage, in case a conversion needs to be performed (Figure 24-3). For cases in which transabdominal suspension of the ovary is going to be performed using an OVE hook or percutaneously placed suspension needle to hold the ovary for a two-port technique, a wider clip needs to be performed. One author states the lateral margins should be approximately 50% of the distance between the ventral and dorsal midline with this technique[8] (Figure 24-4). The OVE hook (Karl Storz Endoscopy, Goleta, CA) is a device with a cutting tip or taper tip surgical needle attached to a weighted handle (Figure 24-5), which keeps the ovary suspended and does not require additional clamps.[8]

A dirty scrub should be performed as for any surgical procedure and the patient moved into the operating room, set up on monitoring equipment, and a final aseptic preparation performed before draping. Patient positioning for these procedures is in dorsal recumbency with the legs tied at all four corners of the table. If a

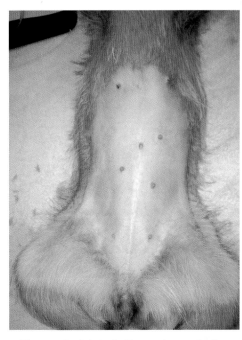

Figure 24-4 Photograph of a hair clip if an ovariectomy hook or needle suspension technique are used. Note that the lateral aspect of the clip must go substantially more dorsal on both sides.

tilt table is available, this greatly facilitates the repositioning of the patient during the procedure. Some descriptions cite a lateral tilt of approximately 15 degrees to be adequate to move intraabdominal organs off of the underlying ovary,[5,8] but in this author's experience, the table is sometimes positioned in a much more acute angle, closer to 25 to 30 degrees, or the patient is manually flipped almost into lateral recumbency[20,23] (Figure 24-6). This is especially true on the left side, where the spleen has a tendency to cover the left kidney and ovary stubbornly. If a tilt table is used, the patient must be *securely* attached to the table to prevent any movement during the

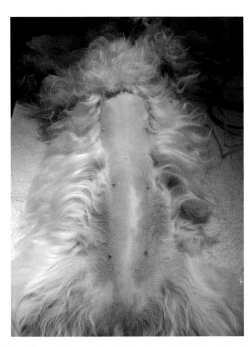

Figure 24-3 Photo of the required hair clip and initial positioning in the operating room for a patient undergoing single-port laparoscopic ovariectomy or three-port ovariohysterectomy.

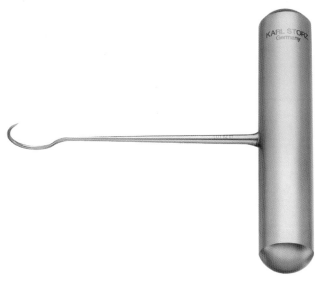

Figure 24-5 A resterilizable ovariectomy hook (Karl Storz Endoscopy, Goleta, CA) can be used in place of a suspension suture for two- or single-port ovariectomy or ovariohysterectomy.

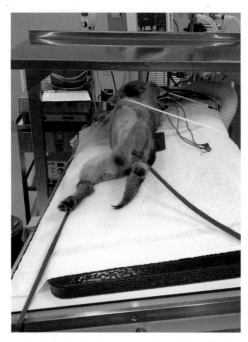

Figure 24-6 Photograph of patient positioned on a tilt table that is used to move organs away from the ovaries during laparoscopic ovariectomy and ovariohysterectomy.

procedure. If a tilt table is not available, then the limbs are loosely attached because the patient will most likely have to be repositioned several times during the procedure. Placing the patient in a Trendelenburg position (head down) has also been discussed in some texts to aid in cranial displacement of the intraabdominal organs.[5]

The positioning of the surgeon will change depending on the side of ovary being removed. For LapOVE, the tower can be set up at the head or back of the table as long as the monitor is easily adjusted. For OVH, the monitor is best at the end of the table because much of the dissection will proceed in a cranial to caudal direction, so this positioning allows the surgeon to look in the direction his or her hands are moving (Figure 24-7).

Portal Placement

Original descriptions of LapOVH describe placement of three or four portals, often with ports placed in paramedian locations. Since that time, there has been a general trend toward fewer ports and placement centered over the linea alba. The four-port technique had one port placed in all four quadrants of the abdomen.[15,17] With this configuration, the telescope portal was always the middle portal, and instruments were passed between the cranial and caudal portal for grasping and dissecting. Early three-portal techniques comprised a telescope portal, which was cranial to the umbilicus, and two portals placed paramedian on both sides in the caudal abdomen.[5,16,18] More recent three median port techniques for LapOVH[22,23] have involved placement of one subumbilical port for the telescope, one port 2 to 3 cm cranial to the umbilicus, and one port 2 to 5 cm cranial to the pubis for eventual removal of the urogenital tract (Figure 24-8). It is very important that this port be placed under visualization because it will be directly overlying the urinary bladder and colon. In 2005, a two-port technique was described using an 11-mm operative laparoscope with an operating channel for insertion of 5-mm instruments.[19] This allowed for one port to be placed at the umbilicus for the telescope and one cannula to be placed 4 to 5 cm cranial to pubis at the midline for eventual extraction of the urogenital tract.

Many different portal positions have been reported for LapOVE, including one median portal at the umbilicus with two lateral portals[24,25] and the three-port technique with all ports on the ventral midline.[6,7,26-29] In 2009, a two median port technique was described in which one port was placed 1 cm caudal to the umbilicus and one port was placed 2 to 5 cm cranial to the pubis (Figure 24-9). This technique used the OVE needle suspension method and was very effective at allowing for dissection while minimizing port numbers.[20] Also in 2009, a technique paper comparing a one- and two-port technique was published.[30] The one-port technique placed a single 12-mm portal 1 to 2 cm caudal to the umbilicus for placement of a 10-mm telescope with an operating channel (often termed an *operating laparoscope*). This technique has also been reported in cats and was safe and feasible but requires considerable skill because there is no triangulation for the graspers and vessel-sealing devices (VSDs).[9,30]

Differences in postoperative pain and surgical time between one-, two-, and three-port techniques have been evaluated, and it

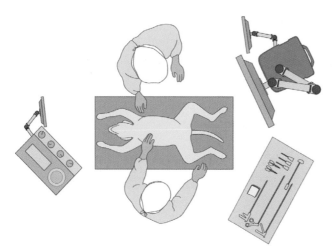

Figure 24-7 The operating room layout for a laparoscopic ovariectomy (LapOVE) or laparoscopic ovariohysterectomy (LapOVH). The endoscopic tower is usually placed at the foot of the patient, especially for LapOVH, but for LapOVE, some surgeons prefer to place the tower at the head of the patient.

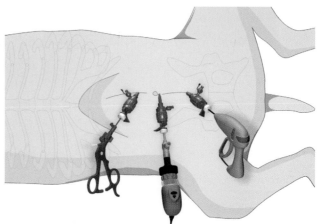

Figure 24-8 Line drawing of three-port ventral midline placement for ovariectomy. The telescope port is placed at the umbilicus, one instrument port 2 to 3 cm cranial to the umbilicus and one instrument port 2 to 5 cm cranial to the pubis.

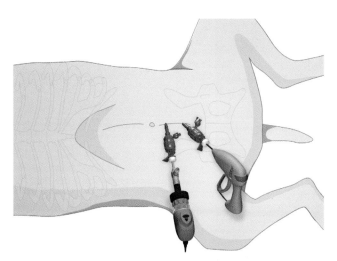

Figure 24-9 Line drawing of two port median placement for ovariectomy used with ovariectomy hook or needle suspension technique. One port is placed 1 cm caudal to the umbilicus, and one port is placed 2 to 5 cm cranial to the pubis.

was found that surgical time was considerably longer for the one-port technique; however, there was no significant difference in complication rates among the groups, and there was no difference in postoperative pain levels between one- and two-port techniques.[31] The authors concluded that a two-port technique resulted in excellent pain control and shorter surgical times compared with one-port techniques. Other single-incision techniques presented include multiple ports placed through a single skin incision[32] and what is more commonly performed today, the use of single-incision multiport devices.[33] These single-incision techniques usually place the incision or port cranial to the umbilicus for LapOVE (Figure 24-10).

Surgical Technique

Instrumentation
Laparoscopic OVE or OVH requires relatively little specific equipment, which includes a telescope (commonly a 5- or 10-mm

telescope is used); laparoscopic Kelly or Babcock forceps for grasping the proper ligament or uterine horn; cannulae or a single-incision multiport device; and most important, some version of a VSD. Many reports have evaluated the differences among ultrasonic and bipolar sealing devices and laser devices and found advantages and disadvantages among them, but it is generally agreed that energy-based devices provide major benefits over endoscopic clips or suture techniques with regards to ease of application, surgical times, and complications.[6,23,24,26-28] Cannula size should be determined based on the patient size and the size of the tissue being extracted; therefore, in large breed dogs with moderate fat surrounding the ovary, 10-mm cannulae are a better choice for ovary extraction.[8] Other than these basic instruments, a large-gauge (usually 1 or 0) suture swaged on a half-circle needle or a resterilizable OVE hook (see Figure 24-5) may be required to suspend the ovary if a transabdominal suspension technique is chosen.

Laparoscopic Ovariectomy
Two-Port Technique
After port placement and pneumoperitoneum have been achieved, the patient should be rotated toward the side of the surgeon approximately 15 to 30 degrees to allow the viscera to move away from the targeted ovary. For the left ovary, the spleen is commonly encountered; for the right ovary, the duodenum and other intestines are often overlying the ovary. A blunt laparoscopic probe or fan retractor can be advanced through the instrument port to help gently guide these organs away from the ovary. At times, it may be necessary to move the patient almost into lateral recumbency to encourage movement of organs off the dorsally placed ovaries. The ovaries will be located directly caudal to the kidneys, so when these organs are identified, the ovaries and uterine horns are usually clearly seen. When the uterine horn is found, the proper ligament is grasped with laparoscopic Kelly or Babcock forceps and held up to the body wall (Figure 24-11). At this point, an OVE hook or needle can be used to suspend the

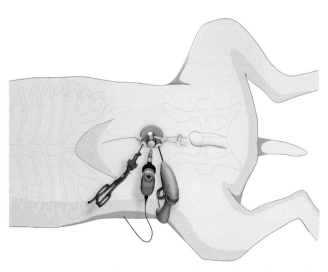

Figure 24-10 Line drawing showing a single-port device placed at the umbilicus for laparoscopic ovariectomy.

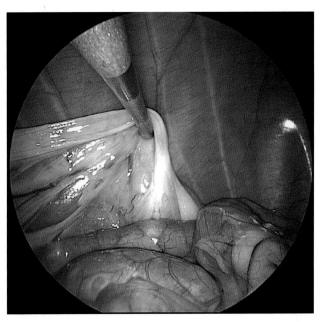

Figure 24-11 Intraoperative view of a blunt probe being used to hold the right uterine horn and ovary up against the body wall in preparation for passage of the transabdominal suspension suture.

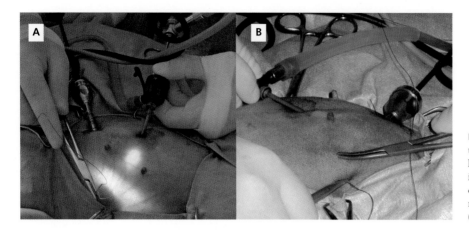

Figure 24-12 The suspension suture is passed under transabdominal illumination to avoid large body wall vessels (**A**). A large needle is required to allow it to pass into the body cavity through the proper ligament and return out of the abdomen at an adjacent site (**B**). (Courtesy of Dr. Philipp Mayhew.)

ovary. The overhead lights should be turned off to illuminate the body wall where the ovary is located and to help illustrate the abdominal vasculature so large vessels are avoided during percutaneous placement of the needle (Figure 24-12). The surgeon should also be able to palpate the hemostats or forceps through the body wall. A half-circle needle is then placed percutaneously through the body wall (see Figure 24-12) under visualization through the proper ligament or cranial uterine horn or mesometrium and then out the body wall again (Figure 24-13). The suture is then pulled tight against the body wall and clamped with mosquito hemostats to hold the ovary suspended (see Figure 24-13). Care must be taken during this procedure not to puncture the ovary or lacerate the pedicle.

With the ovary suspended at the body wall, the hemostats or Babcock forceps can be released and removed from the abdomen and a VSD placed within the abdomen. These instruments should be applied in a line from the suspensory ligament to the proximal uterine horn, staying as close to the uterine body and ovary as is safe to avoid the ureters and large mesometrial vessels (Figure 24-14). It depends on the size of the patient and the positioning of the portals as to which direction the device is driven. In medium to large breed dogs, a caudal to cranial application usually works best. In cats and small dogs, because of the closeness of the portals, a cranial to caudal application may be used. Most times part of the uterine horn is incised and removed with the ovary and does not appear to cause a clinical problem.[8,40] One recent study compared the bursting strengths of a VSD to an encircling suture on the uterine horn and body and found that the failure pressure was high for both techniques in the uterine horn. However, bursting pressure for the uterine body was lower with the VSD and was not recommended in uterine bodies 9 mm or larger in diameter.[40]

The OVE is now complete, and the ovary should be left attached to the body wall by the suture. The VSD is removed and the patient repositioned to dorsal recumbency. The surgeon moves to the opposite side of the table at this point. Instead of removing the caudal port in the middle of the procedure and enlarging the incision, which usually leads to difficulties with reinsufflation or losing the ovary in the abdomen, it is recommended to complete both sides and then remove both ovaries at the end of the procedure. After the procedure has been completed on both sides, the ovary is grasped and brought to the caudal port by releasing or transecting the suture. In the past, the author has seen the sutures left long in case the ovary is dropped during extraction; then the suture can be gently tightened again and the ovary found. After the ovaries have been removed from the caudal incision, the body wall at this site is closed to allow for reinsufflation. A quick exploration is performed to ensure no

ongoing hemorrhage is visible on either pedicle. The cannulae are then removed, and the body wall is closed routinely, being sure to close the muscular fascia of the body wall over each portal site.

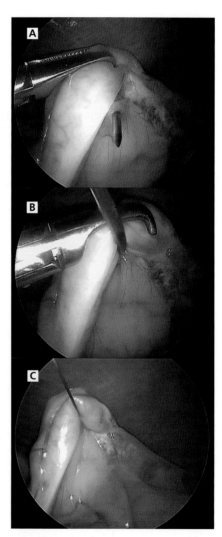

Figure 24-13 Intraoperative view of the percutaneous suspension needle piercing through the mesometrium (**A**). View of suspension needle encircling the proper ligament (**B**). After the needle is passed back out of the abdomen, the suspension suture can be seen anchoring the suture to the body wall (**C**).

One-Port Technique

There are two single-port techniques published for LapOVE. The first describes the use of an operating telescope (10 mm) with an operating channel for 5-mm instruments. Using the operating laparoscope, grasping forceps are placed into the working channel of the laparoscope to grasp and elevate the ovary into position for passage of a transabdominal suspension suture or hook. The grasping forceps are then removed and replaced with a VSD, which is then used to seal and divide the pedicle.[30]

The more popular single incision technique uses a multiport device (e.g., SILS port, Covidien, Mansfield, MA), which allows three cannulae to be placed within the abdomen—one for the telescope, one for the grasper, and one for the VSD. This negates the need for percutaneous ovarian suspension and allows for moderate triangulation (30 degrees), although crosstalk among the instruments can be a frustration. In human medicine, articulating instruments are used commonly with these ports to remove this problem.[34] After transection of the pedicle and uterine horn, the ovary is held by the VSD or forceps while the port is removed (see Figure 24-14). The SILS port is placed using a Hasson technique at

the umbilicus and is easily removed and replaced after each ovary is transected. An important step when removing the SILS port to remove the first ovary is to have whomever is holding the forceps attached to the ovary push safely into the body cavity (usually at the gutter where the ovary was just removed from) while pulling out the port. There will be moderate force required to remove the SILS port even if stay sutures are used to open the body wall incision, and the ovary can be jostled out of the jaws of the graspers if the port is pulled out with the grasping forceps in place. If this happens, *do not move the patient*; instead, replace the SILS port and reinsufflate the abdomen, and almost always the ovary is in clear site. It is wise when first performing these procedures to check each ovary for completeness of dissection to ensure ovarian tissue has not been left behind.

Laparoscopic Ovariohysterectomy
Three-Port Technique

Although many techniques exist, the most commonly performed today is the three-port laparoscopic-assisted technique with all ports placed on the ventral midline (see earlier). The ports are placed as described, and the ovaries are transected cranially as previously described with continued dissection of the mesometrium caudally (Video Clip 24-1). When the uterine body is encountered, the ovary and horn are released, and the surgeon and assistant switch sides of the table to accomplish the same procedure on the opposite side. After the second ovary and horn are transected, the ovary remains in the Kelly or Babcock forceps, which are withdrawn toward the caudal port. The incision is carefully enlarged as necessary, and the port is removed while the forceps are still attached to the ovary, thus exteriorizing it from the peritoneal cavity. The port, forceps, and ovary should be removed as one unit. The uterine horns and ovaries are then gently removed from the incision, and the uterine body is double ligated or sealed and divided in routine fashion (Figure 24-15). The uterine stump is then replaced into the abdomen, the body wall is closed quickly with towel clamps or sutures to allow for reinsufflation, and a brief exploration is performed to ensure no intraabdominal bleeding is present. A totally laparoscopic LapOVH technique can also be performed that involves ligation of the uterine body with a pretied

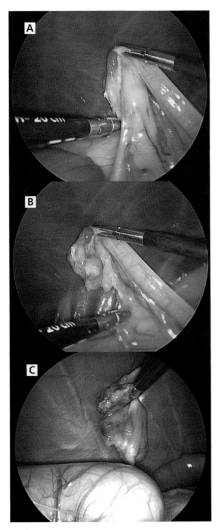

Figure 24-14 Intraoperative view of the vessel-sealing device starting to dissect and seal the ovarian pedicle (**A**). The dissection continues across into the mesometrium (**B**). After complete sectioning through the distal uterine horn, the ovary is being held by laparoscopic Kelly forceps (**C**).

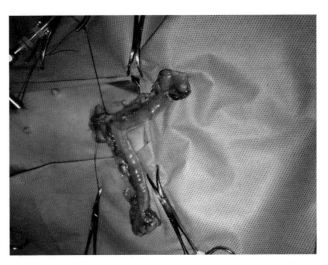

Figure 24-15 The uterine horns and ovaries removed from the abdomen through the caudal port site.

loop ligature (e.g., Endoloop; Ethicon Endosurgery, Cincinnatti, OH) or intracorporeally tied suture. However, because this is technically more challenging and the ovaries and uterus need to be exteriorized through one of the portal incisions anyway, this technique is not frequently performed.

Laparoscopic Ovariohysterectomy for Pyometra

Although pyometra used to be considered a contraindication to laparoscopic procedures, reports have been published describing the use of laparoscopy for pyometra.[15,22] This technique still should only be performed by experienced laparoscopists. Risks associated with the laparoscopic approach to pyometra include the possibility of rupture of the pyometra with trocar or Veress needle insertion, leading to peritonitis and risk of uterine tearing while handling the uterus. One technique described the use of a wound retraction device (Alexis wound retractor; Applied Medical, Rancho Santa Margarita, CA) to create a protected retracted assist incision caudally to remove the enlarged uterine horns and body and ovaries through (Figure 24-16).[22] Patient stability is always of the utmost importance during surgical procedures, and the physiologic effects of endotoxemia from a pyometra are well characterized.[22] Therefore, if a rapid and safe laparoscopic procedure can be performed, a pyometra is not a definitive contraindication.

Challenges Specific to the Technique

Although LapOVE and LapOVH are relatively straightforward procedures, there are always challenges to any laparoscopic surgery. The most common problems encountered are triangulation with the operating telescopes or multiport devices, removal of samples from port incisions, obese patients, and patients in estrus. In one study, obesity was not correlated with a higher fat score of the ovary and ligaments in cats,[27] but in dogs, there has been an association with obesity and difficulty accessing ovaries and longer surgical times.[6,24,29] There has been a connection between number of heat cycles and the occurrence of intraoperative bleeding in dogs as well.[24] As long as appropriate vessel-sealing equipment is available, the procedures can be performed safely. Triangulation causes fewer problems as surgeons become more familiar with the equipment

and more experienced. Articulated instruments decrease the frustration with triangulation but are considerably more expensive than straight instruments. Removal of samples can be problematic if appropriate steps are not taken, including enlarging the port incision or placement of samples into sterile retrieval bags. Because single-port devices are generally placed through larger incisions, exteriorization of reproductive organs is generally facilitated with their use.

Complications

As with any surgical procedure, complications can occur. The complication rate is low, however, with some authors reporting no intraoperative complications.[19,35,36] Complications can be broken down into intraoperative and postoperative. One of the most common intraoperative complications is insertional trauma to intraabdominal organs, most commonly the spleen.[8] Splenic trauma with the initial trocar or Veress needle placement will result in bleeding into the abdominal cavity and has been reported in 5% to 18.7% of cases.[17,18,23,30,31] This bleeding can be brisk depending on the severity of the lesion, but insufflation does help control bleeding by increasing intraabdominal pressure. Any accumulating blood from a splenic laceration may pool in the gutters, making identification of the ovary more difficult. Remember that the magnification of the telescope can create the impression of significant hemorrhage. Other intraoperative complications include puncture of the urinary bladder[41]; bleeding from the pedicle; dropping the ovary, reported in 10% of cases in one paper[33]; burning the peritoneum or other organs with the VSD; leakage of CO_2 from cannulae into subcutaneous tissue (5%)[31]; and burns to drapes or other structures in the operative field by the telescope. Bleeding from the pedicle has been reported more commonly with endoscopic clip techniques (100%) compared with suture (40%) or VSDs (10%) in one study.[23] Regardless of ligation method, the stated incidence of pedicle hemorrhage has been reported in the range of 3% to 30% with most hemorrhage being minor.[6,17,20,24,26,27,30,33] Conversion to laparotomy is not in and of itself considered a complication but a necessary consequence of some of the complications listed in this chapter. There are relatively few times in which conversion is necessary, but the most common cause is uncontrolled hemorrhage from the spleen or pedicle. A methodical technique is the best way to avoid these complications. Another potential reason for conversion is an inability to find a dropped ovary. Conversion has not been reported in any LapOVH performed in patients with normal uterine anatomy. One paper reports a 5% conversion rate (because of splenic laceration) in LapOVE procedures combined with a gastropexy.[34] Complications with LapOVH for pyometra include intraabdominal uterine rupture necessitating conversion and mild bleeding from uterine vessels during retraction.[22] The discovery of a diaphragmatic hernia would be an immediate reason for conversion. Before any laparoscopic procedure, no matter how routine, the owners should always be made aware of the potential for conversion.

Potential postoperative complications include incisional problems including seroma, hematoma at the OVE hook or suspension suture site, port site infection, retained ovarian tissue, intermittent vaginal hemorrhage, herniation of omentum through an incision site, and ongoing bleeding from a pedicle.[6,16,17,24,26,41] An overall postoperative complication rate of 3.9% to 31% has been reported. Incisional complications have been reported in up to 13.4% of cases when the skin was closed with n-butyl-cyanoacrylate, with a significant correlation to complications (dehiscence, swelling, erythema,

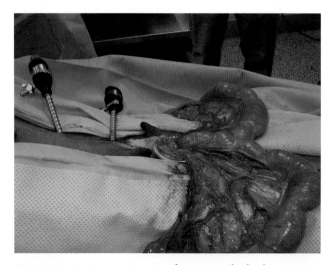

Figure 24-16 An intraoperative view of a pyometra that has been exteriorized through a wound retraction device before ligation of the uterine vessels and body extracorporeally. (Courtesy of Dr. Philipp Mayhew.)

and discharge) and larger port size.[35] Most of these complications are self-limiting and avoidable with appropriate surgical technique and appropriate postoperative instructions, including use of an Elizabethan collar and restriction of normal activity.

A recent study by Pope and Knowles[41] looked at the learning curve associated with LapOVE with four surgeons new to the procedure and evaluated the complication rates as the surgeons progressed. All complications were included in the analysis, and the time for procedure completion was not taken into account because the authors thought that it could be affected by nonsurgical problems (e.g., equipment malfunction). This type of information is quite common in human medicine, especially with laparoscopy, and will aid institutions in setting up appropriate training guidelines. According to this study, a novice surgeon can be proficient and experience a low complication rate after 80 procedures. Although this number seems high, this number can be easily attainable at a busy practice.

Postoperative Care

Postoperative care for LapOVE and LapOVH includes basic pain medication, incision care, and exercise restriction. Although these procedures are considered minimally painful, there has been some work looking at alternative pain control methods such as sprayed intraperitoneal bupivacaine.[36] A recommended postoperative protocol includes opioid (hydromorphone or oxymorphone 0.05 mg/kg IV) pain medication provided as needed every 6 hours with a nonsteroidal antiinflammatory drugs (meloxicam 0.1 mg/kg subcutaneously [SC] orally [PO] every 24 hours or carprofen 2.2 mg/kg SC or PO every 12 hours) administered postoperatively. The patient is usually sent home on the same antiinflammatory drug for 2 to 3 days after surgery as well. Patients stay in the hospital 1 night to be monitored for any signs of discomfort, postoperative bleeding, or trouble urinating. Restricted activity and an Elizabethan collar are recommended for the first week after surgery, and if skin sutures were placed, they should be removed in 7 to 10 days after the procedure.

Choosing between a Laparoscopic Ovariectomy and Ovariohysterectomy

The decision between LapOVE and LapOVH is one that should be made with the owner at the time of initial consult. The reasons animals are usually spayed are to control the population, prevent heat cycles that lead to unwanted behavior, menses, pyometra, and mammary neoplasia. All of these problems are related to the ovarian and not uterine tissue. Some factors to consider when making the decision between these two procedures include ease of the procedure, tissue handling or damage, number of incisions, and potential postoperative complications. This topic of discussion has been contentious at times in the veterinary literature, but a few good reviews have been published illustrating the advantages and disadvantages to both techniques.[11,12,37] The surgeon should be prepared to do either technique in the case of a subclinical pyometra; owner preference; or instability of the patient, necessitating a faster procedure. The surgeon should also be well versed in the literature with regards to occurrence of postoperative pyometra and uterine neoplasia after LapOVE because these are the most commonly asked questions by owners.

LapOVE provides permanent sterilization, as does LapOVH, but veterinarians in the United States have not historically been taught this technique, so many referring veterinarians may not think to discuss it with their clients. In this author's practice, laparoscopic sterilization is done almost exclusively by LapOVE. The reason for this is the ease of the procedure, especially with the advent of single-port devices; the decrease in discomfort because of less tissue manipulation and cauterization[20,38]; decreased number of incisions; and the fact that there has been no statistically significant increase in postoperative complications by leaving the uterine tract in situ.[11,12] Although the surgical time has been shown to be similar for open procedures,[37,39] in the author's experience, LapOVE requires less surgical time than LapOVH. Although no specific studies have compared open OVE versus open OVH or LapOVE and LapOVH in a prospective fashion for differences in signs of pain, it is likely that less tissue dissection and manipulation would lead to decreased postoperative pain. This is an area of ongoing research, and hopefully new insights will emerge soon.

Complications associated with LapOVE vs LapOVH would be expected to be similar except for any complication that arises from the ligation of the uterine body. The incidences of urinary sphincter mechanism incontinence are similar across the procedures because this is a function of loss of the ovaries and not the uterus.[12] Studies in open OVE versus OVH report a similar incidence, 8.7% to 20.8% and 13.6% to 19.1%, respectively.[12] Because inadvertent ligation of the ureters is an uncommon complication but one that holds life-threatening potential, it is important to note that ligation can occur at the proximal ureter, near the ovarian pedicle, or distally at the uterine body. Although OVE does not remove the possibility of proximal ligations, it does negate the possibility of a distal ligation, and some authors have suggested that distal ligations are more common.[11] There have been no published reports of inadvertent ligation or transection of the ureters in a laparoscopic procedure, most likely because of the excellent visualization afforded by the telescope. Ovarian remnant syndrome could occur in either procedure, although inspection of the ovaries is strongly encouraged at the time of dissection to ensure no tissue is left behind. Performance of a LapOVE or LapOVH should decrease the chance of mammary neoplasia as long as it is performed before the third heat cycle because both of these procedures remove the hormonal stimulus to their development.

Studies with long-term follow-up periods have shown no evidence of pyometra in ovariectomized patients.[12] With regards to uterine neoplasia, another potential cause for performance of a LapOVH, many large studies have shown the incidence in dogs to be approximately 0.003% with almost all cases being benign leiomyomas.[12] Additionally, not all uterine tissue is routinely removed during an OVH because the body is usually ligated somewhere distal to the cervix to avoid trauma to the cervix.[8] From those large studies, it also appears that there is a hormonal connection to the development of uterine neoplasia. No dog with the ovaries removed before the age of 2 years had a reported incidence of uterine neoplasia.[12]

In conclusion, there does not appear to be a strong scientific basis for performance of LapOVH over LapOVE for routine sterilization. The decrease in tissue handling, shorter anesthesia time, and lack of substantial risk for long-term complications, if performed correctly, have led most minimally invasive surgeons to prefer LapOVE for routine sterilization.

 All videos cited in this chapter can be found on the book's companion website at **www.wiley.com/go/fransson/ laparoscopy**

References

1 Mayhew, P. (2011) Developing minimally invasive surgery in companion animals. Vet Rec 169:177-178.

2 Parkinson, T.J. (2012) Progress towards less invasive veterinary surgery. Vet Rec 171:67-68.

3 Chittawar, P.B., Magon, N., Bhandari, S. (2013) Laparoscopic single-site surgery in gynecology: LESS is actually how much less? J Midlife Health 4, 46-51.

4 Bogani, G., Cromi, A., Uccella, S., et al. (2014) Laparoscopic versus open abdominal management of cervical cancer: long-term results from a propensity-matched analysis. J Minim Invasive Gynecol 21 (5), 857-862.

5 Twedt, D.C., Monnet, E. (2005) Laparoscopy: technique and clinical experience: ovariohysterectomy. In: McCarthy, T.C. (ed.) Veterinary Endoscopy for the Small Animal Practitioner. Elsevier Saunders, St. Louis, pp. 378-380.

6 van Nimwegen, S.A., Kirpensteijn, J. (2007a) Comparison of Nd:YAG surgical laser and Remorgida bipolar electrosurgery forceps for canine laparoscopic ovariectomy. Vet Surg 36, 533-540.

7 Gower, S., Mayhew, P. (2008) Canine laparoscopic and Laparoscopic-assisted ovariohysterectomy and ovariohysterectomy. Compend Contin Educ Vet 30, 430-440.

8 Hutchinson, R. (2011) Laparoscopic spay of the female canine and feline. In: Tams, T.R., Rawlings, C.A. (eds.) Small Animal Endoscopy, 3rd edn. Elsevier Mosby, St. Louis, pp. 466-477.

9 Kim, Y.K., Lee, S.Y., Park, S.J., et al. (2011) Feasibility of single-portal access laparoscopic ovariectomy in 17 cats. Vet Rec 169, 179-182.

10 Wildt, D.E., Lawler, D.F. (1985) Laparoscopic sterilization of the bitch and queen by uterine horn occlusion. Am J Vet Res 46, 864-869.

11 Van Goethem, B., Schaefers-Okkens, A., Kirpensteijn, J. (2006) Making a rational choice between ovariectomy and ovariohysterectomy in the dog: a discussion of the benefits of either technique. Vet Surg 35, 136-143.

12 DeTora, M., McCarty, R.J. (2011) Ovariohysterectomy versus ovariectomy for elective sterilization of female dogs and cats: is removal of the uterus necessary? J Am Vet Med Assoc 239, 1409-1412.

13 Howard, J.G., Barone, M.A., Donoghue, A.M., et al. (1992) The effect of pre-ovulatory anaesthesia on ovulation in laparoscopically inseminated domestic cats. J Reprod Fertil 96, 175-186.

14 Silva, L.D., Onclin, K., Donnay, I., et al. (1993) Laparoscopic vasectomy in the male dog. J Reprod Fertil 47, 399-401.

15 Minami, S., Okamoto, Y., Eguchi, H., et al. (1997) Successful laparoscopy-assisted ovariohysterectomy in two dogs with pyometra. J Vet Med Sci 59, 845-847.

16 Austin, B., Lanz, O.I., Hamilton, S.M., et al. (2003) Laparoscopic ovariohysterectomy in nine dogs. J Am Anim Hosp Assoc 39, 391-396.

17 Davidson, E.B., Moll, H.D., Payton, M.E. (2004) Comparison of laparoscopic ovariohysterectomy and ovariohysterectomy in dogs. Vet Surg 33, 62-69.

18 Hancock, R.B., Lanz, O.I., Waldron, D.R., et al. (2005) Comparison of postoperative pain after ovariohysterectomy by harmonic scalpel-assisted laparoscopy compared with median celiotomy and ligation in dogs. Vet Surg 34, 273-282.

19 Devitt, C.M., Cox, R.E., Hailey, J.J. (2005) Duration, complication, stress, and pain of open ovariohysterectomy versus a simple method of laparoscopic-assisted ovariohysterectomy in dogs. J Am Vet Med Assoc 227, 921-927.

20 Culp, W.T., Mayhew P.D., Brown, D.C. (2009) The effect of laparoscopic versus open ovariectomy on postsurgical activity in small dogs. Vet Surg 38, 811-817.

21 Fransson, B.A., Ragle, C.A. (2011) Lift laparoscopy in dogs and cats: 12 cases (2008-2009). J Am Vet Med Assoc 239, 1574-1579.

22 Adamovich-Rippe, K.N., Mayhew, P.D., Runge, J.J., et al. (2013) Evaluation of laparoscopic-assisted ovariohysterectomy for treatment of canine pyometra. Vet Surg 42, 572-578.

23 Mayhew, P.D., Brown, D.C. (2007) Comparison of three techniques for ovarian pedicle hemostasis during laparoscopic assisted ovariohysterectomy. Vet Surg 36, 541-547.

24 Van Goethem, B.E.B.J., Rosenveldt, K.W., Kirpensteijn, J. (2003) Monopolar versus bipolar electrocoagulation in canine laparoscopic ovariectomy: a nonrandomized, prospective, clinical trial. Vet Surg 32, 464-470.

25 Rivier, P., Furneaux, R., Viguier, E. (2011) Combined laparoscopic ovariectomy and laparoscopic-assisted gastropexy in dogs susceptible to gastric dilatation-volvulus. Can Vet J 52, 62-66.

26 van Nimwegen, S.A., van Swol, C.F.P., Kirpensteijn, J. (2005) Neodymium:yttrium aluminum garnet surgical laser versus bipolar electrocoagulation for laparoscopic ovariectomy in dogs. Vet Surg 34, 353-357.

27 van Nimwegen, S.A., Kirpensteijn, J. (2007b) Laparoscopic ovariectomy in cats: comparison of laser and bipolar electrocoagulation. J Feline Med Surg 9, 397-403.

28 Ohlund, M., Hoglund, O., Olsson, U., et al. (2011) Laparoscopic ovariectomy in dogs: a comparison of the LigaSure and the SonoSurg systems. J Small Anim Pract 52, 290-294.

29 Van Goethem, B., van Nimwegen, S.A., Akkerdaas, L., et al. (2012) The effect of neuromuscular blockade on canine laparoscopic ovariectomy: a double-blinded, prospective clinical trial. Vet Surg 41, 374-380.

30 Dupre, G., Fiorbianco, V., Skalicky, M., et al. (2009) Laparoscopic ovariectomy in dogs: comparison between single portal and two-portal access. Vet Surg 38, 818-824.

31 Case, J.B., Marvel, S.J., Boscan, P., et al. (2011) Surgical time and severity of postoperative pain in dogs undergoing laparoscopic ovariectomy with one, two, or three instrument cannulas. J Am Vet Med Assoc 239, 203-208.

32 Runge, J.J., Curcillo, P.G. 2nd, King, S.A., et al. (2012) Initial application of reduced port surgery using the single port access technique for laparoscopic canine ovariectomy. Vet Surg 41, 803-806.

33 Manassero, M., Leperlier, D., Vallefuoco, R., et al. (2012) Laparoscopic ovariectomy in dogs using a single-port multiple access device. Vet Rec 171, 69-74.

34 Runge, J.J., Mayhew, P.D. (2013) Evaluation of single port access gastropexy and ovariectomy using articulating instruments and angled telescopes in dogs. Vet Surg 42, 807.

35 Pope, J.F., Knowles, T. (2013) The efficacy of n-butyl-cyanoacrylate tissue adhesive for closure of canine laparoscopic ovariectomy port site incisions. J Small Anim Pract 54, 190-194.

36 Kim, Y.K., Lee, S.S., Suh, E.H., et al. (2012) Sprayed intraperitoneal bupivacaine reduces early postoperative pain behavior and biochemical stress response after laparoscopic ovariectomy in dogs. Vet J 191, 188-192.

37 Peeters, M.E., Kirpensteijn, J. (2011) Comparison of surgical variables and short-term postoperative complications in healthy dogs undergoing ovariohysterectomy or ovariectomy. J Am Vet Med Assoc 238, 189-194.

38 Lee, J.Y., Kim, M.C. (2014) Comparison of oxidative stress status in dogs undergoing laparoscopic and open ovariectomy. J Vet Med Sci 76, 273-276.

39 Harris, K.P., Adams, V.J., Fordyce, P., et al. (2013) Comparison of surgical duration of canine ovariectomy and ovariohysterectomy in a veterinary teaching hospital. J Small Anim Pract 54, 579-583.

40 Barrera, J.S., Monnet, E. (2012) Effectiveness of bipolar vessel sealant device for sealing uterine horns and bodies from dogs. Am J Vet Res 73, 302-305.

41 Pope, J.E., Knowles, T.G. (2014) Retrospective analysis of the learning curve associated with laparoscopic ovariectomy in dogs and associated perioperative complication rates. Vet Surg 43 (6), 668-677.

25 Cryptorchidectomy and Vasectomy

Katie C. Kennedy and Boel A. Fransson

> **Key Points**
>
> - Undescended testes are heritable in nature and lead to poor breeding fitness and a higher incidence of testicular neoplasia or torsion; castration is recommended.
> - Inguinal palpation and assessment of structures entering the inguinal canal can differentiate intraabdominal from inguinal cryptorchid testicles.
> - Laparoscopic or laparoscopy-assisted techniques are most common, performed with a 2 or 3 portal technique, with better visualization than open approaches.
> - Postoperative recovery is shorter with less pain than open techniques.

Preoperative Considerations

Cryptorchid, or undescended, testes are those that have not completed their migration from the retroperitoneal space near the caudal pole of the kidney into the scrotum. This can occur unilaterally, or less commonly, bilaterally.[1-4] When unilateral, the right testicle has sometimes been reported to be more frequently retained.[5-9] The trait is thought to be heritable in dogs and is undesirable because it interferes with breeding fitness.[10] A cryptorchid testis is also up to 13.6 times more likely to develop testicular neoplasms[11] and retained testes have a higher risk of testicular torsion.[12] Because of these factors, castration is the treatment of choice for affected animals.

Normal Testicular Development and Descent

Embryologically, the genital ridge becomes bipotential gonads, which in males differentiate into testicles based on influences from the sex-determining region of the Y chromosome (*SRY* gene) among other genes and hormones. Sertoli cells secrete anti-Mullerian hormone to cause Mullerian structure regression, and Leydig cells begin secreting testosterone to stimulate Wolffian duct differentiation and external virilization.[13]

Testicular descent occurs in two phases: a transabdominal phase and a transinguinal, or inguinoscrotal, phase. Transabdominal descent is largely passive and appears closely related to the descent of the diaphragm with some regulation by insulinlike peptide (INSL3).[14] Within this phase, the gubernaculum, which extends from the caudal pole of the testis through the inguinal canal to the scrotum, increases in volume to expand the inguinal canal. During transinguinal descent, the peritoneum forms the vaginal tunic, and the testis is drawn through the inguinal canal into the scrotum by regression and contraction of the gubernaculum under the influence of androgens and INSL3.[13] This migration is generally completed by 10 days after birth, and a presumptive diagnosis can be made by 8 weeks of age.[15-17] However, because of high testicular mobility in young animals and breed variations, an animal is not typically defined as cryptorchid until 6 months of age, when the inguinal rings of most dogs have closed.[4,10,15,18,19]

Within each testicle, convoluted seminiferous tubules are composed of three different cell types—spermatogenic, Sertoli, and Leydig cells—which are supported by a connective tissue support network. Spermatogenic cells facilitate the production and maturation of spermatozoa. Sertoli cells, or sustentacular cells, control the release of spermatozoa, support their development, and aid in forming the blood–testis barrier. They are stimulated by follicle-stimulating hormone. Leydig cells, or interstitial cells, produce testosterone through stimulation by interstitial cell–stimulating hormone and are inhibited by luteinizing hormone.

Small Animal Laparoscopy and Thoracoscopy, First Edition. Edited by Boel A. Fransson and Philipp D. Mayhew.

© 2015 by ACVS Foundation. Published 2015 by John Wiley & Sons, Inc.

Companion website: www.wiley.com/go/fransson/laparoscopy

Surgical Anatomy

If testicular descent was successful, each cavity of the scrotum contains a testis that has passed through the inguinal canal, with its associated epididymis and distal spermatic cord, and is covered by a vaginal tunic and spermatic fascia. The spermatic cord contains the ductus deferens as well as testicular vessels and nerves. The ductus deferens is the continuation of the tail of the epididymis and ascends the spermatic cord, enters the abdomen through the inguinal canal, crosses ventral to the ureter at the lateral ligament of the bladder, and enters the prostate to open into the urethra. It is accompanied by the artery and vein of the ductus deferens, arising from the prostatic artery, a branch of the internal iliac artery, and internal iliac vein, respectively. The testicular artery arises from the aorta near the fourth lumbar vertebra and anastomoses with the artery of the ductus deferens within the spermatic cord. The testicular vein follows a similar course, but it forms into the pampiniform plexus within the spermatic cord, surrounding the internal spermatic artery, lymphatics, and nerves to create a countercurrent thermal exchange. The right testicular vein drains into the caudal vena cava, and the left drains into the left renal vein. Testicular lymphatics drain into the lumbar lymph nodes. Nervous supply to the testis is largely sympathetic, supplied by the testicular plexus from the fourth to sixth lumbar ganglia.[20] If the testicle is still present within the abdomen, these structures will not have been bundled into the spermatic cord by the vaginal tunic and so will instead course independently from their respective origins.

Pathogenesis of Abnormal Descent

Cryptorchidism is a heritable trait and is suspected to have a sex-linked, autosomal recessive inheritance[9,18,21]; however, its exact etiology is multifactorial and incompletely understood. Its incidence in dogs has been reported between 1.2% and 12.9%.[1,4,5,8,22,23] Although widely reported in purebred and mixed-breed dogs, cryptorchidism is more prevalent in purebred and inbred dogs and more common in small breed compared with large breed dogs.23 Specifically, a high prevalence has been reported in Chihuahuas, miniature Schnauzers, Pomeranians, poodles, Shetland sheepdogs, Siberian huskies, and Yorkshire terriers.[9,10,24] Cryptorchid dogs also have a higher incidence of concurrent congenital defects such as inguinal and umbilical hernias, patellar luxation, and preputial or penile abnormalities.[10,24] Cryptorchidism has been reported in 1.3% to 3.8% of cats, with an increased prevalence in Persians.[2,3,5]

Plasma levels of both INSL3 and testosterone have been shown to be significantly lower in bilateral cryptorchid dogs than normal dogs, although still higher than in castrated dogs. This suggests impairment of Leydig cell function as a contributing factor as well as consequence of cryptorchidism.[25-27] Retained testes are generally smaller with up to 60% reduction in seminiferous tubules compared with a scrotal testis,[27] and even unilaterally affected dogs have decreased testosterone levels and semen quality.[26,27] Although still producing hormones, cryptorchid testicles are sterile because of the adverse effects of core body temperatures on spermatogenesis.[1,3,19] However, a unilaterally affected male remains fertile, albeit less so than a normal male.[1,10] In prepubescent male dogs, hormone treatments with human chorionic gonadotropin (hCG) or gonadotropin-releasing hormone (GnRH) have been used in an effort to encourage testicular descent with only anecdotal reports of success.[10]

Clinical Signs

On physical examination, if one or both of the testes cannot be palpated within the scrotum, it should be considered to be undescended. Testicular aplasia, resulting in monorchism or anorchism, is rare.[2,7] Palpation of the inguinal region, including the inguinal fat pad, should be performed to assess if the testicle has exited through the inguinal canal or if it remains within the peritoneal cavity. This should be performed with the animal standing as well as in dorsal recumbency and may require sedation or general anesthesia because the retained testicle is often smaller and can be difficult to palpate. If the animal is a unilateral cryptorchid, the descended testicle should be manipulated cranially into the prescrotal tissue; during this maneuver, the testis will deviate to one side of the penile shaft, indicating the side from which it has descended and allowing more focused investigation of the contralateral inguinal region. If the testicle cannot be palpated inguinally, it should be assumed to be present within the peritoneal cavity; it is uncommon for the testis to be lodged within the inguinal canal.

Testicular torsion should be considered upon presentation of a cryptorchid male with peracute abdominal pain but also in those with more vague clinical signs (lethargy, anorexia, vomiting) and should be considered a surgical emergency.[12, 28] A palpable inguinal or caudal abdominal mass may be found during evaluation, and on ultrasound examination, the mediastinum testis, a cord of connective tissue running lengthwise through the middle of the testicle, may be poorly defined in either a torsed or neoplastic testicle.[29,30] Given the risk of neoplastic transformation within retained testicles, testicular neoplasia should be considered in any abdominal or inguinal masses in middle-aged to older males. Retained testes in dogs have a 9.2 to 13.6 times higher incidence of neoplasia, with Sertoli cell tumors and seminomas being most common.[11,24,31] Inguinal testes are at twice the risk of neoplasia than intraabdominal testicles.[8,32] The risk of neoplasia also increases 4.7-fold when inguinal hernias are present.[11] Estrogen production, most commonly seen with Sertoli cell tumors, causes feminization syndrome in 16% to 39% of dogs, including bilateral alopecia, prostatic hyperplasia, penile atrophy, gynecomastia, galactorrhea, and myelotoxicosis (anemia, leucopenia, thrombocytopenia).[33-37]

Diagnosis

In the case of suspected bilaterally retained testes with an unknown castration history, other historical and physical examination findings can be used to support presumption of an intact cryptorchid male. This would include behavior typical of an intact male or the typical odor of tom cat urine.[3] In dogs, a well-developed prostate and, in cats, spines along the penile shaft are both androgen-dependent structures that are indirect evidence of the presence of testicular tissue. Plasma testosterone levels can be measured and a stimulation test performed if confirmation of the diagnosis is needed. Basal blood testosterone levels are assessed, and the patient is administered either GnRH (2 or 50 mcg/dog GnRH) or hCG (50 IU/kg hCG intramuscularly), with a second blood sample drawn 60 minutes (GnRH) or 120 minutes (hCG) after injection.[38] A substantial increase in plasma testosterone levels after injection is indicative of the presence of testicular tissue.[39,40]

Diagnostic ultrasonography has been shown to be highly effective at localizing retained testicles in both the inguinal region and intraabdominally. In one study, it carried a 100% positive predicative value compared with surgery and had a 96.6% sensitivity for abdominal testicles and 100% sensitivity for inguinal testicles in the hands of experienced evaluators.[30] Intraabdominal testicles were found anywhere between the kidneys and scrotum, so scanning of the entire ventral abdomen is recommended. Testicles generally maintained their normal sonographic appearance of a coarse, homogenous texture with central hyperechoic mediastinum testis unless they had undergone neoplastic transformation or torsion.[29,30] Magnetic resonance imaging has been reported in humans to search for cryptorchid testicles; however, even though it is more accurate than computed tomography, it had a low diagnostic accuracy.[13]

Patient Preparation

Surgery is generally performed as an elective procedure in young, healthy animals, allowing a minimum preoperative database and standard anesthetic protocols to be used. In older patients, particularly those where neoplastic transformation of the cryptorchid testicle is suspected, a more thorough evaluation such as a complete blood count, serum chemistry, urinalysis, and thoracic radiographs is indicated. Specifically, excess estrogen production by Sertoli cell tumors can result in myelotoxicity, with coagulation assessment and potentially blood transfusions being required.[33-37] Patients should be evaluated for concurrent prostatic disease, necessitating a digital rectal examination, as well as careful testicular palpation when able to assess for bilateral disease (11%–43% incidence with testicular tumors).[8,33,41,42] Because reported metastatic sites include regional lymph nodes, lungs, kidneys, spleen, pancreas, and liver, a complete abdominal ultrasound examination is recommended preoperatively if neoplasia is suspected.[33,42,43] Patients with peracute abdominal pain attributed to a testicular torsion should be stabilized and treated as surgical emergencies, with corresponding anesthetic considerations. Use of a ventilator may be advantageous during anesthesia because of increased intraabdominal pressure with insufflation and abdominal organ compression of the diaphragm if in Trendelenburg position. Perioperative antibiotics should be used at the discretion of the surgeon.

A variety of surgical techniques currently exist for treatment of cryptorchid testicles. Inguinal testes are often removed via a prescrotal, parapreputial, or inguinal incision directly over the palpable testicle. Traditionally, intraabdominal testes are removed via an open approach to the abdomen, either through a ventral midline celiotomy or a paraprepucial laparotomy. For large, neoplastic cryptorchid testicles, this may remain the practical choice because removal will necessitate a large incision. However, poor visualization during limited open approaches has resulted in inadvertent prostatectomy, iatrogenic urethral avulsions, and ureteral trauma.[2,3,44,45] Laparoscopic and laparoscopic-assisted techniques allow visualization and removal through minimally invasive means. A laparoscopic approach minimizes tissue trauma and postoperative incisional complications and decreases pain upon recovery compared to laparotomy. It also provides good visualization of the caudal abdominal and inguinal canals to allow improved surgical technique.[6,7,15]

Laparoscopic cryptorchidectomy is traditionally performed using a positive-pressure capnoperitoneum with a two- or three-portal technique and has been reported in both dogs[6,7,46-48] and cats.[7] A single-port, multiple-access technique has also been reported as feasible and safe.[49] For both cryptorchidectomy and vasectomy, the patient is placed in dorsal recumbency; a 15-degree Trendelenburg position is not required but can be helpful to increase caudal

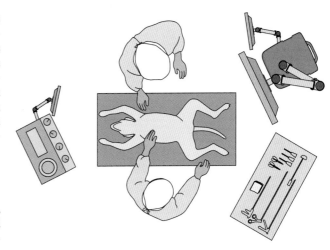

Figure 25-1 Operating room setup. Because a majority of the procedure is performed within the caudal abdomen, the scope tower is placed at the caudolateral end of the table, with the anesthesia machine placed near the head of the patient. The instrument table is placed in the opposing caudolateral corner.

abdominal visualization. A mild lateral obliquity away from the affected side, if unilateral, or use of a tilt table can also be beneficial (Figure 25-1). The entire ventral abdomen is aseptically prepared, from the xyphoid to the pubis and laterally to the mid-abdomen. A rigid laparoscope, instruments, and portals used can be either 5 or 10 mm depending on the equipment available and patient size. Generally, a 30-degree laparoscope is preferred to allow increased visualization of the entire abdominal cavity; however, a 0-degree laparoscope is also sufficient. Maryland or Babcock laparoscopic forceps should be available for tissue manipulation and grasping. If the testicle is suspected to be neoplastic, a specimen retrieval bag should be available to prevent seeding. Torsed testicles have frequently undergone neoplastic transformation and should be treated as such.[12]

Pneumoperitoneum can be induced using either Veress needle or Hasson technique. Insufflation to intraabdominal pressure of 10 to 12 mm Hg is typically sufficient to allow adequate visualization. A camera cannula is established on midline 1 to 2 cm caudal to the umbilicus and the abdominal contents visualized and evaluated as possible. A second cannula for instrument manipulation can be established under direct visualization on the caudal midline (Figure 25-2A) or caudolaterally. A caudal midline cannula should be just cranial to the prepuce or midway between the umbilicus and the brim of the pubis. A caudolateral cannula can be placed parapreputially toward the affected side, being sure to avoid the caudal superficial epigastric and prepucial arteries during placement (the abdominal wall can be transilluminated using the laparoscope to visualize the vasculature). A single caudolateral cannula can be used for bilaterally affected animals, if desired, because both testicles are generally still retrievable. If a three-portal technique is used, either a caudal midline and caudolateral portal or right and left caudolateral portals are established (Figure 25-2B), in addition to the camera portal. Single-incision access can also be used (Figure 25-2C). These instrument portals can be used to facilitate abdominal exploration and identification of the retained testicle. Similar portal placements can be used for laparoscopic vasectomy.

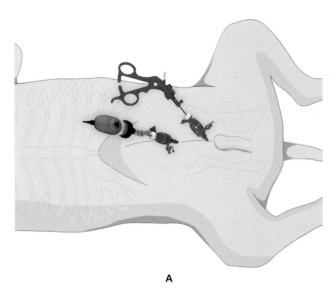

A

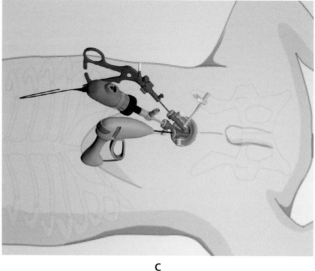

C

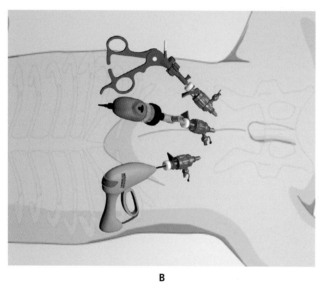

B

Figure 25-2 **A,** Portal placement. Initial visual cannula placement is on midline, 1 to 2 cm caudal to the umbilicus. For a two-portal technique, a second cannula is placed immediately cranial to the prepuce. Alternatively, in unilaterally cryptorchid dogs, the second cannula can be placed in a caudal paramedian position on the side ipsilateral to the testicle. The latter position may be beneficial in laparoscopy-assisted external ligation of a caudally located testicle. **B,** For a three-portal technique, the cannula placements depends on whether the animal is uni- or bilaterally cryptorchid. For bilaterally affected dogs, an umbilical visual cannula is established, and two paramedian cannulas can be placed triangulated with the laparoscope. For unilaterally cryptorchid dogs, the two-portal technique in A can be supplemented with a third cannula placed paramedian on the side of the testicle. **C,** A single-incision, multiple-access portal can be placed in the umbilical region. With bilateral cryptorchid testes, a single access device carries the advantage that reinsufflation after removal of the first testicle is facilitated.

Surgical Techniques

Cryptorchidectomy

To locate the testicle, either the testicular artery and vein can be followed from their craniodorsal origin near the kidney or the ductus deferens can be followed from its insertion into the prostatic urethra. Monorchidism and anorchism are rare (0.1–4% in cats),[2,3] but if present, the ductus deferens and testicular artery and vein will abruptly terminate within the abdominal cavity.[2,7] The gubernaculum can also be followed cranially from the inguinal canal and manipulated to locate the testicle within the abdomen (Figure 25-3). If the testicular artery and vein are visualized, along with the ductus deferens, disappearing within the inguinal canal, then the testicle has completed its transabdominal descent and entered the inguinal canal (see Figure 25-3). Infrequently has the testicle halted within the inguinal canal, so the ipsilateral inguinal region should be closely palpated or surgically explored. The ductus deferens can be grasped using atraumatic forceps and gentle traction applied to facilitate palpation or in an attempt to reduce the testis to within the abdomen.[3] If the testicle can be tractioned back through the inguinal canal into the abdomen, then it can be removed as such.

Alternatively, if the testicle cannot be located extraabdominally, a laparoscopic vasectomy can be performed to achieve sterility. However, this approach does not address androgen-driven conditions or decrease the risk of testicular torsion or neoplastic transformation.

After it is located (Figure 25-4), the testicle(s) can be manipulated using atraumatic forceps applied to the testicle itself or the adjacent spermatic cord. If performing a *laparoscopy-assisted* technique[7] (Video Clip 25-1), the testicle can be brought toward the instrument cannula, the portal enlarged, and the testicle extruded for ligation and transection of the spermatic cord (Figure 25-5). If bilateral, the instrument cannula should then be replaced and the positive-pressure pneumoperitoneum reestablished for visualization of the remaining testicle. This may require partial closure of the enlarged instrument portal, a purse-string suture, or manual pressure using a moistened gauze to help form an air-tight seal. Alternatively, the first testicle can be localized and secured to the abdominal wall using a percutaneous suture with a large-bore needle while the contralateral testicle is located. The contralateral testicle can be located and removed, and the first testicle is then easy to locate and extrude, frequently through the same portal, even

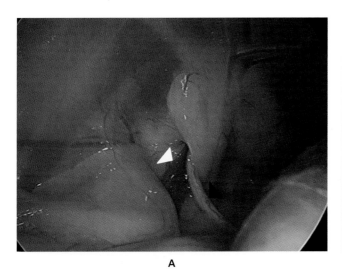

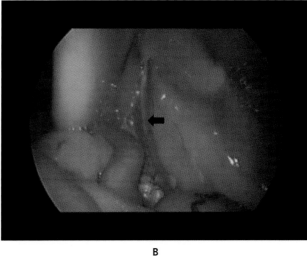

A   **B**

Figure 25-3 Evaluating the inguinal canal. **A,** If the testis has completed its intraabdominal descent and entered the inguinal canal, both the ductus deferens (black arrowhead) and testicular artery and vein (white arrowhead) can be visualized leading into the inguinal canal. **B,** If not, then only the gubernaculum (black arrow) is seen entering the inguinal canal.

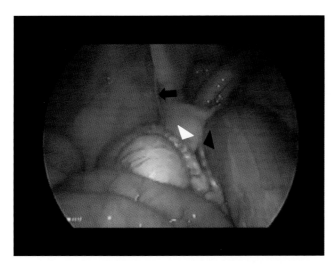

Figure 25-4 Locating an intraabdominal testicle. The gubernaculum (black arrow) or ductus deferens (black arrowhead) can be followed cranially to locate the testicle. The white arrowhead indicates the epididymis immediately adjacent to the testicle.

with compromised insufflation. When each testicle is extruded from the abdominal cavity for ligation, the abdomen should be allowed to collapse to provide less tension on the testicle. Both the ductus deferens and vascular pedicle should be double ligated, similar to an open orchiectomy, and observed for hemorrhage before replacement into the abdomen.

If performing the procedure *laparoscopically*, vascular structures and the ductus deferens can be ligated en bloc or bluntly dissected using Maryland forceps or scissors. Ligation can be achieved using extracorporeal knots, surgical stapling devices,[46] endoclips,[47,48] or a vessel-sealing device. Intracorporeal knots have also been reported,[6] but they are more technically demanding and likely to be more time consuming than the alternatives. To stabilize the testicle during dissection and ligation, two instrument portals can be established, allowing one instrument to grasp the testicle during dissection, or one instrument portal can be used and the testicle secured to the body wall using a percutaneously placed stay suture with a large-bore needle (Figure 25-6). Transabdominal suture fixation may be best used in non-neoplastic testicles. In either instance, the

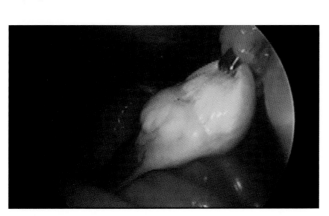

Figure 25-5 Extruding the testicle. If performing a laparoscopy-assisted technique, the instrument portal is enlarged and the testicle extruded from the abdomen for ligation and resection.

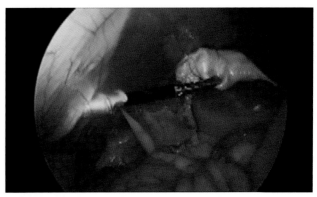

Figure 25-6 Percutaneous suture placement. If bilateral, the first testicle can be located and secured to the body wall using a percutaneous stay suture to allow for easy retrieval after removal of the contralateral testicle. This technique can also be used to secure the testicle for dissection if using a limited access technique.

surgeon should take care to elevate the testicle away from adjacent abdominal contents during dissection and ligation to prevent collateral damage. After ligation, the testicle(s) can be removed from the abdominal cavity by enlarging an instrument portal as needed to be able to extrude the testicle. If desired, and specifically if the testicle is abnormal, enlarged, or thought to be neoplastic, a endoscopic bag should be utilized used during extraction to limit contact of the testicle to the abdominal wall and possible seeding.[47] All removed testicles are submitted for histologic analysis for tissue verification and neoplastic evaluation.

Before routine cannula site closure, the abdominal cavity should be inspected for evidence of hemorrhage or iatrogenic trauma, including possible bowel or organ puncture or laceration. The abdominal cavity should then be decompressed and the entire pneumoperitoneum expelled. This may be accomplished using active suction or simply external compression while tenting open a previous cannula site. Regardless of the technique or portal sizes used, the external rectus sheath should be sutured into apposition to prevent subsequent herniation. If the inguinal canal has been approached or widened, the defect may need to be closed to its original size to prevent herniation. The remainder of the closure is a routine closure, frequently using intradermal closure to decrease irritation and improve cosmesis. In unilaterally affected animals, a standard prescrotal castration can be performed after removal of the retained testicle.

Vasectomy

Methods of sterilization without removal of the testicles have also been described using laparoscopic techniques. *Laparoscopic testicular devascularization* is performed using similar technique as that discussed earlier to identify and isolate the testicular artery and vein, as well as the ductus deferens. These structures are ligated and transected, allowing the ends to retract. Plasma testosterone levels were undetectable at 60 days after surgery. Histopathologic evaluation at 77 days after surgery showed fibrosis and parenchymal loss consistent with testicular ischemia; no spermatozoa were present within the epididymis.[48,50] *Vasectomies* have been similarly described via ligation or transection of the ductus deferens, often with removal of 1 to 2 cm of ductus tissue (Figure 25-7), while preserving the testicular artery and vein. Within the abdominal cavity, the ductus deferens travels apart from the testicular blood supply, so no separation of the structures is needed. This procedure prevents reproduction

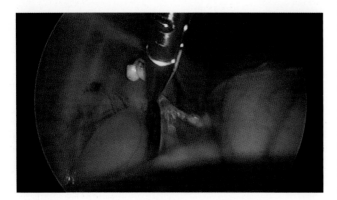

Figure 25-7 Vasectomy. When performing a vasectomy, the ductus deferens and associated vasculature are ligated and the ends allowed to retract or a 1- to 2-cm section removed to decrease the risk of recanalization. The testicular vessels are preserved.

but does not change androgen-driven behaviors or decrease the risk for testicular torsion or neoplasms. *Orchidopexy* involves surgical tractioning of the undescended testicle into the scrotum to secure it in a normal anatomic position.[51-53] Dogs have been extensively studied as experimental models for human orchiopexy and other microvascular procedures. These procedures are not recommended for clinical use in dogs given the heritable nature of the cryptorchid condition and potential detrimental effect on health.

Complications and Prognosis

Surgical complications include infection, hemorrhage, ecchymosis around the incision sites, swelling, and subcutaneous emphysema. In unilaterally affected patients, scrotal hemorrhage or hematomas are possible from castration of the descended testicle. Sperm granulomas after vasectomy have been reported in dog.[54] In the case of neoplastic or torsed testicles, adhesions to adjacent structures can compromise visualization or access for dissection. If the testicle has partially or completely torsed, it should be remove in that position and not derotated to limit reperfusion injury. The prognosis for patients with testicular torsions is good with timely recognition and removal and adequate supportive care.[12,28]

A full abdominal explore should be performed as possible to evaluate for metastasis, with special attention paid to the regional lymph nodes, kidneys, spleen, pancreas, and liver.[33,42,43] Feminization syndrome secondary to Sertoli cell tumors is generally reversible with complete tumor removal and no metastatic disease.[43] Myelotoxicity, however, can be a fatal sequela with a guarded prognosis even with castration.[33-37] Whereas Sertoli cell tumors have a 2.17% to 10% metastatic rate,[41-43] seminomas have been reported to metastasize in 6.38% to 11% of cases.[41,42] Interstitial cell tumors can cause increased testosterone production, leading to an increased incidence of perineal hernias, perianal adenomas, and perianal gland adenocarcinomas.[41] However, only in extremely rare cases do interstitial cell tumors metastasize to regional lymph nodes or lungs. In all testicular tumors, the prognosis is excellent with complete surgical resection and no metastasis.[33,42]

Postoperative Care

Depending on recovery from anesthesia and concurrent health concerns, surgeries can frequently be performed on an outpatient basis. Those undergoing removal for testicular torsions or neoplasm should be evaluated for stability to determine duration of hospitalization. Postoperative recovery should be similar to that of other abdominal surgeries. Animals should be kept exercise restricted for 10 to 14 days after the procedure. An Elizabethan collar or similar method should be used to prevent licking or trauma to the incision sites. Pain is generally well managed with a short course of nonsteroidal antiinflammatory or oral opioid medication (or both).

Plasma testosterone levels have been shown to drop to undectable levels within 2 to 4 hours of castration but can persist for at least 8 days in some animals.[55] Patients are azoospermic within 5 days after castration in dogs.[55] In patients having undergone vasectomy, sperm numbers in the ejaculate rapidly decrease in the first 2 to 3 days,[56,57] but may persist for up to 21 days in dogs.[58] In cats after vasectomy, sperm counts again rapidly decrease for the first 5 to 7 days,[57] but persist for at least 49 days.[59] The persistence of spermatozoa depends on the frequency of ejaculation, as well as other factors, but animals should be separated from prospective breeding partners for at least 10 to 14 days with owners appropriately advised of the risks.

All videos cited in this chapter can be found on the book's companion website at **www.wiley.com/go/fransson/laparoscopy**

References

1 Kawakami E, Tsutsui T, Yamada Y, Yamauchi M. (1984) Cryptorchidism in the dog: occurrence of cryptorchidism and semen quality in the cryptorchid dog. Nihon Juigaku Zasshi 46 (3), 303-308.

2 Millis, D.L., Hauptman, J.G., Johnson, C.A. (1992) Cryptorchidism and monorchism in cats: 25 cases (1980-1989). J Am Vet Med Assoc 200 (8), 1128-1130.

3 Richardson, E.F., Mullen, H. (1993) Cryptorchidism in cats. Compend Contin Educ Pract Vet 15 (10), 1342-1345.

4 Dunn, M.L., Foster, W.J., Goodard, K.M. (1968) Cryptorchidism in dogs: a clinical survey. J Am Vet Med Assoc 4, 180-182.

5 Yates, D., Hayes, G., Heffernan, M., Beynon, R. (2003) Incidence of cryptorchidism in dogs and cats. Vet Rec 152 (16), 502-504.

6 Lew, M., Jalynski, M., Kasprowicz, A., Brzeski, W. (2005) Laparoscopic cryptorchidectomy in dogs—report of 15 cases. Pol J Vet Sci 8 (3), 251-254.

7 Miller, N.A., Van Lue, S.J., Rawlings, C.A. (2004) Use of laparoscopic-assisted cryptorchidectomy in dogs and cats. J Am Vet Med Assoc 224 (6), 875-878, 865.

8 Reif, J.S., Brodey, R.S. (1969) The relationship between cryptorchidism and canine testicular neoplasia. J Am Vet Med Assoc 155 (12), 2005-2010.

9 Cox, V., Wallace, L., Jessen, C. (1978) An anatomic and genetic study of canine cryptorchidism. Teratology 18 (2), 233-240.

10 Memon, M.A. (2007) Common causes of male dog infertility. Theriogenology 68 (3), 322-328.

11 Hayes, H.M. Jr, Pendergrass, T.W. (1976) Canine testicular tumors: epidemiologic features of 410 dogs. International journal of cancer Journal international du cancer. 18 (4), 482-487.

12 Pearson, H., Kelly, D.F. (1975) Testicular torsion in the dog: a review of 13 cases. Vet Rec 97 (11), 200-204.

13 Abaci, A., Cath, G., Anik, A., Bober, E. (2013) Epidemiology, classification and management of undescended testes: does medication have value in its treatment? J Clin Res Pediatr Endocrinol 5 (2), 65-72.

14 Bay, K., Main, K.M., Toppari, J., Skakkebaek, N.E. (2011) Testicular descent: INSL3, testosterone, genes and the intrauterine milieu. Nat Rev Urol 8 (4), 187-196.

15 Mayhew, P. (2009) Laparoscopic and laparoscopic-assisted cryptorchidectomy in dogs and cats. Compend Contin Educ Vet 31 (6), E9.

16 Ashdown, R.R. (1963) The diagnosis of cryptorchidism in young dogs: a review of the problem. J Small Anim Pract 4 (4), 261-263.

17 Kawakami, E., Hirayama, S., Tsutsui, T., Ogasa, A. (1993) Pituitary response of cryptorchid dogs to LH-RH-analogue before and after sexual maturation. J Vet Med Sci 55 (1), 147-148.

18 Rhoades, J.D., Foley, C.W. (1977) Cryptorchidism and intersexuality. Vet Clin North Am 7 (4), 789-794.

19 Romagnoli, S.E. (1991) Canine cryptorchidism. The Veterinary clinics of North America Small animal practice 21 (3), 533-544.

20 Evans, H.E. (1993) Miller's Anatomy of the Dog, 3rd edn. Saunders, Philadelphia.

21 Robinson, R. (1987) Genetic defects in cats. Companion Animal Practice 1 (3), 10-14.

22 Ruble, R.P., Hird, D.W. (1993) Congenital abnormalities in immature dogs from a pet store: 253 cases (1987-1988). J Am Vet Med Assoc 202 (4), 633-636.

23 Priester, W.A., Glass, A.G., Waggoner, N.S. (1970) Congenital defects in domesticated animals: general considerations. Am J Vet Res 31 (10), 1871-1879.

24 Pendergrass, T.W., Hayes, H.M. Jr. (1975) Cryptorchism and related defects in dogs: epidemiologic comparisons with man. Teratology 12 (1), 51-55.

25 Pathirana, I.N., Yamasaki, H., Kawate, N., et al. (2012) Plasma insulin-like peptide 3 and testosterone concentrations in male dogs: changes with age and effects of cryptorchidism. Theriogenology 77 (3), 550-557.

26 Kawakami, E., Tsutsui, T., Yamada, Y., et al. (1987) Spermatogenesis and peripheral spermatic venous plasma androgen levels in the unilateral cryptorchid dogs. Nihon Juigaku Zasshi 49 (2), 349-356.

27 Kawakami, E., Tsutsui, T., Yamada, Y., et al. (1988) Testicular function of scrotal testes after the cryptorchidectomy in dogs with unilateral cryptorchidism. Nihon Juigaku Zasshi 50 (6), 1239-1244.

28 Naylor, R.W., Thompson, S.M.R. (1979) Intraabdominal testicular torsion: a report of two cases. J Am Anim Hosp Assoc 15, 763-766.

29 Hecht, S., King, R., Tidwell, A.S., Gorman, S.C. (2004) Ultrasound diagnosis: intraabdominal torsion of a non-neoplastic testicle in a cryptorchid dog. Vet Radiol Ultrasound 45 (1), 58-61.

30 Felumlee, A.E., Reichle, J.K., Hecht, S., et al. (2012) Use of ultrasound to locate retained testes in dogs and cats. Vet Radiol Ultrasound 53 (5), 581-585.

31 Hayes, H.M. Jr, Wilson, G.P., Pendergrass, T.W., Cox, V.S. (1985) Canine cryptorchism and subsequent testicular neoplasia: case-control study with epidemiologic update. Teratology 32 (1), 51-56.

32 Reif, J.S., Maguire, T.G., Kenney, R.M., Brodey, R.S. (1979) A cohort study of canine testicular neoplasia. J Am Vet Med Assoc 175 (7), 719-723.

33 Dhaliwal, R., Kitchell, B., Knight, B., Schmidt, B. (1999) Treatment of aggressive testicular tumors in four dogs. J Am Anim Hosp Assoc 35 (4), 311-318.

34 Edwards, D.F. (1981) Bone marrow hypoplasia in a feminized dog with a Sertoli cell tumor. J Am Vet Med Assoc 178 (5), 494-496.

35 Morgan, R.V. (1982) Blood dyscrasias associated with testicular tumors in the dog. J Am Anim Hosp Assoc 18 (6), 970-975.

36 Sherding, R.G., Wilson, G.P. 3rd, Kociba, G.J. (1981) Bone marrow hypoplasia in eight dogs with Sertoli cell tumor. J Am Vet Med Assoc 178 (5), 497-501.

37 Suess, R.P. Jr, Barr, S.C., Sacre, B.J., French, T.W. (1992) Bone marrow hypoplasia in a feminized dog with an interstitial cell tumor. J Am Vet Med Assoc 200 (9), 1346-1348.

38 Birchard, S., Nappier, M. (2008) Cryptorchidism. Compend Contin Educ Vet 30 (6), 325-336.

39 Purswell, B.J., Wilcke, J.R. (1993) Response to gonadotrophin-releasing hormone by the intact male dog: serum testosterone, luteinizing hormone and follicle-stimulating hormone. J Reprod Fertil Suppl 47, 335-341.

40 England, G.C.W., Allen, W.E., Porter, D.J. (1989) Evaluation of the testosterone response to hCG and the identification of a presumed anorchid dog. J Small Anim Pract 30 (8), 441-443.

41 Lipowitz, A.J., Schwartz, A., Wilson, G.P., Ebert, J.W. (1973) Testicular neoplasms and concomitant clinical changes in the dog. J Am Vet Med Assoc 163 (12), 1364-1368.

42 Dow, C. (1962) Testicular tumours in the dog. J Comp Pathol 72, 247-265.

43 McNeil, P.E., Weaver, A.D. (1980) Massive scrotal swelling in two unusual cases of canine sertoli-cell tumour. Vet Rec 106 (7), 144-146.

44 Bellah, J.R., Spencer, C.P., Salmeri, K.R. (1989) Hemiprostatic urethral avulsion during cryptorchid orchiectomy in a dog. J Am Anim Hosp Assoc 25 (5), 553-556.

45 Schulz, K.S., Waldron, D.R., Smith, M.M., et al. (1996) Inadvertent prostatectomy as a complication of cryptorchidectomy in four dogs. J Am Anim Hosp Assoc 32 (3), 211-214.

46 Pena, F.J., Anel, L., Dominguez, J.C., et al. (1998) Laparoscopic surgery in a clinical case of seminoma in a cryptorchid dog. Vet Rec 142 (24), 671-672.

47 Spinella, G., Romagnoli, N., Valentini, S., Spadari, A. (2003) Application of the 'extraction bag' in laparoscopic treatment of unilateral and bilateral abdominal cryptorchidism in dogs. Veterinary research communications 27 (suppl 1), 445-447.

48 Mathon, D.H., Palierne, S., Meynaud-Collard, P., et al. (2011) Laparoscopic-assisted colopexy and sterilization in male dogs: short-term results and physiologic consequences. Vet Surg 40 (4), 500-508.

49 Runge, J.J., Mayhew, P., Case, J.B., et al. (2014) Single port laparoscopic cryptorchidectomy in dogs and cats: a multicenter analysis of 25 cases (2009-2014). Presented at the Veterinary Endoscopy Society 11th Annual Meeting, Florence, Italy.

50 Nudelmann, N., Boulouha, L., Rousseau, A., Siliart, B. (1998) Testicular degeneration by devascularization: practical surgical application in the dog. Recueil De Medecine Veterinaire 174 (7-8), 133-1339.

51 Belfield, W. (1975) Canine orchiopexy: surgical fixation, in the scrotum, of an undescended testicle. Vet Med Small Anim Clin 70 (2), 157-161.

52 Kawakami, E., Tsutsui, T., Yamada, Y., et al. (1988) Spermatogenic function in cryptorchid dogs after orchiopexy. Nihon Juigaku Zasshi 50 (1), 227-235.

53 Kawakami, E., Tsutsui, T., Yamada, Y., et al. (1988) Spermatogenic function and fertility in unilateral cryptorchid dogs after orchiopexy and contralateral castration. Nihon Juigaku Zasshi 50 (3), 754-762.

54 Aguirre, A.M., Fernandez, P.G., Muela, M.S. (1996) Sperm granuloma in the dog: complication of vasectomy. J Small Anim Pract 37, 392-393.

55 Taha, M.B., Noakes, D.E., Allen, W.E. (1982) Hemicastration and castration in the beagle dog; the effects on libido, peripheral plasma testosterone concentrations, seminal characteristics and testicular function. J Small Anim Pract 23 (5), 279-285.

56 Schiff, J.D., Li, P.S., Schlegel, P.N., Goldstein, M. (2003) Rapid disappearance of spermatozoa after vasal occlusion in the dog. J Androl 24 (3), 361-363.

57 Wildt, D.E., Seager, S.W., Bridges, C.H. (1981) Sterilization of the male dog and cat by laparoscopic occlusion of the ductus deferens. Am J Vet Res 42 (11), 1888-1897.

58 Pineda, M.H., Reimers, T.J., Faulkner, L.C. (1976) Disappearance of spermatozoa from the ejaculates of vasectomized dogs. J Am Vet Med Assoc 168 (6), 502-503.

59 Pineda, M.H., Dooley, M.P. (1984) Surgical and chemical vasectomy in the cat. Am J Vet Res 45 (2), 291-300.

26 The Role of Laparoscopy in Cancer Staging

Michele A. Steffey

Key Points

- If ports are too high or too low in the dorsoventral direction, dissection of the nodes of the iliosacral lymphatic center will be very challenging.
- Use of electrosurgical units or vessel-sealing devices is very helpful for minimally invasive lymph node biopsy or lymphadenectomy. Even small amounts of hemorrhage may make visualization of nearby normal structures difficult and will slow safe dissection.
- Crush artifact secondary to grasping the tissue with pressure may impact pathologic interpretation and identification of low-volume metastatic disease.
- Surgical oncologic principles should be adhered to, and specimen retrieval devices should be used to minimize risks of port site metastasis.

Advantages of minimally invasive procedures over open surgical procedures have been previously demonstrated in veterinary patients, including reductions in pain and a more rapid return to normal activity.[1,2] However, it is important when choosing a minimally invasive approach to cancer to ensure that the potential benefits of reduced patient discomfort and quicker recovery times that are common to laparoscopic approaches do not result in compromise of oncologic principles and patient outcomes. It has been proposed by some that laparoscopy could worsen oncologic outcomes by fragmenting cancer cells and promoting implantation and spread or that the loss of tactile input during surgery may reduce the quality of the resection that can be achieved. This is an area of ongoing controversy in the human medical field, but it is known that laparoscopic surgery has been shown to cause a less intense inflammatory reaction than traditional surgery, one contributing factor of which seems to be associated with carbon dioxide (CO_2) insufflation.[3,4] Inflammation and neovascularization can be associated with promotion of tumor growth, and a murine model showed that rats with implanted tumor cells exhibited decreased growth of tumor after laparoscopy compared with laparotomy.[5] Further studies are needed to define the relationships between surgical approaches and techniques and oncologic outcomes for the spectrum of neoplastic diseases treated. However, it is likely a more important consideration that operative decisions do not compromise surgical oncologic principles of maintaining appropriate margins and accurate nodal assessment rather than the intrinsic choice of a minimally invasive versus open surgical approach. Appropriate case selection is key.

Diagnostic Laparoscopy and Biopsy

Accurate staging information is an extremely important component of an overall oncologic plan. Although advanced preoperative diagnostic imaging studies have vastly improved our ability to define the disease stage for a given patient, noninvasive imaging can underestimate the tumor burden, especially in cases of peritoneal carcinomatosis or metastatic serosal hemangiosarcoma, smaller multifocal liver metastases from a variety of neoplasms, or micro-metastatic disease to regional lymph nodes. Diffuse or multifocal smaller lesions are very difficult to define on noninvasive imaging modalities such as ultrasonography, computed tomography (CT), or magnetic resonance imaging (MRI). Diagnostic laparoscopy has a place in some patients, providing the staging benefit of identifying metastatic lesions missed by other imaging modalities, identifying locoregional lymph nodes for biopsy, and providing an option for a minimally invasive diagnostic biopsy of the primary lesion or as a preliminary evaluation of lesion resectability. Tissue diagnosis is an important component of an oncologic therapeutic plan, and although other image-guided techniques such as fine-needle aspiration or percutaneous biopsy may also provide minimally invasive options in diagnosis, laparoscopic biopsy provides excellent lesion visualization, the ability to manipulate and possibly minimize

---

Small Animal Laparoscopy and Thoracoscopy, First Edition. Edited by Boel A. Fransson and Philipp D. Mayhew.

© 2015 by ACVS Foundation. Published 2015 by John Wiley & Sons, Inc.

Companion website: www.wiley.com/go/fransson/laparoscopy

injury to nearby viscera, the potential for larger tissue samples, and an improved ability to provide hemostasis.

Lymphatic Staging

The function of the lymphatic system is to drain interstitial fluid back to the venous system. Lymph nodes are junctions throughout this system, between multiple afferent lymphatics and few efferent lymphatics. As such, they form barriers to lymphatic drainage, and in a neoplastic setting, they function as barriers to the lymphatic extension of cancer cells and a rational point of evaluation for metastasis. However, assessing lymph node involvement still remains a challenge in the human and veterinary medical fields.

In concept, locoregional lymph node staging is important in the therapeutic planning of most solid cancers, and identification of metastatic disease within the lymphatic system can significantly alter surgical and adjuvant treatment recommendations. A large body of literature exists evaluating the extent, timing, and methods of surgical lymphatic staging for different neoplastic diseases in humans,[6-10] and there is growing evidence in the veterinary literature for consideration of these techniques in our patients.[11-17] In general, removal of large, grossly abnormal, clearly metastatic lymph nodes is most commonly recommended in veterinary patients for the purpose of overall disease reduction and improved response to adjuvant therapy.[18] The role of surgical sampling of nonenlarged regional lymph nodes in veterinary patients is less clear. Because of their intimate association with the terminal aorta or vena cava and other important blood vessels, abdominal and retroperitoneal lymph nodes can be challenging to sample preoperatively, especially if lymphadenomegaly is not present. However, as micrometastases may take many months to produce palpable lymphadenomegaly, it is conceivable that early histopathologic evaluation of normal-sized lymph nodes could allow for a more accurate assessment of stage. Increased sensitivity in the detection of micrometastasis by lymph node biopsy allows for upstaging of patients who might have been staged as negative for nodal metastasis based on aspiration alone. However, in the case of more superficial tumors in which the draining lymph nodes lie within the abdominal cavity or retroperitoneum, a separate open abdominal approach in addition to the tumor resection can be an unattractive option to many clinicians and clients. A minimally invasive option for biopsy of abdominal lymph nodes when indicated may encourage clients to pursue improved staging of various regional neoplastic diseases, even when lymph nodes are not measurably enlarged. As a profession, the question of which lymph nodes should be sampled and when is a bit of the-chicken-or-the-egg question. How do we justify an invasive procedure to remove a nonenlarged lymph node(s) if we have not demonstrated a reasonably high probability that it will benefit the patient? But how will we obtain that data if we do not remove nonenlarged lymph nodes, assess them for microscopic disease, and correlate that information with survival times and treatment recommendations? Although mechanisms of metastasis are likely to be similar among species, there are noteworthy anatomic differences in lymphatic basins in veterinary patients compared with humans, and lymph node biopsy practices in veterinary patients should be evaluated on their own merits. There is much work to be done in this area in veterinary medicine in general, and minimally invasive approaches may improve our opportunities to answer these questions.

The question of which lymph node(s) to remove for a given tumor may be aided by the technique of sentinel lymph node (SLN) mapping. SLN mapping is based on the concept that lymphatic dissemination from a tumor is an orderly process, with initial involvement of the first lymph node receiving afferent lymphatics from the tumor before dissemination to the remainder of the nodes in the regional lymphatic basin.[6] The SLN is the most likely lymph node to harbor metastatic deposits, and therefore if the pathology of the SLN is negative for metastasis, the nonsentinel nodes in the region should be at minimal risk of harboring metastases. Based on this concept, assessment of the regional lymphatic basin for microscopic metastatic disease via SLN biopsy (even when the lymph nodes in question are palpably unremarkable or normal in appearance on imaging) has become the standard of care in human breast cancer and melanoma patients and is increasing in use for a variety of other neoplasms.[6-9,19] SLN biopsy has been shown to be a highly sensitive and specific indicator of the patient's true metastatic status.[20,21] Increased sensitivity in the detection of micrometastases in SLNs allows for upstaging of patients who might have been staged as negative for nodal metastasis (N0) based on regional lymph node aspirates alone. Human studies have demonstrated up to 30% of patients, previously staged as N0 before SLN evaluation, benefited from upstaging and subsequent adjustments in therapeutic plan after detection of micrometastases.[20,21] The clinical use of SLN mapping is in its infancy in veterinary medicine, but it has been described in a few cohorts of dogs.[13,15] In Worley's study of dogs with mast cell tumor, 42% of patients had additional treatment recommended that would not have otherwise been offered based on findings of micrometastatic disease identified by SLN biopsy.[13] Much experience still needs to be gained on the application of these techniques to veterinary patients, including application to different disease processes, tracer types, tracer doses, and timing.

The most common methods of intraoperative SLN mapping include the use of lymphoscintigraphy; intraoperative vital blue dyes (e.g., isosulfan blue, patent blue V, or methylene blue); or more recently, the use of intraoperative near-infrared fluorescent imaging.[10,13,15,16,20-25] A small volume of the chosen tracer is injected peritumorally (intradermally or subcutaneously at the transition from palpable disease at the tumor margin). Assessment for tracer uptake in the locoregional lymph nodes is then performed. Lymphatic uptake is relatively quick, on the order of seconds to minutes, so SLN assessment must be performed very shortly after injection, or there is a higher likelihood of identification of second- or third-tier lymph nodes, and even possibly missing the true SLN because of tracer washout. In general, the use of scintigraphy and visual vital dyes is most commonly combined in human patients because the combination is more sensitive in SLN identification than using vital blue dyes alone.[26] Although scintigraphy does not discolor the dissection field around the primary tumor, it does not aid in visual identification of the lymph node at surgery. The blue dyes are widely available and do visually identify the lymph node at surgery, but they result in discoloration of the tissues around the primary lesion that can obscure regional anatomy and slow dissection. Near-infrared fluorescence imaging is an emerging modality that in early studies appears to have similar sensitivity and specificity to the combined use of scintigraphy and vital blue dyes and offers the benefit of avoiding patient and surgeon exposure to ionizing radiation.[10,22-25] The main downsides for near-infrared imaging are the need for specialized imaging systems that are not yet widely available and that the most commonly used near-infrared tracer, indocyanine green, is nonspecific and passes very quickly through the lymphatic system, making it prone to highlight second- and third-tier nodes if close attention to timing is not given.

Because, historically, biopsy of the abdominal and retroperitoneal lymph nodes could only be obtained by a major open abdominal procedure, excisional biopsy of these lymph nodes for staging purposes has not commonly been elected in the absence of overtly palpable or ultrasonographically identified lymphadenopathy. In Worley's study of SLN mapping, the two SLNs identified by lymphoscintigraphy that were purposely not extirpated were medial iliac lymph nodes (with the implication that this was because of the intraabdominal location).[13] In a canine experimental study evaluating the utility of various vital dyes for lymphatic mapping, a medial iliac lymph node identified by lymphography as the SLN, received afferent lymphatics from two anatomically divergent injection sites (a dorsal lumbar injection and a hock injection), confirming that the medial iliac lymph node has the potential to be sentinel for a wide variety of tumor locations.[17] Although published clinical data on the minimally invasive removal of cavitary lymph nodes in clinical patients is lacking, a minimally invasive technique for excisional biopsy of the medial iliac lymph nodes using a lateral three-port laparoscopic approach has been described in a cohort of normal dogs.[27] Although this study was performed in a cohort of healthy dogs, anecdotally, this technique has been performed by the author in a clinical setting to obtain lymphatic staging information in dogs presenting for perineal neoplasia.

Preoperative Considerations

Surgical Anatomy

Abdominal lymph nodes can be categorized into regional lymphatic centers including the celiac lymphatic center, the cranial mesenteric lymphatic center, and the caudal mesenteric lymphatic center.[28,29] The celiac lymphatic center encompasses the hepatic lymph node(s) along the portal vein trunk, the splenic lymph node(s) grouped around the splenic vessels, the gastric lymph node found near the pylorus at the lesser curvature of the stomach, and the pancreaticoduodenal lymph node(s) located in the first duodenal flexure.[28,29] The cranial mesenteric lymphatic center encompasses the jejunal lymph nodes, found at the root of the mesentery of the jejunum and ileum, and the colic lymph nodes associated with the ascending and transverse colon.[28,29] The caudal mesenteric lymphatic center encompasses the left colic lymph nodes in the mesocolon of the descending colon, associated with the caudal mesenteric artery.[28,29] In an experimental study in rats, injection of tracers into the peritoneal cavity demonstrated that in these normal animals, the peritoneal space lymphatic drainage went to the celiac and superior (cranial) mesenteric lymphatic centers.[30] In the rat model, there are specific positive and negative nodes within each lymph node group, suggesting a particular lymph node drainage pattern, not merely diffusion into all intraabdominal lymphatics.[30]

Retroperitoneal lymph nodes can also be regionally categorized into iliosacral lymphatic center and the lumbar lymphatic center. The iliosacral lymphatic center encompasses the medial iliac lymph nodes, the median sacral lymph nodes, the lateral sacral lymph nodes, and the hypogastric lymph nodes.[28,29] In general, the iliosacral lymphatic center receives afferent lymphatics from a wide variety of locations, including the skin, subcutis, and fascia caudal to the last rib; the skin of the pelvis and tail; muscles, tendons and joints of the pelvic limbs; the caudal urogenital organs; the peritoneum; the colon, rectum, and anus; and the sacral, hypogastric, iliofemoral, femoral, superficial inguinal, popliteal, and caudal mesenteric lymph nodes.[28,29] The lumbar lymphatic center encompasses the lumbar aortic lymph nodes scattered along the aorta and caudal vena cava from the diaphragm to the iliac arteries and the renal

lymph nodes located near the renal vessels[28,29] and receives afferent lymphatics from the lumbar and abdominal muscles, diaphragm, peritoneum, liver, kidney, adrenal glands, reproductive organs, medial iliac lymph nodes, and caudal mesenteric lymph nodes. The efferent lymphatics from the iliosacral and lumbar lymphatic centers join to form the lumbar trunks and empty into the cisterna chyli.[28,29]

The medial iliac lymph nodes are usually paired structures found at the level of the branching external iliac vessels, although occasionally an additional or accessory medial iliac lymph node may be found slightly cranial to the primary lymph nodes.[28,29] They lie on the lateral aspect of the abdominal aorta and caudal vena cava between the deep circumflex iliac vessels and the external iliac vessels. The deep circumflex iliac vessels, in fact, function as a very useful intraoperative landmark for localization of the medial iliac lymph nodes, which are often buried in fat. The hypogastric lymph node(s) may be single or paired and are generally to be found sitting in the angle of the bifurcating internal iliac vessels. The median sacral lymph nodes are found within the pelvis on dorsal midline, associated with the median sacral artery when this artery is present. The lateral sacral lymph nodes are found within the pelvis, lateral to the midline.

These patterns of afferent and efferent drainage are generalized, and the actual drainage pattern may be different for each individual neoplasm. In Worley's study of SLN mapping, 42% of dogs had SLNs identified that were different from the anatomically predicted regional lymph node,[13] indicating that identification of lymph nodes for sampling based on anatomic descriptions alone may not be sufficiently accurate to ensure that metastatic disease is identified.

Diagnostic Workup and Imaging

Assessment of the lymph nodes of the iliosacral lymphatic center is considered important in the staging of many neoplastic diseases in dogs, including anal sac gland adenocarcinoma in which metastatic disease is identified at diagnosis in 46% to 96% of dogs.[31] Depending on patient size, palpation of the lymph nodes of the iliosacral lymphatic center may be possible per rectum, but in general, consistent identification of these nodes on rectal examination requires gross lymphadenomegaly. Palpation has been shown to be an insensitive indicator of nodal metastasis in dogs in general.[11,12,15] The medial iliac lymph nodes are currently the most commonly assessed lymph nodes for evidence of lymphadenopathy that might indicate metastasis for anal sac adenocarcinoma.[18,32] Because of their more cranial retroperitoneal location, medial iliac lymph nodes are most commonly assessed by ultrasonographic imaging of the abdomen in canine patients, but the hypogastric and sacral lymph nodes are not well assessed by this method, and it is likely for this reason that data are lacking for these lymph nodes. In general, because of their challenging anatomic location in association with the terminal abdominal aorta and vena cava, preoperative sampling of the medial iliac lymph nodes can be challenging, and percutaneous ultrasound-guided aspiration of the medial iliac lymph nodes is often not attempted unless lymphadenomegaly or other indicators of lymphadenopathy are present.

Ultrasonography is widely accessible in veterinary medicine and is most commonly used for imaging assessment of abdominal and retroperitoneal lymph nodes. Ultrasonographic characteristics of normal and neoplastic lymph nodes have been described.[33-38] Ultrasonographic characteristics that are suggestive of nodal invasion by macrometastases include enlargement, round shape, hypoechogenicity, and presence of irregular lymph node contours.[37-39] Advanced cross-sectional imaging modalities such as CT and MRI are becoming increasingly used in the assessment of locoregional lymph nodes in veterinary patients, and imaging characteristics of lymph nodes have been described for these modalities.[40-42] However, with most cross-sectional imaging techniques, nodal size and morphologic characteristics remain insufficient to provide a fully accurate identification. In addition to not distinguishing reactive lymph nodes from malignant lymph nodes well, CT and MRI also do not accurately identify micrometastatic disease. Lymphoscintigraphy is a reliable method to localize SLNs, but it is expensive and requires special considerations in handling of the radiopharmaceutical, and as a result, is not widely available in clinical veterinary practice. Indirect CT or MRI lymphography by peritumoral injections of small-sized iodinated contrast agents that are picked up by local lymphatics and converge toward afferent nodes (similar to the use of radioisotopes) have been described.[43-46] The concept of indirect interstitial CT and MR lymphography matches the concept of intraoperative SLN mapping and may offer alternatives to lymphoscintigraphy in the preoperative determination of which lymph nodes to prioritize for sampling. The author has successfully applied the techniques of CT lymphography to the iliosacral lymphatic center in veterinary patients (Figure 26-1). Functional imaging (positron emission tomography) plays a role in assessment of locoregional lymph node status in humans but is not widely available in veterinary medicine.[47] However, despite the many advances in noninvasive imaging methods, surgical SLN biopsy remains the method of choice to detect metastatic spread in draining lymph nodes in a number of human cancers.

The minimum database for veterinary patients being considered for laparoscopic cancer staging should include complete blood count and serum biochemistry, abdominal ultrasonography (AUS), and any other diagnostic staging recommended based on the patient's underlying disease process or comorbidities. However, in the application of this technique to clinical patients, the author has found the use of contrast-enhanced CT invaluable for the assessment of lymph nodes that are not well visualized with AUS (e.g., the sacral and hypogastric lymph nodes), as well as providing three-dimensional information about regional anatomy relative to lymph node position, vascular invasion, or invasion of other regional structures that can be very helpful in case selection and directing intraoperative dissection. In addition to standard imaging techniques, the author has additionally successfully used preoperative indirect CT lymphography and indirect intraoperative lymphography (using visible methylene blue dye and near-infrared fluorescence lymphography with indocyanine green) for the removal of abdominal and retroperitoneal lymph nodes in clinical veterinary patients.

Patient Selection

Much work remains to be done in determining the limits of application of this technique. To date, the author has performed fully laparoscopic lymph node resections of the medial iliac and hypogastric lymph nodes, as well as laparoscopic-assisted lymph node biopsy of various abdominal lymph nodes. Many abdominal lymph nodes are likely amenable to laparoscopic or laparoscopic-assisted techniques. Laparoscopic-assisted dissections may be performed through small midline incisions as long as the incision is positioned such that the targeted lymph nodes may be sufficiently exteriorized through an Alexis wound retractor (Applied Medical, Rancho Santa Margarita, CA). Patient size may be a limiting factor to successful dissection in laparoscopic lymphadenectomy because of limitations in work-

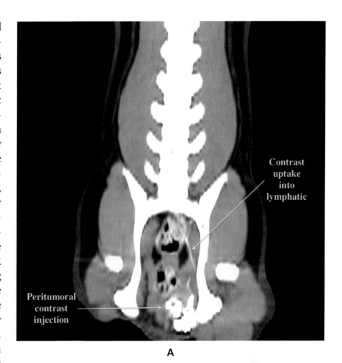

A

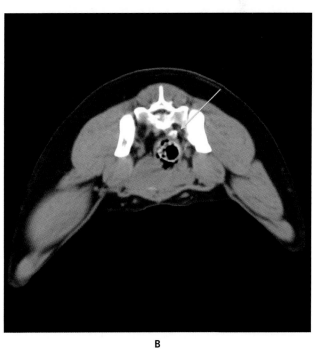

B

Figure 26-1 Computed tomography lymphography of a perineal tumor demonstrating iodinated contrast uptake after peritumoral injection, with contrast highlighting intrapelvic lymphatic drainage (**A**), and first lymph node contrast uptake in the ipsilateral hypogastric lymph node (**B**).

ing space, especially for the more caudally located retroperitoneal lymph nodes, although feline and small dog laparoscopy in general is feasible using smaller ports and instruments. The effect of lymph node size in patient selection remains to be elucidated. Similar to laparoscopic adrenalectomy dissections, there is likely to be an upper limit of size of the lymph node itself for feasible manipulation and dissection. Patients with lymph nodes that exhibit characteristics of retroperitoneal or vascular invasion are not good candidates for a laparoscopic technique. Individual patient comorbidities, such as the presence of a coagulopathy, are contraindications to a minimally invasive technique because visualization or hemostasis may be compromised.

Patient Preparation

Surgical Preparation

A wide clip and standard aseptic preparation encompassing the entirety of the lateral abdomen is recommended. For removal of retroperitoneal lymph nodes, hair is clipped from dorsal midline to ventral midline and from the caudal ribcage to the cranial aspect of the thigh, including the craniomedial aspect of the thigh, so that when the patient is positioned, the entire area may be draped in and anatomic landmarks, especially the wing of the ilium, may be palpated. If desired, preoperative bladder expression or placement of a urinary catheter to drain the bladder of urine to increase the working space in the caudal abdomen can be performed, but the author has not found this to be a requirement for this procedure. For removal of abdominal lymph nodes, the patient should be clipped and aseptically prepared for a ventral midline laparoscopic approach.

Operating Room Setup And Patient Positioning

For removal of abdominal lymph nodes in lateral recumbency, the patient and laparoscopic tower should be positioned in the operating room (OR) according to the diagram in Figure 26-2. For removal of retroperitoneal lymph nodes in sternal recumbency the OR layout is shown in Figure 26-3. A laparoscopic approach to extirpation of the medial iliac lymph node has been described in normal colony dogs.[27] A similar laparoscopic approach to the medial iliac lymph nodes performed with the dog in sternal recumbency has also been evaluated in a cohort of young research colony dogs in which, despite attempts to approach the medial iliac lymph nodes from a variety of body positions (lateral, sternal, and dorsal recumbency), it was found that in this cohort the normal-sized medial iliac lymph nodes could not be consistently identified with the dogs in dorsal recumbency even when optical dyes were

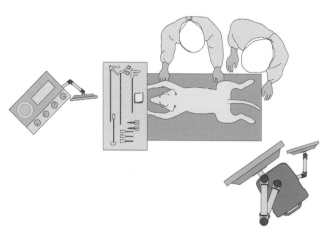

Figure 26-3 Operating room (OR) setup for dissection of the right-sided nodes in sternal recumbency. If the left-sided nodes were to be approached, the OR layout would be similar but with the surgeons and the tower on the opposite sides.

used for indirect lymphography.[48] However, the medial iliac lymph nodes were easily and consistently identified when the dogs were positioned in either lateral or sternal recumbency.[48] As a result, to ensure consistent identification, a laparoscopic approach in lateral or sternal recumbency is recommended.

Lateral Recumbency

If a tilt table is available, the patient should be placed in directly lateral (0 degrees) recumbency. If a tilt table is not available, the patient may be positioned rotated from lateral by 0 to 15 degrees (using towels or sandbags) according to the preference of the surgeon. This procedure is best facilitated if the patient is positioned close to the edge of the surgeon's side of the table. The hindlimbs should be retracted caudally, especially the ipsilateral hindlimb, which should be pulled as far caudal as possible. If it is difficult to fully retract the hip of the ipsilateral hind limb, caudal retraction combined with some external rotation of the leg may improve access to the caudal abdomen for placement of the caudal instrument port.

Sternal Recumbency

The patient should be positioned in the center of the table if a bilateral approach to the iliosacral lymphatic center is elected or may be more lateralized toward the surgeon if a unilateral approach is preferred. The sternum may be supported with towels or sandbags. Rolled-up towels should be placed under the pubis, sufficient to support the pelvis and allow for minimal to no pressure on the abdomen itself. The hindlimbs should be in a relaxed position that mimics a standing position to moderately caudally retracted.

Portal Position and Creation of Working Space

In the previously reported studies in normal colony dogs,[27,48] three 5-mm laparoscopic ports provided adequate access and allowed introduction of appropriate grasping and dissecting laparoscopic instruments for this procedure. However, if desired by the operating surgeon, 10-mm laparoscopic ports may be used. Threaded cannulae are preferred by the author to minimize inadvertent cannula withdrawal during instrument exchanges. Telescope port placement may be performed either using the Hasson technique or with a Veress needle (VN). If a VN is elected, the abdominal wall should be tented well above any underlying abdominal viscera, and care should be exercised in placement. Alternatively, a technique of

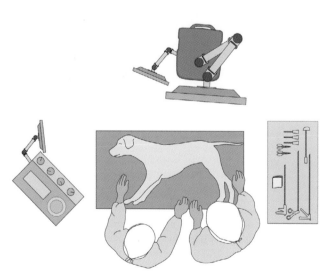

Figure 26-2 Operating room setup for left-sided lymph node dissection in lateral recumbency. If the right-sided nodes were to be approached, the dog would be positioned in a similar fashion but with the right side up.

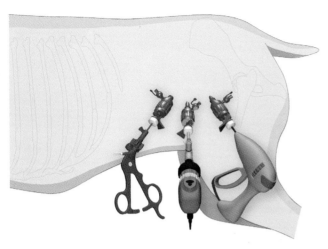

Figure 26-4 Port placement for dissection of the left-sided iliosacral lymphatic center in lateral recumbency. The ports would be placed in a similar location on the right side for dissection of right-sided nodes.

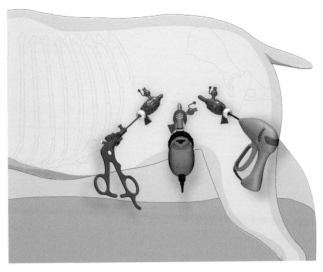

Figure 26-5 Port placement for dissection of the left-sided iliosacral lymphatic center in sternal recumbency. The right-sided nodes could be similarly approached through right-sided ports.

intercostal VN placement has been described that may be used to achieve CO_2 insufflation before port placement.[49]

If the surgeon has elected to perform the procedure with the patient in lateral recumbency, the cannulae should be placed as shown in Figure 26-4. The most important landmark in port placement in a craniocaudal direction is to palpate the cranial edge of the ilial wing and to place the central telescope port directly ventral to very slightly cranial to this landmark. In a dorsoventral plane, the surgeon should be aiming for telescope port placement at the mid-abdominal cavity level (not including the space occupied by the spine and retroperitoneum but rather the peritoneal cavity itself). If the port is too high, dissection will be very challenging; if the port is too low, visualization may be compromised. After the initial port is placed, the laparoscope may be introduced, and the subsequent two instrument ports may be placed under direct visualization according to what positions will allow the most straightforward triangulation to the region of the deep circumflex iliac vessels and the medial iliac lymph node. In practice, this usually means that one port is placed cranial to the camera port and one port is placed caudally. These ports may be at the same dorsoventral position as the central telescope port to slightly more dorsal in position.

In female dogs, the broad ligament may be visualized as a translucent to opaque sheet of tissue that is immediately encountered upon introducing the laparoscope. To proceed with visualization of the medial iliac lymph node, fenestration of the broad ligament is necessary. In general, the abdominal viscera does not impede visualization or dissection with the patient in either lateral or sternal recumbency. The testicular vessels in male dogs and the ureters in both sexes do pass very close to the region of the medial iliac lymph nodes. Usually, with disruption of the peritoneum and gentle manipulation, these structures will fall out of the way sufficiently to allow safe dissection, although the operating surgeon should remain attuned to their position.

If the surgeon has elected to perform the procedure with the patient in sternal recumbency, the port should be placed as shown in Figure 26-5. The approach is similar, but because the patient is rotated 90 degrees toward the operator, the port positions should be very slightly more ventral in the dorsoventral plane to avoid shoulder fatigue.

Surgical Technique
Surgical instrumentation required for laparoscopic lymph node sampling is summarized in Box 26-1.

Abdominal Lymph Node Excisional Biopsy
Completely intracorporeal laparoscopic biopsy of the various abdominal lymph nodes has not yet been reported in the veterinary literature, although in theory, there is no reason that it should not be possible. Laparoscopic-assisted diagnostic biopsy of the mesenteric lymph nodes by exteriorizing the small bowel through a wound retractor[50] is done commonly as part of an abdominal exploration procedure and could be done for minimally invasive staging as indicated. Wound retractor placement would need to be considered based on the lymph node(s) being targeted. A single case each of laparoscopic-assisted biopsy of the medial iliac and ileocolic lymph nodes has been reported, but specific approach dissection details for these cases was not provided.[51]

Medial Iliac Lymph Node Excisional Biopsy
After placement of the initial ports, CO_2 pneumoperitoneum should be maintained at approximately 10 mm Hg. Laparoscopic Babcock forceps, laparoscopic Kelly forceps, and/or laparoscopic right-angled forceps may be used for manipulation and dissection of the retroperitoneal tissue according to the surgeon's preference.

Box 26-1 Instrumentation for Laparoscopic Lymph Note Biopsy or Resection

Instruments Required
30-degree 5 or 10 mm telescope
Laparoscopic Babcock or Kelley grasping forceps
Laparoscopic right-angled dissecting forceps
Specimen retrieval device

Instruments That May Facilitate the Procedure
Monopolar electrosurgical j- or l-hook probe
Vessel-sealing device (LigaSure or Harmonic scalpel)
Suction (with or without irrigation)
Laparoscopic clips

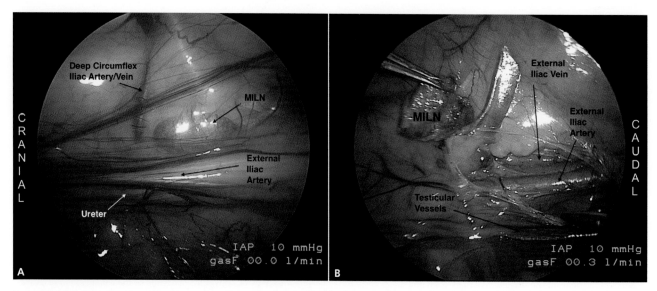

Figure 26-6 Intraoperative image showing predissection regional anatomy with a laparoscopic approach to the left medial iliac lymph node. (Source: Steffey et al. [48]. Reproduced with permission from Wiley.)

Regional anatomy for left-sided and right-sided approaches is shown in Figures 26-6 and 26-7. The peritoneum caudal to the deep circumflex iliac artery and vein and dorsal to the external iliac artery and vein may be incised in a craniocaudal direction. A relatively longer length of disruption of the peritoneum will allow regional structures such as the ureters to more easily fall ventrally away from the area of dissection and improve the safe working space. Attachments of the lymph node to the surrounding retroperitoneum may be disrupted by a combination of blunt and sharp dissection. Use of a monopolar electrosurgical j- or l-hook or vessel-sealing device to provide preemptive hemostasis when sectioning the many small capsular arterioles and venules is very helpful in maintaining appropriate visibility. Laparoscopic clips may also be used as needed for hemostasis, but larger clips may impede dissection. Lymph nodes

should be gently elevated away from the major iliac vessels and the dissection plane safely continued between the lymph node and iliac vessels and circumferentially around the lymph node until it can be extirpated from the retroperitoneal fat. During right-sided approaches, the ventromedial aspect of the medial iliac lymph node will be more closely, although loosely attached, to the right external iliac vein, and during left-sided approaches, the ventromedial aspect of the node will have a closer relationship to the left external iliac artery. Perinodal fat should be grasped with instruments for manipulation of the lymph node whenever possible, rather than directly grasping the node, to minimize crushing of the lymph node parenchyma. Progression of dissection generally varies, but if possible, maintaining the more dorsal retroperitoneal attachments for the majority of dissection, and sectioning them at the end will aid

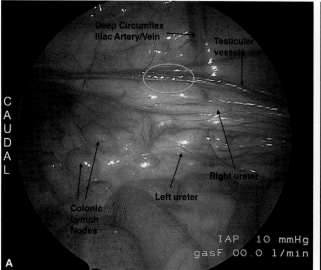
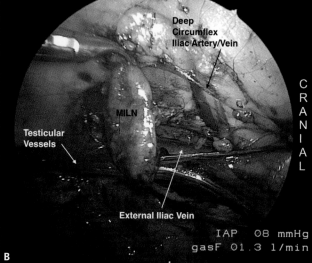

Figure 26-7 Intraoperative image showing predissection regional anatomy with a laparoscopic approach to the right medial iliac lymph node. (Source: Steffey et al. [48]. Reproduced with permission from Wiley.)

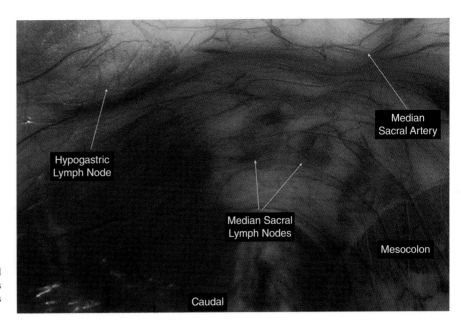

Hypogastric
Lymph Node

Median
Sacral Artery

Median Sacral
Lymph Nodes

Mesocolon

Caudal

Figure 26-8 A view of one hypogastric and two sacral lymph nodes. The endoscope has been introduced through abdominal ports and is viewing caudally into the pelvic canal.

in supporting the lymph node and minimize the amount of direct grasping needed to manipulate the lymph node during dissection. After it has been dissected free from all attachments, protected specimen retrieval should be performed; the exact method should be chosen according to lesion size and surgeon preference. This portion of the procedure is essentially the same, whether the patient is in lateral or sternal recumbency.

When dissection is straightforward, time of laparoscopic medial iliac lymph node removal can be relatively swift. In the laparoscopic removal of medial iliac lymph nodes in normal research colony dogs in lateral recumbency, median dissection times of 13 minutes were reported.[48] These reported dissection times did not include time for port placement and insufflation but did compare favorably with those reported for a cohort of human patients undergoing laparoscopic paraaortic lymphadenectomy for staging of gynecologic cancer in which the mean operative time was 36 minutes for right-sided paraaortic lymphatic basin dissection and 24 minutes for left-sided paraaortic lymphatic basin dissection.[52]

Hypogastric Lymph Node Excisional Biopsy

Extirpation of the hypogastric lymph node(s) can be done through similar port positions as for a medial iliac lymph node removal. The hypogastric lymph nodes tend to be located deeper and more dorsal in the retroperitoneal fat than the medial iliac lymph nodes and when small may be quite difficult to identify. The author has successfully laparoscopically removed hypogastric lymph node(s) in dogs in both lateral and sternal body positions, with and without the use of optical vital dyes.[27,48] With the dog in sternal recumbency, it is necessary to elevate the patient sufficiently away from the table to avoid impeding dissection with long laparoscopic instruments. The hypogastric lymph nodes are most easily accessed from a laparoscopic approach by identification of the medial iliac lymph node ipsilateral to the approach and continuing the retroperitoneal dissection caudally and slightly medially in the plane dorsal to the abdominal aorta and vena cava until the bifurcation of the internal iliac vessels is identified. The hypogastric lymph node will generally be found at this location, sitting in the angle of the bifurcating internal iliac vessels. At this time, there is no literature

documenting attempts at laparoscopic retrieval of the hypogastric lymph nodes in clinical patients, although anecdotally, the author and colleagues have successfully removed both ipsilateral and contralateral hypogastric lymph nodes from patients in lateral recumbency through a single unilateral laparoscopic approach.

Sacral Lymph Nodes

At this time, there is no literature documenting attempts at laparoscopic retrieval of the sacral lymph nodes in dogs, although theoretically this may be possible. The peritoneal reflection occurs very caudally in dogs, allowing for minimally invasive inspection of the pelvic canal with a laparoscope through abdominally placed ports (Figure 26-8). The author has laparoscopically visualized sacral lymph nodes in normal dogs in both lateral (Figure 26-9A) and sternal (Figure 26-9B) body positions, with and without the use of optical vital dyes.[27,48] Lateral recumbency tends to result in collapse of the mesocolon because gravity and in some cases results in increased difficulty in visualizing the median sacral lymph nodes. Laparoscopic removal of the sacral lymph nodes may be possible, but the working space is very tight because of the bony anatomy of the canine pelvis (unlike humans, who have more open pelvic canals). Although use of the port positions as described for medial iliac lymph node retrieval may allow the intrapelvic lymph nodes to be visualized from this approach, the position of the ports optimized to triangulate around the medial iliac lymph node does not allow intrapelvic dissection because of the length and angle of approach of the surgical instruments within the narrow pelvic canal and an essentially 90-degree change in orientation. Although visualization of the lateral sacral and dorsal sacral lymph nodes with the angled telescope is possible, depending on the amount of intrapelvic fat, dissection possibilities from these approaches using standard laparoscopic instrumentation will be limited because of interference between the long instruments and the chest and abdominal wall. If laparoscopic removal of these lymph nodes is to be achieved, it will likely need to be done in sternal recumbency, with the use of specialized articulated instruments for dissection. Additionally, port position as described for the medial iliac lymph nodes will need to be altered (rotation of port position approximately 90 degrees).

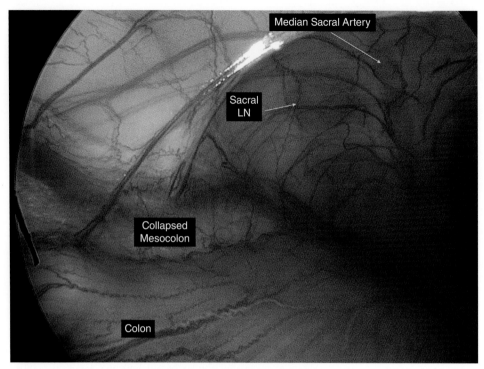

A

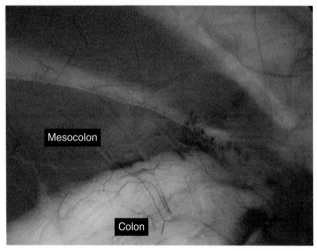

B

Figure 26-9 View of sacral lymph nodes in lateral (**A**) and sternal (**B**) recumbency. Note the collapse of the mesocolon in A compared with B.

Intraoperative Lymphography

Intraoperative lymphography can be very helpful in characterizing which lymph node(s) is or are sentinel for a given tumor. Alternatively, if the desired lymph node to be extirpated is already known based on abnormalities identified on preoperative imaging, intraoperative dyes can be helpful in the operative localization, especially in patients with more intraabdominal fat. The lymphography tracer chosen should be injected peritumorally in a four-quadrant technique in the subcutaneous or intradermal tissue adjacent to the tumor. In veterinary patients, the following vital dyes have been demonstrated experimentally to identify SLNs in dogs: methylene blue (0.1 mL of 5 mg/mL methylene blue injected into each of four quadrants; American Regent Corp., Shirley, NY),[13] patent blue violet (0.5 mL total volume

patent blue violet 2.5%; Fisher Scientific Corp., Fairlawn, NJ),[16,17] and fluorescein disodium (0.5 mL total volume fluorescein 2%; Fischer Scientific Corp).[17] Anecdotally, the author has successfully used both methylene blue under standard white light illumination (Figure 26-10) and the near-infrared fluorescence qualities of indocyanine green (2.5 mg/mL, Akorn, Decatur, IL) (Figure 26-11) for intraoperative lymphatic mapping in the abdomen. Studies in human patients with breast cancer have suggested that the optimal dose for fluorescence SLN mapping with indocyanine green is 0.62 mg (1.6 mL of 0.5-mM solution) injected peritumorally in a four-quadrant technique.[53] Lymphatic uptake is very quick, and highlighting of the SLN(s) with dye will usually occur within a few minutes. If lymphatic uptake is slow, massage of the area of injection may be useful.

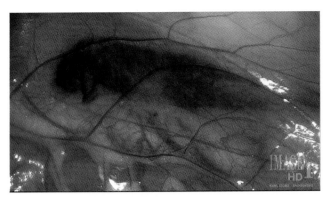

Figure 26-10 Intraoperative indirect lymphography with methylene blue highlights this medial iliac lymph node.

Complications and Challenges

The regional anatomy is complex, and it is necessary for the surgeon to have a good concept of the three-dimensional relationship of the lymph nodes, iliac blood vessels, and other regional structures for laparoscopic lymphadenectomy. Preoperative CT imaging is not required for this procedure but provides a great deal of helpful information regarding lymph node size and position relative to other anatomic structures that can be useful if localization and dissection is difficult. Identification and dissection in older, obese clinical patients is likely to be more challenging and intraoperative lymphography may aid in operative localization of the desired lymph nodes. Iatrogenic trauma to regional structures (e.g., the ureters, iliac vessels, testicular vessels in intact males, uterus in intact females, spleen, bowel, bladder) must be avoided. In particular, both the ipsilateral and contralateral ureter lie in close proximity to the area of dissection for medial iliac lymph nodes and are at risk for iatrogenic surgical trauma. The operating surgeon should remain attuned to their location, but with careful identification and disruption of the peritoneum, they may be reflected ventrally to allow safer dissection of the medial iliac lymph node. The broad ligament present in intact females appears as a sheet of tissue that is immediately visualized upon entry into the abdomen, and it must be fenestrated to perform any visual inspection or dissection of the region of the iliosacral lymphatic center.

A clinical limitation of the lateral and sternal approaches to the medial iliac lymph node is that the contralateral medial iliac lymph node cannot be visualized or excised from the same surgical approach. In the case of the lateral approach, patient repositioning would be required to extirpate both medial iliac lymph nodes. Positioning in sternal recumbency to allow bilateral approaches to these lymph nodes could mitigate this problem. Ports would need to be repositioned on the opposite side of the abdomen after removal of the first lymph node, but time spent repositioning the patient would be saved.

Intraoperative hemorrhage from the retroperitoneal tissue can be a real limitation to safe and expedient removal of the lymph nodes of the iliosacral lymphatic center. Minor hemorrhage from small capsular vessels and vasculature of the retroperitoneal fat during dissection is generally not life threatening but can compromise visibility and increase the risk of injury to other important regional structures, so hemostatic instrumentation (e.g., a vessel sealer or a monopolar electrosurgical hook probe) aids significantly in dissection. In a human study of laparoscopic lymphadenectomy, major vessels were injured during dissection in 7 of 150 patients, of which 4 patients required conversion to laparotomy.[53] No major operative complications were observed in the previously reported experimental cohorts of young, normal dogs,[27,48] but unexpected or unanticipated complications are possible, and the operating surgeon should be prepared to convert to an open technique rather than compromise patient safety. This may be accomplished either by appropriately draping the patient to allow rapid repositioning and conversion to a ventral midline celiotomy or by conversion via a flank laparotomy over the area of the medial iliac lymph node. If a flank laparotomy is elected to convert to an open procedure, care to avoid more superficial branches of the deep circumflex iliac vessels during the approach should be taken.

In general, it can be very difficult to completely avoid direct manipulation of abdominal and retroperitoneal lymph nodes during dissection, but care in handling the lymph nodes is important to prevent capsular tearing during dissection that might lead to regional seeding. The perinodal retroperitoneal or serosal tissue is loose and disrupts easily, but because of the small size of the lymph nodes and their position relative to nearby structures (e.g., the external iliac vessels in the case of medial iliac lymph node dissection, where there is nothing medially to safely push against), at some point in the procedure, some grasping of the lymph node directly becomes required for retraction and dissection. Care must be taken not to crush the tissue in the attempts to

Figure 26-11 Excised hypogastric lymph node from a dog with anal sac gland adenocarcinoma. Indocyanine green was injected peritumorally, and intraoperative near-infrared lymphography identified the hypogastric lymph node as the sentinel lymph node. The lymph node is viewed under standard white light (**A**) and a combination of white light and near-infrared fluorescence (**B**) demonstrating the tracer uptake into the lymph node.

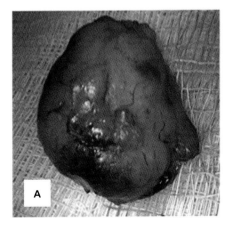
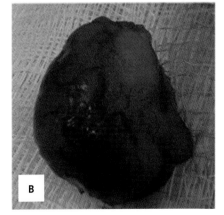

sample it. When histologic artifact of medial iliac lymph nodes that were removed minimally invasively was assessed, the proportion of lymph node cut surface area affected by artifact was generally small.[27] Although this is promising, because the goal of SLN biopsy is to identify low volume micrometastatic disease if present, even minor crush artifact could be clinically important, and care should be taken by the laparoscopic surgeon to minimize handling of the medial iliac lymph node. Protected specimen retrieval must be used to minimize the risk of port site metastasis. Alternative to commercial specimen retrieval bags, use of the finger of a sterile surgical glove allows protected specimen removal of small specimens. In humans, relatively high incidences of port site metastasis (up to 21%) occurring in early reports were probably attributable to inexperience, flaws in technique (excessive tissue manipulation, unprotected specimen extraction), and poor instrumentation.[54] With appropriate oncologic technique, it appears that port site or incisional recurrences are not statistically different between laparoscopic and open groups, both showing approximately 1% occurrence.[54]

To date, the author has only applied these techniques to patients with normal to mildly enlarged medial iliac and hypogastric lymph nodes. Dissections in patients with overt lymphadenopathy are likely to be significantly more challenging because of greater difficulty in visualization of the regional vascular anatomy and ureters in close proximity to the mass effect of the enlarged lymph nodes. Additionally, there is likely to be increased relative difficulty in retraction of grossly enlarged retroperitoneal lymph nodes against the immobile bony anatomy of the spine. Grossly enlarged lymph nodes may be more likely to exhibit characteristics of vascular or retroperitoneal invasion, and at this time, an open approach is recommended for removal of very large lymph nodes and those that exhibit invasive behavior. Use of advanced imaging to assess for local invasion and relative position of nearby structures and careful case selection are needed in extrapolating this technique to clinical patients with grossly enlarged lymph nodes of the iliosacral lymphatic center. Further study is needed to better define the limits of application of this technique to patients with overt lymphadenomegaly.

Postoperative Care

Patient recoveries are usually monitored overnight after laparoscopic lymphadenectomy, with injectable opioid anesthesia provided according to the patient's needs and with discharge from the hospital the following day. If operative procedures and anesthetic recoveries have been uncomplicated and if appropriate analgesia can be provided at home, there is no reason specific to the lymphadenectomy procedure that patients could not be discharged the same day if desired. However, because this procedure may be performed in combination with other surgical procedures that are not minimally invasive (e.g., perineal tumor removal), monitoring and therapeutic needs for these procedures will more likely dictate hospitalization time, analgesic requirements and other treatment recommendations.

References

1 Devitt, C.M., Cox, R.E., Hailey, J.J. (2005) Duration, complications, stress and pain of open ovariohysterectomy versus a simple method of laparoscopic- assisted ovariohysterectomy in dogs. J Am Vet Med Assoc 227, 921-927.

2 Culp, W.T.N., Mayhew, P.D., Brown, D.C. (2009) The effect of laparoscopic versus open ovariectomy on postsurgical activity in small dogs. Vet Surg 38, 811-817.

3 West, M.A., Hackam, D.J., Baker, J., et al. (1997) Mechanism of decreased in vitro murine macrophage cytokine release after exposure to carbon dioxide. Ann Surg 226, 179-190.

4 Kapernik, G., Avinoach, E., Grossman, Y., et al. (1998) The effect of high partial pressure of carbon dioxide environment on metabolism of human peritoneal cells. Am J Obstet Gynecol 179, 1503-1510.

5 Allendorf, J.D., Bessler, M., Kayton, M.L., et al. (1995) Increased tumor establishment and growth after laparotomy vs laparoscopy in a murine model. Arch Surg 130, 649-653.

6 Cochran, A.J., Ohsie, S.J., Binder, S.W. (2008) Pathobiology of the sentinel node. Curr Opin Oncol 20, 190-195.

7 Goyal, A., Mansel, R.E. (2008) Recent advances in sentinel lymph node biopsy for breast cancer. Curr Opin Oncol 20, 621-626.

8 Stojadinovic, A., Nissan, A., Protic, M., et al. (2007) Prospective randomized study comparing sentinel lymph node evaluation with standard pathologic evaluation for the staging of colon cancer: results from the United States Military Cancer Institute Clinical Trials Group Study GI-01. Ann Surg 245, 846-857.

9 Giammarile, F., Vidal-Sicart, S., Valdes Olmos, R.A. (2014) Uncommon applications of sentinel lymph node mapping: urogenital cancers. Q J Nucl Med Mol Imaging 58, 161-179.

10 Takeuchi, H., Kitagawa, Y. (2013) Sentinel node navigation surgery in patients with early gastric cancer. Dig Surg 30, 104-111.

11 Langenbach, A., McManus, P.M., Hendrick, M.J., et al. (2001) Sensitivity and specificity of methods of assessing the regional lymph nodes for evidence of metastasis in dogs and cats with solid tumors. J Am Vet Med Assoc 218, 1428.

12 Williams, L.E., Packer, R.A. (2003) Association between lymph node size and metastasis in dogs with malignant melanoma: 100 cases (1987-2001). J Am Vet Med Assoc 222, 1234-1236.

13 Worley, D.R. (2014) Incorporation of sentinel lymph node mapping in dogs with mast cell tumors: 20 consecutive procedures. Vet Comp Oncol 12, 215-226

14 Szczubial, M., Lopuszynski, W. (2011) Prognostic value of regional lymph node status in canine mammary carcinomas. Vet Comp Oncol 9, 296-303.

15 Balogh, L., Thuroczy, J., Androcs, G., et al. (2002) Sentinel lymph node detection in canine oncological patients. Nucl Med Rev Cent East Eur 5, 139-144.

16 Aquino, J.U., Pinheiro, L.G., Vasques, P.H., et al. (2012) Experimental canine model for sentinel lymph node biopsy in the vulva using technetium and patent blue dye. Acta Cir Bras 27, 102-108.

17 Wells, S., Bennett, A., Walsh, P., et al. (2006) Clinical usefulness of intradermal fluorescein and patent blue violet dies for sentinel lymph node identification in dogs. Vet Comp Oncol 4, 114-122.

18 Hobson, H.P., Brown, M.R., Rogers, K.S. (2006) Surgery of metastatic anal sac adenocarcinoma in five dogs. Vet Surg 35, 267-270.

19 Kitagawa, Y., Takeuchi, H., Takagi Y., et al. (2013) Sentinel node mapping for gastric cancer: a prospective multicenter trial in Japan. J Clin Oncol 31, 3704-3710.

20 Saha, S., Dan, A.G., Beutler, T., et al. (2004) Sentinel lymph node mapping technique in colon cancer. Int Semin Surg Oncol 31, 374-381.

21 Braat, A.E., Oosterhuis, J.W.A., Moll, F.C., et al. (2004) Successful sentinel node identification in colon carcinoma using patent blue V. J Canc Surg 30, 633-637.

22 Xiong, L., Engel, H., Gazyakan, E., et al. (2014) Current techniques for lymphatic imaging: state of the art and future perspectives. Eur J Surg Oncol 40, 270-276.

23 Yuasa, Y., Seike, J., Yoshida, T., et al. (2012) Sentinel lymph node biopsy using intraoperative indocyanine green fluorescence imaging navigated with preoperative CT lymphography for superficial esophageal cancer. Ann Surg Oncol 19, 486-493.

24 Guo, W., Zhang, L., Ji, J., et al. (2014) Breast cancer sentinel lymph node mapping using near-infrared guided indocyanine green in comparison with blue dye. Tumor Biol 35, 3073-3078.

25 Jewell, E.L., Huang, J.J., Abu-Rustum, N.R., et al. (2014) Detection of sentinel lymph nodes in minimally invasive surgery using indocyanine green and near-infrared fluorescence imaging for uterine and cervical malignancies. Gynecol Oncol 133, 274-277.

26 Motomura, K., Inaji, H., Komoike Y., et al. (2001) Combination technique is superior to dye alone in identification of the sentinel node in breast cancer patients. J Surg Oncol 76 (2), 95-99.

27 Steffey, M.A., Radlinsky, M.G., Padgett, K., et al. (2014) Operative assessment of pelvic lymphatic drainage and laparoscopic surgical access to the iliosacral lymphatic center of the dog: preliminary results of preclinical studies. Proceedings of the 11th Annual Meeting of the Veterinary Endoscopy Society, Florence, Italy.

28 Rogers, K.S., Barton, C.L., Landis, M. (1993) Canine and feline lymph node: part 1. Compend Contin Educ Pract Vet 15, 397-400.

29 Evans, H.E. (2012) The lymphatic system. In: Evans, H.E., De Lahunta, A. (eds.) Miller's Anatomy of the Dog, 4th edn. Saunders, St. Louis.

30 Parungo, C.P., Soybel, D.I., Colson, Y.L., et al. (2007) Lymphatic drainage of the peritoneal space: a pattern dependent on bowel lymphatics. Ann Surg Oncol 14, 286-298.

31 Buracco, P. (2012) Alimentary tract: colorectal and perianal tumors. In: Kudnig, S.T., Seguin, B. (eds.) Veterinary Surgical Oncology. Wiley-Blackwell, Ames, IA.

32 Poulton, G.A., Brearly, M.J. (2007) Clinical stage, therapy, and prognosis in canine anal sac gland adenocarcinoma. J Vet Intern Med 21, 274-280.

33 Spaulding, K.A. (1997) A review of sonographic identification of abdominal blood vessels and juxtavascular organs. Vet Radiol Ultrasound 38, 4-23.

34 Llabres-Diaz, F.J. (2004) Ultrasonography of the medial iliac lymph nodes in the dog. Vet Radiol Ultrasound 45, 156-165.

35 Mayer, M.N., Lawson, J.A., Silver, T.I. (2010) Sonographic characteristics of presumptively normal canine medial iliac and superficial inguinal lymph nodes. Vet Radiol Ultrasound 51, 638-641.

36 Agthe, P., Caine, A.R., Posch, B., et al. (2009) Ultrasonographic appearance of jejunal lymph nodes in dogs without clinical signs of gastrointestinal disease. Vet Radiol Ultrasound 50, 195-200.

37 Kinns, J., Mai, W. (2007) Association between malignancy and sonographic heterogeneity in canine and feline abdominal lymph nodes. Vet Radiol Ultrasound 48, 565-569.

38 De Swarte, M., Alexander, K., Rannou, B. (2011) Comparison of sonographic features of benign and neoplastic deep lymph nodes in dogs. Vet Radiol Ultrasound 52, 451-456.

39 Tregnaghi, A., De Candia, A., Calderone M., et al. (1997) Ultrasonographic evaluation of superficial lymph node metastasis in melanoma. Eur J Radiol 24, 216-221.

40 Ballegeer, E.A., Adams, W.M., Dubielzig, R.R., et al. (2010) Computed tomography characteristics of canine tracheobronchial lymph node metastasis. Vet Radiol Ultrasound 51, 397-403.

41 Beukers, M., Grosso, F.V., Voorhout, G. (2013) Computed tomographic characteristics of presumed normal canine abdominal lymph nodes. Vet Radiol Ultrasound 54, 610-617.

42 Anderson, C.L., Mackay, C.S., Roberts, G.D., et al. (2013) Comparison of abdominal ultrasound and magnetic resonance imaging for detection of abdominal lymphadenopathy in dogs with metastatic apocrine gland adenocarcinoma. Vet Comp Oncol DOI: 10.1111/vco.12022. (Epub ahead of print)

43 Suga, K., Ogasawara, N., Yuan, Y., et al. (2003) Visualization of breast lymphatic pathways with an indirect computed tomography lymphography using a nonionic monometric contrast medium iopamidol: preliminary results. Invest Radiol 38, 73-84.

44 Suga, K., Yuan, Y., Ueda, K., et al. (2004) Computed tomography lymphography with intrapulmonary injection of iopamidol for sentinel lymph node localization. Invest Radiol 39, 313-324.

45 Motomura, K., Sumino, H., Noguchi, A., et al. (2013) Sentinel nodes identified by computed tomography-lymphography accurately stage the axilla in patients with breast cancer. BMC Medical Imaging 12, 42-48.

46 Notohamiprodjo, M., Weiss, M., Baumeister, R.G. (2012) MR lymphangiography at 3.0T: correlation with lymphoscintigraphy. Radiology 264, 78-87.

47 Barranger, E., Grahek, D., Antoine, M., et al. (2003) Evaluation of fluorodeoxyglucose positron emission tomography in the detection of axillary lymph node metastases in patients with early-stage breast cancer. Ann Surg Oncol 10, 622-627.

48 Steffey, M.A., Daniel, L., Mayhew, P.D., et al. (2014) Laparoscopic extirpation of the medial iliac lymph nodes in normal dogs. Vet Surg Jun 5. doi: 10.1111/j.1532-950X.2014.12207.x. (Epub ahead of print)

49 Fiorbianco, V, Skalicky, M., Doerner, J., et al. (2012) Right intercostal insertion of a Veress needle for laparoscopy in dogs. Vet Surg 41, 367-373.

50 Mayhew, P. (2009) Surgical views: techniques for laparoscopic and laparoscopic assisted biopsy of abdominal organs. Compend Contin Educ Pract Vet 31, 170-176.

51 Case, J.B., Ellison, G. (2013) Single-incision laparoscopic-assisted intestinal surgery (SILAIS) in 7 dogs and 1 cat. Vet Surg 42, 629-634.

52 Possover, M., Krause, N., Plaul, K., et al. (1998) Laparoscopic para-aortic and pelvic lymphadenectomy: experience with 150 patients and review of the literature. Gynecol Oncol 71, 19-28.

53 Verbeek, F.P.R., Troyan, S.L., Mieog, J.S.D., et al. (2014) Near infrared fluorescence sentinel lymph node mapping in breast cancer: a multi-center experience. Breast Cancer Res Treat 143, 333-342.

54 Are, C., Talamini, M.A. (2005) Laparoscopy and malignancy. J Laparoendosc Adv Surg Tech 15, 38-47.

27 Diaphragmatic and Inguinal Herniorrhaphy

Eric Monnet and Boel A. Fransson

Key Points

- Minimally invasive surgery (MIS) is used in acute and relatively cardiopulmonary stable cases of diaphragmatic hernia.
- Diaphragmatic herniorrhaphy is accomplished by low-pressure pneumoperitoneum (3 mm Hg).
- The spleen is challenging to reduce by an MIS technique.
- Barbed suture is very advantageous in diaphragmatic and inguinal herniorrhaphy.
- For small inguinal hernias, a simple laparoscopy-assisted technique can be used.

Preoperative Considerations

Anatomy and Physiology of the Diaphragm

The diaphragm is a musculotendinous plate separating the thoracic from the abdominal cavity. The triangular central tendon occupies approximately 21% of the diaphragm and is surrounded completely by the muscular parts on all sides (Figure 27-1). Through it, the caval foramen transmits the caudal vena cava.

The muscular diaphragm consists of the lumbar and the costal parts. The costal part has a 40% greater cross-sectional area and exerts 60% more force than the crural parts.[1] Both show a mixed population of slow- and fast-twitch fibers allowing for continuous cycles of activity and an ability to respond to intermittent high ventilatory loads. The crura close to the esophageal hiatus show high density of slow-twitch fibers, which are associated with a sphincter function.[2] In cats, the lower esophageal sphincter and the crural diaphragm are anatomically superimposed.[3]

The lumbar part of the diaphragm is formed by the right and left crura (Figure 27-2) between which the aortic hiatus is enclosing the aorta, the azygos and hemiazygos veins, and the thoracic duct. In dogs, the right crus is larger than the left. The thick (5–6 mm) medial aspect of the right lumbar crus is surrounding the esophageal hiatus, which transmits the two vagal nerve trunks together with esophagus and its vessels.

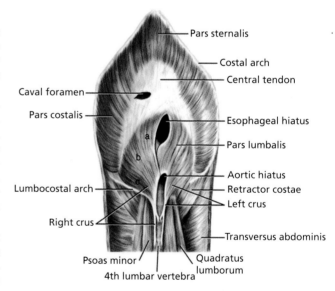

Figure 27-1 Diaphragm, abdominal surface. a, medial; b, intermediate; c, lateral portions of pars lumbalis. (Source: Hermanson [4]. Reproduced with permission from Elsevier.)

Small Animal Laparoscopy and Thoracoscopy, First Edition. Edited by Boel A. Fransson and Philipp D. Mayhew.

© 2015 by ACVS Foundation. Published 2015 by John Wiley & Sons, Inc.

Companion website: www.wiley.com/go/fransson/laparoscopy

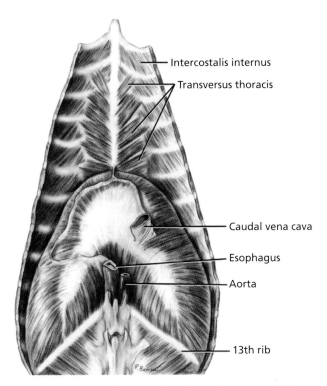

Figure 27-2 Diaphragm, thoracic surface. (Source: Hermanson [4]. Reproduced with permission from Elsevier.)

The costal part consists of muscle fibers radiating from the costal wall to the central tendon. The muscle arises from the medial proximal part of the 13th rib, the distal 12th rib, and the costochondral junction of the 11th rib, as well as from the entire length of the 9th and 10th ribs.

The diaphragm is innervated by the phrenic nerves, arising from the fifth through seventh cervical nerves. The right branch reaches the muscle within the plica vena cava. The left phrenic nerve lies in its own fold in the ventral mediastinum. The phrenico-pericardial ligament attaches to the diaphragm near the midline.[4] This arrangement contrasts to humans, in whom the pericardial sac itself attaches to the diaphragm, enabling traumatically acquired peritoneopericardial hernias, which are not seen in small animals.

The diaphragm protrudes as a cupola into the chest cavity. The active muscle contraction flattens the cupola, leading to inspiration of lungs. It is considered the prime mover of tidal air,[3] and both muscular parts contract during respiration. However, the diaphragm also has important functions associated with swallowing and emesis. In swallowing, the esophageal distension leads to reflex relaxation of crural diaphragm, allowing the bolus to pass. In vomiting, the diaphragm first contracts strongly as a single muscle during retching. During expulsion, the crura relaxes by central non-vagal mechanisms while the costal diaphragm remains contracted.[3] It has been suggested that the crural contraction during inspiration may be due less to respiration but more to increase the pressure on the esophagus, thus minimizing reflux.[3]

Congenital Diaphragmatic Hernia

Peritoneal-pericardial diaphragmatic hernia (PPDH) is a common congenital anomaly in dogs and cats. Cats are more often affected than dogs, with prevalences in one study of 0.062% and 0.015% in cats and dogs, respectively.[5] Of small animal diaphragmatic hernias (DHs), PPDH constitutes around 15%.[6] Weimaraners and domestic long hair cats have been overrepresented.[5,7] The direct underlying developmental abnormality has not been determined.

Surgical herniorrhaphy of PPDH has mainly consisted in primary closure of the defect.[5,7] In one dog with partial agenesis of the diaphragm, reconstruction using the pericardium was performed.[5]

Adhesions between herniated organs to the pericardium and heart have been noted in 19 of 83 (23%) of cats,[5,7,8] but in none of 27 dogs in two studies.[5,7] However, adhesions may occur in dogs as well. When present, dissection of adhesions may add significantly to surgical morbidity.[7] Chest tubes may not be routinely indicated after PPD herniorrhaphy, but if the pleural cavity has been entered because of adhesion dissection, their use has been recommended.[5,7]

The perioperative mortality rate has ranged between 5.1% and 14%,[5,7,8] with lower fractions in more recent studies. In conservative management of primarily nonclinical disease, 16 of 24 (67%) died during the study period,[5] all from reasons supposedly unrelated to PPDH. Two animals with clinical signs of PPDH, in which the owners declined surgery, survived the study period with no clinical signs at the end of the study.[5]

Minimally invasive herniorrhaphy has not yet been reported in PPDH but is likely to be in the future, similar to that in traumatic DH. If adhesions or diaphragmatic agenesis is encountered, conversion to open surgery may be indicated.

Acquired Diaphragmatic Hernia

The vast majority of DHs in dogs and cats, between 77% and 85%, are of traumatic origin.[6] Vehicular trauma has been noted as the most common underlying reason.[6,9] Dyspnea was seen in a majority of cats (72%) at time of admission, but in dogs, only 41% showed dyspnea, and gastrointestinal signs were often seen.[9] Importantly, 30% to 40% of animals also sustained other soft tissue traumatic injury,[9] and surgical treatment needs to include careful assessment in order to not overlook concurrent trauma.

Radiographic evaluation is commonly diagnostic for DH (Figures 27-3 and 27-4), and pleural effusion may be indicative of a

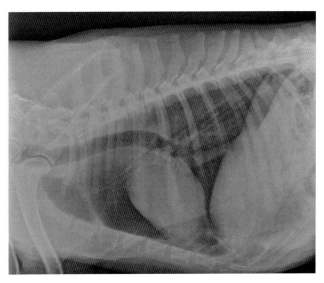

Figure 27-3 Thoracic radiograph of a 4 year-old German shepherd hit by a car 5 hours earlier. Right lateral recumbency. The chest cavity did not show obvious signs of trauma.

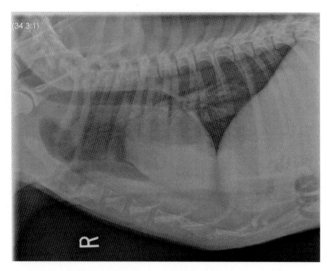

Figure 27-4 Thoracic radiograph in right lateral recumbency of the same dog in Figure 27-3 48 hours later. A large soft tissue opacity, containing a marginated structure, is present in the left caudal thorax. A 7-cm left ventral radial diaphragmatic tear was found during surgery, and the hernia was containing spleen and omentum.

more extensive rupture.[10] Ultrasonography was accurate in diagnosing DH in 93% of cases.[11] The most commonly herniated organs include the liver, stomach, and small intestines.[6,10] The large intestine and spleen were shown to be herniated less frequently, in 12% to 38% of cases.[6,10] Assessment of a patient before minimally invasive herniorrhaphy may benefit from computed tomography (CT) to better outline the extent of the DH and concurrent soft tissue trauma before surgery (Figure 27-5). Animals with extensive traumatic injury may be less ideal candidates for minimally invasive surgery (MIS).

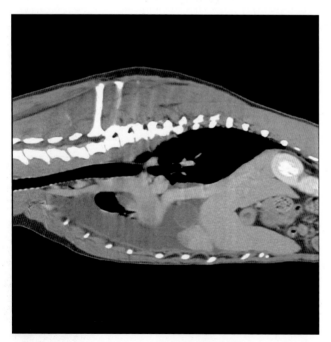

Figure 27-5 Sagittal plane of contrast-enhanced computed tomography image of a 3-year-old German shorthair pointer with a 4-week history of pleural effusion. The gallbladder and right liver lobe are herniated into the thoracic cavity through a 4-cm right ventral diaphragmatic defect.

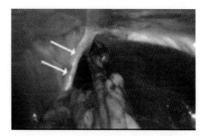

Figure 27-6 The fibrous tissue forming in the chronic diaphragmatic hernia defect (white arrows) will lead to stricture and narrowing, which makes laparoscopic reduction of organs more challenging.

Diaphragmatic hernias frequently occur in the costal muscles and less often in the central tendon; the crural muscles are seldom ruptured.[6] Orientation of tears of the pars costalis in surgery are 40% radial, 40% circumferential, and 20% a combination of the two.[12] Adhesions are rare and have not been seen in acute acquired DH.[12]

The mean survival rate for dogs and cats undergoing open surgical repair has varied between 79% to 89% in the past 2 decades.[9,13] Historically, survival rates were reported as low as 56%.[12] Older studies considered survival rates being dependent on the timing of surgical intervention after trauma, with early surgery (within 24 hours) leading to a poor outcome.[14,15] However, with improvements in critical care, the timing of surgery is no longer a critical factor.[9] Chronic DH, defined as DH lasting longer than 2 weeks, was historically considered more challenging than acute DH, but more recent studies showed a 79% resolution rate with surgical treatment.[13]

Indication and Case Selection for Minimally Invasive Herniorrhaphy

Successful DH repair by MIS has been completed in cases with acute hernias. In these, fibrous tissue was not present on the edges of the hernia, and debridement was not necessary. Also, with a recent trauma, the hernia port has not started to heal and to stricture, compressing the herniated organs and compromising attempts at reduction (Figure 27-6).

The spleen seems to be the most difficult organ to reduce with MIS technique because it is difficult to grasp without inducing severe hemorrhage from the parenchyma. Liver lobes can also represent a challenge, but they can usually be reduced with minimal blunt manipulation. A dual, thoracoscopic and laparoscopic, approach may be advantageous for hernia reduction. Organs can be pushed from the thoracic cavity while simultaneously traction is applied from the abdominal cavity. The stomach and loops of intestine are easily reduced during the procedure.

It is not possible to decide from any imaging modality which hernia will be reducible or repairable with laparoscopy. It is necessary to explore each case with laparoscopy to be able to make a decision on the possibility of MIS herniorrhaphy. If the reduction or the repair is too difficult, the laparoscopy will have to be converted to an open approach. Large hernias are difficult to close with laparoscopy because of the amount of tension on a conventional suture. The knotless sutures with unidirectional barbs have helped tremendously in the repair of DH.

Surgical Technique: Diaphragmatic Herniorrhaphy

Dogs are placed in dorsal recumbency in a reverse Trendelenburg position for gravitational help in reduction of the hernia. Similar to any DH repair, the patient is placed on a ventilator during the

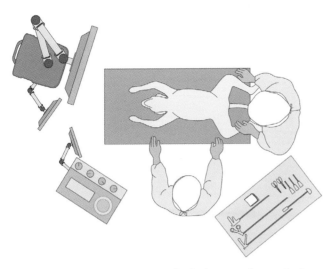

Figure 27-7 The operating room setup for diaphragmatic herniorrhaphy.

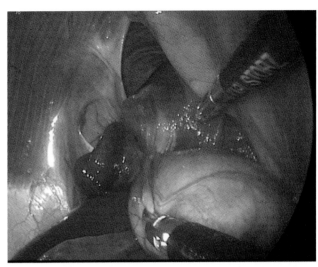

Figure 27-9 Fine-toothed, atraumatic, grasping forceps is used to apply traction to reduce loops of the intestine and the gallbladder when herniated.

procedure (Figure 27-7). DH repair is a three-cannula procedure (Figure 27-8). A fourth cannula can be used to help the reduction of the hernia. A midline approach caudal to the umbilicus is used for placement of the telescope cannula. One other cannula can be placed on the midline cranial to the umbilicus. Other cannulas are placed on either side of midline for triangulation and to facilitate suturing. Because the diaphragm is opened, a capnoperitoneum of more than 3 mm Hg may severely compromise pulmonary compliance and venous return. Fortunately, the ribs help to support the cranial abdomen and create a sufficient work space.

After placement of the cannulas, the herniated organs are reduced. Traction and lifting of the organ are used to get the organs over the dorsal ridge of the hernia into the abdominal cavity. Fine-toothed grasping forceps is used to pull on loops of the intestine and the gallbladder when herniated (Figure 27-9). Liver lobes and the spleen are better manipulated with blunt palpation probes, and a fan retractor is used to scoop the organs into the abdomen from the thoracic cavity.

Before starting the closure of the hernia, a chest tube is placed in an intercostal space. The placement is visualized with the endoscope across the diaphragm. The DH is then closed. If a ring of fibrous tissue is present, it will need to be resected to improve healing of the diaphragm after closure. An intracorporeal suture technique is used. Staples (Endo Hernia Stapler; Covidien, Mansfield, MA) exist and are designed for closure of hernia but mainly for patch repairs using mesh. These staples can be used as primary repair if limited tension across the hernia allows apposition of the edges of the hernia while the staples are applied. Knotless unidirectional barb sutures facilitate the surgery because the barb sutures maintain the tension on their own (Figure 27-10). Also, the knotless sutures have an Endostitch version (Endostitch, Covidien), making suturing easier. The suture is started at the most dorsal part of the hernia and is continued in a simple continuous fashion toward the most ventral part. If barbed knotless suture is used, the suture line is anchored in the start by placing the suture through the welded loop. The end of the suture line is anchored by two suture bites in opposing direction. Size 2-0 unidirectional barbed suture (VLoc 180, Covidien) has experimentally been showing equal biomechanical strength as

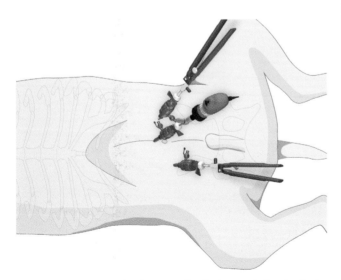

Figure 27-8 Three-cannula placement for diaphragmatic herniorrhaphy. The endoscope cannula and one of the instrument cannulae are placed on ventral midline. The third portal is placed ipsilateral to the hernia location.

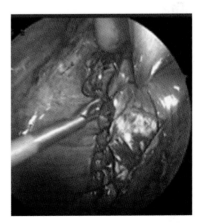

Figure 27-10 After each stitch, barbed suture maintains the edges of the defect in contact without the need for tension applied to the suture strand. This greatly helps in intracorporeal continuous suturing.

conventionally sutured canine diaphragm samples.[16] The surgeon must avoid trauma to the vena cava at the level of the caval foramen.

After closure of the diaphragm, the pleural space is evacuated through the thoracostomy tube. The cannulas are removed, and the cannula defects are closed routinely.

Aftercare

In the postoperative period, the pleural space is evacuated every hour for 4 hours and then every 6 hours. If fluid production has been minimal and if no air has been produced within the first 4 hours after surgery, the thoracostomy tube should be removed.

Analgesia should be administered intravenously and in the pleural space with the thoracostomy tube. This author (EM) has had success with lidocaine and bupivacaine (1.5 mg/kg each) delivered every 6 hours until the tube is removed.

Blood gas analysis is performed every 4 to 6 hours after surgery to make sure the patient is ventilating adequately and that the atelectasis of the lung is resolving. If the patient is hypoxemic with adequate ventilation or hyperventilation, supplemental oxygen should be provided until the lung function improves.

Preoperative Considerations for Inguinal Hernia

Anatomy and Pathophysiology

The superficial inguinal ring in dogs is a slit opening in the aponeurosis formed from the external abdominal oblique muscle. It is located at the level of the femoral triangle just cranial to the iliopubic eminence. The deep inguinal ring is formed by the inguinal ligament laterally and caudally, the caudal border of the internal abdominal oblique muscle cranially, and the lateral border of the rectus abdominis muscle medially.[4]

The caudal inguinal canal transmits the external pudendal vessels and the genitofemoral nerve in both genders. In males, the vessels, muscle, and spermatic cord associated with the descended testicles passes through the inguinal canal.

Congenital inguinal hernia develops more often in male dogs than females. Breed predisposition has mainly included small- and medium-sized breeds.[17,18] In cats, inguinal hernia has been reported infrequently, with both genders equally represented.

Acquired hernias are fairly common in middle-aged female dogs. In one study of dogs with inguinal hernia, 16 of 22 (73%) dogs older than 2 years were female.[19] Systemic clinical signs are unusual unless intestine is strangulated within the hernia. Vomiting for 2 to 6 days was predictive of nonviable strangulated small intestine.[19] A majority (4 of 5; 80%) of the nontraumatic inguinal hernia containing nonviable small intestine were young male dogs. Only one of 19 (5%) female dogs with nontraumatic inguinal hernia had nonviable intestine in the hernia.[19]

Patient Selection and Preparation for Laparoscopic Inguinal Herniorrhaphy

The case selection for laparoscopic herniorrhaphy includes cases with no or minimal systemic clinical signs. Dogs with a history of vehicular trauma or vomiting before diagnosis may best be explored by conventional open surgery. Also, dogs with abdominal effusion or signs of sepsis at time of diagnosis should undergo open surgery. The ideal case for laparoscopic herniorrhaphy is a nontraumatic case with a small to moderate hernia sac, which is easily reducible and does not need to be amputated.

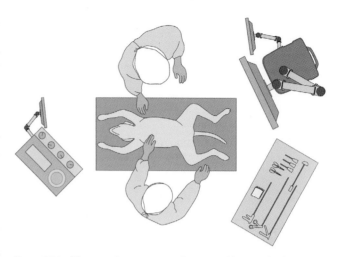

Figure 27-11 The operating room setup for inguinal herniorrhaphy.

Surgical Technique

Laparoscopic Inguinal Herniorrhaphy

The patient is placed in Trendelenburg position, and after laparoscopic access is achieved, the intraabdominal pressure is maintained at 8 to 12 mm Hg. Cannulas are placed triangulated with the surgeon facing caudally (Figure 27-11). For a three-cannula technique in a left-sided hernia, the telescope cannula is placed on midline cranial to the umbilicus or slightly craniolateral to avoid falciform ligament. The right-hand cannula is placed under visualization on the midline, caudal to the umbilicus, but ideally 15 cm cranial to the planned suture site and the left hand cannula in left lateral abdominal wall at a similar level as the right cannula (Figure 27-12). For bilateral herniorrhaphy, cannulas 2 and 3 are placed symmetrically in the left and right body walls. For left-sided hernias, the right-hand instrument cannot be placed parallel to the axis of suture line, which may make needle driving from right to left difficult. The surgeon may need to drive the needle with the left hand instrument or use an automated suture device (VLoc Endostitch).

Laparoscopic repair of inguinal hernia has not yet been reported in a series of dogs or cats. However, laparoscopic suturing with barbed

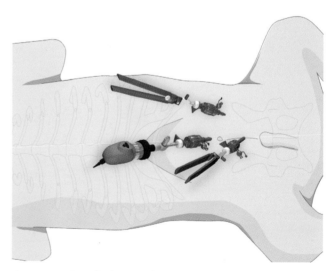

Figure 27-12 Cannula placement for a unilateral (left-sided) hernia. If bilateral, instrument cannulas are spaced symmetrically to the telescope cannula, slightly more cranially, bilaterally in the abdominal wall. For left-sided hernias, the left-hand cannula is best positioned for needle driving.

suture has been reported in a horse,[20] and a similar technique is reasonable in dogs. Single-incision laparoscopic site (SILS) suturing has been reported in people but is considered very challenging because the instruments cross paths because of the proximity of the cannulas. SILS suturing may be more feasible with an automated device.

The hernia is reduced by traction applied with atraumatic grasping forceps and aided by applying external digital pressure on the hernia sac. If the hernia is not easily reducible, it can be enlarged by incising the cranial hernia ring using scissors or electrocautery hook dissector in a craniomedial direction. If intestine is involved in the hernia, it needs to be protected from dissection devices or serious trauma, including perforation, can occur. Fat obscuring the suture site needs to be carefully dissected to expose the deep inguinal ring. The caudal 10 to 12 mm of the deep inguinal ring is not dissected in order to avoid trauma to the pudendal vessels.

An early report of laparoscopic inguinal herniorrhaphy in dogs used staples with satisfactory outcomes.[21] However, stapled herniorrhaphy was significantly weaker than sutured repairs in an experimental model.[22]

Barbed sutures are knotless and do not require tension on the suture between bites, two features that greatly facilitate continuous intracorporeal suturing. Different barbed sutures are available and have individual requirements. This authors favor VLoc suture size 2-0 or 3-0 of 6-inch length for a continuous suture of up to 5 cm length. VLoc has unidirectional barbs and a welded loop on the end and may be best passed through a cannula incision by temporary removal of one cannula. The suture can be inserted through the cannula if a 10 to 12 mm cannula is used. Suturing ensues from the cranial aspect of the deep inguinal ring, engaging internal rectus fascia medially and inguinal ligament laterally. With VLoc, the first suture bite is taken, and the needle passed through the end loop for anchoring. Thereafter, the deep inguinal ring is closed in a simple continuous pattern, which is ended with two suture bites in opposing direction. At least 10 to 15 mm of inguinal ring needs to remain open in order to not compromise the pudendal vessels and genitofemoral nerve.

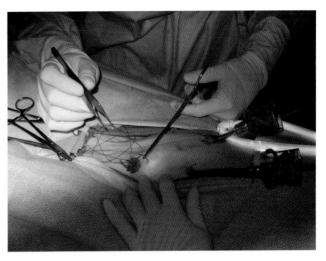

Figure 27-13 A two-cannula laparoscopy-assisted technique for closing small inguinal hernias. (Courtesy of Drs. Bonnie G. Campbell and Andreas Bachelez.)

Laparoscopic-Assisted Technique

A laparoscopic-assisted herniorrhaphy has been performed at Washington State University (personal Communication, Drs. Bonnie G. Campbell and Andreas Bachelez). With the patient in a mild Trendelenburg position, a two-port technique was used with the telescope portal on ventral midline and a lateral portal for an atraumatic grasping forceps (Figure 27-13). After reduction of the hernia, a small skin incision was performed over the inguinal ring, and a regular suture was placed through the incision and guided by intraabdominal visualization around the hernia sac. The needle was exiting the abdomen outside the stab incision but when it was partially exiting the body wall, the needle was grabbed by its tip, and the swage was pushed through the subcutaneous tissue back into the original skin stab, where the suture was tied (Figure 27-14).

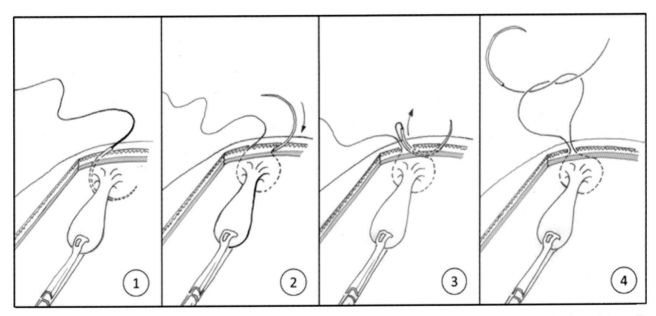

Figure 27-14 Laparoscopy-assisted inguinal herniorrhaphy. (1) The hernia sac is reduced into the abdomen by traction. A suture is placed transabdominally through a small stab incision, partially exiting the abdominal wall. (3) The needle is directed through the subcutaneous tissue with the swaged on end first to exit in the stab incision. (4) The suture is tied. (Original artwork courtesy of Dr. Sabrina Barry.)

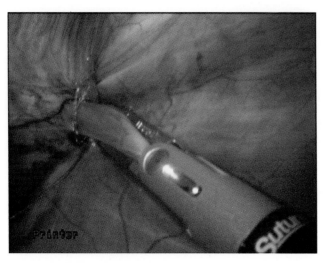

Figure 27-15 Barbed suture closure of an inguinal hernia in a gelding using an automated suture device (Endostitch; Covidien, Mansfield, MA). (Courtesy of Dr. Claude A. Ragle.)

Prognosis: Comparative Aspects

Laparoscopic repair of inguinal hernias is frequently performed in men. Primary repair was historically associated with high recurrence rates, of 15% or more,[23] and therefore tension-free repairs with mesh application is considered gold standard in humans. Conversely, in dogs, inguinal hernias are most commonly repaired by using the patient's own tissues, and only in patients with large traumatic defects or recurrent hernias has mesh reinforcement been considered indicated.[17] The prognosis is generally good to excellent.

Similar to the case in dogs, primary repair of inguinal hernia is standard in foals and geldings. In stallions, a peritoneal overlay technique is favored. Primary transperitoneal laparoscopic repair using barbed suture was recently reported in a gelding with an inguinal hernia (Figure 27-15).[20]

References

1 Farkas, G.A., Rochester, D.F. (1988) Functional characteristics of canine costal and crural diaphragm. J Appl Physiol (1985) 65 (5), 2253-2260.
2 Gordon, D.C., Hammond, C.G., Fisher, J.T., Richmond, F.J. (1989) Muscle-fiber architecture, innervation, and histochemistry in the diaphragm of the cat. J Morphol 201 (2), 131-143.
3 Pickering, M., Jones, J.F. (2002) The diaphragm: two physiological muscles in one. J Anat 201 (4), 305-312.
4 Hermanson, J.W. (2013) The muscular system. In: Evans, H.E, de Lahunta, A.E. (eds.) Miller's Anatomy of the Dog, 4th edn. WB Saunders, St. Louis, pp. 185-280.
5 Burns, C.G., Bergh, M.S., McLoughlin, M.A. (2013) Surgical and nonsurgical treatment of peritoneopericardial diaphragmatic hernia in dogs and cats: 58 cases (1999-2008). J Am Vet Med Assoc 242 (5), 643-650.
6 Wilson, G.P. 3rd, Hayes, H.M. Jr. (1986) Diaphragmatic hernia in the dog and cat: a 25-year overview. Semin Vet Med Surg Small Anim 1 (4), 318-326.
7 Banz, A.C., Gottfried, S.D. (2010) Peritoneopericardial diaphragmatic hernia: a retrospective study of 31 cats and eight dogs. J Am Anim Hosp Assoc 46 (6), 398-404.
8 Reimer, S.B., Kyles, A.E., Filipowicz, D.E., Gregory, C.R. (2004) Long-term outcome of cats treated conservatively or surgically for peritoneopericardial diaphragmatic hernia: 66 cases (1987-2002). J Am Vet Med Assoc 224 (5), 728-732.
9 Gibson, T.W., Brisson, B.A., Sears, W. (2005) Perioperative survival rates after surgery for diaphragmatic hernia in dogs and cats: 92 cases (1990-2002). J Am Vet Med Assoc 227 (1), 105-109.
10 Hyun, C. (2004) Radiographic diagnosis of diaphragmatic hernia: review of 60 cases in dogs and cats. J Vet Sci 5 (2), 157-162.
11 Spattini, G., Rossi, F., Vignoli, M., Lamb, C.R. (2003) Use of ultrasound to diagnose diaphragmatic rupture in dogs and cats. Vet Radiol Ultrasound 44 (2), 226-230.
12 Garson, H.L., Dodman, N.H., Baker, G.J. (1980) Diaphragmatic hernia. Analysis of fifty-six cases in dogs and cats. J Small Anim Pract 21 (9), 469-481.
13 Minihan, A.C., Berg, J., Evans, K.L. (2004) Chronic diaphragmatic hernia in 34 dogs and 16 cats. J Am Anim Hosp Assoc 40 (1), 51-63.
14 Boudrieau, R.J., Muir, W.W. (1987) Pathophysiology of traumatic diaphragmatic hernia in dogs. Compend Contin Educ Pract 9 (4), 379-385.
15 Sullivan, M., Reid, J. (1990) Management of 60 cases of diaphragmatic rupture. J Small Anim Pract 31 (9), 425-430.
16 Templeton, M.M., Krebs, A.I., Kraus, K.H., Hedlund, C.S. (2013) Ex vivo biomechanical comparison of V-Loc 180° absorbable wound closure device and standard Polyglyconate suture for diaphragmatic herniorrhaphy in a canine model. Presented at the 12th Annual Scientific Meeting of the Society of Veterinary Soft Tissue Surgery, June 13-15, Grand Haven, MI.
17 Smeak, D.D. (2012) Abdominal wall reconstruction and hernias. In: Tobias, K.M., Johnston, S.A. (eds.) Veterinary Surgery Small Animal, 1st edn. Saunders, Elsevier, St. Louis, pp. 1353-1379.
18 Strande, A. (1989) Inguinal hernia in dogs. J Small Anim Pract 30 (9), 520-521.
19 Waters, D.J., Roy, R.G., Stone, E.A. (1993) A retrospective study of inguinal hernia in 35 dogs. Vet Surg 22 (1), 44-49.
20 Ragle, C.A., Yiannikouris, S., Tibary, A.A., Fransson, B.A. (2013) Use of a barbed suture for laparoscopic closure of the internal inguinal rings in a horse. J Am Vet Med Assoc Jan 242 (2), 249-253.
21 Ger, R., Monroe, K., Duvivier, R., Mishrick, A. (1990) Management of indirect inguinal hernias by laparoscopic closure of the neck of the sac. Am J Surg 159 (4), 370-373.
22 Fugazzi, R.W., Fransson, B.A., Davis, H.M., Gay, J.P. (2013) Biomechanical strength of two laparoscopic herniorrhaphy techniques in a cadaveric diaphragm and in a neoprene model. Vet Comp Orthop Traumatol 26 (3), 198-203.
23 Neumayer, L., Giobbie-Harder, A., Jonasson, O., et al. (2004) Open mesh versus laparoscopic mesh repair of inguinal hernia. N Engl J Med 350 (18), 1819-1827.

28 Advanced Surgical Platforms: NOTES and Robotic Surgery

Lynetta Freeman and Heather A. Towle Millard

Key Points

- Natural Orifice Translumenal Endoscopic Surgery (NOTES) procedures in animals should be considered experimental and therefore performed under a supervised research protocol with signed client consent.
- Veterinarians performing NOTES procedures should be familiar with both surgery and therapeutic endoscopy or work with team members who have these skills.

Natural Orifice Translumenal Endoscopic Surgery (NOTES)

An ultimate goal of surgery is "scarless" surgery, not only because of the improved cosmetic outcome but also because the "stress" of surgery appears to be less when it is possible to minimize or avoid incisions in the skin and body wall. Natural Orifice Translumenal Endoscopic Surgery (NOTES) involves performing surgical procedures using a flexible endoscope passed through a natural orifice (mouth, vulva, urethra, anus) and then through an opening in the trachea, esophagus, stomach, vagina, bladder, or colon.[1] When the surgical procedure is performed only with a single point of access and a flexible endoscope, it is considered "pure" NOTES. When the endoscope is through a natural orifice and combined with a laparoscopic approach, the surgical procedure is considered a "hybrid" NOTES technique.

History of NOTES

NOTES grew out of the merger of two technologies in human medicine: laparoscopic surgery and interventional endoscopy. Surgeons performing less invasive surgery and gastroenterologists performing therapeutic endoscopic procedures (e.g., percutaneous endoscopic gastrostomy [PEG] tube placement, drainage of pancreatic cysts and necrosis, ultrasound-guided fine-needle aspirates) merged the tools and techniques to develop what is now known as NOTES. The first NOTES procedure was presented in 2000 at Digestive Disease Week by Dr. Anthony Kalloo, a gastroenterologist, and it involved a transgastric approach to the peritoneal cavity in swine to perform peritoneoscopy, obtain liver biopsy samples with a flexible endoscope, and close the gastrotomy with endoscopic clips.[2] Two years later, the first human case of transgastric NOTES appendectomy was presented at the same meeting by Drs. Rao and Reddy from India. Researchers around the world have performed experimental NOTES tubal ligation, cholecystectomy, splenectomy, intestinal anastomosis, gastrojejunostomy, nephrectomy, lymphadenectomy, thoracic access, and colon resection in swine[3] and hybrid transvaginal ovariohysterectomy,[4,5] ovariectomy (OVE),[6] cecectomy,[7] inguinal hernia repair,[8] thoracic surgery,[9,10] gastroenterostomy,[11] nephrectomy,[12] cholecystectomy,[13] and prostatectomy[14] in dogs. By these studies, NOTES instrumentation was developed, the safety of translumenal access and infection control methods were established, and the physiology of NOTES procedures and closure of the access means were investigated.[2] These animal studies provided a strong foundation for clinical trials of NOTES procedures in humans.[3] In recent years, the evolution of NOTES in human surgery has been away from transgastric approaches in favor of transvaginal and hybrid approaches.[15]

Advantages and Disadvantages of NOTES

Theoretical advantages of NOTES over open and laparoscopic surgery include less postoperative pain, decreased wound complications, and fewer adhesions and faster recovery mediated through a decreased inflammatory reaction, as well as improved cosmesis.[16] A recent review of experimental and clinical studies determined no significant advantage or disadvantage to NOTES over laparoscopy

Small Animal Laparoscopy and Thoracoscopy, First Edition. Edited by Boel A. Fransson and Philipp D. Mayhew.
© 2015 by ACVS Foundation. Published 2015 by John Wiley & Sons, Inc.
Companion website: www.wiley.com/go/fransson/laparoscopy

in regards to the pulmonary, cardiovascular, and immunologic systems.[17] In animal and human studies, NOTES procedures appear to elicit less postoperative pain than laparoscopic or open surgery.[4,18-20] Although there have been no large studies of complication rates in animals, the German registry of NOTES observed that cholecystectomy performed via transvaginal or laparoscopic approaches in humans resulted in equivalent complication and conversion rates to open surgery.[21]

As for disadvantages, the availability and limitations of endoscopic equipment and lack of familiarity with therapeutic gastroenterology present challenges for wide utilization of NOTES in veterinary medicine. The natural orifice must be prepared properly to prevent infection and of sufficient diameter to accept the endoscope. Poor visualization and issues with navigation, maneuverability, grasping or tissue extraction, and lumen closure are additional issues that must be addressed. The learning curves for NOTES techniques in veterinary medicine are quite steep.[22] The pure NOTES procedures nearly always result in longer operative times, and our studies have shown that transgastric access requires approximately 10 OVE procedures to be performed by the same team before approaching proficiency.[22] This does not appear to be the case with hybrid transvaginal OVH procedures performed in dogs because operative times are relatively short.[5,23]

Instrumentation

Pure NOTES approaches use primarily endoscopic equipment. When a hybrid approach is used, both flexible endoscopy equipment and laparoscopic equipment are needed. Figure 28-1 demonstrates the typical operating room (OR) setup for NOTES procedures in dogs.[16] For transgastric access, a 12.8-mm outer diameter dual channel therapeutic endoscope (Olympus GIF 2T-160; Olympus America; Center Valley, PA) works well for dogs weighing more than 15 kg. A mouth speculum or overtube (US Endoscopy, Mentor,

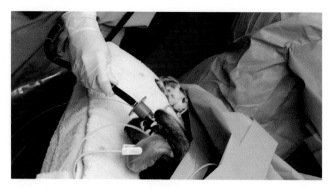

Figure 28-2 The endoscope is passed through an overtube in the dog's mouth (orange arrow). In this case, the dog is being maintained under deep sedation with propofol, and no endotracheal tube is passed. A polypropylene catheter (blue arrow) is positioned in the trachea to provide supplemental oxygen.

OH) (Figure 28-2) facilitates repeated endoscope insertion into the esophagus and prevents damage to the scope if the anesthesia level becomes too light during the procedure. Basic endoscopic accessories may include grasping forceps with alligator-type jaws, teeth, or two or three-prong jaws (Polygrab Tripod; Olympus Endoscopy, Center Valley, PA). Snares are available in a variety of sizes ranging from 25 to 60 mm and in oval, hexagonal, and crescent configurations (AcuSnare; Cook Medical, Bloomington, IN) (Figure 28-3) An endoscopic needle knife or sphincterotome (Huibregtse Triple Lumen Needle Knife, Cook Medica) is needed if tissue cutting is anticipated, and endoscopic scissors are needed to cut suture. A method of achieving monopolar coagulation is needed for dissection and hemostasis. The 0.035-inch guidewire (Tracer Metro Direct Wire Guide, Cook Medical) and several types of over-the-wire disposable balloon dilators (CRE Esophageal/Colonic Wire-guided Balloon, Boston Scientific Corporation, Natick, MA) are available. A pressure-monitored injection means (Cook Inflation Device, Cook Medical) is needed if balloons are to be used.

After access, a means of closing the site must be provided.[24] Sutures, staples, endoscopic clips or tacks, suturing devices,

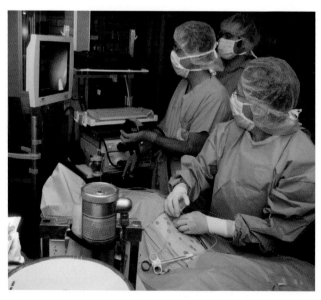

Figure 28-1 The typical operative setup for performing transgastric pure Natural Orifice Translumenal Endoscopic Surgery (NOTES) surgery. The gastroenterologist is at the head of the table and uses the endoscopy equipment. The sterile surgeon presides over the sterile field to perform the percutaneous maneuvers.

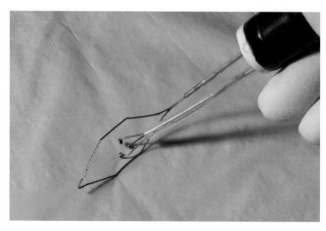

Figure 28-3 Demonstration of the use of a dual-channel endoscope with hexagonal snare and tripod grasping forceps being used in a coaxial manner. Before performing procedures, it is important to ensure that the outside diameters of the endoscopic instruments are appropriate for diameter of the working channels of the endoscope.

T-fasteners and tissue anchors, rivets, bioabsorbable plugs, surgical glue, and occlusion devices have been tried experimentally; however, few are commercially available. Gastropexy, submucosal tunneling, and omental sealing have been used to achieve lumen closure in experimental NOTES procedures; however, reliable lumen closure remains a significant unmet need in NOTES procedures.[25]

For transvaginal access to OVE, a hybrid approach is most often used in dogs, with the need for laparoscopic instrumentation, tower, insufflation, and monitor.[5,23,26] Vaginoscopy is performed before insertion of the vaginal trocar to determine the best site for port entry. The laparoscope is inserted at the umbilicus and monitors entry of the trocar from the vagina into the abdominal cavity and subsequent introduction of the bipolar instruments for electrocoagulation of the ovarian pedicles and broad ligament in performing an OVH.

Preoperative Preparation

One of the concerns with translumenal access is the potential for introduction of pathogenic microorganisms into the abdominal or thoracic cavity. When investigators first began to perform the transgastric NOTES procedures in swine, systemic antibiotics were administered.[27] Because infections were noted in early studies, efforts were then directed toward sterilizing the instruments that would be used during the procedure. It now appears that when sterile instruments are used, local lavage with povidone-iodine or systemic antibiotics is effective in addressing the potential for infection in NOTES procedures.[28] For transgastric procedures, cefazolin 1 g in 200 cc of saline is instilled into the stomach, allowed to dwell for 10 minutes, and then aspirated before the procedure.[6,18] For transvaginal approaches, the vagina is lavaged with povidone-iodine solution for 2 minutes followed by flushing with saline.[5] In addition, a wide surgical prep is used, and the OR is prepared so that rapid conversion to an open or laparoscopic procedure is possible if needed.

Anesthesia

Laparoscopic procedures and all endoscopic procedures in small animals are routinely performed under general inhalation anesthesia. This is necessary to minimize movement, ensure a patent airway, and assist with ventilation if necessary during the procedure. Because insufflation levels are generally lower than routine laparoscopy and procedures are thought to be less painful in NOTES procedures, the feasibility of using conscious sedation for NOTES procedures was investigated in dogs undergoing transgastric NOTES OVE.[1] There were no airway emergencies and no episodes of oxygen desaturation, and the outcomes were comparable to those of inhalant anesthesia.

Access

Although there are many potential routes of access to the abdominal and thoracic cavity, the two most commonly used in small animals are the transgastric and transvaginal approaches.

Transgastric

Endoscopists are very familiar with the techniques for PEG tube placement and using air to distend an organ for proper examination. Transgastric access is gained by inflating the stomach with air via a flexible endoscope, transilluminating the abdominal wall, applying pressure with a fingertip, and observing it with an endoscope.[16,29]

A catheter and guidewire are introduced percutaneously into the stomach (similar to the technique for performing PEG tube placement) at the safe site and grasped with a snare passed through the accessory channel of the endoscope. One technique involves using a dual-channel endoscope and keeping the guidewire through one channel while passing a needle knife through the other channel and using the needle knife to make an incision in the gastric wall close to the guidewire. Another technique uses an endoscopic sphincterotome passed over the guidewire to enlarge the opening around the guidewire. Both of these techniques are potentially associated with electrocautery injury to the abdominal wall or internal organs. The safest technique appears to involve creating a loop with the guidewire inside the peritoneal cavity (between the stomach and body wall) and passing a balloon dilator over the guidewire to traverse the gastric wall. The 20-mm balloon is inflated to 6 atm pressure and held for approximately 2 minutes. As the balloon is deflated, the endoscope is advanced so that it follows the balloon into the abdominal cavity. The balloon is then deflated and withdrawn from the scope, leaving the guidewire in place (Video Clip 28-1). An alternative to using the looping technique is to use blind insertion of a Veress needle to inflate the abdomen with carbon dioxide (CO_2) and then using a needle knife to create the opening in the stomach at a safe location.[30]

Transvaginal

Although "pure" techniques have been performed,[31] the most common means to approach the abdominal cavity is a hybrid technique that involves transvaginal access under laparoscopic monitoring. After the primary laparoscopic cannula is placed at the umbilicus, a 5-mm cannula is introduced through the vagina under laparoscopic monitoring. To protect the bladder, it is drained before surgery, and the patient is tilted to right or left lateral recumbency during cannula insertion.[5,23,26,31]

Insufflation

Insufflation is necessary to create an optical cavity in which to perform NOTES procedures (Figure 28-4). Air is instilled through the flexible endoscopes, but the pressure is not regulated. Therefore,

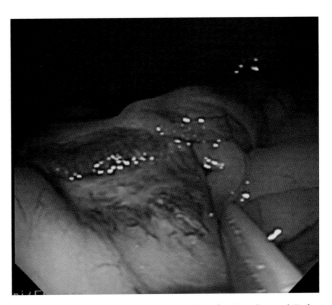

Figure 28-4 Intraoperative view of a Natural Orifice Translumenal Endoscopic Surgery (NOTES) ovariectomy showing the location of the ovary.

several studies have evaluated air versus CO_2 and the intraabdominal pressures in NOTES procedures.[32-34] Air may support combustion when lasers or electrocautery is used. When it was shown that peak intraabdominal pressures with endoscopic air are higher than with regulated CO_2 via laparoscopy,[34,35] surgeons began using pressure-controlled insufflation during NOTES procedures. In hybrid procedures, the CO_2 tubing is attached to the laparoscopic trocar. In pure NOTES, CO_2 is instilled via a catheter or an attachment to the endoscope.

Exposure and Navigation

In pure NOTES procedures, both working channels of the endoscope are used to introduce instruments to perform the procedure. Usually, the guidewire is left in place, and the endoscope is introduced into the abdominal cavity beside the guidewire. In hybrid procedures, visualization is provided by a laparoscope. If the cannula is used for insertion of an instrument (e.g., a stapler or clip applier), then visualization is provided by the endoscope. Procedures are technically much easier with a hybrid approach because rigid and larger diameter traditional laparoscopic instruments can be used. Similar to laparoscopy, additional exposure in NOTES procedures is gained by tilting the table to allow gravity retraction of internal structures.

Closure

Closure of the access site remains the most challenging aspect of NOTES procedures in veterinary medicine, primarily because of the lack of commercially available devices.[33] In the authors' opinion, the lack of an acceptable closure means has hindered widespread adoption of transgastric NOTES procedures in humans. Tissue apposition, prevention of infection, and sealing of the opening against leakage are critical factors in the healing of incisions. Pairs of T-fasteners were used in one of the author's studies for the transgastric closure, and the outcomes were favorable (Figure 28-5).[1,6,36,37] The omentum appears to play a role in sealing the incisions. Despite considerable experience with using the T-fastener device, the time required for gastric closure accounts for a major portion of overall operative time (Video Clip 28-2).[22]

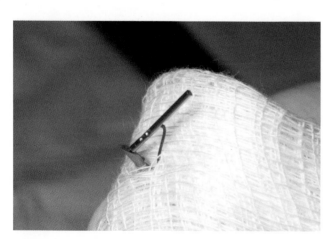

Figure 28-5 A T-fastener has suture swaged to the middle of a hollow shaft stored inside a larger needle. After the needle penetrates tissue (in this case, a surgical sponge), the T-fastener is deployed in the tissue. After deployment, slight traction is applied to the suture, which causes the T-tag to toggle into place.

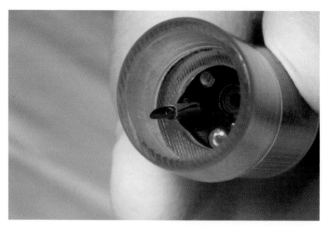

Figure 28-6 A beveled cap is placed on the end of the gastroscope. The cap is placed in contact with the gastric mucosa, and vacuum is applied to suction tissue into the cap so that the needle tip can be deployed safely without injury to underlying structures.

One of the limitations to the use of T-fasteners is that the tip may incorporate tissue on the outside of the stomach if it penetrates too deeply during deployment. Utilization of a clear cap on the end of the endoscope helps to avoid injury to adjacent tissue during closure (Figure 28-6). Judging by early assessment of histologic healing and postoperative outcomes, the closure is secure; however, others have found that clips may result in improved healing.[37] The vaginal incision is not closed in dogs. Minor vaginal bleeding has been noted in the postoperative period.[4,5]

Specific Procedures

Canine Transgastric NOTES Ovariectomy
Preoperative Considerations

Patients are fasted for 12 to 20 hours but given access to water. A nonsteroidal antiinflammatory drug is given subcutaneously for analgesia followed by general anesthesia. Intravenous (IV) propofol is given for anesthetic induction followed by endotracheal intubation and maintenance anesthesia with isoflurane and oxygen. IV fluids are given, and the animal is placed in dorsal recumbency on a warming blanket and monitored with indirect blood pressure, SpO_2, end-tidal CO_2, electrocardiography, and temperature probe. The abdomen is prepared for aseptic surgery. A perioperative antimicrobial is given every 90 minutes. The overtube is placed in the esophagus. After endoscopic examination and cleansing of residual food particles, an antimicrobial, such as cefazolin, 1 g in 200 mL of saline, is instilled into the stomach and allowed to remain for 10 minutes.

Surgical Technique

A standard PEG technique is used to introduce a 0.035-inch guidewire through a 16-gauge catheter from the patient's left side. A balloon-tipped through-the-scope catheter is introduced over the guidewire to traverse the stomach wall. The balloon is inflated to 6 atm pressure for approximately 2 minutes to dilate the opening in the stomach to 2 cm around the guidewire (Figure 28-7). The balloon and endoscope are passed into the abdominal cavity. The balloon is deflated and withdrawn, and the endoscope is removed and reinserted beside the guidewire into the abdominal cavity. To provide an adequate optical cavity, air or CO_2 is instilled to create a pneumoperitoneum. For access to the left ovary, the table is tilted to the right.

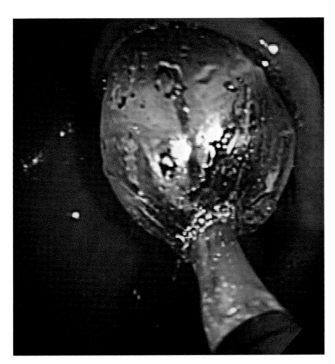

Figure 28-7 Endoscopic view of the balloon being used to dilate the gastrotomy site for introduction of the endoscope into the abdominal cavity during Natural Orifice Translumenal Endoscopic Surgery (NOTES) procedures in a dog.

For a "pure NOTES" OVE (meaning that no supplemental laparoscopic ports are used), each ovary is elevated with grasping forceps through a monopolar snare (Figure 28-8, Video Clip 28-3). Energy is applied to the snare as it is closed and ultimately transects the tissue. The ovary is then grasped with both the snare and the endoscopic forceps and withdrawn with the endoscope (Video Clip 28-4). After the

ovary has been examined to ensure complete removal, the endoscope is reintroduced, and the surgical site is inspected to ensure hemostasis. To access the right ovary, the table is tilted left. The endoscope is passed and retroflexed cranially from the right inguinal area to visualize the right ovary. Ligation and transection of the right ovary with the monopolar snare is performed, and the ovary and endoscope are removed. The guidewire is left in place during the procedure to assist in identifying the gastric incision.

The gastrotomy is closed with two sets of T-fasteners positioned at 12 and 6 o'clock and 3 and 9 o'clock, each held together by a suture clip. A beveled cap is secured to the outside of the gastroscope and the scope is passed into the stomach (Video Clip 28-5). A T-fastener is loaded into a delivery device and passed through the working channel of the endoscope so that the tip is visualized inside the cap. The gastrotomy is identified by the guidewire, and the cap is positioned on gastric mucosa adjacent to the incision. Vacuum is applied to pull gastric mucosa into the cap. The needle is quickly advanced into the gastric submucosa, and the T-fastener is deployed. The tissue is inspected as vacuum is released, and a slight tug is applied to ensure that the T-fastener is correctly located (Figure 28-9). The scope is then withdrawn, and a second T-fastener is applied on the opposite side of the incision. The two free ends of suture exit the endoscope working channel. Outside the body, the two suture strands are captured in a loop threaded through the suture clip. The clip is positioned against the tissue, and the inside plug is advanced to trap the sutures and appose the gastric incision. Endoscopic scissors are used to cut the sutures. The guidewire is removed. After two pairs are placed, the stomach is inflated with air, and the abdomen is monitored for tympany. Any residual air in the abdominal cavity is evacuated by a 16-gauge catheter.

Complications and Prognosis

A feasibility and technique development study was undertaken in 10 research dogs.[6] The mean operative time was about 2.5 hours, and no dogs died. The ovaries were incompletely excised in three dogs, and inadequate access to the right ovary required conversion

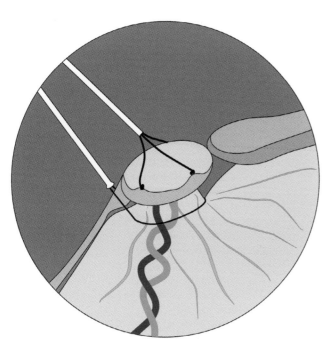

Figure 28-8 Diagram showing an ovary as it is being cauterized with a monopolar snare.

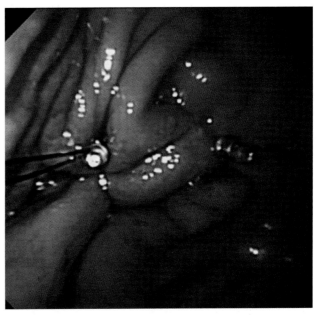

Figure 28-9 Endoscopic view of the gastric mucosa after the gastrotomy has been closed with two pairs of T-fasteners secured with clips.

an open procedure in one. Necropsy at 2 weeks revealed uneventful healing of the surgical sites with no significant damage to surrounding organs, no significant growth on bacterial cultures, and no evidence of peritonitis. A prospective comparison study was then conducted in 30 dogs that underwent NOTES, laparoscopic, or open OVE.[18] Surgical times for the NOTES procedure were longer, but the dogs demonstrated less evidence of pain in the postoperative period. Since then, NOTES OVE was performed in 19 dogs.[1] Ten dogs were performed under inhalant anesthesia and nine with propofol sedation. There were five operative failures with no difference between the anesthetic methods used. Four were related to inadequate hemostasis of the ovarian pedicle because of incorrect power setting of the electrosurgical device, and there was one conversion to an open procedure because of an unusually large uterus that was too heavy to lift with endoscopic instruments. Surgical times were significantly longer than with open or laparoscopic OVE; however, the pain scores were lower with the NOTES approach.[18] Evaluation of the time required to perform each procedural step revealed that gastrotomy closure required the most time.[12,22] All of the animals recovered well after surgery, and no immediate postoperative complications were apparent.

Transvaginal-Assisted Laparoscopic Ovariectomy or Ovariohysterectomy

Hybrid techniques have been performed by veterinarians in Iran, Brazil, and Russia (personal communication with Alex Chernov, DVM, May 2014).[4,5,23] The patient size is limited by pelvic canal diameter and length of cannula that are available. The vagina is prepared by 2-minute lavage with 10% povidone-iodine followed by saline flush.[5] A laparoscope is placed at the umbilicus and, under direct visualization, a 5-mm cannula is introduced through the vagina into the abdominal cavity. Standard laparoscopic instruments are then introduced through the vaginal port for ligation and transection of the ovarian pedicle and the laparoscope provides visualization during the procedure. The ovary and uterine horns are extracted through the vaginal port, and the uterine body is ligated externally. No attempt is made to close the colpotomy. A pure NOTES approach to OVH was performed in five dogs through an 11-mm cannula inserted transvaginally.[31] An operating laparoscope was used, and bipolar forceps were inserted through the working channel to seal and transect the ovarian pedicles. The uterine horn was exteriorized, and the uterine arteries and body of the uterus were ligated or coagulated externally. The uterine stump was then returned to the abdomen. The vaginal incision was not closed, and the animals recovered without major complications. Comparative studies with traditional laparoscopy and open OVH suggest that the patients undergoing the hybrid NOTES procedures are less painful than those undergoing traditional surgery.[4,26] The operative times in the hybrid studies were similar to or slightly longer than for the laparoscopic approach.[4,5,26]

Postoperative Care

Dogs undergoing NOTES OVE procedures are usually given a single dose of analgesic and monitored for pain. They are fed the evening of surgery. In most cases, additional analgesia is not required, and the patients are discharged the day after surgery.

Canine NOTES Gastropexy
Preoperative Considerations

A NOTES approach to endoscopic gastropexy might offer an advantage in lessening the invasiveness of a surgical procedure to create a permanent adhesion between the stomach and right lateral body wall in dogs at risk for gastric dilatation and volvulus (GDV); however, the NOTES procedure introduced new questions that were addressed by research studies. An experimental study in 10 research dogs was followed by a clinical study in 15 client-owned animals.[16,36] Studies involving client-owned animals used laparoscopic monitoring for safety with a 5-mm laparoscope placed through a cannula just caudal to the umbilicus. Because the laparoscope was only used for safety monitoring and the procedure was performed with the flexible endoscope, the technique was considered a pure NOTES approach.

Patient Preparation

Anesthesia and preoperative preparation were similar to canine transgastric NOTES OVE procedures.

Surgical Technique

A dual-channel endoscope was passed into the stomach, and the proposed gastrotomy site was identified in the antral portion of the stomach midway between the greater and lesser curvature on the ventral (anterior) aspect of the stomach. The site was adjacent to the incisura angularis, a narrow fold that divides the pyloric antrum from the lesser curvature of the gastric body (Video Clip 28-6).

A 19-gauge, 5-inch stylet-loaded catheter was inserted through the right lateral body wall just inferior to the 13th rib and directed into the antral portion of the stomach. The stylet was removed, and a 0.035-inch guidewire was inserted and pulled through the scope using a standard 11-mm snare. A through-the-scope, sequential dilating balloon was used to directly dilate the gastrostomy to 20 mm. The endoscope was then passed through the gastrotomy into the peritoneal cavity. Insufflation was provided through CO_2 connected to the cannula at the umbilicus.

The site of guidewire penetration through the abdominal musculature, which marks the location of the gastropexy, was identified. A needle knife electrode or wire loop cautery device was then used to create one or several incisions in the abdominal musculature surrounding the guidewire. A generous incision or a series of incisions, approximately 50 mm long, was made (Figure 28-10). Monopolar

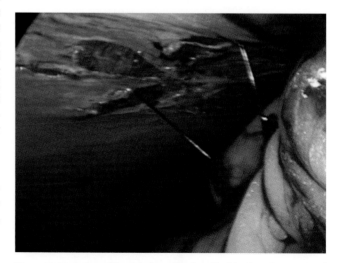

Figure 28-10 A view of the right lateral body wall of the dog after a series of incisions make with an endoscopic needle knife deployed through the flexible endoscope. The guidewire maintains alignment of the gastrotomy and the gastropexy site. Two nylon sutures are placed, and this is the view before the suture clips are applied to bring the tissue in apposition.

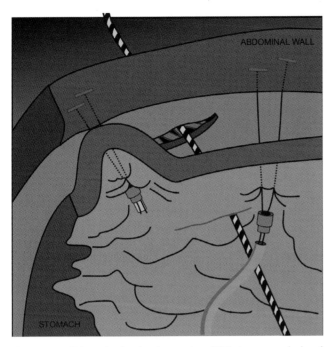

Figure 28-11 Schematic showing how pairs of T-fasteners are deployed from inside the stomach to create the Natural Orifice Translumenal Endoscopic Surgery (NOTES) gastropexy. (Reproduced with permission from Freeman, L.J., Pader, K. (2012) NOTES Application in Veterinary Medicine. In: Kalloo, A.N., Marescaux, J., Zorron, R. (eds.) Natural Orifice Translumenal Endoscopic Surgery Textbook & Video Atlas. Wiley-Blackwell, Oxford.)

electrocautery was used to coagulate and cut the peritoneum and abdominal musculature. The site was examined to ensure adequate hemostasis and further cauterized if needed.

Keeping the guidewire in place, the endoscope was removed and reinserted into the stomach beside the guidewire. To obtain adequate insufflation of the stomach to permit dilation of the stomach to the body wall, it was necessary to first close the gastric incision around the guidewire. The T-fastener suturing device was used to place one or two sutures through the gastric mucosa to close the incision. The intraabdominal pressure was lowered to 4 to 6 mm Hg to permit the stomach to move closer to the abdominal wall. A series of sutures was placed through the gastric mucosa into the abdominal wall to secure the gastropexy for 360 degrees around the incision in the abdominal wall. During placement of each suture, the abdominal wall was palpated until the tip of the T-fastener was felt within the subcutaneous tissue before deployment. Digital palpation caused the tip of the fastener to toggle and remain in the subcutaneous tissue just beneath the skin. Approximately six sets of sutures were placed and joined with surgical clips to secure an intact gastropexy (Figure 28-11). The laparoscope was used to ensure that no other organs become entrapped in the gastropexy site. After final examination, excess air was removed from the stomach, and the endoscope was removed from the stomach. The abdomen was desufflated, the laparoscope and cannula were removed, and the site closed with sutures.

Complications and Prognosis

Transgastric NOTES gastropexy procedures were successfully performed in 25 dogs, and all survived.[16] There were no known postoperative complications. Median operative times were 75 minutes (range, 52–182) for the feasibility study and 148 minutes (range, 104–229) for the clinical study.[36] In the feasibility study, only 6 of 10 animals had significant gastric adhesions. The gastropexy technique was then modified to increase the number of incisions in the peritoneum and the numbers of fasteners used and to include laparoscopic safety monitoring. In the clinical study, ultrasonographic examination indicated that 15 of 15 gastropexy sites were intact and there was no evidence of gastritis. The number of fasteners visible on gastric endoscopic examination decreased over time in dogs in the clinical study. None of the animals developed GDV during the 1-year follow-up period. These studies showed that the technique is feasible and results in a durable adhesion with minimal morbidity; however, operative times are long using the T-fasteners for gastric closure.

Postoperative Care

Postoperatively, each animal was recovered from general anesthesia and, upon extubation, were given hydromorphone 0.05 mg/kg IV for pain. The dogs were released with the owners with instructions to restrict activity for 2 weeks to prevent disruption of adhesions. Animals were returned for endoscopic and ultrasound evaluations of the gastropexy sites at 4, 8, and 12 months and were clinically healthy at the time of follow-up.

Complications of NOTES

Complications of NOTES, similar to laparoscopy, lead to prolonged operative time and are best avoided when possible. Iatrogenic trauma can occur during access when the stomach is not properly inflated or the initial percutaneous needle placement is incorrect. Issues with overinflation can lead to subcutaneous emphysema or cardiorespiratory instability. The coaxial nature of using the two-channel endoscope prevents triangulation, leading to restricted range of motion and less tactile feedback.[16] Even minor bleeding can be difficult to control and may lead to conversion to a hybrid technique because of the lack of equipment that can be used through the endoscope.

Conclusion

The positive outcomes associated with NOTES procedures in animals suggest that NOTES may be an alternate means of performing abdominal procedures in the future when proper equipment is available to reduce procedure times.

Robotic Surgery

Human and veterinary surgeons have answered the call to improve upon intra- and postoperative morbidity, cosmesis, and pain while reducing hospitalization stays with minimally invasive surgery (MIS). This has brought about a new era in the treatment of surgical disease with a fast evolution in human medicine and a slower evolution in veterinary medicine beginning with laparoscopic-assisted surgery followed by multiple-port laparoscopic surgery, single-port laparoscopic surgery, and NOTES.[38-40]

The challenge was then placed on surgeons in human medicine and innovators to improve upon this already significant advancement from traditional open surgery,[41] partly because specific aspects of several commonly performed human laparoscopic surgeries were lacking. Other shortcomings of minimally invasive laparoscopic surgery included that surgeons are limited by two-dimensional vision, awkwardness of instruments, lack of complete simulation of a surgeon's wrist movements, tremor magnification, and surgeon fatigue. Robotic surgery has addressed these limitations and more.[38,39]

Robotic surgery entered the human surgical arena more than 20 years ago. The technology first began with 'fixed' anatomic procedures in orthopedics and neurosurgery. With the advancement of minimally invasive laparoscopic procedures and a coinciding new interest in telepresence technology, visceral robotic surgery emerged through the collaborative efforts of the Department of Defense, Stanford Research Institute, and the National Aeronautics and Space Administration.[39,42]

One of the earliest systems was Aesop (Computer Motion, Goleta, CA). This single robotic arm was voice activated, and its primary role was to operate the camera during laparoscopic procedures and thus serve as an assistant to the surgeon. This system evolved into Zeus (Computer Motion), which had three robotic arms and a robotic console, and for the first time allowed the surgeon to be distant from the operating table.[39] The da Vinci System (Intuitive Surgical, Sunnyvale, CA) improved on three-dimensional technology and allowed the surgeon to feel immersed in the "operating field," while providing four robotic arms, as well as improved instrument ergonomics that more completely simulate the wrist movements of surgeons. In 2003, the two manufacturers of Zeus and da Vinci merged, and Zeus, along with other Computer Motion robots, were discontinued.[38]

In brief, the da Vinci System is composed of four main parts, a vision cart; patient-side robot; robotic master console; and most recently a second console that allows novice surgeons to be coached by a mentor at the master console, which increases patient safety.[39,42] Ultimately, the master console controls the patient-side robot with multiple hand and foot controls. The hand controls operate the camera or all instrument manipulations, and the foot pedals control camera movement, camera focus, and cautery. The master console also has a stereoscopic viewer that provides the surgeon with a three-dimensional image of the operating field. A bedside human assistant provides suction, irrigation, suture introduction and retrieval, instrument exchanges, and any additional retraction[39] (Figure 28-12).

Robots in Action

In 2012, an estimated 450,000 human surgical procedures were performed with the da Vinci System.[38] The three most common procedures were OVH, prostatectomy, and nephrectomy.[38] As with any new technology, it must be reviewed in terms of security, efficiency, and reproducibility. At this time, there have been few randomized studies comparing robotic surgery with laparoscopic surgery. In addition, there will be an expected learning curve that will initially affect operative times, complication rates, and outcomes, and, of course, there is an increase in cost compared with older technologies.[38,43]

Innovators will respond to skeptics and improve existing technology as studies delineate the issues. For instance, in a study by Sarlos et al.,[44] 95 patients were randomized to robotic or laparoscopic OVH. Robotic operating times were significantly longer ($P < 0.001$), and this was largely because of increased docking times. Kho et al.[44] showed that with experience, docking times can be reduced to less than 5 minutes.[45] As with initial laparoscopic procedures, initial robotic studies showed that blood loss and conversion to open surgery were higher; new studies have improved outcomes.[44] Wright et al.[46] found no difference in blood transfusions, reoperation, death, or intra- or postoperative complications when comparing open, vaginal (NOTES), laparoscopic, and robotic OVH.

In another study of 688 OVHs, blood loss was reduced, and there were no conversions to open surgery with robotics; the laparoscopic conversion rate was 2.82%.[47] In prostatic surgery, robotic surgery offers a distinct advantage over laparoscopy in that surgeons can more easily maneuver the robotic instruments deep in the pelvis.[38] Recent studies have also demonstrated a slight but significant improvement in urinary function at 12 months and a trend toward improved potency, urinary continence, and blood loss, as well as reduced operative times in favor of robotics.[38,48] Recent studies in nephrectomy patients showed that robotic, compared with laparoscopic, surgery was superior in terms of reduced operative time, blood loss, and warm ischemia time, and patients undergoing robotic surgery did not require any long-term dialysis.[38,49]

Results from recent randomized clinical studies are promising, but long-term studies are needed. The issues of cost, training, safety, and performance validation have yet to be thoroughly addressed in human medicine.[38] The cost of the average da Vinci System is approximately $1.4 to $1.6 million in addition to annual maintenance fees and the cost of instrumentation.[39] Similar issues, albeit not quite as high costs, were encountered when laparoscopic surgery was introduced in addition to open surgery. As with MIS, these limitations will likely be overcome with time.

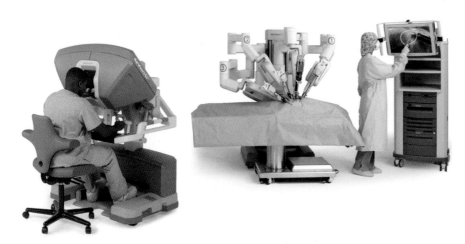

Figure 28-12 Components of the Table-da Vinci Si Surgical System. (© 2014 Intuitive Surgical, Inc.)

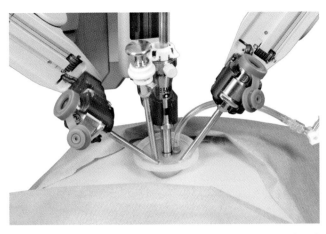

Figure 28-13 Single-Site final docked position. (© 2014 Intuitive Surgical, Inc.)

Future Applications of Robotic Surgery

Robotic surgery was initially explored for the purpose of telemedicine with the goal of performing surgery on wounded soldiers or in areas with inadequate health care by "dropping" a robot to the operating area while the surgeon operates from a remote, safe location.[38,39,50,51] This concept may seem like it is far in the future, but Marescaux et al.[52] have successfully performed a transatlantic robotic-assisted laparoscopic cholecystectomy. Additional studies are sure to be on the horizon as the technology continues to improve. Another application, given its real-time communication system, is that a local, novice laparoscopic surgeon could be guided through an advanced procedure by a distant mentor who manipulates the robotic arms.[53] Also, as with laparoscopic surgery, there is a movement from multiple-access ports to single-site access ports (Figure 28-13). Another robotic technology that will lead medical robotics into the next millennium will require a "quantum leap" in current technology. Stoianovici et al.[54] recently discussed the idea of developing robots that can operate inside a computed tomography or magnetic resonance image scanner. This could improve the mapping between volumetric image and the patient and thus further improve precision and patient outcomes.

Conclusion

Although robotic technology has not made its way into the clinical arena of veterinary medicine, as with advanced laparoscopic and thoracoscopic procedures, it undoubtedly is a matter of time and patience. There are many skeptics in the human field regarding robotic surgery compared with laparoscopic surgery, just as there are in veterinary medicine regarding laparoscopic surgery compared with conventional open surgery. Human laparoscopic surgery offered improved cosmesis and clear benefits that allowed distinct advantages over traditional open surgery. These benefits are still difficult for many veterinary surgeons to accept, but veterinary medicine is very slowly overcoming the critics. It is our belief that robotic surgery will do the same, especially as learning curves are conquered; cost decreases; and more prospective, randomized studies with long-term clinical outcomes are documented in human medicine. "Surgical innovation is necessary . . . and the future of robotic surgery may be bright . . ., but currently, caution is advisable."[55]

Acknowledgments

We are deeply grateful for the gastroenterologists and surgeons at the Indiana University School of Medicine and to the Veterinary Clinical Sciences department at Purdue University School of Veterinary Medicine and to NOSCAR, the Collie Health Foundation, the American College of Veterinary Surgeons, and the Indiana Equine Research Foundation for funding our basic research. Cook Endoscopy and Boston Scientific provided disposable endoscopic products used in our studies. Without these groups, this work would not have been possible.

All videos cited in this chapter can be found on the book's companion website at **www.wiley.com/go/fransson/ laparoscopy**

References

1 Al-Haddad, M., McKenna, D., Ko, J., et al. (2012) Deep sedation in natural orifice transluminal endoscopic surgery (NOTES): a comparative study with dogs. Surg Endosc 26, 3163-3173.

2 Kalloo, A.N., Singh, V.K., Jagannath, S.B., et al. (2004) Flexible transgastric peritoneoscopy: a novel approach to diagnostic and therapeutic interventions in the peritoneal cavity. Gastrointest Endosc 60, 114-117.

3 Flora, E.D., Wilson, T.G., Martin, I.J., et al. (2008) A review of natural orifice transluminal endoscopic surgery (NOTES) for intra-abdominal surgery: experimental models, techniques, and applicability to the clinical setting. Ann Surg 247, 583-602.

4 Luz, M.J., Ferreira, G.S., Santos, C.L., et al. (2011) Ovariohysterectomy in dogs by transvaginal hybrid NOTES (Natural Orifice Transluminal Endoscopic Surgery): prospective comparison with laparoscopic and open techniques. Proceedings of the 8th annual meeting of the Veterinary Endoscopy Society, San Pedro, Belize.

5 Bakhtiari, J., Khalaj, A.R., Aminlou, E., et al. (2012) Comparative evaluation of conventional and transvaginal laparoscopic ovariohysterectomy in dogs. Vet Surg 41, 755-758.

6 Freeman, L.J., Rahmani, E.Y., Sherman, S., et al. (2009) Oophorectomy by natural orifice transluminal endoscopic surgery: feasibility study in dogs. Gastrointest Endosc 69, 1321-1332.

7 Lee, S.I., Park, J.H., Park, C.W., et al. (2010) Transgastric cecectomy in canine models: natural orifice transluminal endoscopic surgery (NOTES). Surg Endosc 24, 2387-2392.

8 Sherwinter, D.A., Gupta, A., Eckstein, J.G. (2011) Natural orifice transluminal endoscopic surgery inguinal hernia repair: a survival canine model. J Laparoendosc Adv Surg Tech A 21, 209-213.

9 Liu, C.Y., Chu, Y., Wu, Y.C., et al. (2013) Transoral endoscopic surgery versus conventional thoracoscopic surgery for thoracic intervention: safety and efficacy in a canine survival model. Surg Endosc 27, 2428-2435.

10 Chen, W.H., Chu, Y., Wu, Y.C., et al. (2012) Endoscopic closure of a tracheal access site using bioglue after transtracheal thoracoscopy in a nonsurvival canine model. Eur Surg Res 48, 26-33.

11 Luo, H., Pan, Y., Min, L., et al. (2012) Transgastric endoscopic gastroenterostomy using a partially covered occluder: a canine feasibility study. Endoscopy 44, 493-498.

12 Isariyawongse, J.P., McGee, M.F., Rosen, M.J., et al. (2008) Pure natural orifice transluminal endoscopic surgery (NOTES) nephrectomy using standard laparoscopic instruments in the porcine model. J Endourol 22, 1087-1091.

13 Sugimoto, M., Yasuda, H., Koda, K., et al. (2009) Evaluation for transvaginal and transgastric NOTES cholecystectomy in human and animal natural orifice translumenal endoscopic surgery. J Hepatobiliary Pancreat Surg 16, 255-260.

14 Krambeck, A.E., Humphreys, M.R., Andrews, P.E., et al. (2010) Natural orifice transluminal endoscopic surgery: radical prostatectomy in the canine model. J Endourol 24, 1493-1496.

15 Sankaranarayanan, G., Matthes, K., Nemani, A., et al. (2013) Needs analysis for developing a virtual-reality NOTES simulator. Surg Endosc 27, 1607-1616.

16 Freeman, L.J., Pader, K. (2012) NOTES applications in veterinary medicine. In: Kalloo, A.N., Marescaux, J., Zorron, R. (eds.) Natural Orifice Transluminal Endoscopic Surgery Textbook & Video Atlas. Wiley-Blackwell, Oxford, pp. 215-231.

17 Bingener, J., Moran, E., Gostout, C.J., et al. (2011) Randomized study of natural orifice transluminal endoscopic surgery and endoscopy shows similar hemodynamic impact in a porcine model. Surg Endosc 25, 1065-1069.

18 Freeman, L.J., Rahmani, E.Y., Al-Haddad, M., et al. (2010) Comparison of pain and postoperative stress in dogs undergoing natural orifice transluminal endoscopic surgery, laparoscopic, and open oophorectomy. Gastrointest Endosc 72, 373-380.

19 Wood, S.G., Dabu-Bondoc, S., Dai, F., et al. (2014) Comparison of immediate postoperative pain after transvaginal versus traditional laparoscopic cholecystectomy. Surg Endosc 28, 1141-1145.

20 Bulian, D.R., Trump, L., Knuth, J., et al. (2013) Less pain after transvaginal/transumbilical cholecystectomy than after the classical laparoscopic technique: short-term results of a matched-cohort study. Surg Endosc 27, 580-586.

21 Lehmann, K.S., Ritz, J.P., Wibmer, A., et al. (2010) The German registry for natural orifice translumenal endoscopic surgery: report of the first 551 patients. Ann Surg 252, 263-270.

22 Freeman, L., Rahmani, E.Y., Burgess, R.C., et al. (2011) Evaluation of the learning curve for natural orifice transluminal endoscopic surgery: bilateral ovariectomy in dogs. Vet Surg 40, 140-150.

23 Brun, M.V., Silva, M.A., Mariano, M.B., et al. (2011) Ovariohysterectomy in a dog by a hybrid NOTES technique. Can Vet J 52, 637-64030.

24 Sun, G., Yang, Y., Zhang, X., et al. (2013) Comparison of gastrotomy closure modalities for natural orifice transluminal surgery: a canine study. Gastrointest Endosc 77, 774-783.

25 Sodergren, M.H., Coomber, R., Karimyan, V., et al. (2010) What are the elements of safe gastrotomy closure in NOTES? A systematic review. Surg Innov 17, 318-321.

26 de Souze, F.W., Brun, M.V., de Oliveira, M.T., et al. (2014) Ovariohysterectomy for videosurgery (hybrid vaginal NOTES), celiotomy or mini-celiotomy in bitches. Ciência Rural 44, 510-516.

27 Giday, S.A., Dray, X., Magno, P., et al. (2010) Infection during natural orifice transluminal endoscopic surgery: a randomized, controlled study in a live porcine model. Gastrointest Endosc 71, 812-816.

28 Nau, P.N., Hazey, J.W. (2012) Infection control in NOTES. In: Kalloo, A.N., Marescaux, J., Zorron, R. (eds.) Natural Orifice Translumenal Endoscopic Surgery Textbook & Video Atlas. Wiley-Blackwell, Oxford, pp. 29-38.

29 Bonin, E.A., Goustout, C.J. (2012) NOTES access techniques. In: Kalloo, A.N., Marescaux, J., Zorron, R. (eds.) Natural Orifice Translumenal Endoscopic Surgery Textbook & Video Atlas. Wiley-Blackwell, Oxford, pp. 39-58.

30 Ko, C.W., Shin, E.J., Buscaglia, J.M., et al. (2007) Preliminary pneumoperitoneum facilitates transgastric access into the peritoneal cavity for natural orifice transluminal endoscopic surgery: a pilot study in a live porcine model. Endoscopy 39, 849-853.

31 Silva, M., Augusto, M., Toniollo, G.H., et al. (2012) Pure-transvaginal natural orifice transluminal endoscopic surgery (NOTES) ovariohysterectomy in bitches: a preliminary feasibility study. Ciênca Rural 42, 1237-1242.

32 Bingener, J., Johnson, A.M. (2012) Physiology of NOTES. In: Kalloo, A.N., Marescaux, J., Zorron, R. (eds.) Natural Orifice Translumenal Endoscopic Surgery Textbook & Video Atlas. Wiley-Blackwell, Oxford, pp. 19-28.

33 Bergstrom, M., Swain, P., Park, P.O. (2007) Measurements of intraperitoneal pressure and the development of a feedback control valve for regulating pressure during flexible transgastric surgery (NOTES). Gastrointest Endosc 66, 174-178.

34 Meireles, O., Kantsevoy, S.V., Kalloo, A.N., et al. (2007) Comparison of intraabdominal pressures using the gastroscope and laparoscope for transgastric surgery. Surg Endosc 21, 998-1001.

35 Reider, E., Swanstrom, L.L. (2012) NOTES closure techniques. In: Kalloo, A.N., Marescaux, J., Zorron, R. (eds.) Natural Orifice Translumenal Endoscopic Surgery Textbook & Video Atlas. Wiley-Blackwell, Oxford, pp. 59-69.

36 Freeman, L.J., Al-Haddad, M., McKenna, D.M., et al. (in press) Feasibility and clinical evaluation of transgastric NOTES gastropexy in dogs.

37 Dray X, Krishnamurty DM, Donatelli G., et al. (2010) Gastric wall healing after NOTES procedures: closure with endoscopic clips provides superior histological outcome compared with threaded tags closure. Gastrointest Endosc 72, 343-350.

38 Brody, F., Richards, N.G. (2014) Review of robotic versus conventional laparoscopic surgery. Surg Endosc 28, 1413-1424.

39 Visco, A.G., Advincula, A.P. (2008) Robotic gynecologic surgery. Obstet Gynecol 112, 1369-1384.

40 Mayhew, P.D. (2014) Recent advances in soft tissue minimally invasive surgery. J Small Anim Pract 55, 75-83.

41 Qadam, M., Curet, M.J., Wren, S.M. (2014) The evolving application of single-port robotic surgery in general surgery. J Hepatobiliary Pancreat Sci 21, 26-33.

42 Pugin, F., Bucher, P., Morel, P. (2011) History of robotic surgery: from AESOP and ZEUS to da Vinci. J Visc Surg 148, e3-e8.

43 Duran, H., Ielp, B., Caruso, R., et al. (2014) Does robotic distal pancreatectomy surgery offer similar results as laparoscopic and open approach? A comparative study from a single medical center. Int J Med Robot 10 (3), 280-285.

44 Sarlos, D., Kots, L., Stevanovic, N., et al. (2012) Robotic compared with conventional laparoscopic hysterectomy: a randomized controlled trial. Obstet Gynecol 120, 604-611.

45 Kho, R.M., Hilger, W.S., Hentz, J.G., et al. (2007) Robotic hysterectomy: technique and initial outcomes Am J Obstet Gynecol 197, 332.

46 Wright, K.N., Jonsdottir, G.M., Jorgensen, S., et al. (2012) Costs and outcomes of abdominal, vaginal, laparoscopic and robotic hysterectomies. JSLS 16, 519-524.

47 Wright, J.D., Ananth, C.V., Lewin, S.N., et al. (2013) Robotically assisted vs laparoscopic hysterectomy among women with benign gynecologic disease. JAMA 309, 689-698.

48 Moran, P.S., O'Neill, M., Teljeur, C., et al. (2013) Robot-assisted radical prostatectomy com- pared with open and laparoscopic approaches: a systematic review and meta-analysis. Int J Urol 20, 312-321.

49 Panumatrassamee, K., Autorino, R., Laydner, H., et al. (2013) Robotic versus laparoscopic partial nephrectomy for tumor in a solitary kidney: a single institution comparative analysis. Int J Urol 20, 484-491.

50 Senapati, S., Advincula, A.P. (2005) Telemedicine and robotics: paving the way to the globalization of surgery. Int J Gynecol Obstet 91, 210-216.

51 Bergeles, C., Yang, G. (2014) From passive tool holders to microsurgeons: safer, smaller, smarter surgical robots. IEEE Trans Biomed Eng 61, 1565-1576.

52 Marescaux, J., Leroy, J., Rubino, F., et al. (2002) Transcontinental robot- assisted remote telesurgery: feasibility and potential applications. Ann Surg 235, 487-492.

53 Drasin, T., Dutson, E., Gracia, C. (2004) Use of a robotic system as surgical first assistant in advanced laparoscopic surgery. J Am Coll Surg 199, 368-373.

54 Stoianovici, D. (2000) Robotic surgery. World Journal of Urology 18, 289-295.

55 Whiteside, J.L. (2008) Robotic gynecologic surgery. A brave new world? Obstet Gynecol 112, 1198-2000.

Fundamental Techniques in Thoracoscopy

29 Anesthesia for Thoracoscopy

Peter J. Pascoe and Philipp D. Mayhew

Key Points

- Although many thoracoscopic procedures can be performed using the working space provided by a pneumothorax, some procedures may require additional working space and necessitate the use of one-lung ventilation (OLV) techniques or thoracic insufflation.
- OLV can be induced using endobronchial blockers, double-lumen endobronchial tubes, or selective intubation. No one of these three techniques is suitable for all patients, so gaining experience with all three techniques is recommended to maximize success.
- OLV causes numerous physiological abnormalities, including significant ventilation/perfusion mismatching.

As minimally invasive procedures have increased in popularity in veterinary medicine in recent years, more complex surgeries have been described, including a growing number of thoracic procedures. With this trend has come the need to adapt anesthetic techniques to the needs of the surgeon in order to provide adequate working space for these approaches to be used within the closed confines of the thoracic cavity. Manipulation of ventilation during open chest pneumothorax, creation of one-lung ventilation (OLV), and thoracic insufflation have all been advocated for thoracoscopic procedures, but all have advantages and disadvantages. Knowledge of the physiological consequences of these techniques as well as the logistical challenges in obtaining them is key to achieving favorable outcomes; for example, failure of OLV is reported to be the primary cause of conversion to an open thoracotomy rather than complications or challenges of the surgical procedure.[1,2]

Pathophysiology of One-Lung Anesthesia

Surgical intervention in thoracoscopy often involves the collapse of one lung to provide enough space for the surgeon to visualize the lesion or to be able to work with abnormal pulmonary tissue. Under these circumstances, one would normally expect to see a hypoxic pulmonary vasoconstriction (HPV) response in the isolated lung. This diverts blood flow away from the hypoxic lung to the ventilated/perfused lung to minimize the amount of blood with a low oxygen tension mixing with the oxygenated blood. If the lung is collapsed during the procedure, the reexpansion of the lung at the end

of surgery may be associated with a risk of reexpansion pulmonary edema and reperfusion injury and subsequent release of reactive oxygen species (ROS).

Hypoxic Pulmonary Vasoconstriction

This is a normal physiologic mechanism that is present in the pulmonary circulation to increase resistance in areas of hypoxia. During embryonic life, the pulmonary circulation has a high resistance in order to divert blood to the systemic circulation through the ductus arteriosus. When animals or humans reach high altitudes, HPV increases pulmonary vascular resistance, which in turn increases pulmonary arterial pressure and may lead to pulmonary edema. Animals and humans that are adapted to higher altitudes have a weaker HPV than those who are not. HPV is often shown to have two phases with the first, immediate, response involving local circulatory influences on the pulmonary vasculature and a secondary phase that involves hypoxia-inducible factors (HIFs).[3,4] The low oxygen tensions are detected in the pulmonary vasculature, and a response can occur in less than 1 minute, although the peak response may take up to 1 hour.[5] There is some controversy over the sensing mechanisms for low oxygen tensions, but it appears that the mitochondria in the pulmonary arterial smooth muscle cells are the most likely site with an increased production of ROS during hypoxia.[6]

Hypoxic pulmonary vasoconstriction is affected by many factors, so the clinical result may be difficult to predict (Table 29-1). In dogs, a number of reports have identified "normal" dogs that

---

Small Animal Laparoscopy and Thoracoscopy, First Edition. Edited by Boel A. Fransson and Philipp D. Mayhew.

© 2015 by ACVS Foundation. Published 2015 by John Wiley & Sons, Inc.

Companion website: www.wiley.com/go/fransson/laparoscopy

Table 29-1 Effect of Different Factors on Hypoxic Pulmonary Vasoconstriction

Factor or Drug	Effect on Hypoxic Pulmonary Vasoconstriction	References
Increasing PA or LA pressures	Attenuates HPV response because of the relatively weak musculature being overcome by the increased pressure	Lejeune et al.[89]
PEEP or CPAP	Reduces the effect of HPV	Lejeune et al.[90]
Body temperature	HPV decreases with hypothermia; <50% of the response at 31°C compared with normothermia	Benumof and Wahrenbrock[91]
Acidosis or alkalosis	HPV is depressed by metabolic and respiratory alkalosis; hypercapnic and metabolic acidosis may enhance HPV, but this is not consistent across studies	Lloyd[92] and Silove et al.[93]
Acepromazine	α Blockade attenuates the response, but there are no data on acepromazine itself	Brimioulle et al.[9]
α2 Agonists	Dexmedetomidine in humans during one-lung anesthesia did not appear to alter oxygenation	Kernan et al.[94]
Opioids	Minimal effect	Bjertnaes[12,13]
IV lidocaine	Minimal effect	Bindslev et al.[95]
Propofol	Enhanced response in dogs	Nakayama and Murray[14]
Ketamine	Minimal effect but could decrease the response because of increases in PA pressure	Nakayama and Murray[14]
Thiopental and other barbiturates	Minimal effect	Bjertnaes[13]; Carlsson et al.[96]
Inhalants	Dose-dependent effect to reduce HPV in vitro; sevoflurane and desflurane may have less effect than isoflurane, but at low doses (1 MAC), little effect on HPV is observed	Benumof and Wahrenbrock[97]; Lejeune et al.[89]; Lennon and Murray[98]; Lesitsky et al.[99]
Nitrous oxide	Decreases HPV	Bindslev et al.[95]
Nitric oxide	Abolishes HPV when delivered to the hypoxic lung	Sustronck et al.[100]
Calcium channel blockers	Abolish HPV by blocking the calcium channels involved in creating the constriction	Nakazawa and Amaha[101]
NSAIDs	COX-1 inhibition tends to enhance HPV; COX-2 inhibition may decrease HPV	Lennon and Murray[98]; Kylhammar and Radegran[102]

COX, cyclooxygenase; CPAP, continuous positive airway pressure; HPV, hypoxic pulmonary vasoconstriction; IV, intravenous; MAC, minimum alveolar concentration; LA, left atrial; PA, pulmonary artery; PEEP, positive end-expiratory pressure; NSAID, nonsteroidal antiinflammatory drug.

appear to have a very poor HPV response (nonresponders), and it is not clear what factors are involved, but the proportion of nonresponders reported was up to 50%.[7,8] Because the smooth muscles in the pulmonary vasculature are relatively weak, it would be expected that increases in pulmonary arterial pressure or left atrial pressure could attenuate the response. The elastance of the vessels is also limited, so increases in blood flow also tend to increase pressure and decrease HPV. By the mechanisms described, it is clear that HPV is not under parasympathetic or sympathetic control, so it is not surprising that acepromazine and dexmedetomidine appear to have minimal effect on HPV.[9,10] The opioids also appear to have minimal effect.[11,12] The injectable anesthetics have generally been reported to have no inhibitory effect, and in one report, propofol was reported to enhance HPV.[13,14] Given that the inhalants are thought to inhibit HPV, it has been suggested that the use of a propofol infusion rather than an inhalant would provide better oxygenation during one-lung anesthesia. However, in reviewing randomized clinical trials that have tested this hypothesis, the results are not supportive.[15]

Nevertheless, it probably makes sense to limit the concentration of inhaled anesthetic by using a balanced technique with drugs such as opioids or systemic lidocaine that have minimal effect on HPV.

Reexpansion of the Lung

The incidence of postoperative complications after prolonged one-lung anesthesia in humans is relatively high.[16] During one-lung anesthesia, if the side that is collapsed is left untreated, the lung will be hypoperfused because of HPV. At the end of the procedure, this may then lead to a type of reperfusion injury and the release of ROS into both the pulmonary and systemic circulation. In laboratory studies, it has been shown that the reexpansion is associated with an acute inflammatory response; this has been demonstrated in human patients as well.[17] Reexpansion may be associated with

overt pulmonary edema, but this is not a common sequela in clinical practice. However, it is likely that there is neutrophil recruitment to the affected lung with increased myeloperoxidase (MPO) release, and increased concentrations of cytokines such as interleukin (IL) -6, -1α, -1β, -8, and -10; tumor necrosis factor-α (TNF-α); macrophage inflammatory protein-1α (MIP-1α); pulmonary and activation-regulated chemokine (PARC); and soluble intercellular adhesion molecule-1 (sICAM-1) in alveoli or serum.[18,19] An experiment in rats has confirmed that the injury is attributable to reexpansion.[20] In this experiment, some rats had the right mainstem bronchus clamped, and some of the rats were euthanized without reinflating the lung; others had their lungs reinflated and ventilated for a period of time before sacrifice. The lungs that were occluded but not reexpanded showed no more changes than the lungs that were ventilated throughout, but the lungs that were reexpanded had an increase in pulmonary protein extravasation, increased MPO in the pulmonary tissue, and increased IL-1β and TNF-α in fluid washed from the lung, increased IL-10 in the serum, and increased IL-6 in both. This experiment also evaluated the effect of time, with one group being collapsed for 1 hour and the other for 3 hours, and showed that the longer occlusion time was associated with greater changes in the above parameters; this is also supported in clinical studies in humans.[21,22] The release of these inflammatory mediators has also been shown to affect other tissues. In an experiment in rats, malondialdehyde (MDA, an end product of lipid peroxidation) and MPO were examined in liver and ileum.[23] This study showed significant increases in MDA and MPO in both tissues after 2 but not 1 hour of one-lung collapse. Hepatic leakage enzymes, alanine aminotransferase (ALT), and aspartate aminotransferase (AST) were also increased with the 2-hour collapse.

A number of studies in humans have evaluated the effect of different anesthetics on these responses. Propofol is supposed to have some ability to attenuate the production of ROS, and its molecular structure is somewhat similar to α-tocopherol (vitamin E), which is a well-known antioxidant.[24,25] However, despite this effect on ROS,[25] human studies show that the production of cytokines and the effect on the alveolar leukocytes seem to be less pronounced with the inhalants than with propofol.[22,26] In a rabbit study, propofol caused a lower increase in pulmonary cytokines than midazolam, but inhalant anesthesia was not tested in this study.[27]

Another factor that may decrease the inflammatory response is hypercapnic acidosis (HCA). In a number of animal studies, HCA has been shown to decrease neutrophil endothelial cell adhesion,[28] decrease nuclear factor-κβ,[29] decrease release of TNF-α from alveolar macrophages,[30] inhibit production of xanthine oxidase and thereby reduce free radical production,[31] decrease IL-8 production,[32] decrease nitric oxide release, and inhibit production of nitric oxide synthase.[33] In acute lung injury, HCA has provided some protection[30] and improved survival times in humans.[34] In contrast to these studies, HCA did not change the outcome in a ventilator-induced lung injury[35] and caused injury to alveolar epithelial cells in vitro.[36]

A number of individual studies have looked at methods of attenuating the inflammatory response, but these methods do not appear to have been adopted widely. Corticosteroids have been applied systemically (methylprednisolone) and by inhalation (budesonide) to reduce the inflammatory response and improve lung function.[19,37,38] Simvastatin treatment has also been shown to decrease some of the inflammatory markers associated with one-lung anesthesia.[39] The release of cytokines was also reduced if continuous positive airway pressure (CPAP) (5 cm H_2O) was applied to the collapsed lung using oxygen.[19] It should be recognized that this approach may decrease surgical exposure, and even during the study, the CPAP had to be removed in a number of patients to improve visibility.

Ventilation

In recent years, there has been further emphasis on the injury that can occur with excessive ventilation of the lungs.[40] This can be divided into injury caused by excessive volume, or volutrauma; injury associated with atelectasis, or atelectrauma; and injury associated with ROS caused by hyperoxemia.

Volutrauma

That volume, and not pressure, was the major factor was illustrated in an experiment in which the expansion of the lungs was limited by external binding and showing that despite high airway pressures, no injury ensued, compared with allowing a large volume to be delivered with unrestricted expansion, which resulted in injury.[41] This has led to the use of low tidal volumes and higher breathing rates in order to provide "lung-protective" ventilation. Such a strategy has been applied in humans during surgery and appears to be associated with less inflammatory response[42] and lower postoperative pulmonary complications.[43] In humans, the low tidal volume used is usually around 6 mL/kg. Using allometric scaling values, the normal resting tidal volume for the dog would be of the order of 8 to 10 mL/kg.[44] This would require respiratory rates of 25 to 70 breaths/min, with the higher rates being applied to smaller patients, to achieve normal minute ventilation.[45]

Atelectrauma

With current practices of using very high inspired concentrations of oxygen, it is common to see atelectasis in dogs and cats after relatively short periods of anesthesia.[46,47] These areas of atelectasis create shear forces between the inflated and uninflated lung that can

lead to tissue damage. This is exacerbated by the repeated cycling that is inherent to typical intermittent positive-pressure ventilation (IPPV). In conjunction with this, because the atelectatic areas are not expanding, the aerated parts of the lung will expand to a greater extent than normal, and this could lead to volutrauma in those regions. The management of this situation is to try to prevent the formation of atelectasis and to minimize ongoing airway collapse. The first approach is to apply positive end-expiratory pressure (PEEP) to the lung to prevent airway collapse.[47,48] It has been shown that even when high tidal volumes are used, the addition of PEEP decreases pulmonary injury.[41] As PEEP is increased, it transmits pressure to the thoracic cavity, and this decreases venous return in a pressure-dependent manner.[49] If venous return is decreased, then cardiac output and oxygen delivery to the tissues will be decreased. At a PEEP of 5 cm H_2O cardiac output is reduced marginally, but at 20 cm H_2O, it is decreased by nearly 50% in dogs.[49] It is also thought that PEEP may have an effect on ventricular distensibility, further limiting cardiac output.[50] However, if the PEEP improves uptake of oxygen by decreasing atelectasis, it may improve oxygen delivery despite the reduced cardiac output. This has led to the concept of ideal PEEP whereby oxygen delivery is measured (cardiac output x oxygen content of blood) as PEEP is increased in a stepwise manner. The point at which oxygen delivery is maximized is the ideal PEEP under those particular conditions. Because it is not routine, in a clinical environment, to measure cardiac output, it would be difficult to make this titration. However, a correlation has been found for the difference between end-tidal (PE′CO_2) and arterial CO_2 (PaCO_2) tensions such that the point of lowest difference corresponds to "ideal" PEEP for that animal. This could be achieved by stepwise increases in PEEP and the measurement of serial blood gases at each step to compare the values for PaCO_2 with PE′CO_2.[51] This approach may not work well when significant pulmonary pathology is present.

The second approach is to reduce the inspired oxygen concentration ($F_I O_2$) such that there is an insoluble gas, such as nitrogen, in the alveoli and lower airways that will not get absorbed and thus prevent absorption atelectasis. This is a really important factor because the combination of small tidal volumes and high $F_I O_2$s fosters absorption atelectasis. The addition of a nitrogen "splint" helps to reduce the likelihood of atelectasis. This has been demonstrated in both dogs and cats using an $F_I O_2$ of 0.4 and looking for areas of atelectasis with computed tomography (CT).[46,52] When doing procedures on animals when only one lung is being ventilated, there is invariably a decrease in the PaO_2.[53-55] If the lung that is being ventilated has some pathology, then this decrease will be greater, and it may be very difficult to decrease the $F_I O_2$ and maintain adequate oxygen delivery. Ideally, the animal should not be exposed to pure oxygen so that some nitrogen is maintained in the lung, but this is often unavoidable if hypoxemia is to be prevented during the manipulations required to isolate the lungs. If the animal has been exposed to pure oxygen, it may be necessary to apply a recruitment maneuver to minimize atelectasis. This term is very vaguely defined in the literature but essentially involves applying high pressures to the lung for a defined period of time. To sustain the opening of the airways, it is best if the recruitment maneuver is followed by the application of PEEP, a reduction in the $F_I O_2$, or both. In the past, many anesthesiologists have "sighed" patients by applying a 15- to 25-cm H_2O pressure for one breath every 5 to 10 minutes. This "recruitment" maneuver appears to be ineffective, and pressures of about 35 to 50 cm H_2O held for 20 to 60 seconds are needed to open the lung.[48,56] This may depend on the individual characteristic of the lung, but this author suggests starting with 40 cm H_2O held for 20 to 30 seconds.[48] This should be followed by a PEEP of at least 5 cm H_2O.

Anesthesia

These patients should be worked up in routine fashion with further testing appropriate for the signs shown. If cardiac signs are part of the clinical picture, it may be best to do an echocardiogram to fully define the lesion before anesthesia. This will allow the anesthetist to make appropriate choices for the condition involved. Ideally, a baseline arterial blood gas (ABG) analysis should be obtained to define any limitations to gas exchange, although this is not always possible.

Given the information provided, it appears that the drugs used for premedication and induction are not greatly important, although higher doses of both opioids and α_2 agonists may be associated with increased pulmonary arterial pressures that could decrease HPV.[57,58] For the maintenance of anesthesia, a technique using an inhalant in combination with adjuncts such as opioids, ketamine, or lidocaine would seem to be prudent to limit the effect of the inhalant dose on HPV. Pretreating the patient with a corticosteroid may be beneficial, but clinical evidence for this is currently lacking. After the animal is endotracheally intubated, it should be started on a gas mixture with an F_1O_2 of 0.4 and IPPV instituted with PEEP to minimize atelectasis. The F_1O_2 can be titrated to achieve adequate oxygenation while trying to limit the exposure to F_1O_2s less than 0.9. The information presented earlier suggests that low tidal volumes with higher rates should be used to limit lung injury and aim for hypercapnia rather than eucapnia. However, this strategy has not been proven to be beneficial in a clinical setting,[59] and more work needs to be done to prove the superiority of this approach. It is important that PEEP is used with a low tidal volume strategy because there has been an association reported between low tidal volumes and increased 30-day mortality rates in humans when minimal PEEP was used.[60]

Monitoring

These patients need to be monitored intensively because of the risks of hypoxemia resulting from the initial disease and the significant reduction in pulmonary exchange area associated with the isolation of each lung.

Pulse Oximetry

This is a noninvasive continuous monitor that estimates the saturation of arterial hemoglobin (SpO_2). It is an essential monitor for these cases because of the significant risk of desaturation associated with OLV. The reliability of these monitors is still not ideal in that they often give readings that are inaccurate, but in these cases, a low SpO_2 reading should not be disregarded with a supposition that it is just an erroneous reading.

Capnography

The capnograph is also a noninvasive continuous monitor that provides essential information about the state of ventilation ($PECO_2$) and can also provide information about the circulation (e.g., sudden decrease in cardiac output) and the equipment being used (rebreathing indicated by a rise in inspired CO_2). In conjunction with the measurement of $PaCO_2$, it may also be used to optimize the ventilation strategy being used (see earlier).

Arterial Blood Pressure

Ideally, for these cases, this should be measured directly with the placement of an arterial catheter. This then provides a continuous measurement, allowing the anesthetist to see and respond to rapid changes in circulation.

With any intrathoracic procedure, there is a risk of manual compression or puncture of large vessels with a resulting sudden decrease in blood pressure. Noninvasive techniques (Doppler or oscillometric) may show such reduced pressures, but because the measurement is intermittent, they may not allow a rapid enough response to prevent serious consequences. A direct arterial line will also allow the measurement of systolic pressure variation (SPV) that is an indicator of hypovolemia. With the low tidal volume approach advocated earlier, the SPV has been shown to be predictive of fluid responsiveness.[61] It is recognized that placing an arterial catheter is not feasible in all patients, so the most appropriate noninvasive technique should be used for these animals.

Electrocardiography

Electrocardiography is continuous and noninvasive and is the only monitor that allows the diagnosis of arrhythmias. Manual stimulation of the heart during surgery may precipitate an arrhythmia, and it will be beneficial to the patient if this can be accurately and immediately diagnosed and managed appropriately.

Blood Gases

Although a pulse oximeter does provide a gross estimate of desaturation, if it occurs, it does not allow the accurate titration of F_1O_2 that is beneficial for these cases. Ideally, ABG analysis should be obtained from the catheter placed to measure blood pressure. This will provide the best information with regard to changes in oxygenation occurring with the onset of OLV. In dogs, it is well established that lingual venous samples can be used to approximate arterial values,[62] if an arterial line cannot be placed. However, the relationship between lingual venous and arterial PaO_2 is not reliable on an individual sample, so this is not an ideal approach for these cases.

Spirometry

Several monitors now provide the capability of measuring flow and pressure of the gases during ventilation, allowing the machine to provide integrated outputs of pressure–volume and flow–volume loops and make calculations of compliance and resistance. These loops are helpful in looking at immediate changes in airway dynamics and in monitoring the expected changes in compliance associated with OLV. Such monitors usually have a function that allows a loop to be captured and remain visible on the screen. It is helpful to do this at each stage of the procedure so that changes over time can be compared with the starting point.

Body Temperature

These cases often require imaging before the procedure, during which they may lose heat rapidly. Because hypothermia will decrease the HPV response, it is important to monitor body temperature throughout the procedure and provide external heat to maintain normothermia.

Support

To maintain anesthesia in these patients, it is ideal to have the ability to run a constant-rate infusion, and it is essential to be able to ventilate the animal.

Ventilator

Ideally, the ventilator used for these cases should be volume limited and have a setting to allow PEEP to be added to the ventilation. Being able to use a volume rather than a pressure setting to control tidal volume allows the anesthetist to provide a protective ventilator strategy in order to limit the volutrauma to the lung. A pressure-limited ventilator can also be used in conjunction with spirometry to allow measurement and adjustment of the tidal volume. PEEP can be added in any circumstance by simply submersing the expired limb of the breathing circuit under water to the depth desired for the PEEP (e.g., submersing the tubing 10 cm under water will provide 10 cm H_2O of PEEP). However, it can be difficult to capture the gas from the fluid, so it is much easier if a PEEP valve can be attached to the expired side of the circuit. Such valves come in fixed increments (e.g., 2.5, 5 or 10 cm H_2O) and can either be spring-loaded or use a weighted ball. For the latter, the valve must be kept in the vertical position for the ball to seat properly in its mounting; the spring-loaded valves can be oriented in any direction. The valve must be connected in the direction specified by the manufacturer, or it may cause complete obstruction of the outlet, which could lead to death of the patient. Modern electronic and some older pneumatic ventilators may have a PEEP setting that allows the anesthetist to set an exact value in increments of 1 cm H_2O. This is obviously the most convenient approach because it can be adjusted very rapidly as determined by the clinical needs of the patient. If a recruitment maneuver is required, it usually needs to be done manually, so it is helpful if the ventilator can be switched in and out of the circuit rapidly.

Anesthetic Machine

Most machines provide the essentials of a variable flow of oxygen and a precision vaporizer to deliver the anesthetic. For these cases, it is also helpful to be able to vary the F_1O_2, so the addition of a compressed air source, an air flowmeter, and a method to measure the resulting concentration of oxygen in the mixture would be useful.

One-Lung Ventilation

The requirement with thoracoscopic surgery is to be able to view the lesion and to have enough space that surgical manipulation can be carried out. In a procedure carried out in lateral recumbency, it may be sufficient to block the airway to the nondependent lung and ventilate the dependent lung. For procedures carried out in dorsal recumbency, it may be best to be able to ventilate one side or the other depending on surgical requirements. These differences give rise to the two basic approaches to isolating the lung: block one bronchus with a balloon tipped catheter or use a double-lumen tube to separate the ability to ventilate one side or the other. The use of bronchial blockers appears to be associated with a lower incidence of sore throat after use in humans.[63] In patients with fluid-filled masses in their pulmonary tissue, isolation of the lung is imperative before surgery to prevent that fluid (especially if it is pus) from flowing from the surgical site down the airway and into the opposite lung.

Tracheobronchial Dimensions

These are important because the equipment currently available is designed for people. The tracheas of dogs are longer and wider than that humans of similar weight, so the equipment designed for humans is not easily applicable to all of our canine patients. The length of the trachea in a dog has been described by the formula $6.2 \times (BW\ [kg])^{0.4}$ and the diameter as $4.1 \times (BW\ [kg])^{0.39}$,[64] where BW is body weight. However, this does not seem to fit well with dogs at the high and low ends of the spectrum of size, and based on some other measurements,[65] a better formula for tracheal diameter might be $5.1 \times (BW)^{0.34}$. This and further information give the data presented in Table 29-2 for tracheal and bronchial internal

Table 29-2 Tracheal and Bronchial Dimensions in Dogs*

Weight (kg)	Tracheal Diameter (mm)	Left Mainstem Bronchus (mm)	Right Mainstem Bronchus (mm)	Length from Incisors to Carina (cm)
1.0	5.1	3.9	4.6	15.6
5.0	8.8	6.7	8.0	26.9
10.0	11.1	8.5	10.1	34.0
15.0	12.8	9.8	11.6	39.0
20.0	14.1	10.8	12.7	42.9
25.0	15.2	11.7	13.7	46.3
30.0	16.2	12.4	14.6	49.2
35.0	17.0	13.1	15.4	51.9
40.0	17.8	13.7	16.1	54.3
45.0	18.6	14.2	16.8	56.5
50.0	19.2	14.7	17.4	58.5
55.0	19.9	15.2	18.0	60.4
60.0	20.5	15.7	18.5	62.2
65.0	21.0	16.1	19.0	63.9
70.0	21.6	16.5	19.5	65.5
75.0	22.1	16.9	20.0	67.1
80.0	22.6	17.3	20.4	68.6
85.0	23.1	17.7	20.8	70.0
90.0	23.5	18.0	21.2	71.3
95.0	23.9	18.3	21.6	72.7
100.0	24.4	18.7	22.0	73.9

*Based on the formulas:
Diameter = $5.09 \times$ body weight $(kg)^{0.39}$
Left mainstem bronchus length = $3.9 \times$ body weight $(kg)^{0.34}$
Right mainstem bronchus length = $4.6 \times$ body weight $(kg)^{0.34}$
Tracheal length from the incisors to the carina = $15.631 \times$ body weight $(kg)^{0.3374}$

diameters and length related to weight. The lengths presented from the incisors to the carina were measured by the author from CT scans of dogs weighing 2.6 to 44 kg. There may be significant variations in these values between breeds. English Bulldogs are the most likely to have a much smaller airway than expected for their weight. In cats and small dogs, the airway is small enough that it is very difficult to use standard approaches developed for humans. There are currently no double-lumen endotracheal tubes (DLTs) available for these small patients, so the bronchial blockers or selective intubation of one bronchus with a standard endotracheal tubes (ETT) are the only choices.

Endobronchial Blockers

Fogarty Catheter (Edwards Lifesciences Corp., Irvine, CA) (Figure 29-1)

This catheter was developed as an embolectomy device to help remove clots from vessels. It is a balloon-tipped catheter and can be placed in a mainstem bronchus and the balloon inflated to occlude the airway. These have largely been supplanted by the Arndt bronchial blocker but may still be used in larger dogs because they are manufactured in lengths up to 120 cm.

Arndt Endobronchial Blocker (Cook Medical Inc. Bloomington, IN) (Figure 29-2)

This is an advance on the Fogarty catheter because it was designed specifically for OLV. These are available in 5-, 7-, and 9-French sizes that are 50, 65, and 78 cm in length, respectively. For the 9-French catheters, there are two balloon types, an elliptical and a round balloon. In humans, the round balloon is used for the right bronchus and the elliptical one for the left bronchus. In dogs, neither shaped balloon will spare the blockade of the right apical lobe if the balloon is placed in the right bronchus. The elliptical balloon has been less likely to back out of the bronchus in our hands. These catheters come with a loop of nylon that runs down the central channel of the catheter. This loop is used to snare the endoscope to assist with placement of the blocker. The best way to do this is to pass the fiberoptic bronchoscope (FOB) and blocker through the adapter and pass the loop over the FOB before attaching the adapter to the ETT

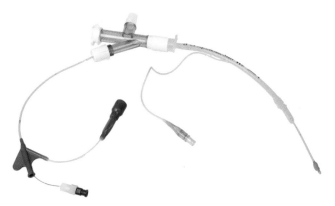

Figure 29-2   Arndt endobronchial blocker. The loop in the distal end has been withdrawn so the end hole of the catheter is exposed. The endobronchial blocker has been passed through the side arm of the adapter and is shown passing through an endotracheal tube. The endoscope would be advanced through the straight part of the adapter and the breathing circuit attached to the side port. After the endobronchial blocker was in place, the cap on the adapter would be tightened to seal the port around the catheter.

(Figure 29-3); this is much easier than trying to snare the FOB inside the adapter with everything connected. The FOB is then advanced into the relevant bronchus, and then the loop is loosened and the blocker slid off the end of the FOB into that bronchus (Figure 29-4). The FOB is then withdrawn into the trachea, the blocker is positioned, and the balloon inflated using the FOB to confirm its location (Figure 29-5). The cap on the adapter is then tightened, closing the silicone plug around the catheter, thus locking the catheter in place and creating a seal around it at the adapter. The loop of the Arndt blocker should also be withdrawn so that it does not get incorporated into the surgical site.[66] The FOB can now be removed, but it is best to keep it nearby until the end of the procedure so that it can be used again if the catheter needs to be replaced. In human studies, the endobronchial blockers are more likely to be displaced during surgery than double-lumen endotracheal tubes (DLTs) with prevalences

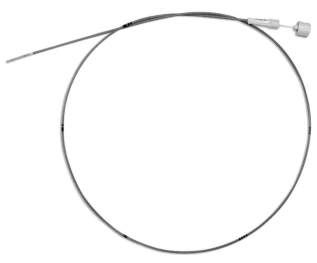

Figure 29-1 Fogarty catheter with a catheter-tipped balloon and a lockable inflation port.

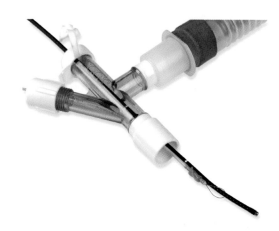

Figure 29-3 Arndt endobronchial blocker showing the endoscope passed though its port and the loop from the Arndt endobronchial blocker passed over the endoscope and tightened on to it (arrow). This is best done before attaching it to the endotracheal tube.

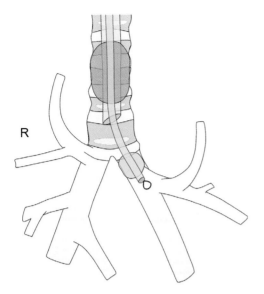

Figure 29-4 Diagram of the placement of the endobronchial blocker. The balloon is placed in the left mainstem bronchus in this diagram, so the left lung would be collapsed and the right lung ventilated.

of 30% to 100%.[67,68] Collapse of the lung takes longer using a blocker than a DLT, and in humans, it is much more likely that the anesthetist will have to apply suction to collapse the lung. If the lung does not need to be fully collapsed, then CPAP can be applied to the lung using a flowmeter and CPAP valve. At the end of the procedure, the bronchial blocker can be deflated and the catheter pulled back into the adapter, but it is better not to try to remove it completely because it will be difficult to then create a seal without removing the whole adapter, and there is a case report of the balloon being torn and pieces of the balloon passing into the ETT.[69] The use of the Arndt blocker has been reported in a few dogs undergoing thoracoscopy for persistent right aortic arch (3.7 kg) and pericardial fenestration (24 kg).[70,71]

If the airway is too small to allow the passage of the FOB and the catheter at the same time, it may be feasible to pass the catheter down the side of the ETT. This is achieved by placing the catheter in the airway before the ETT is introduced. Having this tube in between the tracheal wall and the endotracheal cuff may

make it difficult to achieve a sealed airway. It may also be necessary to deflate the cuff at the time the blocker is being advanced into a bronchus to make the catheter slide more easily. When the cuff is reinflated, it will help to hold the catheter in place. In a study performed by the authors' group in cats, because there is no space to pass the FOB through the ETT, we administered a propofol infusion and provided high-frequency (3-Hz) jet ventilation with oxygen.[72] We loaded an ETT onto the blocker (5 French) and then inserted the blocker into the airway. This was followed by the FOB, and that was then used to guide the blocker into the relevant bronchus. The FOB can then be used to place the blocker correctly, or the FOB can be removed and the ETT slid over the blocker into the trachea. If the latter method is used, it is important to advance the catheter deep into that bronchus to avoid getting it displaced during intubation. Under thoracoscopic guidance (observing differential lung ventilation in the thorax), the balloon on the blocker can be inflated and withdrawn until none of the lung on that side of the animal is inflating. To ensure that all lung lobes in both hemithoraces are visible, it is necessary to break down the mediastinal attachments to the sternum to allow inspection of the contralateral hemithorax. In our study, we had difficulty maintaining adequate oxygenation when the right lung was blocked despite increasing CPAP and tidal volumes, and in one cat, we could not achieve stable oxygenation when blocking either side.

Cohen Blocker (Cook Medical Inc. Bloomington, IN) (Figure 29-6A)

This device has a wire down the middle and a wheel on the proximal end that can be used to tighten the wire such that a bend is created at the distal end of the catheter. This is engineered so that it will only displace in one direction, so locating the blocker into the correct bronchus depends on tightening the wire to create the bend and then twisting the catheter until it is oriented toward the relevant bronchus. It is then advanced into the opening using FOB guidance. In a trial using this blocker, it took about the same length of time to set it into the right location as the Arndt device, but it displaced less often.[68] It also provided better lung collapse, possibly because the distal end of the catheter has multiple holes rather than just one in the Arndt. A major disadvantage for this catheter in veterinary patients is that it is only supplied as a 9-French, 65-cm catheter.

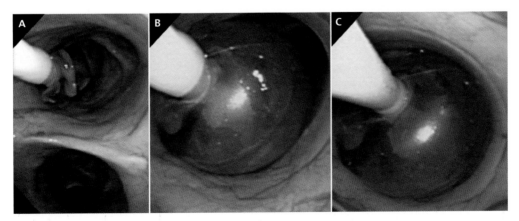

Figure 29-5 **A**, End of the endobronchial blocker placed in the left mainstem bronchus. **B**, Partial inflation of the balloon; note that one can still see beyond the balloon into the bronchus. **C**, Full inflation of the balloon, creating airway occlusion.

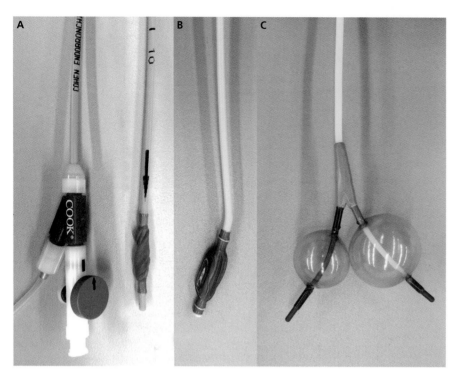

Figure 29-6 **A**, Cohen endobronchial blocker showing the wheel at the proximal end that can be used to bend the distal end of the catheter to facilitate placement. **B**, Coopdech endobronchial blocker showing the angled end of the catheter. **C**, E-Z blocker showing the two arms at the end of the catheter. Only one of the balloons would be inflated at a time in a patient.

Coopdech Blocker (Daiken Medical Co., Osaka, Japan) (Figure 29-6B)

This is similar to the Cohen blocker except that the bend at the end of the catheter is preformed, and there is no wire to control the amount of bend.

E-Z Blocker (Teleflex Medical Inc., Research Triangle Park, NC) (Figure 29-6C)

This catheter has a fork at the distal end with a balloon on each side. The catheter is advanced into the airway such that one side of the catheter is in each major bronchus. This allows the anesthetist to block one side or the other as needed for the surgery. It also means that one side could be blocked for surgery on that side, and then the balloon could be deflated, the lung reexpanded, and the opposite side blocked without having to reposition the catheter. Each of the ends has a central lumen, so gas can be removed from the lung or PEEP or CPAP can be applied to the lung as needed. This catheter is only supplied as a 75-cm, 7-French version.

Univent and Fuji Uniblockers (Fuji Systems Corp.,Tokyo, Japan) (Figure 29-7)

The Univent tubes are ETTs that have a separate lumen for a endo bronchial blocker, which comes as part of the tube. The blocker is similar to the Coopdech version in that it has a preformed bend at the end of the catheter, allowing it to be directed to one side or the other by twisting the proximal end of the blocker. The tubes are supplied as 6-to-9 mm inner diameter (ID) tubes in 0.5-mm increments, so they can be useful for dogs in the 15- to 25-kg range. There are also a 3-mm ID uncuffed version and a 4.5-mm cuffed tube (but no 5- or 5.5-mm ID tubes). The bronchial blockers that are supplied with these two smaller sizes do not have end holes, so they do not allow for lung collapse after the balloon is inflated. The Univent tubes are slightly oval in cross-section so that the outside diameter is slightly greater than that of a comparable regular ETT

(Table 29-3). The endo bronchial blockers that the company (Uniblocker) produces come in 5- and 9-French sizes that are 30 and 51 cm in length, respectively. This makes these catheters rather short for dogs, and even with the longer version, it can be hard to get the catheter into place. Because of the D shape of the internal lumen of the ET, a smaller FOB is needed to be able to visualize the tip of the catheter in the bronchus. The construction of the tube also means that for an equivalent external diameter, the tube has a much higher resistance to airflow than either a regular ETT or a DLT.[73]

To place a Univent tube, the wires within the tube and blocker should be removed first. The cuffs on both the tube and the blocker should be checked for leaks and then fully deflated. The blocker should be pulled back into the channel within the ETT before it is inserted into the patient. As the ETT is advanced into the patient, the distal tip of the tube should be at least 2 to 3 cm

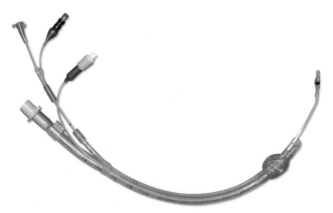

Figure 29-7 Univent endotracheal tube with incorporated endobronchial blocker. Note the angled distal end of the endobronchial blocker to assist with placement.

Table 29-3 Comparison of Univent Tubes with Regular Endotracheal Tubes

Univent or Portex ETT ID	Maximum Univent OD	Portex ETT OD	Equivalent French Size to Univent	Maximum FOB diameter (mm)
>3 uncuffed				
4.5				3.6
6	11.5	8.2	36	3.6
6.5	12	8.8	38	3.6
7	12.5	9.6	39	3.8
7.5	13	10.2	41	4.2
8	13.5	11.0	42	5.0
8.5	14	11.6	44	5.0
9	14.5	12.2	46	5.5

ETT, endotracheal tube; ID, inner diameter; OD, outside diameter.

above the carina to allow enough room for the placement of the blocker. An adapter can then be attached to the proximal end of the ETT to allow passage of an FOB while maintaining connection to the breathing circuit. After the FOB is in place and the anatomic landmarks identified, the endo bronchial blocker is advanced into the appropriate bronchus. If rotation of the blocker does not allow for the correct angle, it may be helpful to rotate the ETT to place the channel on the same side as the bronchus to be blocked. When the blocker is in the correct location, the balloon can be inflated and visually inspected before the FOB is removed. The cuffs on these blockers are high-pressure, low-volume cuffs, and the measured internal cuff pressures measured using a model bronchus were more than 120 mm Hg, but the contact pressure after just sealing the cuff was less than 5 mm Hg in all tests.[74] A study in dogs (23 ± 6 kg) using the Univent blocker to block the left main bronchus showed a significant decrease in PaO_2. The dogs were ventilated with a tidal volume of 10 mL/kg on 98% oxygen, and the respiratory rate was increased to try to control $PaCO_2$. PaO_2 decreased from about 360 to 190 mm Hg, but the cardiac index did not change, so it is unlikely that there was a decrease in oxygen delivery.[53]

Troubleshooting Positional Problems with Endobronchial Blockers

No matter which endobronchial blocking device is used, all have the potential to be placed incorrectly or to move out of their correct position because of motion and traction on the device during patient repositioning or traction on tissues during the procedure. Ideally, blockers should be placed after final positioning of the patient on the surgical table because subsequent repositioning will invariably lead to tube movement.[1] During initial placement, several common problems are seen. Incomplete filling of the balloon, resulting in residual partial ventilation of the blocked lung, is common and can be easily detected thoracoscopically. Increasing the amount of air in the balloon will usually resolve this problem. Prolapse of the balloon into the trachea during placement can also occur because of the challenging nature of resting the balloon in the short space aborad to the carina but orad to the cranial lobar bronchus in dogs and cats. This is especially common in smaller patients, where this space is very limited. During the procedure, prolapse of the blocker into the trachea can also occur. This usually has the effect of causing acute airway obstruction and must be noticed immediately. In some cases, placement of the blocker into the incorrect bronchus will have the effect of blocking the incorrect hemithorax. Both of these latter complications can be remedied by repositioning of the tube with the help of the FOB.

Double-Lumen Endotracheal Tubes

These are made by a variety of different companies and have slightly different conformations and types. Tubes that have been "named" include the Carlens, Robertshaw (Portex, Keene, NH; Rüsch, Teleflex Medical, Research Triangle Park, NC), and White tubes, and then there are different manufacturers with the Sher-I-Bronch, (Teleflex Medical Inc., Research Triangle Park, NC), Broncho-Cath (Covidien Inc., Mansfield, MA), and Silbroncho (Teleflex Medical Inc., Research Triangle Park, NC) tubes. Some of these come in right- and left sided conformations to manage the difference between the left and right mainstem bronchi (Figure 29-8). All of them consist of two D-shaped tubes welded together with one tube being longer than the other. The longer tube is expected to sit in the bronchus and has a cuff very near the end of the tube (see Figure 29-8). The second tube is designed to end in the trachea and usually has a beveled end with a cuff proximal to the opening that, when inflated, will seal against the trachea. The proximal ends of the tubes and the cuffs are color coded so that the respective end can be

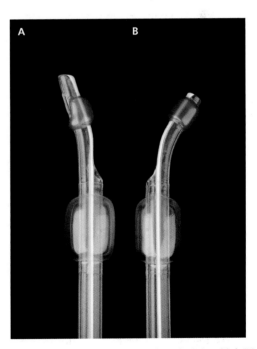

Figure 29-8 Double-lumen tubes showing the right (A) and left (B) bronchial blockers. The tube on the left has a horseshoeshaped balloon and slit to allow for the right apical bronchus.

identified. Each tube can be attached to the breathing circuit separately or an adapter can be added that joins them together.

Carlens

This was the first tube described and was only designed to be placed in the left mainstem bronchus. It has a spur above the bronchial tube that is designed to engage the carina and prevent the tube being advanced too far.

Dr. White

This is effectively the right-sided version of the Carlens tube. It has a cuff that is circumferential proximally but continues down the medial side of the tube to seal the bronchus without blocking the opening to the cranial lobe bronchus. It also has a spur to help with placement.

Robertshaw[75]

There are right- and left-sided Robertshaw tubes (Portex, Keene, NH; Rüsch, Teleflex Medical, Research Triangle Park, NC) with cuffs that are similarly designed to the above. The right-sided version has an end and side hole in the bronchial tube. The bronchial parts of these tubes are angled at their distal ends with the right one being at 20 degrees and the left at 40 degrees to the main axis. Both left- and right-sided versions have a slight bevel on the end of the bronchial tube to facilitate insertion through the larynx. There is no spur on these tubes. They are manufactured in 28- to 41-French sizes. The Portex version (Figure 29-9) has the longest useable length, but it also has the longest cuff on the bronchial tube and the longest distance from the top of the cuff to the end of the tube, making it more difficult to place without partially blocking off more of the left lung. The Rüsch version has a short cuff and a shorter distance from the cuff to the end of the tube (Table 29-4).

Sher-I-Bronch (Sheridan)

The right-sided version of this has two cuffs and an opening in the side and at the end of the bronchial lumen. The bronchial tube in the left sided version is at 34 degrees to the axis. It is made in 28- to 41-French sizes. The cuff length and the distance from the cuff to the end of the tube are intermediate (see Figure 29-9 and Table 29-4).

Broncho-Cath (Mallinckrodt)

The right-sided version of this has an S-shaped cuff and a slot in the tube that is supposed to open to the right cranial lobe bronchus. There is no bevel on the end of the right-sided bronchial

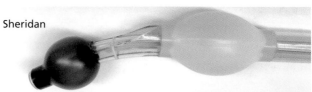

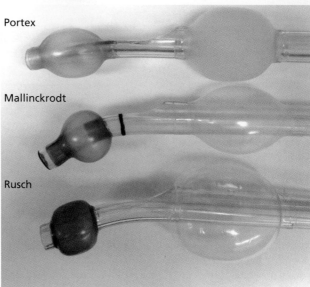

Figure 29-9 Robertshaw double-lumen endotracheal tubes from four different manufacturers. Note the relative sizes of the upper and lower balloons (blue).

segment. The left-sided version has a bronchial tube at an angle of 45 degrees to the axis, and there is a bevel on this segment. It is available in 28- to 41-French sizes and can be purchased with or without a carinal hook. The cuff length and the distance from the cuff to the end of the tube are intermediate (see Figure 29-9 and Table 29-4).

Silbroncho (Fuji)

Whereas the other tubes are all made of polyvinyl chloride (PVC), this version is made of silicone. It has a wire-reinforced bronchial component, making it easy to see on radiographs. It is made in right and left versions, and the bronchial tube of the left-sided version is beveled. The balloon on the right-sided version is S shaped, and there is a slot in the side of the tube for the right cranial lobe. The ODs are measured in millimeters.

Table 29-4 Details of Left Double-Lumen Tubes

Manufacturer	Material	Size range (French)	ID range (mm)	OD (mm)	Bronchial Part OD (mm)	Bronchial Cuff Length (mm)*	Distance from Top of Left Bronchial Cuff to End of Left-Sided Tube (mm)	Useable Length from Upper Amalgamation of the Tubes to the Top of the Cuff (cm)
Portex	PVC	28–41		9–13	9.8–11.7*	23–30	35	36.5
Rusch	PVC	26–41		9–13	9.4–11.5*†	14–21	32†	31
Mallinckrodt	PVC	28–41		9–13	7.5–10.6†	12–21	29†	29
Sheridan	PVC	28–41		9–13	8.5–10.7†	22–23	30†	
Fuji	Silicone	33–39	4.1–5.3‡	12.3–15.3	10.8–12‡	13‡	18.8–19.3‡	

*35- to 41-French sizes only.
†Benumof et al.[103]
‡Lohser and Brodsky.[77]
ETT, endotracheal tube; ID, inner diameter; OD, outer diameter; PVC, polyvinyl chloride.

In tests on some of these tubes, there seemed to be considerable variation in the lengths and diameters of the bronchial segments, and as can be seen from Table 29-4, the relative size of the bronchial tube may not change much relative to the overall size of the tube.[76,77] These tubes have the shortest distance from the top of the cuff to the end of the tube (see Table 29-4).

All of these DLTs are manufactured for use in humans; consequently, they are not entirely appropriate for dogs and cats. In dogs, the right cranial lobe bronchus is almost invariably above the carina. In most canine CT images, the right cranial lobe bronchus appears before the septum at the bifurcation of the trachea as one scrolls back through tracheal cross-sections. Hence, the right-sided endobronchial tubes do not work well because the cuff will almost invariably block the entrance to this lobe when the cuff is inflated. The lengths of the primary bronchi are also shorter than in humans (the left main bronchus is about 50% as long as in humans with equivalent sizes), so any tube beyond the cuff may get lodged in another bronchus and isolate more lung than expected. In humans, the margin of safety for placement of a DLT is defined as the distance between the end of the tube and the first bronchial branch when the top of the cuff is at the carina. This means that, as seen in the numbers in Tables 29-2, the length of the canine left mainstem bronchus is always shorter than the distance from the top of the cuff to the end of the tube. Last, the length of the mouth and trachea together seem to be comparatively longer in dogs, so these DLTs are generally suitable only in dogs weighing less than 30 kg. In medium-sized dogs, there seemed to be no advantage to the presence of the carinal hook on the Carlens and Dr. White tubes, and the Robertshaw was placed with the most accuracy.[78]

We have used the left-sided Robertshaw tubes in our practice, and our usual approach is to intubate with a radiolucent ETT first if the animal requires a CT scan or radiographs. When the animal is ready for surgery or no imaging is required, the DLT would be placed into the trachea but not advanced to the carina. The tracheal balloon would be inflated as for a normal ETT until any leak ceased. The two tubes would be joined together at the proximal end, and the animal would breathe from a single circuit (Figure 29-10). After the animal has been positioned for surgery, an adapter would be attached to the tracheal tube and the circuit reattached while an FOB is advanced into the airway. The tracheal balloon may be deflated for repositioning the tube, but this is not essential if the cuff has just been inflated to stop the leak. After the left bronchus

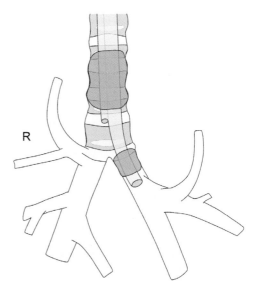

Figure 29-11 Diagram showing the placement of the proximal and distal balloons in the trachea and left mainstem bornchus, respectively.

has been identified, the tube is advanced until the bronchial part of the tube is well seated in the left bronchus. While the surgeon is still observing with the FOB, the cuff is inflated and the position adjusted if necessary as judged by visual inspection (Figure 29-11). The seal on the cuff can be confirmed as below or the surgeon can observe the inflation of the lungs on either side. The circuit can then be attached to one side, and the other side can be allowed to collapse. If it does not interfere with the surgery, a CPAP valve can be applied to the collapsed lung with 50% to 100% oxygen to improve the effective exchange area and decrease the chance of reinflation injury later. The single lung should be ventilated as discussed earlier, and end-tidal CO_2 and arterial hemoglobin saturation (SpO_2) should be monitored carefully for signs of poor ventilation or desaturation. Thoracoscopy may entail the use of CO_2 insufflation to push the lung out of the way. The start of insufflation may be accompanied by a sudden increase in $PECO_2$. At the end of the procedure, some people will remove the Robertshaw tube and replace it with a regular ETT just to ensure that extubation is not made more difficult with the DLT. The success of placement of either a DLT or bronchial blocker is definitely related to experience. In a study in humans using senior residents or faculty who used fewer than two lung isolation techniques per month, the failure rate was greater than 30%, and success was related to the anesthesiologist's knowledge of bronchoscopic anatomy.[79]

There are few reports of the use of DLT in clinical cases in dogs, but they have been reported for the removal of thymomas, primary lung tumors, a lung bulla, and for pericardectomy.[72,80-82] In the seven dogs undergoing pericardectomy, the DLT was used to provide ventilation of one side or the other depending on surgical need, and there were problems with tube placement in four of seven dogs.[81] The recorded PaO_2 values were lower when the right lung was being ventilated compared with the left, which is expected in dogs, given the larger volume of the right lung. In the two dogs with thymoma, one case was fairly uneventful, but the second dog had a low PaO_2 before the onset of OLV and became hypoxemic even with the use of 98% oxygen and 2 to 4 cm H_2O PEEP. In the primary lung tumor series, 10 of 22 dogs were intubated with a DLT, and a number of patients had complications related to placement or displacement of the DLT.[72]

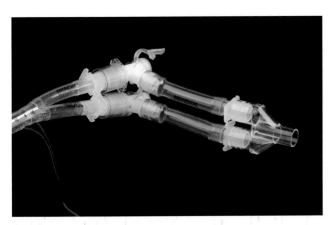

Figure 29-10 Proximal end of a Robertshaw tube with a connector to allow both sides of the tube to be attached to a single circuit. This picture also shows the ports to allow the passage of an endoscope.

Methods Used to Confirm a Seal on a Bronchial Blocker or Double-Lumen Tube

- Visual inspection: During the inflation of the cuff under observation with the FOB, one often sees bubbles emanating from around the balloon until the cuff is inflated enough to prevent gas entering that side of the lung and deflating during expiration.
- Positive-pressure test: With bronchial blockers that have an end hole or DLTs, the proximal end is attached to some tubing, the end of which is submerged under about 1 cm of water. As the cuff is being inflated, air will bypass the cuff into the lung, and egress through the bronchial lumen will be seen as bubbles under the water. When the cuff seals, the bubbles stop.[74]
- Negative-pressure test: An ascending bellows ventilator is attached to the circuit, which is attached to the tracheal lumen. Without turning on the ventilator, suction is applied to the bronchial lumen of the blocker or DLT. Before the cuff is inflated, this will result in the bellows descending, but after the cuff is sealed, the bellows will not move. This needs to be done very carefully because the suction with the bronchial blocker may create a negative pressure beyond the balloon and suck the catheter into the lung.[74]
- Ventilator test: This is the same as above, but no negative suction is applied to the bronchial lumen. As soon as the cuff seals the airway, the bellows will no longer descend because the cuff should break the connection between the trachea and the bronchial opening of the DLT or blocker.[74]
- End-tidal CO_2: The capnograph is attached to the bronchial lumen and the trace examined as the cuff is inflated. The cuff is sealed when the capnographic trace is a flat line with no variation. This requires the use of a sidestream capnograph and is not very easy to use because of the delay in the time from sampling to reading.[74]

Troubleshooting Positional Problems with DLTs

During initial placement of DLTs, the most common problem seen is excessively deep positioning of the tube within the bronchus, resulting in lack of blockade of the cranial lobes.[78] This is usually easily remedied by slow withdrawal of the tubes under thoracoscopic visualization. As soon as blockade of the cranial lobes occurs, the tube is assumed to be positioned correctly. Prolapse of the bronchial balloon into the trachea is also common, and similar to the situation with endobronchial blockers, can result in complete airway obstruction in some cases. Placement of the bronchial tip of the tube into the incorrect side can result in reversal of the expected ventilation patterns. On some occasions, it may be possible to proceed with the planned intervention by simply switching the attachment of the circuit from the ventilator to the other lumen of the tube, but in other cases, this may be unsuccessful.

Single-Lumen Bronchial Intubation

In dogs that are too big for the use of conventional bronchial blockers or DLTs, the only other alternative is to use a small ETT and advance it into one bronchus. This is best achieved using an FOB down the ETT and directing the FOB into the required bronchus followed by the ETT. However, this does not allow good estimation of the depth of insertion, and it would be best if the tube is advanced as far as possible, and then the cuff is inflated and the tube withdrawn until ventilation of the lung expands all of that side as gauged by visual inspection through the thoracoscope. It may also be possible to pass the FOB into the trachea and then intubate. The tube can then be manipulated into the correct bronchus and the cuff inflated while this is observed with the FOB. Because this requires very long ETTs, usually only the silicone veterinary tubes will work for this. They are manufactured as 55-cm (22-inch) tubes in sizes 9 to 12 and 14 mm ID. The cuffs on these tubes are quite long, so the ideal position may leave part of the cuff in the trachea. The major disadvantage with this technique is that there is no access to the unventilated lung that may be needed for suction or supply of oxygen.

Changing from Double-Lung Ventilation to One-Lung Ventilation

Ideally, both lungs have been ventilated with an F_IO_2 of 0.5 or less using a volume limited ventilator with tidal volumes of around 7 to 8 mL/kg and a PEEP of about 5 cm H_2O. When the shift is made to ventilating one lung, the tidal volume may be decreased a little (e.g., 5-6 mL/kg) but not decreased to half the original value. As in humans, the right lung is bigger than the left lung, so slightly higher tidal volumes may be used for the right than the left lung. PEEP should be maintained or increased depending on the resulting changes in oxygenation.

Managing Hypoxemia During One-Lung Ventilation

In an animal with normal pulmonary function before OLV, it should be possible to maintain oxyhemoglobin saturations above 90% without too much difficulty. Saturations decreasing below this level are more likely attributable to technique than inherently poor exchange. If the patient has abnormal pulmonary function, as evidenced by low PaO_2s preoperatively or during double-lung ventilation, it may require the use of more aggressive techniques to maintain saturation (see later). The five causes of hypoxia usually described are:

1. Decreased F_IO_2
2. Hypoventilation
3. Diffusion impairment
4. Vascular shunting: a functional or anatomic shunting of blood from the venous to the arterial side bypassing the gas exchange area
5. Ventilation/perfusion mismatch

In using OLV, each of these may play a role and can therefore be treated accordingly.

In this case, if we are ventilating with an F_IO_2 of less than 1, then an easy treatment may be to just increase the F_IO_2 until the hypoxia disappears. This may be a temporary measure while the cause of the hypoxia is investigated.

Hypoventilation will only cause hypoxia directly if the increase in CO_2 reduces the effective alveolar oxygen tension to something that will contribute to the low oxygen tensions. In most circumstances, when the F_IO_2 is greater than 0.5, it would be very difficult to increase $PaCO_2$ enough to cause hypoxia on its own. An F_IO_2 of 0.5 would give an inspired oxygen tension of the order of 355 mm Hg at sea level, so $PaCO_2$ would have to exceed 200 in order to reduce the F_IO_2 to a value less than when the animal was breathing room air. However, when combined with other factors, it certainly may contribute to further reducing PaO_2, and the minute ventilation of the patient may need to be adjusted to decrease $PaCO_2$. The starting F_IO_2 will be affected by altitude because the PAO_2 will decrease at higher elevations. Hypoventilation or low tidal volumes might contribute to atelectasis, especially if the F_IO_2 is close to 1. If there is some airway closure and no reexpansion with the next breath, any oxygen distal to the collapse will be absorbed, leading to atelectasis.

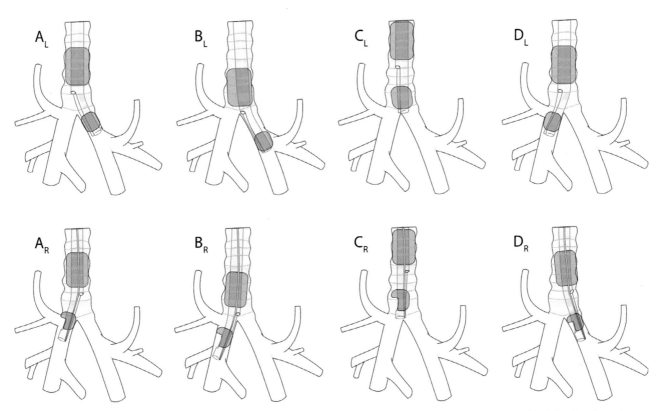

Figure 29-12 Diagram showing correct and incorrect placement of left and right Robertshaw tubes. A_L, Correct placement of the left Robertshaw tube. B_L, Excessively deep placement of the DLT with exclusion of the apical lobe of the left lung. C_L, The bronchial segment has slipped back into the trachea; this may be associated with tracheal occlusion. D_L, Left-sided tube misplaced into the right side. A_R, correct placement of the right Robertshaw tube; B_R, Excessively deep placement of the double-lumen tube with exclusion of the apical lobe of the right lung. In this diagram, the right apical lobe would be ventilated from the tracheal lumen. C_R, The bronchial segment has slipped back into the trachea; this may be associated with tracheal occlusion. D_R, Right-sided tube misplaced into the left side. (From Karzai, W., Schwarzkopf, K. (2009) Hypoxemia during one-lung ventilation: prediction, prevention, and treatment. Anesthesiology 110, 1402-1411.)

This can be treated by using the recruitment maneuver described earlier. Hypoventilation may also be a result of poor positioning of the bronchial tube or blocker. This appears to be the case in a significant proportion of these patients, so further investigation using an FOB or thoracoscopic approach will help to determine if the tube or blocker needs to have its position adjusted (Figure 29-12).[83] As noted earlier, hypoventilation with an accompanying HCA may be beneficial to the patient. This can be achieved by limiting the minute ventilation, adding CO_2 to the inspired gas or the insufflation of CO_2 into the pleural space. Using the latter approach, in a study in children, there were increases in heart rate, cardiac output, and PaO_2 at insufflation pressures over 4 mm Hg, allowing $PaCO_2$ to rise to about 60 mm Hg.[84]

Diffusion impairment is already occurring because only one lung is being ventilated, so we have removed almost half of the diffusion surface by starting OLV. This can be counteracted by providing oxygen to the collapsed lung and applying some pressure (CPAP) to the airway. This may improve oxygenation but may not be tenable for the surgical team, especially in dogs with low thoracic depth-to-width ratios. A CPAP of as little as 3 cm H_2O may provide enough oxygen to the lung to mitigate the hypoxia without expanding the lung excessively and interfering with the surgical field.[85]

Vascular shunting will occur because there is bound to be some flow through the unventilated lung, and it may be worsened if the HPV reflex has been reduced or abolished. At present, there seems to be little clinical evidence for manipulating the anesthetic protocol (see earlier) to minimize the effect on HPV, but the simple reduction of inhalant concentrations by the addition of injectable drugs may help.

Ventilation/perfusion mismatching is again expected with this procedure, but within the lung that is being ventilated, the recruitment and PEEP are helpful to minimize the mismatching that occurs.

Pain Management

It is expected that minimally invasive procedures will decrease the pain associated with surgery.[86] Consequently, these patients may be quite comfortable with the use of an opioid as part of premedication and another dose administered at the end of the procedure in addition to a nonsteroidal antiinflammatory drug administered at the end of the procedure. This author prefers to administer the opioid intramuscularly 10 to 20 minutes before the end of the procedure (depending on the pharmacokinetics of the chosen drug) and typically uses either carprofen or meloxicam administered intravenously. Many patients are hypothermic at the end of a procedure and undergo some sympathetic activation during recovery, both of which may cause dermal vasoconstriction and thus limit the uptake of drugs administered subcutaneously. In one study, the administration of buprenorphine subcutaneously at the end of a procedure provided less analgesia than either intramuscular or intravenous administration.[87] In a study in dogs after ovariohysterectomy, the time to peak plasma concentration of carprofen after subcutaneous administration ranged from 1 to 8 hours, showing the great variation associated with this method of administration.[88]

Local anesthetics infiltrated into the wounds or used as intercostal or paravertebral blocks may also benefit the patient, although no studies in veterinary medicine have examined the efficacy or utility of these approaches. Epidural analgesia is used widely in humans and would be a useful adjunct for some thoracoscopic procedures.

References

1 Lansdowne, J.L., Monnet, E., Twedt, D.C., et al. (2005) Thoracoscopic lung lobectomy for treatment of lung tumors in dogs. Vet Surg 34, 530-535.

2 Mayhew, P.D., Hunt, G.B., Steffey, M.A., et al. (2013a) Evaluation of short-term outcome after lung lobectomy for resection of primary lung tumors via video-assisted thoracoscopic surgery or open thoracotomy in medium- to large-breed dogs. J Am Vet Med Assoc 243, 681-688.

3 Semenza, G.L. (2012) Hypoxia-inducible factors in physiology and medicine. Cell 148, 399-408.

4 Shimoda, L.A., Laurie, S.S. (2014) HIF and pulmonary vascular responses to hypoxia. J Appl Physiol (1985) 116, 867-874.

5 Glasser, S.A., Domino, K.B., Lindgren, L., et al. (1983) Pulmonary blood pressure and flow during atelectasis in the dog. Anesthesiology 58 225-231.

6 Sylvester, J.T., Shimoda, L.A., Aaronson, P.I., et al. (2012) Hypoxic pulmonary vasoconstriction. Physiol Rev 92, 367-520.

7 Vachiery, J.L., Lejeune, P., Hallemans, R., et al. (1990) Atrial natriuretic peptides in canine hypoxic pulmonary vasoconstriction. Cardiovasc Res 24, 352-357.

8 Brimioulle, S., Lejeune, P., Vachiery, J.L., et al. (1994) Stimulus-response curve of hypoxic pulmonary vasoconstriction in intact dogs: effects of ASA. J Appl Physiol (1985) 77, 476-480.

9 Brimioulle, S., Vachiery, J.L., Brichant, J.F., et al. (1997) Sympathetic modulation of hypoxic pulmonary vasoconstriction in intact dogs. Cardiovasc Res 34, 384-392.

10 Kernan, S., Rehman, S., Meyer, T., et al. (2001) Effects of dexmedetomidine on oxygenation during one-lung ventilation for thoracic surgery in adults. J Minim Access Surg 7, 227-231.

11 Gibbs, J.M., Johnson, H. (1978) Lack of effect of morphine and buprenorphine on hypoxic pulmonary vasoconstriction in the isolated perfused cat lung and the perfused lobe of the dog lung. Br J Anaesth 50, 1197-1201.

12 Bjertnaes, L., Hauge, A., Kriz, M. (1980) Hypoxia-induced pulmonary vasoconstriction: effects of fentanyl following different routes of administration. Acta Anaesthesiol Scand 24, 53-57.

13 Bjertnaes, L.J. (1977) Hypoxia-induced vasoconstriction in isolated perfused lungs exposed to injectable or inhalation anesthetics. Acta Anaesthesiol Scand 21, 133-147.

14 Nakayama, M., Murray, P.A. (1999) Ketamine preserves and propofol potentiates hypoxic pulmonary vasoconstriction compared with the conscious state in chronically instrumented dogs. Anesthesiology 91, 760-771.

15 Modolo, N.S., Modolo, M.P., Marton, M.A., et al. (2013) Intravenous versus inhalation anaesthesia for one-lung ventilation. Cochrane Database Syst Rev 7, CD006313.

16 Misthos, P., Katsaragakis, S., Theodorou, D., et al. (2006) The degree of oxidative stress is associated with major adverse effects after lung resection: a prospective study. Eur J Cardiothorac Surg 29, 591-595.

17 Lee, J.J., Kim, G.H., Kim, J.A., et al. (2012) Comparison of pulmonary morbidity using sevoflurane or propofol-remifentanil anesthesia in an Ivor Lewis operation. J Cardiothorac Vasc Anesth 26, 857-862.

18 Wang, L.J., Gu, L.B., Jiang, D.M., et al. (2013) Ketamine inhalation before one-lung ventilation for perioperative lung protection in thoracic surgery patients. Zhonghua Yi Xue Za Zhi 93, 832-836.

19 Verhage, R.J., Boone, J., Rijkers, G.T., et al. (2014) Reduced local immune response with continuous positive airway pressure during one-lung ventilation for oesophagectomy. Br J Anaesth 112, 920-928.

20 Leite, C.F., Calixto, M.C., Toro, I.F., et al. (2012) Characterization of pulmonary and systemic inflammatory responses produced by lung reexpansion after one-lung ventilation. J Cardiothorac Vasc Anesth 26, 427-432.

21 Misthos P, Katsaragakis S, Milingos N., et al. (2005) Postresectional pulmonary oxidative stress in lung cancer patients. The role of one-lung ventilation. Eur J Cardiothorac Surg 27, 379-382 discussion 382-373.

22 Sugasawa, Y., Yamaguchi, K., Kumakura, S., et al. (2012) Effects of sevoflurane and propofol on pulmonary inflammatory responses during lung resection. J Anesth 26, 62-69.

23 Yulug, E., Tekinbas, C., Ulusoy, H., et al. (2007) The effects of oxidative stress on the liver and ileum in rats caused by one-lung ventilation. J Surg Res 139, 253-260.

24 Cheng, Y.J., Wang, Y.P., Chien, C.T., et al. (2002) Small-dose propofol sedation attenuates the formation of reactive oxygen species in tourniquet-induced ischemia-reperfusion injury under spinal anesthesia. Anesth Analg 94, 1617-1620, table of contents.

25 Huang, C.H., Wang, Y.P., Wu, P.Y., et al. (2008) Propofol infusion shortens and attenuates oxidative stress during one lung ventilation. Acta Anaesthesiol Taiwan 46, 160-165.

26 De Conno, E., Steurer, M.P., Wittlinger, M., et al. (2009) Anesthetic-induced improvement of the inflammatory response to one-lung ventilation. Anesthesiology 110, 1316-1326.

27 Bae, H.B., Li, M., Lee, S.H., et al. (2013) Propofol attenuates pulmonary injury induced by collapse and reventilation of lung in rabbits. Inflammation 36, 680-688.

28 Serrano, C.V. Jr, Fraticelli, A., Paniccia, R., et al. (1996) pH dependence of neutrophil-endothelial cell adhesion and adhesion molecule expression. Am J Physiol 271, C962-C970.

29 Contreras, M., Ansari, B., Curley, G., et al. (2012) Hypercapnic acidosis attenuates ventilation-induced lung injury by a nuclear factor-kappaB-dependent mechanism. Crit Care Med 40, 2622-2630.

30 De Smet, H.R., Bersten, A.D., Barr, H.A., et al. (2007) Hypercapnic acidosis modulates inflammation, lung mechanics, and edema in the isolated perfused lung. J Crit Care 22, 305-313.

31 Shibata, K., Cregg, N., Engelberts, D., et al. (1998) Hypercapnic acidosis may attenuate acute lung injury by inhibition of endogenous xanthine oxidase. Am J Respir Crit Care Med 158, 1578-1584.

32 Coakley, R.J., Taggart, C., Greene, C., et al. (2002) Ambient pCO2 modulates intracellular pH, intracellular oxidant generation, and interleukin-8 secretion in human neutrophils. J Leukoc Biol 71, 603-610.

33 Adding, L.C., Agvald, P., Persson, M.G., et al. (1999) Regulation of pulmonary nitric oxide by carbon dioxide is intrinsic to the lung. Acta Physiol Scand 167, 167-174.

34 Kregenow, D.A., Rubenfeld, G.D., Hudson, L.D., et al. (2006) Hypercapnic acidosis and mortality in acute lung injury. Crit Care Med 34, 1-7.

35 Park, C.M., Lim, S.C., Kim, Y.I., et al. (2005) Does hypercapnic acidosis, induced by adding CO2 to inspired gas, have protective effect in a ventilator-induced lung injury? J Korean Med Sci 20, 764-769.

36 Lang, J.D. Jr, Chumley, P., Eiserich, J.P., et al. (2000) Hypercapnia induces injury to alveolar epithelial cells via a nitric oxide-dependent pathway. Am J Physiol Lung Cell Mol Physiol 279, L994-L1002.

37 Theroux, M.C., Olivant, A., Lim, D., et al. (2008) Low dose methylprednisolone prophylaxis to reduce inflammation during one-lung ventilation. Paediatr Anaesth 18, 857-864.

38 Ju, N.Y., Gao, H., Huang, W., et al. (2014) Therapeutic effect of inhaled budesonide (Pulmicort(R) Turbuhaler) on the inflammatory response to one-lung ventilation. Anaesthesia 69, 14-23.

39 Shyamsundar, M., McAuley, D.F., Shields, M.O., et al. (2014) Effect of simvastatin on physiological and biological outcomes in patients undergoing esophagectomy: a randomized placebo-controlled trial. Ann Surg 259, 26-31.

40 Marini, J.J. (2001) Ventilator-induced airway dysfunction? Am J Respir Crit Care Med 163, 806-807.

41 Dreyfuss, D., Soler, P., Basset, G., et al. (1988) High inflation pressure pulmonary edema. Respective effects of high airway pressure, high tidal volume, and positive end-expiratory pressure. Am Rev Respir Dis 137, 1159-1164.

42 Wolthuis, E.K., Choi, G., Dessing, M.C., et al. (2008) Mechanical ventilation with lower tidal volumes and positive end-expiratory pressure prevents pulmonary inflammation in patients without preexisting lung injury. Anesthesiology 108, 46-54.

43 Hemmes, S.N., Serpa Neto, A., Schultz, M.J. (2013) Intraoperative ventilatory strategies to prevent postoperative pulmonary complications: a meta-analysis. Curr Opin Anaesthesiol 26, 126-133.

44 Stahl, W.R. (1967) Scaling of respiratory variables in mammals. J Appl Physiol 22, 453-460.

45 Bide, R.W., Armour, S.J., Yee, E. (2000) Allometric respiration/body mass data for animals to be used for estimates of inhalation toxicity to young adult humans. J Appl Toxicol 20, 273-290.

46 Staffieri, F., Franchini, D., Carella G.L., et al. (2007) Computed tomographic analysis of the effects of two inspired oxygen concentrations on pulmonary aeration in anesthetized and mechanically ventilated dogs. Am J Vet Res 68, 925-931.

47 Henao-Guerrero, N., Ricco, C., Jones, J.C., et al. (2012) Comparison of four ventilatory protocols for computed tomography of the thorax in healthy cats. Am J Vet Res 73, 646-653.

48 De Monte, V., Grasso, S., De Marzo, C., et al. (2013) Effects of reduction of inspired oxygen fraction or application of positive end-expiratory pressure after an alveolar recruitment maneuver on respiratory mechanics, gas exchange, and lung aeration in dogs during anesthesia and neuromuscular blockade. Am J Vet Res 74, 25-33.

49 MacDonnell, K.F., Lefemine, A.A., Moon, H.S., et al. (1975) Comparative hemodynamic consequences of inflation hold, PEEP, and interrupted PEEP: an experimental study in normal dogs. Ann Thorac Surg 19, 552-560.

50 Dorinsky, P.M., Whitcomb, M.E (1983) The effect of PEEP on cardiac output. Chest 84, 210-216.

51 Murray, I.P., Modell, J.H., Gallagher, T.J., et al. (1984) Titration of PEEP by the arterial minus end-tidal carbon dioxide gradient. Chest 85, 100-104.

52 Staffieri, F., De Monte, V., De Marzo, C., et al. (2010) Effects of two fractions of inspired oxygen on lung aeration and gas exchange in cats under inhalant anaesthesia. Vet Anaesth Analg 37, 483-490.

53 Cantwell, S.L., Duke, T., Walsh, P.J., et al. (2000) One-lung versus two-lung ventilation in the closed-chest anesthetized dog: a comparison of cardiopulmonary parameters. Vet Surg 29, 365-373.

54 Riquelme, M., Monnet, E., Kudnig, S.T., et al. (2005) Cardiopulmonary changes induced during one-lung ventilation in anesthetized dogs with a closed thoracic cavity. Am J Vet Res 66, 973-977.

55 Riquelme, M., Monnet, E., Kudnig, S.T., et al. (2005) Cardiopulmonary effects of positive end-expiratory pressure during one-lung ventilation in anesthetized dogs with a closed thoracic cavity. Am J Vet Res 66, 978-983.

56 Jeon, K., Jeon, I.S., Suh, G.Y., et al. (2007) Two methods of setting positive end-expiratory pressure in acute lung injury: an experimental computed tomography volumetric study. J Korean Med Sci 22, 476-483.

57 Copland, V., Haskins, S., Patz, J. (1987) Oxymorphone: cardiovascular, pulmonary, and behavioral effects in dogs. Am J Vet Res 48, 1626-1630.

58 Pypendop, B.H., Barter, L.S., Stanley, S.D., et al. (2011) Hemodynamic effects of dexmedetomidine in isoflurane-anesthetized cats. Vet Anaesth Analg 38, 555-567.

59 Roze, H., Lafargue, M., Perez P., et al. (2012) Reducing tidal volume and increasing positive end-expiratory pressure with constant plateau pressure during one-lung ventilation: effect on oxygenation. Br J Anaesth 108, 1022-1027.

60 Levin, M.A., McCormick, P.J., Lin, H.M., et al. (2014) Low intraoperative tidal volume ventilation with minimal PEEP is associated with increased mortality. Br J Anaesth 113, 97-108.

61 Lee, J.H., Jeon, Y., Bahk, J.H., et al. (2011) Pulse pressure variation as a predictor of fluid responsiveness during one-lung ventilation for lung surgery using thoracotomy: randomised controlled study. Eur J Anaesthesiol 28, 39-44.

62 Pang, D.S., Allaire, J., Rondenay, Y., et al. (2009) The use of lingual venous blood to determine the acid-base and blood-gas status of dogs under anesthesia. Vet Anaesth Analg 36, 124-132.

63 Zhong, T., Wang, W., Chen, J., et al. (2009) Sore throat or hoarse voice with bronchial blockers or double-lumen tubes for lung isolation: a randomised, prospective trial. Anaesth Intensive Care 37, 441-446.

64 Calder, W.A. (1984) Size, Function, and Life History. Harvard University Press, Cambridge, MA.

65 Woldehiwot, Z., Horsfield, K. (1978) Diameter, length and branching angles of the upper airways in the dog lung. Respir Physiol 33, 213-218.

66 Levionnois, O.L., Bergadano, A., Schatzmann, U. (2006) Accidental entrapment of an endo-bronchial blocker tip by a surgical stapler during selective ventilation for lung lobectomy in a dog. Vet Surg 35, 82-85.

67 Campos, J.H., Kernstine, K.H. (2003) A comparison of a left-sided Broncho-Cath with the torque control blocker Univent and the wire-guided blocker. Anesth Analg 96, 283-289, table of contents.

68 Narayanaswamy, M., McRae, K., Slinger, P., et al. (2009) Choosing a lung isolation device for thoracic surgery: a randomized trial of three bronchial blockers versus double-lumen tubes. Anesth Analg 108, 1097-1101.

69 Prabhu, M.R., Smith, J.H. (2002) Use of the Arndt wire-guided endobronchial blocker. Anesthesiology 97, 1325.

70 MacPhail, C.M., Monnet, E., Twedt, D.C. (2001) Thoracoscopic correction of persistent right aortic arch in a dog. J Am Anim Hosp Assoc 37, 577-581.

71 Bauquier, S.H., Culp, W.T., Lin, R.C., et al. (2010) One-lung ventilation using a wire-guided endobronchial blocker for thoracoscopic pericardial fenestration in a dog. Can Vet J 51, 1135-1138.

72 Mayhew, P.D., Pascoe, P.J., Shilo-Benjamini, Y., et al. (2013a) Effect of one-lung ventilation with or without low-pressure carbon dioxide insufflation on cardiorespiratory parameters in cats undergoing thoracoscopy. Vet Surg DOI: 10.1111/j.1532-950X.2014.12272.x

73 Slinger, P.D., Lesiuk, L. (1998) Flow resistances of disposable double-lumen, single-lumen, and Univent tubes. J Cardiothorac Vasc Anesth 12, 142-144.

74 Guyton, D.C., Besselievre, T.R., Devidas, M., et al. (1997) A comparison of two different bronchial cuff designs and four different bronchial cuff inflation methods. J Cardiothorac Vasc Anesth 11, 599-603.

75 Robertshaw, F.L. (1962) Low resistance double-lumen endobronchial tubes. Br J Anaesth 34, 576-579.

76 Russell, W.J., Strong, T.S. (2003) Dimensions of double-lumen tracheobronchial tubes. Anaesth Intensive Care 31, 50-53.

77 Lohser, J., Brodsky, J.B. (2006) Silbronco double-lumen tube. J Cardiothorac Vasc Anesth 20, 129-131.

78 Mayhew, P.D., Culp, W.T., Pascoe, P.J., et al. (2012) Evaluation of blind thoracoscopic-assisted placement of three double-lumen endobronchial tube designs for one-lung ventilation in dogs. Vet Surg 41, 664-670.

79 Campos, J.H., Hallam, E.A., Van Natta, T., et al. (2006) Devices for lung isolation used by anesthesiologists with limited thoracic experience: comparison of double-lumen endotracheal tube, Univent torque control blocker, and Arndt wire-guided endobronchial blocker. Anesthesiology 104, 261-266, discussion 265A.

80 Mayhew, P.D., Friedberg, J.S. (2008) Video-assisted thoracoscopic resection of noninvasive thymomas using one-lung ventilation in two dogs. Vet Surg 37, 756-762.

81 Mayhew, K.N., Mayhew, P.D., Sorrell-Raschi, L., et al. (2009) Thoracoscopic subphrenic pericardectomy using double-lumen endobronchial intubation for alternating one-lung ventilation. Vet Surg 38, 961-966.

82 Adami, C., Axiak, S., Rytz, U., et al. (2011) Alternating one lung ventilation using a double lumen endobronchial tube and providing CPAP to the non-ventilated lung in a dog. Vet Anaesth Analg 38, 70-76.

83 Karzai, W., Schwarzkopf, K. (2009) Hypoxemia during one-lung ventilation: prediction, prevention, and treatment. Anesthesiology 110, 1402-1411.

84 Mukhtar, A.M., Obayah, G.M., Elmasry, A., et al. (2008) The therapeutic potential of intraoperative hypercapnia during video-assisted thoracoscopy in pediatric patients. Anesth Analg 106, 84-88, table of contents.

85 Hogue, C.W. Jr. (1994) Effectiveness of low levels of nonventilated lung continuous positive airway pressure in improving arterial oxygenation during one-lung ventilation. Anesth Analg 79, 364-367.

86 Walsh, P.J., Remedios, A.M., Ferguson, J.F., et al. (1999) Thoracoscopic versus open partial pericardectomy in dogs: comparison of post-operative pain and morbidity. Vet Surg 28, 472-479.

87 Giordano, T., Steagall, P.V., Ferreira, T.H., et al. (2010) Postoperative analgesic effects of intravenous, intramuscular, subcutaneous or oral transmucosal buprenorphine administered to cats undergoing ovariohysterectomy. Vet Anaesth Analg 37, 357-366.

88 Lascelles, B.D., Cripps, P.J., Jones, A., et al. (1998) Efficacy and kinetics of carprofen, administered preoperatively or postoperatively, for the prevention of pain in dogs undergoing ovariohysterectomy. Vet Surg 27, 568-582.

89 Lejeune, P., De Smet, J.M., de Francquen, P., et al. (1990) Inhibition of hypoxic pulmonary vasoconstriction by increased left atrial pressure in dogs. Am J Physiol 259, H93-H100.

90 Lejeune, P., Vachiery, J.L., De Smet, J.M., et al. (1991) PEEP inhibits hypoxic pulmonary vasoconstriction in dogs. J Appl Physiol (1985) 70, 1867-1873.

91 Benumof, J.L., Wahrenbrock, E.A. (1977) Dependency of hypoxic pulmonary vasoconstriction on temperature. J Appl Physiol Respir Environ Exerc Physiol 42, 56-58.

92 Lloyd, T.C. Jr. (1966) Role of nerve pathways in the hypoxic vasoconstriction of lung. J Appl Physiol 21, 1351-1355.

93 Silove, E.D., Inoue, T., Grover, R.F. (1968) Comparison of hypoxia, pH, and sympathomimetic drugs on bovine pulmonary vasculature. J Appl Physiol 24, 355-365.

94 Kernan, S., Rehman, S., Meyer, T., et al. (2001) Effects of dexmedetomidine on oxygenation during one-lung ventilation for thoracic surgery in adults. J Minim Access Surg 7, 227-231.

95 Bindslev, L., Cannon, D., Sykes, M.K. (1986) Reversal of nitrous oxide-induced depression of hypoxic pulmonary vasoconstriction by lignocaine hydrochloride during collapse and ventilation hypoxia of the left lower lobe. Br J Anaesth 58, 451-456.

96 Carlsson, A.J., Bindslev, L., Santesson, J., et al. (1985) Hypoxic pulmonary vasoconstriction in the human lung: the effect of prolonged unilateral hypoxic challenge during anaesthesia. Acta Anaesthesiol Scand 29, 346-351.

97 Benumof, J.L., Wahrenbrock, E.A (1975) Local effects of anesthetics on regional hypoxic pulmonary vasoconstriction. Anesthesiology 43, 525-532.

98 Lennon, P.F., Murray, P.A. (1996) Attenuated hypoxic pulmonary vasoconstriction during isoflurane anesthesia is abolished by cyclooxygenase inhibition in chronically instrumented dogs. Anesthesiology 84, 404-414.

99 Lesitsky, M.A., Davis, S., Murray, P.A. (1998) Preservation of hypoxic pulmonary vasoconstriction during sevoflurane and desflurane anesthesia compared to the conscious state in chronically instrumented dogs. Anesthesiology 89, 1501-1508.

100 Sustronck, B., Van Loon, G., Deprez, P., et al. (1997) Effect of inhaled nitric oxide on the hypoxic pulmonary vasoconstrictor response in anaesthetised calves. Res Vet Sci 63, 193-197.

101 Nakazawa K, Amaha K. (1988) Effect of nicardipine hydrochloride on regional hypoxic pulmonary vasoconstriction. Br J Anaesth 60, 547-554.

102 Kylhammar, D., Radegran, G. (2012) Cyclooxygenase-2 inhibition and thromboxane A(2) receptor antagonism attenuate hypoxic pulmonary vasoconstriction in a porcine model. Acta physiologica 205, 507-519.

103 Benumof, J.L., Partridge, B.L., Salvatierra, C., et al. (1987) Margin of safety in positioning modern double-lumen endotracheal tubes. Anesthesiology 67, 729-738.

30 Patient Positioning, Port Placement, and Access Techniques for Thoracoscopic Surgery

Philipp D. Mayhew and William T.N. Culp

Key Points

- Most thoracoscopic procedures are initiated using either a subxiphoid or intercostal approach.
- Despite major morbidity being possible during thoracoscopic entry, because most cases are performed without insufflation, there is no need to maintain a tight seal around the port sites as is necessary for laparoscopy.
- Optical entry provides a very reliable and safe access technique for thoracoscopic procedures.

To achieve optimal results, thoracoscopic surgeons need to consider operating room (OR) setup, patient positioning, safe and efficient thoracic cavity access, and port type and configuration necessary to accomplish the goals of the procedure. The major difference between access to the thoracic and peritoneal cavities is that many procedures can be performed without gas insufflation. The ribs form a rigid frame that maintains working space if a pneumothorax is allowed to form. Because unrestricted gas flow in and out of the thorax causes no loss of working space, there is no need to maintain a tight seal around thoracoscopic cannulae as there is in laparoscopy. For this reason, obtaining access for thoracoscopy is often less problematic than for laparoscopy, in which loss of pneumoperitoneum intraoperatively results in a loss of working space. However, thoracoscopic access can still be associated with major morbidity because many vital structures reside close to commonly used port positions. Maintenance of good technique during access is imperative to avoid complications. In this chapter, important potential pitfalls of thoracoscopic access are discussed.

Operating Room

With two to four surgeons, an endoscopic tower, an instrument table, and one or two electrosurgical units, as well as anesthesia personnel and equipment, a considerable logistical challenge is present during most minimally invasive surgical procedures. Although many human centers now operate in custom-designed minimally invasive procedure suites, where ceiling-mounted booms house most of the required components used in these procedures, these facilities are not widely available in veterinary medicine. Integrated minimally invasive surgery suites often have the advantage of incorporating multiple viewing screens, allowing surgeons and surgical assistants to maintain a straight viewing angle to the area of interest and on to the viewing screen. The ability to always maintain this direct line of vision is key to maintaining good hand–eye control. Because only one viewing screen is available in most ORs and is generally located on top of the endoscopic tower, the position of the tower is key.

Thoracoscopic procedures performed in dorsal recumbency usually involve placement of a subxiphoid telescope portal that is used to visualize more cranially located structures. Therefore, positioning the endoscopic tower and monitor at the head of the patient with the anesthesia machine and personnel moved slightly to one or the other side of the patient is recommended (Figure 30-1). It is helpful with patients in dorsal recumbency to not encumber the lower end of the operating table by draping in instrument tables or having cords attached in that location so that the surgeons can move freely around the caudal end of the patient. This can allow a surgeon to lean over the patient in order to handle surgical instrumentation entering through right- and left-sided intercostal portals if necessary as well as allowing the surgeon an obstructed path to move to either side of the patient if required.

Small Animal Laparoscopy and Thoracoscopy, First Edition. Edited by Boel A. Fransson and Philipp D. Mayhew.
© 2015 by ACVS Foundation. Published 2015 by John Wiley & Sons, Inc.
Companion website: www.wiley.com/go/fransson/laparoscopy

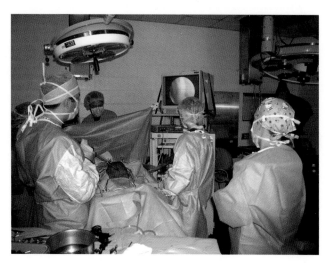

Figure 30-1 For thoracoscopic procedures performed in dorsal recumbency with a subxiphoid telescope portal, the endoscopic tower is placed at the head of the patient to ensure that a straight line can be maintained from the surgeon to the lesion being operated to the video monitor.

For patients that are positioned in lateral or sternal recumbency, the surgeon generally positions the endoscopic tower on the contralateral side of the patient. This is commonly the case for lung lobectomy, thoracic duct ligation, a pericardial window performed in lateral recumbency, or for dissection of the tracheobronchial lymph nodes. This allows the surgeon to look across the patient, observe the monitor, and maintain a straight viewing angle. For cases in lateral recumbency, in which a structure is being operated in either the cranial or caudal thorax, the endoscopic tower is generally moved to a slightly more cranial (for cranially located lesions) or more caudal location. This is often the case when a cranial or caudal lung lobe is being removed.

Patient Positioning

Proper patient positioning is critical to success in thoracoscopic surgery to allow gravity to aid in visualization and organ retraction during surgery. In general, patients are positioned one of three ways for thoracoscopic interventions: lateral, dorsal, or sternal recumbency. Broadly speaking, procedures that are usually approached by an open intercostal thoracotomy are approached thoracoscopically in lateral recumbency with intercostally placed telescope and instrument ports. Open procedures performed by median sternotomy are usually positioned in dorsal recumbency for thoracoscopy using a paraxiphoid telescope portal. Sternal recumbency has been used exclusively for performance of thoracic duct ligation at this time but may be used for other procedures in the future.[1]

For patients in lateral recumbency, the forelimbs are pulled in a cranial direction and secured to allow access to the most cranial intercostal spaces if required. The hindlimbs are tied caudally. Straps or 2-inch medical tape can be used to secure the patient to the surgical table to avoid any patient movement during table tilting. The entire lateral thorax (cranially to the scapula) and cranial half of the abdomen are surgically clipped from the ventral midline to close to the dorsal midline. The entire abdomen can be clipped if any ancillary abdominal procedures are planned during the procedure. This entire clipped area is aseptically prepared for surgery.

For procedures performed in dorsal recumbency, the forelimbs are retracted cranially using limb ties to allow access to the cranial intercostal spaces if required. The hindlimbs are more loosely tied cau-

dally. Sandbags or a vacuum-based surgical positioning device can be used to secure the patient from rolling off the table. Devices that would be placed high up on the thoracic wall are discouraged because they may interfere with surgeon movement during instrument and telescope manipulation. A strap or length of 2-inch surgical tape can be used to strap across the abdomen and lower neck area to provide additional stabilization. This is especially important to avoid patient movement or falling off the operating table in cases where lateral table tilting or Trendelenburg or reverse Trendelenburg positioning may be used intraoperatively. The patient is clipped for surgery widely from the midneck area to the umbilicus caudally or even farther if any access to the abdominal cavity is required for adjunctive procedures. Laterally, the surgical clip should extend up to the dorsal third of the thoracic wall. This entire area is aseptically prepared for surgery.

For procedures in sternal recumbency (see Chapter 36 for further details), positioning devices have been placed under the pubis to stabilize the pelvis and ensure that the abdomen is suspended, allowing gravity-induced ventral positioning of the organs away from the mediastinal root.[1] For this position, wide clipping of the hair from near the ventral midline to the dorsal midline and from the scapular spine to the mid-abdominal region is advised. Some authors have also used a bilateral thoracoscopic approach for access to the thoracic cavity for optimal viewing of the thoracic duct for ligation (see Chapter 36). If bilateral access is performed, similar clipping and aseptic preparation are performed bilaterally.

Thoracic Access Techniques

Just as in laparoscopy, access to the thoracic cavity for thoracoscopic procedures needs to be obtained in a safe and efficient manner. This can be achieved in a number of different ways. The advantages and disadvantages to these different techniques have not been well evaluated in human or veterinary medicine, so the choice of which technique to use is currently largely down to surgeon preference and may be influenced by the available equipment. In all cases, it is advised that a blunt-tipped trocar or trocarless cannula is used for initial establishment of telescope access in all cases.

Open Technique

The traditional open technique is similar to the Hasson technique used for laparoscopy in that a small incision is made either in a subxiphoid or intercostal location, and dissection down through the deeper tissue layers is continued until the parietal pleura is penetrated. Dissection can be pursued either using a combination of blunt and sharp dissection or with the aid of monopolar electrosurgery. Many surgeons like to perform this deeper dissection using blunt dissection with a mosquito hemostat. Penetration of the actual pleura itself with electrosurgery is avoided to prevent iatrogenic injury to the lung tissue beneath. After penetration of the pleura is complete, the incision is widened to allow passage of the cannula. Correct cannula placement can be confirmed by passing the telescope down the cannula to allow visualization of intrathoracic structures. Using an initial subxiphoid telescope portal, final cannula penetration into the pleural cavity is usually performed at least partially with the trocar–cannula assembly because penetration through the most ventral part of the diaphragm is challenging with surgical instruments due to the deep location.

Optical Entry

Optical entry involves the process of visualizing penetration of the thoracic wall tissues with the telescope as cannula placement is occurring. This necessitates the use of either a trocarless cannula (e.g., Ternamian EndoTip cannula; Karl Storz Veterinary Endoscopy, Goleta, CA) or a specialized disposable optical entry cannula (e.g., Versaport Bladeless Optical trocar; Covidien, Mansfield, MA or Kii Fios First Entry; Applied Medical, Rancho Santa Margarita, CA). Optical entry is gaining widespread use in the human field and is usually performed using specialized disposable cannulae that incorporate a translucent trocar with a lumen that can accommodate the telescope. An initial 1.0 to 1.5-cm incision is made in the desired location of the portal. The subcutaneous tissues can be incised although penetration into the deeper layers is achieved by advancement of the cannula–trocar assembly during placement. Placement of the cannula is initiated just until the cannula starts to become "seated" in the deeper tissues. After this has occurred, the telescope is placed into the cannula (or trocar–cannula assembly in the case of disposable versions), and the cannula is advanced into the thorax by firm pressure combined with a twisting motion around the telescope. This can be done both for subxiphoid cannula placement (Video Clip 30-1) or intercostal placement (Video Clip 30-2). During this procedure, the telescope is able to visualize penetration of the deeper muscle layers as it occurs (Video Clip 30-3). Additionally, penetration of the visceral pleura is seen as soon as it happens, thus avoiding placement of the cannula into an excessively deep position. This technique is currently the preferred technique of the authors and is performed very effectively using the trocarless EndoTip cannulae in veterinary species. Use of disposable cannulae for this technique is also very successful, although the cost of these specialized cannulae can be high.

Veress Needle Technique

Veress needles (VNs), used commonly in laparoscopic surgery are rarely used in veterinary access to the thorax because the open and optical entry techniques mentioned earlier are generally very safe and effective access techniques. However, in human thoracoscopic procedures, VNs that incorporate an expandable sleeve (e.g., Versastep, Covidien) have been used for thoracic access with success. In these cases, the VN is used to penetrate the thoracic cavity, and a pneumothorax is allowed to form. The needle component is then withdrawn, leaving the expandable sheath in place. A blunt-tipped trocar–cannula assembly can then be placed within the expandable sheath, which will dilate a tissue plane within the thoracic wall musculature as it is advanced into the thorax.

Thoracic Port Types, Placement, and Position

A variety of techniques can be used for achieving safe and efficient access into the thoracic cavity. Because positive-pressure insufflation is not used in most cases, closed cannulae that maintain a seal against gas leakage are not necessary. This facilitates access considerably and means that very simple cannula designs can be used that simply form a protective sleeve against iatrogenic damage to structures in the vicinity of the cannula. Commercially available disposable thoracic cannulae (e.g., Thoracoport, Covidien) are little more than plastic cylinders without incorporation of a one-way valve to prevent gas leakage. Thoracic cannulae have even been fashioned out of small syringe casings in very small patients.[2] The author regularly uses resterilizable trocarless EndoTip cannulae for thoracoscopy in which the one-way valve is simply unscrewed and left off to allow free passage of room air in and out of the thorax during the procedure (Figure 30-2). Despite it being possible to perform thoracoscopic procedures without the use of cannulae, their use is encouraged to avoid iatrogenic damage to thoracic wall tissues

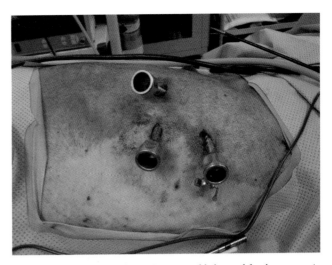

Figure 30-2 Nondisposable cannulae can readily be used for thoracoscopic access if the one-way valve is removed to allow free movement of room air in and out of the thorax to allow a pneumothorax to form.

during repeated instrument exchanges. In cases in which carbon dioxide is to be insufflated into the thorax, closed cannulae, used routinely for laparoscopy can be used interchangeably for thoracic access.

Subxiphoid Port Placement

With the patient positioned in dorsal recumbency, a trocar–cannula assembly or trocarless cannula (EndoTip, Karl Storz) can be placed into either the right or left hemithorax. An initial 0.5- to 1.0-cm incision is made over the subxiphoid area. Subcutaneous tissues are bluntly dissected using Metzenbaum scissors (down to the level of the underlying muscle), or monopolar electrosurgical dissection can be used to incise down to the muscle layer. Further dissection is generally not necessary because the trocar–cannula assembly will be used to penetrate deeper tissues. To achieve successful entry into the thorax, the cannula must be forcefully pushed in a cranial direction, angled at 45° to the sagittal and perpendicular planes as well as 45 degrees to the ventral midline (see Video Clip 30-1). This orientation helps to ensure clean passage through the most ventral aspect of the diaphragm and into the hemithorax of choice. Surgeons need to ensure that some force is used during the process of screwing the cannula into position and that the cannula remains wedged into the triangle formed by the angle of the 13th rib and the xiphoid cartilage. The cannula must be passed under (dorsal) to the rib to avoid it passing too superficially. Several frustrations can arise during attempts at subxiphoid port placement. In cases in which the cannula is not driven in a cranial enough position, it may be possible to enter the abdominal cavity, in which case the caudal aspect of the diaphragm may be visible upon entry in addition to one or more liver lobes (Figure 30-3). If the cannula is positioned too parallel to the ventral midline and not angled sufficiently laterally, it is possible to enter the mediastinal attachment to the sternum. In these cases, the mediastinal tissue is generally dragged with the cannula, and it may be challenging or impossible to penetrate the desired hemithorax. If this occurs, the cannula should be withdrawn and repositioned in a more lateral-oriented trajectory. Another scenario that can occur if the cannula is insufficiently directed laterally from the ventral midline is that the cannula may enter the pleural reflection where the accessory lung lobe resides. In these cases, the

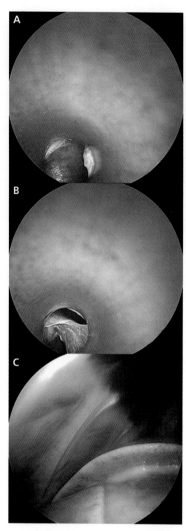

Figure 30-3 In this case, the thoracic port was placed too caudally, and the abdominal cavity has been inadvertently been penetrated. The liver can be seen initially (**A**). To achieve thoracic access in this case, the cannula was simply partially withdrawn and redirected cranially at which point the tip of the cannula could be seen passing the diaphragm (**B**) and finally entering the thorax, where normal intrathoracic structures could be recognized (**C**).

pericardium over the apex of the heart along with the accessory lobe may be seen upon entry, but the right or left hemithorax may not have been entered (Figure 30-4). In some cases, the camera can be gently pushed through a thin part of the pleural reflection to gain access to one or the other hemithorax. However, in other cases, withdrawal and redirection may also be necessary when this happens. Care needs to be taken not to damage the phrenic nerve, which runs over the pleural reflection in this area (see Figure 30-4). In some dogs, a cannula with significant length (>8–10 cm) may be required to fully penetrate the hemithorax from the subxiphoid approach, However, in the authors' experience, the 6.5-cm EndoTip cannulae are of sufficient length in most cats and medium to large breed dogs.

Intercostal Port Placement

Initial port placement for procedures performed in lateral recumbency is by placement of an intercostal port. Surgeons might also choose in some cases to initiate thoracic access using an intercostal port for some procedures performed in dorsal recumbency. All

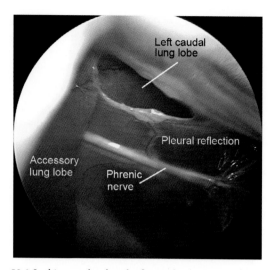

Figure 30-4 In this case, the pleural reflection has been entered from a subxiphoid approach instead of normal penetration of the pleural cavity. The accessory lung lobe can be seen as well as the pleural reflection over which the phrenic nerve can be seen running.

procedures performed in sternal recumbency are initiated using intercostal port placement because access to the sternal area is not possible with this approach. The choice of which intercostal space to initiate access to and whether to gain access in the more dorsal or more ventral aspect of the space will be dictated by the procedure to be performed. A 0.5- to 1.0-cm incision is made in the mid to caudal aspect of the intercostal space, and the subcutaneous fat is dissected bluntly or incised using monopolar electrosurgery. Deeper incision into the deeper muscle layers is usually unnecessary because they can be penetrated by placing pressure on the trocar–cannula assembly (see Video Clip 30-2). Care should be taken to avoid the more cranial aspect of the intercostal space during port placement in order to avoid iatrogenic damage to the intercostal neurovascular bundle. During placement of intercostal ports, it should be noted that the intercostal musculature is not very thick, especially in smaller patients, so penetration of the thoracic cavity occurs relatively rapidly. Use of an optical entry approach (as described earlier) or frequent checking with the telescope to detect penetration into the thorax when it has occurred is prudent. The choice of cannula diameter is important especially when intercostal ports are placed. Larger diameter cannulae may be required for use with larger diameter telescopes and instruments; however, the larger the cannula, the less maneuverability the surgeon will have within the space because of progressive impingement on the ribs as cannula size increases. It is therefore advised that the smallest diameter cannulae that will accommodate the instrumentation to be used is chosen to allow maximal possible angulation of the cannula intraoperatively. Some species such as pigs have very narrow intercostal spaces, making angulation of the cannulae very challenging during surgery, and this is exacerbated when larger cannulae are used.

Thoracic Inlet Approach

This approach is used very uncommonly and should not be used as a primary telescope port placement technique because there may be a greater chance of iatrogenic damage to the many vital structures located close to the thoracic inlet.[3] A skin incision is made close to the thoracic inlet lateral to the trachea and medial to the first rib. A blunt trocar or trocarless cannula is used to penetrate into the cranial thorax under direct observation with the telescope. It is imperative to avoid damage to the internal thoracic arteries, the carotid arteries, and the vagosympathetic trunk. Despite this approach being potentially useful for dissection of cranially located lesions, there are few indications for this approach in veterinary patients.

Placement of Instrument Portals

After telescope access has been obtained, additional instrument ports must be placed for insertion of surgical instruments and hemostatic devices. Instrument ports are almost always placed in intercostal locations no matter what approach was used for obtaining thoracoscopic access. Because a telescope has already been introduced, the great advantage of instrument port placement is the ability to directly observe these cannulae being passed into the thorax; this allows the surgeon to minimize the chances of iatrogenic damage to thoracic structures during cannula insertion (Figure 30-5). Additionally, because a pneumothorax has been allowed to form, there is usually a space between the lung and the thoracic wall, making iatrogenic damage to lung during entry much less common. The location of instrument portals is largely dictated by the procedure being performed. In cases operated in dorsal recumbency in which bilateral hemithorax access is anticipated, the first instrument portal is usually positioned in the same hemithorax into which the telescope was initially passed. If the contralateral hemithorax is entered, visualization of the instrument cannula will usually be obscured by the intact mediastinal tissue that remains suspended from the sternum. After the intercostal instrument portal has been placed, a vessel-sealing device can usually be used to penetrate the contralateral hemithorax, thus allowing complete exploration of both sides of the thorax and placement of further instrument portals into the contralateral hemithorax if required. The vessel-sealing device can then be used to completely remove the mediastinal tissues from the sternum. The number and type and size of instrument portals that are established are also dictated by the procedure and the availability of instrumentation and are discussed in the chapters on the individual thoracoscopic procedures. However, it is helpful to consider several factors. The anticipated size of instrumentation that will be required be complete a procedure should be carefully considered. As an example, thoracoscopic lung lobectomy usually requires the placement of a surgical stapler such as the EndoGIA

(Covidien). These staplers are generally 12-mm devices requiring the placement of at least one cannula that can accommodate 12-mm instrumentation. Another variable that needs to be considered is the ideal trajectory that will optimize dissection of a lesion because this will influence instrument port location. For some aspects of a procedure, surgeons are able to work from a variety of angles (even with straight instruments), but for others, the angle of trajectory is vital. The example of thoracoscopic lung lobectomy is useful here as well because the angle at which the stapler enters the thorax may only be optimal from only a certain limited area.

Complications of Thoracic Access

Both in the human and veterinary literature, little information exists on the complications associated with thoracoscopic access. This may be due to the inherently lower level of morbidity associated with entering the thorax in a minimally invasive fashion, but it is also possible that access-related morbidity is underreported. The low level of thoracic access-related morbidity is, however, in contrast to the significant body of literature describing laparoscopic access-related morbidity.

During placement of subxiphoid portals, major morbidity has not been reported in the veterinary literature, probably because few major vascular structures exist in this area. Penetration of the ventral aspect of the diaphragm almost certainly occurs in many cases during this approach. However, the small defect that may result appears to be inconsequential, and these authors have not seen associated complications. Injuries to the lung or cardiac structures are conceivable during subxiphoid port placement, although with careful technique and attention to detail, this appears to be exceedingly rare from this approach. Entry into the abdomen from the subxiphoid approach can occur; however, this complication is usually easily dealt with by withdrawal of the cannula and redirection into a more cranial trajectory unless penetration into the liver or another abdominal organ occurs.

When telescope portals or instrument portals are placed intercostally, incising in the middle of the intercostal space is imperative to avoid iatrogenic damage to the intercostal neurovascular bundle, which runs parallel and caudal to each rib. Hemorrhage from these vessels can be very profuse and can occur during placement, intraoperatively, or after withdrawal of the cannula at the end of the procedure (Figure 30-6).[4-6] For this reason, it is always recommended

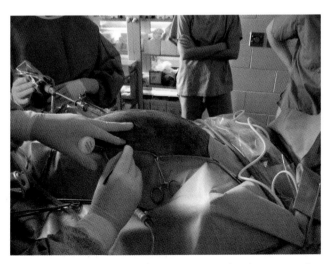

Figure 30-5 During placement of instrument ports, the telescope is used to visualize cannula entry from inside the pleural cavity.

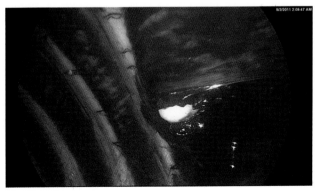

Figure 30-6 A bleeding intercostal vessel can be seen in this image. Intercostal vessel bleeding can be profuse and should never be ignored. In this image, the normal neurovascular bundles of the more caudal intercostal spaces can be seen running down the caudal aspect of the rib.

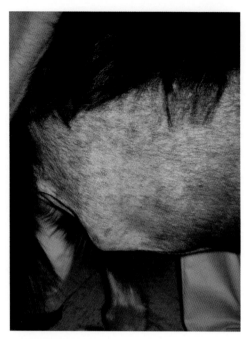

Figure 30-7 A seroma can be seen in this dog associated with one of the thoracoscopic port incisions.

that before final removal of the telescope, each portal site is briefly inspected for hemorrhage after the cannula removal. Attempts can be made to achieve hemostasis in these cases using vessel-sealing devices or hemostatic clips; however, the vessels are located so close to the periosteum of the rib that achieving hemostasis using these methods is not always successful.[6] In these cases, placement of a circumcostal suture proximal and distal to the bleeding vessel may be necessary.

Iatrogenic injury to lung parenchyma can occur during initial telescope placement, especially in cases in which adhesion of lung lobes to the thoracic wall has occurred. The presence of adhesions can be difficult to predict preoperatively from diagnostic imaging studies, and an awareness on behalf of the surgeon that these may be present is required. In the authors' experience, this is especially common in animals with chronic pleural effusions and is a further reason why direct observation of all subsequently placed instrument ports is so vital. To avoid iatrogenic lung damage, blunt trocars or trocarless cannulae should always be used. It is unknown whether iatrogenic access-related morbidity is more or less likely with the methods of obtaining access for thoracoscopy described in this chapter, and further studies are required to investigate this question.

Postoperative complications at thoracoscopic port sites are also possible and can include port site infections, seromas, and port site metastasis. Herniation of intrathoracic structures is less likely because of the anatomically less mobile nature of most thoracic organs. This is in contrast to the peritoneal cavity, where herniation of omentum, intestines, and other structures through port sites can occur readily when peritoneal closure is not performed correctly. Seromas occur at thoracoscopic port site incisions readily, especially in cases in which pleural effusions are ongoing after surgery (Figure 30-7). These are usually easily managed conservatively with warm compression and rarely become large. Port site infections are rare occurrences that might require drainage or antibiotic administration based on the results of bacterial culture and sensitivity testing.[7] Port site metastasis is also a rare occurrence but has been reported after extraction of pericardial tissue[8] and has been seen by the authors group after thoracoscopic resection of a thymoma. Port site metastasis occurs because of complex interplay of factors involving direct tumor cell inoculation, aerosolization of tumor cells during surgery, and the local immune response. To minimize the risk of this complication, surgeons should attempt to prevent perforation of any tumor capsules during surgery and use specimen retrieval bags to remove potentially neoplastic lesions through small port incisions.

 All videos cited in this chapter can be found on the book's companion website at **www.wiley.com/go/fransson/ laparoscopy**

References

1 Allman, D.A., Radlinsky, M.G., Ralph, A.G., et al. (2010) Thoracoscopic thoracic duct ligation and pericardectomy for treatment of chylothorax in dogs. Vet Surg 39, 21-27.

2 MacPhail, C.M., Monnet, E., Twedt, D.C. (2001) Thoracoscopic correction of a persistent right aortic arch in a dog. J Am Anim Hosp Assoc 37, 577-581.

3 Potter, L., Hendrickson, D.A. (1999) Therapeutic video-assisted thoracic surgery. In: Freeman, L.J. (ed.) Veterinary Endosurgery, 1st edn. Mosby, St. Louis, pp. 169-191.

4 Radlinsky, M.G., Mason, D.E., Biller, D.S., et al. (2002) Thoracoscopic visualization and ligation of the thoracic duct in dogs. Vet Surg 31, 138-146.

5 Lansdowne, J.L., Monnet, E., Twedt, D.C., et al. (2005) Thoracoscopic lung lobectomy for treatment of lung tumors in dogs. Vet Surg 34, 530-535.

6 Mayhew, P.D., Hunt, G.B., Steffey, M.A., et al. (2013) Evaluation of short-term outcome after lung lobectomy for resection of primary lung tumors via video-assisted thoracoscopic surgery or open thoracotomy in medium- to large-breed dogs. J Am Vet Med Assoc 243, 681-688.

7 Mayhew, P.D., Freeman, L., Kwan, T., et al. (2012) Comparison of surgical site infection rates in clean and clean-contaminated wounds in dogs and cats after minimally invasive versus open surgery: 179 cases (2007-2008). J Am Vet Med Assoc 240, 193-198.

8 Brisson, B.A., Reggeti, F., Bienzle, D. (2006) Portal site metastasis of invasive mesothelioma after diagnostic thoracoscopy in a dog. J Am Vet Med Assoc 229, 980-983.

31 Thoracoscopic Contraindications, Complications, and Conversion

J. Brad Case and Jeffrey J. Runge

Key Points

- Thoracoscopic complications can be rapidly life threatening if not diagnosed promptly and managed appropriately.
- Prospective thoracoscopic surgeons need to be experienced in open thoracic surgery in order to manage complications and conversions appropriately.
- Creation of adequate working space using pneumothorax, one-lung ventilation, or carbon dioxide insufflation are critical to the safe completion of thoracoscopic procedures.
- If deemed necessary, surgeons should view conversion of a thoracoscopic procedure to an open thoracotomy as a sign of good surgical judgment rather than a complication.

Thoracoscopy or video-assisted thoracic surgery (VATS) was first described in 1910 by H.C. Jacobaeus as a minimally invasive method for diagnosing and treating humans with pulmonary adhesions secondary to tuberculosis. Jacobaeus recognized very early the unique advantages of thoracoscopy and wrote: "Without doubt, the predominant value of endoscopy centres around the examination of the pleural cavities, the so-called thoracoscopy." At the time, exploratory thoracotomy was not performed because of the exceptionally high morbidity associated with an open thorax. Jacobaeus went on to explain: "With regard to the chest cavity there is as we know, nothing corresponding to exploratory laparotomy."[1] Since the time of Jacobaeus, thoracoscopy has evolved immensely and is now described for a myriad of diagnostic and therapeutic procedures in both human and veterinary surgery. Furthermore, the indications in veterinary medicine for VATS compared with traditional invasive procedures are constantly evolving. That said, specific indications and contraindications for VATS procedures are lacking in the veterinary literature. In human VATS, few explicit contraindications exist. These include diffuse body wall neoplasia, diffuse pleural adhesions, and lack of cardiopulmonary reserve to tolerate lung collapse.[2] Currently, in veterinary surgery, patients are candidates for VATS if they are hemodynamically stable, have a disease that can be treated effectively and safely with VATS methodology, and have owners that have been counseled on the risks and potential for conversion to thoracotomy. Clearly, subjectivity exists when defining a patient as suitable for a particular VATS procedure because guidelines in veterinary medicine do not exist. The experience and training of the surgeon and surgery team, facilities and equipment, and capabilities for intraoperative as well as postoperative support further complicate the decision-making process.

Strategies to Avoid Complications

Preoperative Assessment

Dogs and cats undergoing VATS should have a thorough preoperative evaluation, including a complete physical and neurologic examination, complete blood count, serum chemistry, urinalysis, and thoracic imaging. Fluid, electrolyte, and acid–base abnormalities should be addressed before anesthesia. Anemic dogs should be transfused with erythroid-rich blood (packed red blood cells or whole blood) to maximize oxygen-carrying capacity before anesthesia and VATS. Significant *hemorrhage* or preoperative *anemia* can complicate the procedure and compromise the patient during VATS. Because oxygen delivery (CO × O$_2$ content) to tissues is dependent on the oxygen content of blood (Hg × SPO$_2$ × 1.34 + PaO$_2$ × 0.003), most significantly hemoglobin, patients undergoing thoracoscopic surgery should have a minimum preoperative hematocrit of 30% and blood transfusion should be considered in patients with marked intraoperative hemorrhage. A cross-match should be performed ahead of surgery, and donor blood should be readily available if needed in an emergency. Rupture of a great thoracic

Small Animal Laparoscopy and Thoracoscopy, First Edition. Edited by Boel A. Fransson and Philipp D. Mayhew.
© 2015 by ACVS Foundation. Published 2015 by John Wiley & Sons, Inc.
Companion website: www.wiley.com/go/fransson/laparoscopy

vessel may result in the near-immediate death of the patient if not dealt with rapidly, and the surgeon must avoid this complication by judicious preparation, careful attention to technique, and possessing the ability to convert to thoracotomy rapidly.

Depending on the underlying pathology or suspected pathology, survey thoracic radiography, echocardiography, contrast-enhanced computed tomography, or magnetic resonance imaging (MRI) may be indicated. In general, dogs with pericardial effusion should undergo echocardiography in addition to survey radiography and electrocardiography before VATS pericardectomy and pericardoscopy. If diastolic function is compromised by cardiac tamponade, pericardiocentesis should be performed before surgery. Echocardiography is more sensitive in detecting epicardial masses if pericardial fluid is present.[3] MRI does not appear to be reliable in differentiating neoplastic from non-neoplastic causes of pericardial disease in dogs.[4] In dogs with a pronounced pneumothorax or pleural effusion, preoperative thoracocentesis or placement of a thoracic drain should be accomplished before VATS. Thorough preoperative assessment facilitates patient selection for a VATS approach and therefore reduces the risk for conversion to thoracotomy and allows for more accurate surgical planning.

Patient Preparation and Conversion

Dogs and cats undergoing VATS are prepared similarly to those undergoing traditional thoracotomy. This is because general surgical principles apply to both open and VATS operations and because VATS may require elective or emergent conversion to an open thoracotomy if complications such as inability to complete the procedure or major hemorrhage occur. It is therefore mandatory that the minimally invasive thoracic surgeon has a secondary site prepared for an open conversion for all VATS procedures. Finochietto retractors, electrosurgical capabilities, vascular forceps and clip applicators, vessel-sealing devices, and staplers normally used for open thoracic surgery should be made available in the operating suite ready for immediate use.[5] For patients in which a median sternotomy may be used for conversion, an oscillating saw should be present. After the VATS patient is induced, a wide surgical clip is completed, which includes the regions that may be needed if conversion becomes necessary. Thoracic surgical site infections have the potential to progress to pyothorax if not detected early and treated effectively. Thus, careful attention to surgical asepsis and patient preparation should be considered paramount in patients undergoing thoracic surgery even if a minimal VATS approach is used.

Antimicrobial Prophylaxis

Perioperative antibiotic administration is recommended in VATS patients just as it is recommended in patients undergoing open thoracic surgery to reduce the risk of surgical wound infection.[6] All surgical wounds are contaminated by bacteria, but only a small fraction of these become infected. VATS is likely associated with a reduced risk of surgical site infection compared with thoracotomy or median sternotomy.[7] The risk of developing a postoperative infection varies greatly with the nature of the operation and the characteristics of the patient undergoing the procedure. The optimal timing for the preoperative dose of antibiotics is within 30 to 60 minutes of the start of the surgical incision.[8,9] In human surgery, repeat intraoperative antimicrobial dosing is recommended to ensure adequate serum and tissue concentrations of the antibiotic if the duration of the procedure exceeds two half-lives of the drug or if there is excessive blood loss during the procedure.[8] In veterinary

surgery, several different protocols have been suggested with most surgeons using preoperative cefazolin at 22 mg/kg intravenously and then every 90 minutes for the remainder of the procedure.[10,11] The prophylactic antibiotic need not be administered beyond 24 hours postoperatively unless a major break in sterile technique or a change in contamination classification indicates that a therapeutic course of antimicrobials should be prescribed.

Exposure and Working Space

The initial requirement for any VATS procedure is an active *pneumothorax*. However, in some cases, increasing the amount of working space beyond that created by the initial pneumothorax may be necessary or beneficial for safe completion of a VATS procedure. Numerous factors play a role in limiting the actual amount of *operable* space during VATS, including patient size and morphology, positioning, instrumentation, and attributes of the patient's underlying disease (e.g., adhesions, effusion, tumor size). Various techniques have been used to circumvent these limitations, including patient tilting or repositioning, organ retraction, intermittent ventilation, pleural space CO_2 insufflation, and one-lung ventilation (OLV).

Pneumothorax causes retraction of the pulmonary parenchyma away from the thoracic wall, which generates the initial exposure and working space necessary to evaluate the pleural space. Pneumothorax also limits pulmonary expansion and therefore gas exchange at the blood–gas interface of the alveoli. Consequently, *hypoventilation* and *hypoxemia* will result if the patient is not adequately supported. Gas exchange is further impaired by positioning of the patient, use of pleural insufflation with CO_2, and use of one-lung ventilation techniques.[12-16] However, the addition of positive end-expiratory pressure ventilation may minimize some of these untoward effects.[13]

One of the simplest and safest methods for increasing working space in the thoracic cavity is by specific positioning or tilting of the patient. Trendelenburg principles also apply to the thoracic cavity during VATS. Using a mechanical tilt table, patients can easily be positioned into lateral-oblique, Trendelenburg, or reverse Trendelenburg recumbency during the procedure. Slight lateral tilting (~20 degrees) of the patient while in dorsal recumbency is often helpful in shifting the heart and lungs to provide increased exposure in the thoracic cavity. However, the primary author of this chapter has seen acute desaturation because of bronchial obstruction of the ventilated lung in a dog that was tilted while undergoing OLV with a double-lumen endobronchial tube in place.[17] This complication can also occur if an endobronchial blocker is used and becomes dislodged during patient positioning. It is therefore recommended that endobronchial blockers be placed after the patient has been positioned for surgery. Blockers that become dislodged or malpositioned during the procedure can be quickly addressed if a bronchoscope is available in the operating room to aid in rapid repositioning under direct visualization. Complete airway obstruction can be detected early by visualization of acute atelectasis and by a *decremental* or *zero* reading on capnometry. Working space in the thoracic cavity can also be improved through tissue retraction using instruments such as a fan retractor, blunt probe, or atraumatic tissue grasper. The pulmonary parenchyma is especially susceptible to iatrogenic damage (Figure 31-1), which can result in postoperative pneumothorax.[5] Thus, extreme caution should be exercised during manipulation of the lung (Video Clip 31-1).

Several other options exist to help reduce the pleural space volume occupied by the lungs including intermittent ventilation,

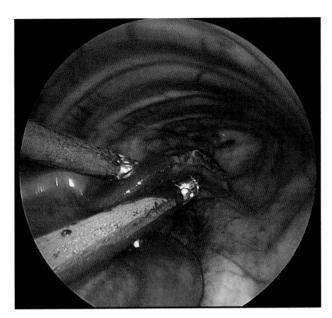

Figure 31-1 Intraoperative image of a thermally injured lung lobe during video-assisted thoracic surgery. Notice the discolored injured cuff of lung parenchyma. Saline was applied to this tissue during a breath hold to ensure that no evidence of rupture was present.

intrathoracic CO_2 insufflation, and OLV. Intermittent ventilation is a safe method commonly used for many types of VATS procedures, but this method is labor intensive and is generally not practical for prolonged procedures.[18] Unfortunately, studies have shown that intrathoracic CO_2 insufflation is not well tolerated in clinically normal dogs even at low intrathoracic pressures because of significant cardiorespiratory compromise.[19] It is for these reasons that OLV has generally been favored to increase working space within the thoracic cavity. OLV in veterinary surgery is becoming more common and has been used for a number of VATS procedures.[12,20-23] There are three main methods for achieving OLV: selective bronchial intubation,[24] endobronchial blockade,[12,20,24] and double-lumen endobronchial tubes (DLT).[18,22] Selective intubation is a simple method of achieving OLV and is accomplished by placing the cuff of a long endotracheal tube into the mainstem bronchus of the selected lung. Endobronchial blockade requires tracheobronchoscopy to guide and position an inflatable balloon in the bronchus of the lung to be excluded. The lung is then blocked by inflating the balloon within the bronchus. Potential complications associated with this technique include overinflation of the balloon, resulting in obstruction of the contralateral bronchus at the carina,[22] and entrapment of the guidewire within the surgical stapler.[25,26] DLTs facilitates gas flow directly to a selected bronchus isolated from the contralateral lung by a dedicated lumen and an inflatable bronchial cuff. The contralateral lung is ventilated via a *Murphey eye* style opening and an independent lumen, which is positioned craniad to the endobronchial portion of the tube.[16,18,27] The angled endobronchial tip can be positioned in either the left or right mainstem bronchus. After it has been positioned correctly, both cuffs (tracheal and bronchial) are inflated, and gas inflow is directed into either or both of the individual lumens as indicated by the particular VATS procedure.[18] A dedicated anesthesiologist should be present to monitor and support the patient during OLV procedures, and time of OLV should be limited to the time required to complete the surgical dissection.[16,21] OLV techniques have the ability to dramatically improve

intrathoracic working space but can be associated with significant complications if not performed and monitored properly. It is therefore strongly advised that the minimally invasive surgeon and anesthesiologist work together to perform these procedures to improve patient safety and clinical outcome. For a more detailed discussion of anesthetic techniques for VATS procedures see chapter 29.

Complications

Port Placement

Appropriate port placement is critical to the success of a VATS procedure. In some instances, an exploratory thoracoscopy may be necessary before a definitive procedure such as lung lobectomy, or a targeted procedure such as lung lobectomy may be planned based on preoperative imaging. Regarding the former, ports should initially be placed to allow for triangulated evaluation of the major cardiopulmonary structures. After the target organ has been identified, additional ports can be placed as needed to perform the definitive treatment. If the definitive organ and procedure are known in advance, then the patient's position and ports should be placed to best create triangulation around the region of interest. Inappropriate patient and port positioning may result in the inability to complete the VATS procedure and will increase the risk of complications.

In general, portal placement for VATS procedures requires incision through the rectus and transversus abdominis muscles, the sternal diaphragmatic muscle, and the intercostal musculature depending on the procedure being performed. Ports located in the transdiaphragmatic location run the risk of perforation and hemorrhage from the cranial superficial epigastric and musculophrenic branches (Figure 31-2) of the internal thoracic artery.[28] Careful visualization and hemostasis during selection and insertion of the transdiaphragmatic port will minimize the risk of hemorrhage. Intercostal arteries and veins run in a dorsoventral direction and are intimately associated with the caudal aspect of the ribs. Rupture of the intercostal vasculature can occur during port insertion, during the procedure, and after port removal. Rupture of the intercostal vasculature may not be visible until the port is removed at the end of the procedure. Close inspection of the port sites on insertion and removal is critical because significant hemorrhage from

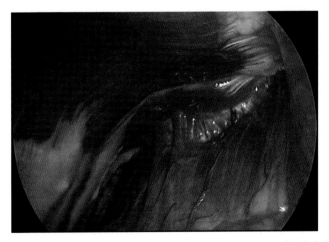

Figure 31-2 Intraoperative video-assisted thoracic surgery image of the left diaphragmatic crus and its sternal and costal muscular attachments. Notice the musculophrenic branches of the internal thoracic artery and vein.

the intercostal vessels can be life threatening if not diagnosed until the animal is recovered from anesthesia.[20] Intercostal hemorrhage (Video Clip 31-2) can be controlled with pressure, radiofrequency electrosurgery, vascular clips, suture ligation, or vessel-sealing devices.[5] Postoperative complications associated with port sites can include seroma, incisional infection, and port site metastasis caused by leakage of malignant effusions.[29] Use of endoscopic specimen retrieval bags (Video Clip 31-3) or a sterile glove is advised to reduce the risk of *extraction-associated*, port site neoplasia. Although the risk of extraction or port site metastasis is unknown with VATS procedures in veterinary surgery, the risk appears to be quite low (0.26%) in human VATS as long as surgical oncologic principles are adhered to.[30] This is likely true for veterinary patients as well.

Pericardial

One the most commonly performed VATS procedure in dogs is pericardectomy.[12,16,25,27,31,32] The pericardium is a collagenous structure, which has both a visceral and parietal mesothelial surface and is contiguous with the epicardium. The pericardium contains both phrenic nerves, which run in a *cranial-to-caudal* direction at the level of the *dorsal third* of the heart. The phrenic nerves are a critical landmark for surgeons performing pericardectomy because transection may result in paresis or plegia of the associated hemidiaphragm. With chronic effusions, the pericardium can become severely thickened, and some dogs may have excessive pericardial fat that may obscure visualization of the phrenic nerves and increase the risk of inadvertent transection.[22,27] The surgeon must therefore be aware of their general location and maintain visualization as best as is possible during VATS pericardectomy to reduce this risk.

The epicardium is a thin mesothelial lining that lies directly over the myocardium. The epicardium and structures within the pericardial space are visible after the pericardium has been incised, but visibility of epicardial structures depends on the particular pericardial pathology as well as the size and location of the pericardectomy.[34] An important decision that the surgeon must make when performing a pericardectomy is how much pericardium to excise. In palliative cases such as with mild hemorrhagic neoplastic effusions, a 4 × 4 cm pericardial window appears to be adequate.[27,31] When an underlying cause of the effusion is not known, *presumed idiopathic*, a thorough *pericardioscopic assessment* is necessary to reduce the chance of a missed diagnosis.[31] The goals of *pericardoscopy* are to further characterize the extent of disease affecting epicardial and other pericardial structures and to obtain diagnostic biopsy samples when possible. Because masses are common on the right auricle and heart base, the surgeon must have a comfortable understanding of the pericardial anatomy before performing pericardoscopy, auriculectomy,[32,33] or epicardial biopsy.[34]

The aortic root and cranial vena cava can easily be visualized at the cranial aspect of the pericardial space after subphrenic pericardectomy. In some cases, vaso vasorum or neoplastic tissue may obscure visibility in this region. This is a common location for small nodules in dogs with mesothelioma[3] and can be biopsied in many cases (Video Clip 31-4), although hemorrhage is possible. The right auricle is visible in the cranial and right lateral aspect of the pericardial space and may sometimes be infiltrating or compressing the right atrium. With normal atrial appendages or those with small apically located masses, the auricle can be displaced away from the epicardium for evaluation and possible resection.[32] Again, severe hemorrhage may result with overzealous

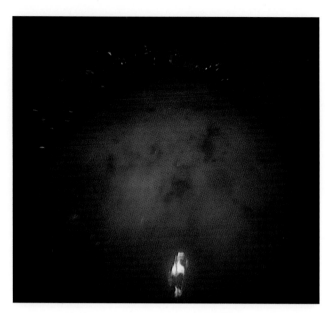

Figure 31-3 Cardiac apex in a dog undergoing VATS pericardectomy for chronic idiopathic pericardial effusion. Notice the lack of visible myocardial vessels as a result of epicardial thickening.

manipulation or with auriculectomy.[32] Another consideration is the location of the myocardial vessels, which are often obscured by a thickened epicardium (Figure 31-3) in dogs with chronic pericardial effusion. The paraconal and ventricular branches of the left coronary artery are the easiest myocardial vessels to identify in dogs undergoing pericardoscopy. These vessels are visible running between the right and left ventricles over the cardiac apex (Figure 31-4). If epicardial biopsy is to be considered in this region, these vessels should be identified first and avoided during biopsy.

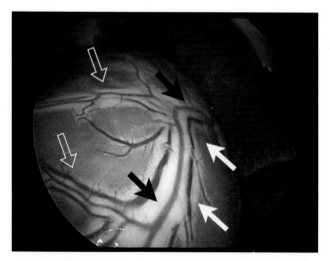

Figure 31-4 The paraconal interventricular branch of the left coronary artery (black arrows), seen coursing toward the apex alongside the great coronary vein (white arrows) in the interventricular groove; left ventricular branches lie to the right of the image and right ventricular branches to the left (open white arrows). (Source: Skinner et al. [34]. Reproduced with permission from Wiley.)

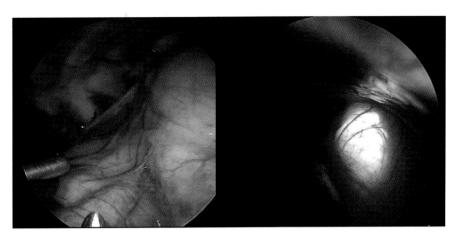

Figure 31-5 Intraoperative image of a puppy undergoing video-assisted thoracic surgery of the left hemithorax with a clinical and radiographic diagnosis of vascular ring anomaly. Notice the dilated esophagus positioned dorsally to a normal left aortic arch. An endoscope was used intraoperatively to confirm the location of the extraluminal constriction. The puppy was repositioned to left lateral recumbency for ligation and division of the aberrant right subclavian artery.

Vascular

A number of other vascular structures are at increased risk for hemorrhage during VATS procedures. For example, dogs undergoing video-assisted patent ductus arteriosus (PDA) ligation are at particular risk for severe hemorrhage from the ductus arteriosus. The PDA is nestled tightly between the aorta and pulmonary artery and can exist with variable morphology and diameters. Preoperative knowledge of the particular size and morphology of the PDA is important to better guide patients potentially amenable to this approach. Dogs with large (>1 cm), type 3 PDAs are likely not candidates for this procedure because the surgical clips need to be large enough to ligate the entire diameter of the ductus, and type 3 PDAs do not taper.[35,36] Additionally, the risk of residual ductal flow may be high with this approach. Hemorrhage is also a concern in dogs with vascular ring anomalies undergoing ligamentum arteriosum transection if the ligamentum is patent or if an aberrant left subclavian is present and inadvertently transected. Approaching the left side in a puppy with an aberrant right subclavian artery or double aortic arch in which the right aorta is atretic is another potential complication if preoperative advanced imaging is not performed (Figure 31-5). Therefore, computed tomography angiography (CTA) and esophagoscopy are usually necessary to determine the vascular anatomy in dogs with vascular ring anomalies before considering a VATS approach.

VATS thymectomy is another procedure that involves substantial risk for hemorrhage, and the authors of this chapter consider preoperative MRI or CTA to be a requirement in patient selection and preoperative planning.[21] Thymomas are usually located in the mediastinum of the cranioventral thorax, but their extension can be quite variable. They can be invasive or noninvasive based on the degree of vascular invasion, involvement with regional structures, and metastatic behavior.[37,38] Dogs with relatively small (<5 cm) and noninvasive thymic masses may be candidates for VATS thymectomy.[21] However, the operating surgeon must exercise caution during dissection, especially dorsally as the cranial vena cava and brachycephalic artery are typically adjacent to the thymoma when in dorsal recumbency (Figure 31-6) regardless of invasiveness. It is also not uncommon for noninvasive thymomas to be associated with the internal thoracic arteries on their cranial margin, which requires dissection during VATS thymectomy (Video Clip 31-5). If large cystic lesions are encountered associated with the thymus, fluid removal may prove beneficial in reducing its size to enable thoracoscopic excision and identification of adjacent vasculature.

The thoracic duct in dogs runs predominantly on the dorsolateral right side of the aorta in the caudal thorax. Ligation requires dissection among the thoracic aorta, costal arteries, and azygous vein, which can be technically challenging.[39] Proper identification of the thoracic duct and its surrounding structures is vital to reduce the chances of damaging the adjacent vasculature. Recently, near-infrared fluorescence imaging has been used for thoracic duct ligation and may improve anatomic identification of the duct and reduce the risk of inadvertent tissue injury (Figure 31-7).

Pulmonary

The lungs present a substantial challenge to minimally invasive surgeons because they occupy a large volume of the pleural space, are under cyclic motion, and are easily injured (see Video Clip 31-1). Iatrogenic pulmonary injury from an intercostal cannula and thermal sealing device (see Figure 31-1) was reported in two dogs undergoing lung lobectomy in one study.[22] Lung laceration and postoperative pneumothorax have also been reported with VATS pericardectomy.[25,27]

VATS lung lobectomy is becoming more common in dogs with pulmonary neoplasia and spontaneous pneumothorax.[20,22,23,40]

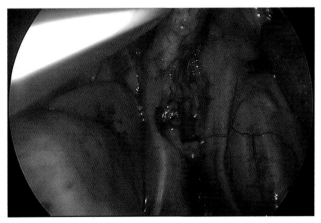

Figure 31-6 The craniodorsal mediastinal defect after VATS thymectomy in a dog with a thymoma. Notice the dissection plane immediately adjacent to the cranial vena cava, brachycephalic artery, phrenic nerves, and costocervical vein. The thymoma must be retracted ventrally away from these structures during dorsal dissection.

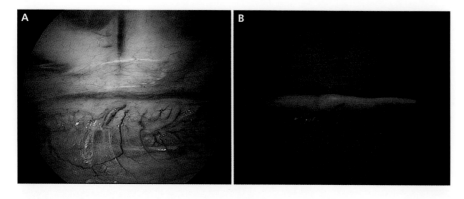

Figure 31-7 **A,** Thoracoscopic image of the mediastinum during a thoracic duct ligation procedure. The patient is in sternal recumbency, and the camera is directed at the caudal dorsal region of the chest with the azygos vein in direct view. **B,** The same thoracoscopic view in the same patient now with fluorescence imaging activated. Note fluorescence of the thoracic duct in blue after injection of a mesenteric abdominal lymph node with the tracer indocyanine green.

However, VATS lung lobectomy appears to be associated with a moderate risk for conversion to thoracotomy,[20,22,23] which ranges from 10% to 50%. The reported reasons for conversion include intraoperative loss of OLV,[20,22] hemorrhage from intercostal arteries,[20] inability to access or assess specific lung lobes,[20,23] and large size of a pulmonary tumor.[22] Suggested guidelines for VATS lung lobectomy include lung tumor diameter less than 8 cm or tumor volume less than 150 cm^3 in dogs weighing more than 30 kg,[22] although further studies with larger numbers of cases need to be performed to evaluate these criteria further. If OLV is not available or if the patient's size or size of the pulmonary mass precludes safe VATS lung lobectomy, a mini-thoracotomy can be used to exteriorize the affected lung lobe during VATS resection. This approach may mitigate some of the difficulties encountered in smaller patients or in patients with larger masses.[41]

It has been recommended that dogs undergoing lung lobectomy for neoplastic disease should have histopathologic evaluation of the regional hilar lymph nodes to better guide adjunctive treatment and for prognostic evaluation.[22,42] Thoracoscopic tracheobronchial lymph node extirpation has been described in dogs with normal-size tracheobronchial lymph nodes.[43] Dissection at the level of the pulmonary hilus can be facilitated with OLV techniques,[20,22] but tissue dissection in this region can be challenging. These lymph nodes can be very small (<1–2 mm) and are surrounded by the pulmonary vein and artery. Thus, dissection runs a high risk of hemorrhage if the minimally invasive surgeon is inexperienced.

Evaluation for pulmonary leaks or ruptures is required in dogs with spontaneous pneumothorax. With a VATS approach, the dog is positioned in dorsal recumbency, and the lung parenchyma explored and submerged in saline to check for the affected lobe or lobes (Video Clip 31-6). After the affected lobe or lobes are identified, they are removed partially or completely. If a leaking pulmonary lesion is not identified or if the lungs cannot be adequately submerged and evaluated, then conversion to median sternotomy is necessary.[23] In a recent study, only 5 of 11 dogs with a spontaneous pneumothorax had an active pulmonary leak identified during VATS.[23] If a leaking lesion is missed, persistent pneumothorax will occur, and revision surgery will be necessary. Submerging large lung lobes completely while administering positive-pressure ventilation is exceptionally challenging with a VATS approach. This is because the limited space available within the thoracic cavity; interference from other ventilated lung lobes; and mobility of individual lung lobes, especially the cranial lobes.

The thoracic cavity is an exceptionally complicated area both physiologically and anatomically. Furthermore, there is significant variability in the thoracic morphology and physiologic status of

veterinary patients. Thus, the onus of selecting patients potentially suitable for a VATS approach falls on the operating surgeon. Conversion to intercostal thoracotomy or median sternotomy is indicated when VATS procedures cannot be performed effectively and safely and when emergent complications arise. All owners should be counseled on the possibility of conversion before surgery. Conversion should not be seen as a surgical failure but rather as a necessary aspect of performing more advanced and refined surgical procedures.

Postoperative Surveillance

All patients undergoing a VATS procedure should be supported and monitored postoperatively as if they had undergone an intercostal thoracotomy or median sternotomy. Before closure of the thorax, the World Health Organization Surgical Safety Checklist should be implemented.[44] This checklist has been validated and demonstrated to reduce patient morbidity and mortality in human surgery.[44,45] All VATS surgery sites should be addressed for hemorrhage and treated appropriately before thoracic closure. All pulmonary parenchymal surgical sites should be inspected for air leakage either by submersion in warm saline or by pouring of saline over the affected lobe during a positive-pressure breath hold. Any pulmonary leaks should be resolved before thoracic closure. All VATS cases should have a thoracostomy tube placed to create negative pleural pressure before recovery and for monitoring of the pleural space for postoperative complications such as pneumothorax, pyothorax, and hemorrhage. The thoracostomy tube should not be placed through one of the existing cannula portals, and it is helpful to place it under direct video observation (Video Clip 31-7). All thoracostomy tubes should be anchored with at least a 2-0 suture at the base of the incision and secured using a *finger trap* pattern, including at least four throws around the tube.[46] Thoracostomy tubes should be monitored at least hourly for the first few hours after VATS. Quantification and characterization of the fluid and air produced should be documented in the medical record and assessed for trends. In the event of large or increasing volumes of hemorrhage, consideration for reoperation should be made based on the status of the patient and the severity of the hemorrhage. Increasing volumes or nonresolving air accumulation after a VATS procedure may be the result of pulmonary leakage or transthoracic air movement, usually because of an inappropriately placed thoracostomy tube. As such, the housing and insertion site of the tube should be assessed for compromise. If the thoracostomy tube device is not compromised and significant air accumulation persists, continuous evacuation from the pleural space using a continuous drainage system (e.g.,

Pleur-evac; Teleflex, Research Triangle Park, NC) may be indicated. If the pneumothorax fails to resolve after 2 or 3 days with continuous pleural drainage, the patient may require reexploration to resolve the pneumothorax.[47] Patients with chronic effusive disease or who are at risk for recurrent postoperative effusion may benefit from placement of a subcutaneous thoracic access port.[48] These ports enable fluid removal without the need for transthoracic thoracocentesis, potentially reducing the chance of iatrogenic lung injury and discomfort.

The authors of this chapter believe that the most significant benefit of VATS is the clinically apparent improvement in postoperative recovery compared with dogs undergoing intercostal thoracotomy or median sternotomy.[12] Postoperative pain and complications involving the pleural space, including pneumothorax, fluid accumulation, and atelectasis, appear to be improved, although this has not been demonstrated objectively in veterinary surgery as it has been in human surgery.[12,49,50] Furthermore, complications, including postoperative pneumonia, sepsis, and death, were reduced in patients that had undergone a VATS procedure compared with those who underwent an intercostal thoracotomy.[49,50] Local and regional analgesia using preoperative epidurals, intraoperative intercostal nerve blocks, systemic opioids, and nonsteroidal drugs enhance and function in concert with the hypalgesia accomplished with minimally invasive thoracic surgery and should be administered regardless of whether or not a minimally invasive approach was used.[12]

 All videos cited in this chapter can be found on the book's companion website at **www.wiley.com/go/fransson/ laparoscopy**

References

1 Jacobaeus, H.C. (1923) The cauterization of adhesions in artificial pneumothorax treatment of pulmonary tuberculosis under thoracoscopic control. Proc R Soc Med 16 (Electro Ther Sect), 45-62.

2 Demmy ,T.L. (2001) Overview and general considerations for video-assisted thoracic surgery. In: Video-Assisted Thoracic Surgery (VATS), 1st edn. Landes Bioscience, Texas, pp. 1-24.

3 MacDonald, K.A., Cagney, O., Magne, M.L. (2009) Echocardiographic and clinicopathologic characterization of pericardial effusion in dogs: 107 cases (1985-2006). J Am Vet Med Assoc 235, 1456-1461.

4 Boddy, K.N., Sleeper, M.M., Sammarco, C.D., et al. (2011) Cardiac magnetic resonance in the differentiation of neoplastic and nonneoplastic pericardial effusion. J Vet Intern Med 25, 1003-1009.

5 Radlinsky, M.G. (2009) Complications and need for conversion from thoracoscopy to thoracotomy in small animals. Vet Clin North Am Small Anim Pract 39, 977-984.

6 Classen, D.C., Evans, R.S., Pestotnik, S.L., et al. (1992) The timing of prophylactic administration of antibiotics and the risk of surgical-wound infection. N Engl J Med 326, 281-286.

7 Mayhew, P.D., Freeman, L., Kwan, T., et al. (2012) Comparison of surgical site infection rates in clean and clean-contaminated wounds in dogs and cats after minimally invasive versus open surgery: 179 cases (2007-2008). J Am Vet Med Assoc 240, 193-198.

8 Bratzler, D.W., Dellinger, E.P., Olsen, K.M., et al. (2013) Clinical practice guidelines for antimicrobial prophylaxis in surgery. Am J Health Syst Pharm 70, 195-283.

9 Hansen, E., Belden, K., Silibovsky, R., et al. (2014) Perioperative antibiotics. J Orthop Res 32 (suppl 1), S31-S59.

10 Petersen, S.W., Rosin, E. (1995) Cephalothin and cefazolin in vitro antibacterial activity and pharmacokinetics in dogs. Vet Surg 24, 347-51.

11 Rosin, E., Uphoff, T.S., Schultz-Darken, N.J., et al. (1993) Cefazolin antibacterial activity and concentrations in serum and the surgical wound in dogs. Am J Vet Res 54, 1317-1321.

12 Walsh, P.J., Remedios, A.M., Ferguson, J.F., et al. (1999) Thoracoscopic versus open partial pericardectomy in dogs: comparison of postoperative pain and morbidity. Vet Surg 28, 472-479.

13 Kudnig, S.T., Monnet, E., Riquelme, M., et al. (2003) Effect of one-lung ventilation on oxygen delivery in anesthetized dogs with an open thoracic cavity. Am J Vet Res 64, 443-448.

14 Cantwell, S.L., Duke, T., Walsh, P.J., et al. (2000) One-lung versus two-lung ventilation in the closed-chest anesthetized dog: a comparison of cardiopulmonary parameters. Vet Surg 29, 365-373.

15 Riquelme, M., Monnet, E., Kudnig, S.T., et al. (2005) Cardiopulmonary changes induced during one-lung ventilation in anesthetized dogs with a closed thoracic cavity. Am J Vet Res 66, 973-977.

16 Mayhew, K.N., Mayhew, P.D., Sorrell-Raschi, L., et al. (2009) Thoracoscopic subphrenic pericardectomy using double-lumen endobronchial intubation for alternating one-lung ventilation. Vet Surg 38, 961-966.

17 Case, J.B., Garcia-Pereira, F.L. (2013) Complication of selective, double-lumen endobronchial intubation in a dog undergoing lung lobectomy. Proceedings of the Veterinary Endoscopy Society Annual Meeting. Key Largo, FL, p. 9.

18 Mayhew, P.D., Culp, W.T., Pascoe, P.J., et al. (2012) Evaluation of blind thoracoscopic-assisted placement of three double-lumen endobronchial tube designs for one-lung ventilation in dogs. Vet Surg 6, 664-670.

19 Daly, C.M., Swalec-Tobias, K., Tobias, A.H., et al. (2002) Cardiopulmonary effects of intrathoracic insufflation in dogs. J Am Anim Hosp Assoc 38, 515-520.

20 Lansdowne, J.L., Monnet, E., Twedt, D.C., et al. (2005) Thoracoscopic lung lobectomy for treatment of lung tumors in dogs. Vet Surg 34, 530-535.

21 Mayhew, P.D., Friedberg, J.S. (2008) Video-assisted thoracoscopic resection of noninvasive thymomas using one-lung ventilation in two dogs. Vet Surg 37, 756-762.

22 Mayhew, P.D., Hunt, G.B., Steffey, M.A. et al. (2013) Evaluation of short-term outcome after lung lobectomy for resection of primary lung tumors via video-assisted thoracoscopic surgery or open thoracotomy in medium- to large-breed dogs. J Am Vet Med Assoc 243, 681-688.

23 Case, J.B., Mayhew, P.D., Singh, A. (2014) Evaluation of video-assisted thoracic surgery for the treatment of spontaneous pneumothorax and pulmonary bullae in dogs. Vet Surg DOI: 10.1111/j.1532-950X.2014.12288.x

24 Radlinsky, M.G., Mason, D.E., Biller, D.S., et al. (2002) Thoracoscopic visualization and ligation of the thoracic duct in dogs. Vet Surg 31, 138-146.

25 Dupre, G.P., Corlouer, J.P., Bouvy, B. (2001) Thoracoscopic pericardectomy performed without pulmonary exclusion in 9 dogs. Vet Surg 30, 21-27.

26 Levionnois, O.L., Bergadano, A., Schatzmann, U. (2006) Accidental entrapment of an endo-bronchial blocker tip by a surgical stapler during selective ventilation for lung lobectomy in a dog. Vet Surg 35, 82-85.

27 Jackson, J., Richter, K.P., Launer, D.P. (1999) Thoracoscopic partial pericardiectomy in 13 dogs. J Vet Intern Med 13, 529-533.

28 Evans, H.E. (1993) The digestive apparatus and abdomen. In: Miller's Anatomy of the dog, 3rd edn. Saunders, Philadelphia, pp. 441-444.

29 Brisson, B.A., Reggeti, F., Bienzle, D. (2006) Portal site metastasis of invasive mesothelioma after diagnostic thoracoscopy in a dog. J Am Vet Med Assoc 229, 980-983.

30 Parekh, K., Rusch, V., Bains, M., et al. (2001) VATS port site recurrence: a technique dependent problem. Ann Surg Oncol 2, 175-178.

31 Case, J.B., Maxwell, M., Aman, A., et al. (2013) Outcome evaluation of a thoracoscopic pericardial window procedure or subtotal pericardectomy via thoracotomy for the treatment of pericardial effusion in dogs. J Am Vet Med Assoc 242, 493-498.

32 Ployart, S., Libermann, S., Doran, I., et al. (2013) Thoracoscopic resection of right auricular masses in dogs: 9 cases (2003-2011). J Am Vet Med Assoc 242, 237-241.

33 Crumbaker, D.M., Rooney, M.B., Case, J.B. (2010) Thoracoscopic subtotal pericardectomy and right atrial mass resection in a dog. J Am Vet Med Assoc 237, 551-554.

34 Skinner, O.T., Case, J.B., Ellison, G.W., et al. (2014) Pericardioscopic imaging findings in cadaveric dogs: comparison of an apical pericardial window and subphrenic pericardectomy. Vet Surg 43, 45-51.

35 Borenstein, N., Behr, L., Chetboul, V., et al. (2004) Minimally invasive patent ductus arteriosus occlusion in 5 dogs. Vet Surg 33, 309-313.

36 Miller, M.W., Gordon, S.G., Saunders, A.B., et al. (2006) Angiographic classification of patent ductus arteriosus morphology in the dog. J Vet Cardiol 8, 109-114.

37 Bellah, J.R., Stiff, M.E., Russell, R.G. (1983) Thymoma in the dog: two case reports and review of 20 additional cases. J Am Vet Med Assoc 183, 306-311.

38 Withrow, S.J. (2006) Thymoma. In: Withrow, S.J., Vail, D.M. (eds.) Withrow and McEwan's Small Animal Oncology, 4th edn. Saunders, Philadelphia, pp. 795-799.

39 Allman, D.A., Radlinsky, M.G., Ralph, A.G. et al. (2010) Thoracoscopic thoracic duct ligation and thoracoscopic pericardectomy for treatment of chylothorax in dogs. Vet Surg 39, 21-27.

40 Brissot, H.N., Dupre, G.P., Bouvy, B.M., et al. (2003) Thoracoscopic treatment of bullous emphysema in 3 dogs. Vet Surg 32, 524-529.

41 Wormser, C., Singhal, S., Holt, D.E. (2014) Thoracoscopic-assisted pulmonary surgery for partial and complete lung lobectomy in dogs and cats: 11 cases (2008-2013). J Am Vet Med Assoc 245, 1036-1041.

42 Flores, R.M. (2010) Video-assisted thoracic surgery (VATS) lobectomy: focus on technique. World J Surg 34, 616-620.

43 Steffey, M.A., Daniel, L., Mayhew, P.D., et al. (2014) Video-assisted thoracoscopic extirpation of the tracheobronchial lymph nodes in dogs. Vet Surg 2014 Jun 2. doi: 10.1111/j.1532-950X.2014.12204.x. [Epub ahead of print]

44 Haynes, A.B., Weiser, T.G., Berry, W.R., et al. (2009) A surgical safety checklist to reduce morbidity and mortality in a global population. N Engl J Med 360, 491-499.

45 Levy, S.M., Senter, C.E., Hawkins, R.B., et al. (2012) Implementing a surgical checklist: more than checking a box. Surgery 152, 331-336.

46 Song, E.K., Mann, F.A., Wagner-Mann, C.C. (2008) Comparison of different tube materials and use of Chinese finger trap or four friction suture technique for securing gastrostomy, jejunostomy, and thoracostomy tubes in dogs. Vet Surg 37, 212-221.

47 Radlinsky, M.G. (2011) Thoracoscopy: postoperative care. In: Tamms, T.R., Rawlings, C.A. (eds.) Small Animal Endoscopy, 3rd edn. Elsevier Mosby, Oxford, p. 495.

48 Cahalane, A.K., Flanders, J.A. (2012) Use of pleural access ports for treatment of recurrent pneumothorax in two dogs. J Am Vet Med Assoc 241, 467-471.

49 Whitson, B.A., Andrade, R.S., Boettcher, A., et al. (2007) Video-assisted thoracoscopic surgery is more favorable than thoracotomy for resection of clinical stage I non-small cell lung cancer. Ann Thorac Surg 83, 1965-1970.

50 Villamizar, N.R., Darrabie, M.D., Burfeind, W.R., et al. (2009) Thoracoscopic lobectomy is associated with lower morbidity compared with thoracotomy. J Thorac Cardiovasc Surg 138, 419-425.

SECTION VI

Thoracoscopic Surgical Procedures

32 Thoracoscopic Lung Biopsy and Lung Lobectomy

Eric Monnet

> **Key Points**
>
> - Small masses located peripherally in the lung lobe can be removed with thoracoscopy.
> - One-lung ventilation is required to facilitate lung lobectomy with thoracoscopy in dogs.
> - Lateral recumbency in an oblique position improves visualization of the hilus of the lung for the placement of the stapling equipment.
> - Lung biopsies are collected with either loop ligatures or stapling equipment.

Lung biopsy and lung lobectomy can be performed with video-assisted thoracoscopic surgery (VATS) in dogs. The minimal invasiveness of the procedure, the rapid patient recovery, and diagnostic accuracy make VATS an ideal technique over other more invasive procedures for the resection of small primary lung tumors. It can also be used for surgical treatment of spontaneous pneumothorax. Diffuse lung disease may require the collection of a peripheral lung biopsy for culture and histology. Lung biopsy can be collected with VATS with minimal morbidity for the patient. Also, lymph node biopsies for staging purposes can be collected at the same time.

Complete or partial lung lobectomy can be completed under VATS or with a thoracoscopic-assisted procedure. One-lung ventilation (OLV) may be required for lung lobectomy.

Preoperative Considerations

Patient Selection

Thoracoscopic or thoracoscopic-assisted resection of lung disease is especially appropriate for the resection of small lung lesions at the periphery of the lung lobes (Figures 32-1 and 32-2).[1,2] Primary lung tumor is the most common indication for lung lobectomy, but resection of single lung metastasis has also been performed.

Adenocarcinomas are the most commonly reported lung tumors in dogs.[3-5] Squamous cell carcinomas and anaplastic carcinoma are less frequently seen in dogs.[4] Primary mesenchymal lung neoplasms, osteosarcoma, fibrosarcoma, and hemangiosarcoma are rarely reported in dogs and cats.[4] In young dogs, benign lympho-matous granulomatosis has been reported; however, they are very rare. Malignant histiocytosis is a large tumor which metastasize very quickly; it is reported most commonly in Bernese mountain dog. Primary lung tumors are usually aggressive tumors that metastasize to the lungs, lymph nodes, and pleural space.[6-8] They have been reported to metastasize to the skeletal muscles, liver, kidney, and heart.[9] Transitional cell carcinoma, hemangiosarcoma, thyroid carcinoma, melanoma, and osteosarcoma have a tendency to metastasize to the lungs.

Dogs with primary lung tumors are on average 10 to 12 years of age, and no sex or breed predisposition has been reported. Dogs with primary lung tumors are asymptomatic early in the disease process. Lethargy, inappetence, weight loss, and exercise intolerance could be present in dogs with primary lung tumors. Nonproductive cough can be reported by the owners. Hypertrophic osteopathy inducing severe lameness has been observed in several dogs with primary lung tumors.[3] Lung sounds may be decreased at the level of the lung mass or if effusion is present in the pleural space.

Three-view radiographs are required for the diagnosis of primary lung tumors and identification of metastasis.[3] Primary lung tumors more commonly appear as a one solid mass in a caudal lung lobe but may occur in any lung lobe (see Figure 32-1). Computed tomography (CT) is another alternative to further identify primary lung tumors, small metastasis, and lymph node involvement (see Figure 32-2).[10,11]

The size of the tumor (<5 cm), lymph node involvement, and clean margin at the time of surgery have been established as determinants for long-term outcome in dogs with primary lung tumors.[5,12]

Small Animal Laparoscopy and Thoracoscopy, First Edition. Edited by Boel A. Fransson and Philipp D. Mayhew.

© 2015 by ACVS Foundation. Published 2015 by John Wiley & Sons, Inc.

Companion website: www.wiley.com/go/fransson/laparoscopy

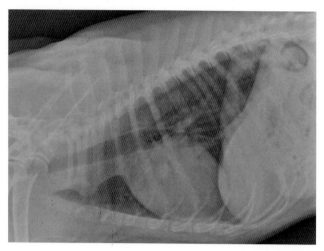

Figure 32-1 Radiograph of a dog with a solitary lung mass in the right middle lung lobe. The mass is small and located peripheral to the hilus, making it an ideal case for thoracoscopic lung lobectomy.

The median survival time was 26 days for dogs with lymph node involvement versus 452 days without lymph node involvement in a study on 67 cases of primary lung tumor in dogs.[5] Dogs with a well-differentiated tumor had longer survival time (790 days) than dogs with a poorly differentiated tumor (5 days).[5] The tumor stage is also a prognostic indicator with T1 (solitary noninvasive) tumor having a 790-day median survival time and T3 (locally invasive) tumor 81 days.[5] The median survival time for adenocarcinoma was 19 months versus 8 months for squamous cell carcinoma.[13]

In a mass larger than 5 to 7 cm in diameter, VATS is of questionable value because a large thoracotomy at the end of the surgery is required for tumor extraction, and the benefit of the minimally invasive approach will be lost. Dogs with a large mass in the lung

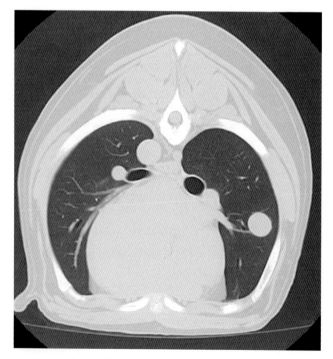

Figure 32-2 Computed tomography of the same mass as in Figure 32-1.

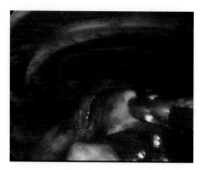

Figure 32-3 Biopsy of hilar lymph nodes are often indicated in dogs with video-assisted thoracoscopic surgery lung lobectomy.

parenchyma or a mass close to the hilus are not good candidates for thoracoscopic surgery. A large mass makes the manipulation required for lung hilus visualization and staples placement difficult. Also, if the mass is close to the hilus, safe placement of staples is difficult.[1] In addition, a clean margin might be difficult to obtain if the mass is located close to the hilus. A thoracoscopic-assisted procedure can be performed but the thoracotomy to extract the lung lobe has to be large enough to safely remove the lung lobe.

Spontaneous pneumothorax occurs in dogs without evidence of trauma. Spontaneous pneumothorax caused by a ruptured lung bullae can be explored and treated with VATS.[14] However, an evaluation of the entire lung parenchyma is not always possible with either a transdiaphragmatic or an intercostal approach, making the utilization of VATS for treatment of spontaneous pneumothorax questionable.

Diagnosis and Imaging

Exploration of the entire lung parenchyma can be very challenging in dogs even with OLV. CT has been used for localizing bullae and bleb,[15,16] but the ruptured bullae or bleb may not be visible if located in atelectatic tissue.

In dogs with lung tumor, the size and location of the mass are important criteria for selection of patients. Therefore, thoracic radiographs and CT of the thorax are important imaging modalities. For tumors in the cranial lung lobe, it can be difficult to determine if the mass is in the left or right cranial lung lobe on radiographic examination. Therefore, CT may help to further define the location of the mass and in deciding the side for intercostal VATS.[10]

A CT scan will also help to evaluate the hilar lymph nodes. If any hilar lymph node looks reactive on CT scan, an effort to biopsy it during VATS will be important (Figure 32-3). Lymph node metastasis is an important prognostic indicator for long-term survival.[5,12]

Patient Evaluation and Preparation

Patient Preparation

Spontaneous pneumothorax is usually severe and requires placement of a thoracostomy tube for effective treatment before surgery. Continuous pleural suction is often necessary to keep the pleural space evacuated, especially in the early treatment period. After evacuation of the pleural space, thoracic radiographs, including both lateral views, and CT scan should be examined for primary or secondary causes of pneumothorax. Pulmonary bullae may be

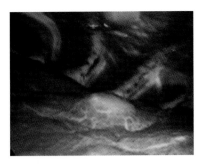

Figure 32-4 Intraoperative view of a mass in the left caudal lung lobe. The lung parenchyma is not inflated around the mass because of one-lung ventilation.

visible on thoracic radiographs. Pulmonary blebs usually are not visible.[15,16]

Creation of Working Space: One-Lung Ventilation

One-lung ventilation is important for performance of lung lobectomy. OLV improves visualization of the mass and the hilus of the lungs and increases the amount of space in the thoracic cavity available for instrumentation (Figure 32-4). Stapling equipment is used during lung lobectomy or lung biopsy and requires a large space for instrument manipulation.

One-lung ventilation can be achieved with different procedures. Selective intubation of the lung lobe that will remain ventilated, with either a double-lumen endotracheal tube or a long endotracheal tube, has been used.[17,18] Use of a double-lumen endotracheal tube allows for selective or alternating ventilation of the left or right lung lobes. This technique has mostly been used for resection of cranial mediastinal masses or subtotal pericardectomy.[17-19] Placement of an endobronchial blocker to exclude the lung lobe to be resected is another option.[20] Both techniques require a bronchoscope for correct placement of the double-lumen endotracheal tube or the endobronchial blocker. When an endobronchial blocker is used, it is important to inflate the balloon at the end of the blocker appropriately. If the balloon is not inflated enough, it may create a one-way valve, allowing oxygen to pass around the balloon during positive-pressure ventilation but not allowing gas escape passively during expiration. Consequently, overinflation of the lung may lead to barotrauma.

One-lung ventilation induces atelectasis of the nonventilated (dependent) lung, which result in a ventilation/perfusion (V/Q) mismatch with hypoxemia.[20,21] The dependent lung receives more blood flow than the nondependent one because of the patient's lateral recumbency for most of the lung lobectomy, leading to a low V/Q ratio. Conversely, the dependent lung is in a high V/Q situation, which cannot compensate for the low V/Q situation of the nondependent lung. The dependent lung under the pressure of the heart will gradually get atelectatic, which exacerbates the hypoxemia.[20,21] To prevent or correct the atelectasis of the dependent lung, the application of positive end-expiratory pressure (PEEP) has been recommended. In normal dogs with OLV, PEEP of 2.5 and 5.0 cm H_2O was studied.[20,21] PEEP was able to maintain arterial oxygen saturation without interfering with cardiac output. Therefore, any gain in percent of oxygen saturation will translate to an increase of oxygen delivery during the procedure.

When an endobronchial blocker is used to induce ventilation, it is important to avoid dislodgment of the blocker. If the endobronchial

blocker is dislodged into the carina, a complete obstruction of the lower airway is induced, and the end-tidal CO_2 reads zero on the capnograph. If this occurs, the balloon of the endobronchial blocker has to be deflated immediately. Bronchoscopy is required for appropriate replacement of the occluder. The risk of dislodgment of the blocker is the greatest when the patient is moved in the operating room and on the surgical table. Therefore, it is paramount to not induce OLV until the patient is positioned on the surgery table.

Surgical Techniques

Lung Biopsy
Lung biopsy for chronic lung disease can be performed effectively with a minimally invasive technique.

Approach
A transdiaphragmatic subxiphoid approach with the patient in dorsal recumbency may be the most appropriate approach for a lung biopsy because of diffuse lung disease. This approach allows examination of both sides of the thoracic cavity and biopsy of the lungs on the right and left sides. However, with this approach, hilar lymph nodes will not be seen, but sternal and mediastinal lymph nodes will be easily accessible for biopsy.

If the pathology is unilateral, an intercostal approach with the patient in lateral recumbency would be appropriate, and the hilar lymph nodes would be visible. With a lateral approach, a thoracoscopic-assisted approach can be used to collect biopsies from a cranial or middle lung lobe. Caudal lung lobes are not really amenable to a thoracoscopic-assisted approach because of their attachment dorsally in the thoracic cavity by the pulmonary ligament.

Surgical Technique
Key points for lung biopsy include:
- Dorsal recumbency
- Transdiaphragmatic approach
- EndoGIA 45 (EndoGIA stapling device; US Surgical, Norwalk, CT) 3.5 mm
- Loop ligatures
- Vessel-sealing device (VSD) for small biopsy

Lung biopsies can be collected with loop ligature, a stapling device, or a VSD device.[22,23] Loop ligatures are commercially available or made at the surgical table with a Roeder or a modified Roeder knot and provide a good seal for biopsies taken as far as 3 cm from the edges of the lung lobe.[23] EndoGIA with 2.5-mm staples were shown to inconsistently provide a good seal, and some samples leaked at a pressure lower than 20 cm H_2O.[23] A VSD did not provide a reliable pneumatoseal for large lung biopsies, and several samples leaked at pressure as low as 10 cm H_2O.[23] In a study in which smaller biopsies were taken, the seal seemed adequate using a VSD.[22]

If a loop ligature is used, the device is introduced in the thoracic cavity through one of the cannulas. A grasping forceps is then introduced through another cannula and passed through the loop. The tip of a lung lobe is grasped and pulled into the loop. The distal extremity of the loop ligature is broken and the slip knot tightened around the lung parenchyma. The knot pusher is used to direct the suture to where it should be positioned for the biopsy. Usually, monofilament loop ligatures are easier to work with because they are stiffer. The lung biopsy is then cut with Metzenbaum scissors, making sure 0.5 cm of tissue is left passed the suture. If leakage

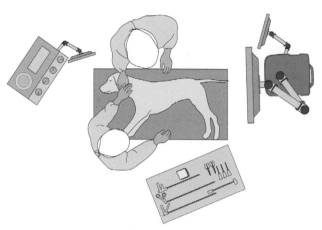

Figure 32-5 Operating room setup for thoracoscopic lung lobectomy of a caudal lung lobe.

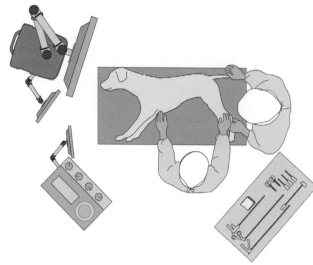

Figure 32-6 Operating room setup for thoracoscopic lung lobectomy of a cranial lung lobe.

is observed on the line of incision, a second loop ligature can be applied. The suture can then be cut.

If a solid mass is present in the center of a lung lobe, biopsy forceps could be used to biopsy the center of the mass. A palpation probe can be used to provide tamponade to help control bleeding. Also, hemostatic absorbable foam can be applied into the biopsy site to help control bleeding.

If the lung lobe is completely consolidated with no ventilation, the biopsy could be harvested with a biopsy forceps on the edges of the lobes. This technique is not recommended if the lung lobe is still ventilated because it may increase the risk of pneumothorax after surgery.

A chest drain is placed at a site away from all portals, operative and telescope cannulas are removed, and the portals are closed routinely.

Complete Lung Lobectomy
Approach
Lateral recumbency with intercostal cannula placement is the preferred technique for complete lung lobectomy.[1] The patient is placed in an oblique position with the dorsal part of the thoracic cavity elevated (Figures 32-5 and 32-6). In this position, gravity displaces the thoracic organ toward the sternum, which improves visualization of the hilus of the lungs. This positioning combined with OLV optimizes the surgical field for placement of the endoscopic staplers.

Three to four cannulas are required for a lung lobectomy (Figures 32-7 to 32-9). If a retractor is required to increase exposure of the hilus of the lung, four cannulas are used. If three cannulas are used, they can be placed in the same intercostal space to minimize pain after surgery. The fourth cannula, if required, is placed one intercostal space cranial or caudal to the space with the three cannulas. Portals are ideally placed in the ventral third of the intercostal space. If a cranial lung lobe is resected, the cannulas are placed in the eighth or ninth intercostal space. If a caudal lung lobe or the right middle lung is resected, the cannulas are placed in the third or fourth intercostal space.

Surgical Technique
Key points include:
- Lateral recumbency in an oblique position
- Intercostal approach
- Endobronchial blocker or tube for selective intubation

- Induce OLV in the operating room
- EndoGIA 45 and 60 mm 3.5 mm
- Sterile retrieving pouch

Lung lobectomy can be performed for any lung lobe. The accessory lung lobe is more difficult to access, but its resection can be performed. For lung lobectomy, it is important to place the staple line as perpendicular as possible to the hilus of the lung to optimize the length of the cartridge of staples. Therefore, the cannula used to introduce the stapling device will be placed last, after visualization of the hilus of the lung, to place it in an appropriate position. The EndoGIA stapler is articulated, and its positioning can be adjusted even if the cannula is not in a perfect position (Figure 32-10).

Individual structures of the hilus do not need to be isolated for minimally invasive lung lobectomy. For caudal lung lobes and the accessory lung lobe, the pulmonary ligament is divided to free the lung lobe for manipulation. The dorsal ligament is dissected with

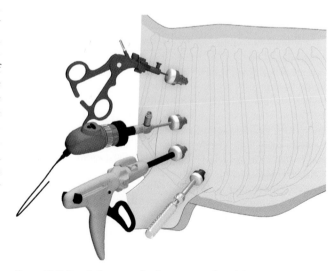

Figure 32-7 Portal placement for thoracoscopic lung lobectomy of a caudal lung lobe.

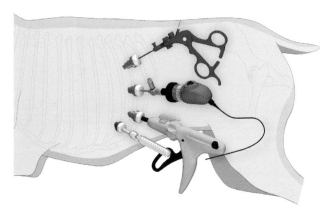

Figure 32-8 Portal placement for thoracoscopic lung lobectomy of a cranial lung lobe.

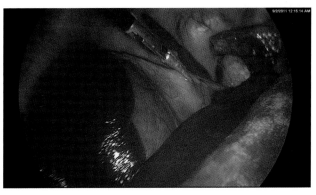

Figure 32-11 The dorsal pulmonary ligament of a caudal lung lobe. (Courtesy of Dr. Philipp Mayhew, University of California, Davis.)

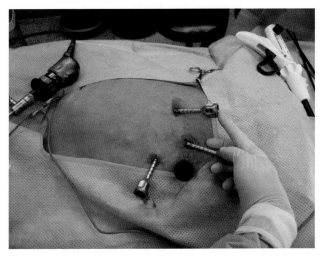

Figure 32-9 Portals placement in the 9th and 10th intercostal spaces for a cranial lung lobectomy. One port is 12 mm in diameter, and the other ports are 5 mm. Port 4 is optional for a retractor. (Courtesy of Dr. Philipp Mayhew, University of California, Davis.)

Metzenbaum scissors, a hook mounted with electrocautery, or a VSD (Figure 32-11). It seems easier to dissect from caudal to cranial, being careful not to damage the pulmonary vein.

After localization of the appropriate lung lobe hilus, the cannula for the stapler is placed. It has to be placed as far as possible from the hilus to allow complete opening of the staple cartridge in the thoracic cavity before it reaches the hilus of the lung. A 45- or 60-mm-long EndoGIA stapling cartridge with 3.5-mm staples is commonly used across the hilus of the lobe (Figure 32-12).

Before releasing the staples, it is important to make sure that no other structures (e.g., the phrenic nerve) than the hilus of the lung are caught in the stapler equipment. An angled telescope makes this

step easier. The stapling cartridge must be long enough to include the entire hilus to be stapled (Figure 32-13). A 60-mm-long cartridge is most commonly used for this purpose.

After releasing the staples (Figure 32-14), the resected lung lobe is placed in a sterile retrieving bag to prevent seeding of the thoracic wall with tumor cells (Figure 32-15). A cannula site is enlarged to permit exteriorizing the lung lobe in the retrieving bag (Figure 32-16). Enlarged hilar lymph nodes should be biopsied or removed. If a lymph node is biopsied, a combination of sharp and blunt dissection is used to isolate the lymph node. Electrosurgical assistance and clip application can be used for hemostasis. Before removal of the telescope, the hilus is observed for air leakage or bleeding. A chest drain is placed at a site away from all portals, the operative and telescope cannulas are removed, and the portals are closed.

Surgical Technique: Thoracoscopically Assisted Lung Lobectomy

A lung lobectomy can be performed with a thoracoscopically assisted technique. The telescope is introduced through a cannula placed distant from the hilus of the prospective lung lobe. A mini-thoracotomy is then performed at the level of the hilus of the lung to remove. A regular thoracoabdominal stapling device (TA stapling device, US Surgical) is introduced in thoracic cavity through the mini-thoracotomy. The telescope is used to visualize the appropriate placement of the stapling device at the hilus of the lung. After firing of the staples, a scalpel blade is used to detach the

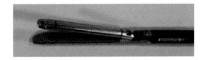

Figure 32-10 EndoGIA staple cartridge (US Surgical, Norwalk, CT) used for lung lobectomy.

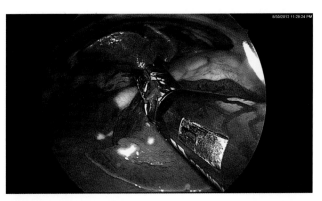

Figure 32-12 EndoGIA (US Surgical, Norwalk, CT) applied to the hilus of a caudal lung lobe. (Courtesy of Dr. Philipp Mayhew, University of California, Davis.)

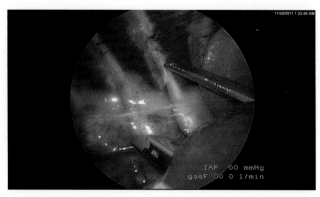

Figure 32-13 The EndoGIA staple cartridge (US Surgical, Norwalk, CT) needs to be long enough to encompass the entire hilus. During transection, the EndoGIA tends to push the parenchyma toward the opening of the cartridge, and several millimeters of cartridge extending beyond the tissue margin is required. (Courtesy of Dr. Philipp Mayhew, University of California, Davis.)

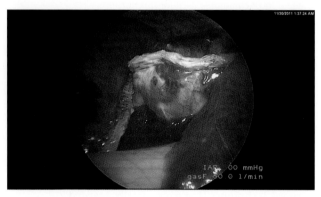

Figure 32-14 The stapled hilus after lung lobe removal. (Courtesy of Dr. Philipp Mayhew, University of California, Davis.)

lung lobe under visualization with the telescope. Then the lung lobe is removed through the mini-thoracotomy. This technique requires a larger thoracotomy for the placement and manipulation of the stapling device than with a thoracoscopic procedure. The mini-thoracotomy is closed in a routine fashion.

Alternatively, the lung lobe is exteriorized, and a partial lung lobectomy to remove the lesion is performed (Figure 32-17).

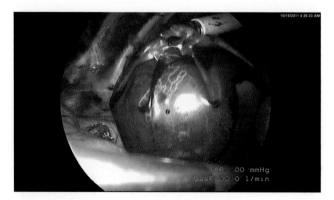

Figure 32-15 Lung lobe positioned in a retrieval bag. (Courtesy of Dr. Philipp Mayhew, University of California, Davis.)

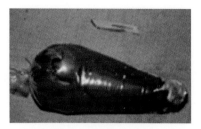

Figure 32-16 A retrieval bag containing a lung lobe after removal from the thoracic cavity.

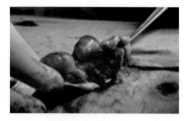

Figure 32-17 A thoracoscopic-assisted technique can be used for peripherally located lesions or for biopsies. The affected area is exteriorized through a mini-thoracotomy and can be stapled with a thoracoabdominal stapler.

Surgical Technique: Lymph Node Biopsy

Biopsy of the hilar lymph nodes is important for the staging of the patient. Lymph node involvement is an important prognostic indicator for dogs[5] with lung tumor. Hilar lymph nodes, especially if they are reactive, can be biopsied during VATS with a cup biopsy forceps or completely dissected from the mediastinum.

Sentinel lymph nodes can be identified with fluorescent markers. The most common marker used is indocyanine green. After injection of indocyanine green in a tumor in the lung, it will diffuse through the lymphatic into the hilar lymph nodes. Near-infrared light induces fluorescence from the indocyanine green, which helps identify and dissect hilar lymph nodes (Figure 32-18).

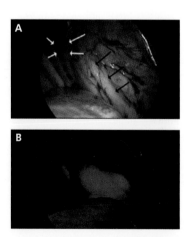

Figure 32-18 A, Hilar lymph node of the cranial lung lobe in a dog with normal light indocyanine green has been injected the left cranial lung lobe. Black and white arrows outline the margins of the lymph nodes. **B,** Same view as in A but with near-infrared light. The hilar lymph node is now fluorescent and easily located.